Statistical Methods for Rates and Proportions

THIRD EDITION

Statistical Methods for Rates and Proportions

Third Edition

JOSEPH L. FLEISS
BRUCE LEVIN
MYUNGHEE CHO PAIK

Department of Biostatistics
Mailman School of Public Health
Columbia University

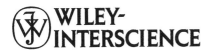

A JOHN WILEY & SONS, INC., PUBLICATION

For general information on our other products and services please contact our Customer Care Department within the U.S. at 877-762-2974, outside the U.S. at 317-572-3993 or fax 317-572-4002.

Wiley also publishes its books in a variety of electronic formats. Some content that appears in print, however, may not be available in electronic format.

Library of Congress Cataloging-in-Publication Data

Fleiss, Joseph L.
  Statistical methods for rates and proportions.-- 3rd ed. / Joseph L. Fleiss, Bruce Levin, Myunghee Cho Paik.
    p. cm.-- (Wiley series in probability and statistics)
  Includes bibliographical references and indexes.
  ISBN 0-471-52629-0 (cloth : acid-free paper)
    1. Analysis of variance. 2. Sampling (Statistics) 3. Biometry. I. Levin, Bruce. II. Paik, Myunghee Cho. III. Title. IV. Series.

QA279.F58 2003
519.5'38--dc21   2002191005

Printed in the United States of America

10 9 8 7 6 5

To Isabel, Betty, and Yi Hyon

and

To Joe, who passed away as this book went to press

Contents

Preface

Much has happened in the twenty-two years since the publication of the second edition. The explosive development of personal computing and statistical software has removed the main impediment to sophisticated analyses of data. Indeed, these developments have brought the ability to carry out such analyses out of the sole possession of the specialist and into the hands of every researcher. Logistic, Poisson, and other generalized linear regression models have taken their rightful place as standard analytic methods. Our clinical and public health colleagues no longer view the odds ratio as an inscrutable version of the rate ratio—they understand and use odds ratios all the time. Generalized estimating equations and empirical Bayes methods have become powerful tools to deal with complex data. Exact methods and other computational challenges like conditional likelihood analysis have gone way beyond the Fisher-Irwin exact test for 2×2 tables. Correct ways to deal with missing data can no longer be ignored. The randomized clinical trial and the special role statisticians play in safeguarding the validity of the trial's conduct and findings have come of age in dramatic ways.

This means we can no longer content ourselves with methods that require only a desktop or pocket calculator, which was a hallmark of the second edition. Anyway, the limitations that those devices once represented no longer exist. Yet the elegance of simple, clear, and common-sense methods, which was another hallmark of the previous editions, must never be allowed to take second place to useless complexity. Meeting these requirements has been something of a challenge because, tragically, time has also brought a disabling form of Parkinson's disease to the first author. Joe's inimitable writing style—direct, friendly, honest, sensible, authoritative, and prescriptive in the best sense of the word—hopefully has been allowed to shine through our attempts to bring the book up to date for both students and researchers engaged in the analysis of their data.

Our approach has been to leave much of the original material intact with clarifications, corrections, and streamlining only as necessary, while covering new material at two levels. The first introduces methods with only as much complexity as is required to give a clear presentation. The mathematical prerequisites continue to be a knowledge of high school algebra and an ability to take logarithms and extract square roots. A familiarity with computers in everyday use is now assumed.

The second level is, admittedly, aimed at students of biostatistics and specialists in data analysis, and requires a level of mathematical preparation equivalent to a first and second course in statistics. These sections have been marked with an asterisk to indicate that full comprehension may require some familiarity with matrix algebra, multivariate statistical concepts, or asymptotic methods. Our suggestion to novice readers is to skim these sections in order to get the lay of the land without getting lost in the thicket of details.

We have added many new problems, some numerical and some theoretical. The numerical problems all have answers at the back of the book, as in the second edition. Many of the theoretical problems have cogent hints to guide students to a successful solution and, we hope, an increase in their understanding and level of expertise. We have tried to bear in mind, and cannot resist paraphrasing here, Stanislaw Lem's humbling definition of an expert, given in *His Masters Voice*: An *expert* is a barbarian with an uneven level of ignorance. Our hope is that we can move the level without exacerbating Lem's characterization.

The statistical analysis of single-sample data, such as a prevalence study, now occupies an entire early chapter. We took this as an opportunity to introduce a few technical definitions of a two-tailed p-value for asymmetrical discrete distributions, notions which arise in the exact analysis of categorical data. Armed with such tools, we have fully reinstated exact and approximate-yet-accurate confidence intervals as appropriate statements of statistical uncertainty, notwithstanding Joe's initial reluctance to promulgate their routine use in the first edition. Again, modern computing enables us to recommend them while respecting Joe's warning that a properly constructed confidence interval is frequently more complicated than simply the point estimate plus or minus a multiple of its standard error.

Regarding other foundational issues of statistical inference, we have continued Joe's unabashed preference for frequentist methods. The reader will see, however, that in key places we take an empirical Bayes approach. This occurs, for example, in the new sections on the analysis of many proportions with an element of randomness (Section 9.6*), random effects meta-analysis (Section 10.9.1), tests of odds ratio homogeneity in the large-sparse case (Section 10.9.2), overdispersion in Poisson regression (Section 12.3*), and extensions of logistic regression for correlated binary data (Section 15.5*). In these applications, the empirical Bayes approach provides the most natural analytic framework while avoiding the abuses of subjectivism that underpinned Joe's original distaste for Bayesian methods. Of course, Bayes' theorem, being the fundamental means to pass between conditional probabilities, is used throughout the book. The reader will also notice the likelihood ratio highlighted for its fundamental role in the weighing of statistical evidence, in addition to its frequentist use as a hypothesis test statistic. This, however, is as close as we come to a frank Bayesian approach.

There is new material on sample size calculations in Chapter 4 (formerly Chapter 3) and some insights about why the sample size tables in the second edition work as well as they do. As mentioned above, exact statistical methods are now presented in a formal and routine manner throughout the first half of the book, where they can be feasibly applied. There is new material on randomization in clinical trials (Chapter 5) and factors relating to statistical power in randomized clinical trials (Section 8.3). The Mantel–Haenszel procedure and its generalizations for combining the evidence across several cross-classification tables plays a prominent role starting in Chapter 10 and recurs in several subsequent chapters. We have included entirely new chapters on logistic regression (both binary and polytomous, in Chapter 11), Poisson regression (Chapter 12), regression models for matched samples (Chapter 14), the analysis of correlated binary data (Chapter 15), and methods for analyzing fourfold tables with missing data (Chapter 16). The chapters on the effects of, control of, and adjustment for errors of misclassification from the previous editions have been consolidated into one (Chapter 17), with new material on these issues in logistic regression. Chapter 18 on the measurement of interrater agreement has a new section connecting this topic with that of Chapter 15.

We are most grateful to the colleagues and students who helped us with critical review and constructive suggestions. We especially want to thank Melissa Begg for helpful comments; Ann Kinney for her massive and masterful editing; Boanerges Dominguez and Amy Murphy, who assisted us in teaching "The Analysis of Categorical Data" course at Columbia University with preliminary versions of this edition; Cheng-Shiun Leu and Mei-Yin Chen for reading and computing; Jennie Kline for allowing us to use her spontaneous abortion data and her epidemiologic guidance as to their interpretation; and Ralph Sacco for the NOMASS data on risk factors for stroke. We thank James Walkup for kindly updating the citations to the psychiatric literature—Joe's knowledge of this field in the earlier editions was immense and no doubt contributed to their success. We are also indebted to Michael Finkelstein for his insight into applied statistics and for stimulating us to think about how to present technical material to nontechnical audiences during the writing of *Statistics for Lawyers*. We thank Steve Quigley and Heather Haselkorn for their utterly endless patience during this project. And we are forever grateful to our spouses, Betty and Yi Hyon, and our families, who, like Joe's wife Isabel, now departed, have been a constant source of inspiration and forbearance during the writing of this book.

BRUCE LEVIN
MYUNGHEE CHO PAIK

New York, New York and
Bear River, Nova Scotia
August 2002

Preface to the Second Edition

The need for a revised edition became apparent a few years after the publication of the first edition. Reviewers, researchers, teachers, and students cited some important topics that were absent, treated too briefly, or not presented in their most up-to-date form. In the meantime, the field of applied statistics continued to develop, and new results were obtained that deserved citation and illustration.

Of the several topics I had omitted from the first edition, the most important was the construction of confidence intervals. In the revision, interval estimation is treated almost as extensively as hypothesis testing. In fact, the close connection between the two is pointed out in the new Section 1.4. The reader will find there, in the new Section 5.6, and elsewhere realizations of the warning I gave in the Preface to the first edition that a properly constructed confidence interval is frequently more complicated than simply the point estimate plus or minus a multiple of its standard error.

Another important topic missing from the first edition was the planning of comparative studies with unequal sample sizes. This is treated in the new Section 3.4.

Several other topics not covered in the first edition are covered here. The Fisher-Irwin "exact" test for a fourfold table is described in the new Section 2.2. Attributable risk, an important indicator of the effect of exposure to a risk factor, is discussed in the new Sections 5.7 and 6.4. The Cornfield method for making inferences about the odds ratio is presented in the new Sections 5.5 and 5.6.

A number of topics touched on superficially or not dealt with adequately in the first edition have, I hope, now been covered properly. The analysis of data from a two-period crossover study is described in an expansion of Section 7.2. A more appropriate method for analyzing data from a study of matched pairs when the response variable is qualitatively ordered is presented in Section 8.2. The comparison of proportions from several matched samples in Section 8.4 has been expanded to include the case of quantitatively ordered samples. A method for comparing data from several fourfold tables that has been found capable of yielding erroneous results has been relegated to the section (now Section 10.7) on methods to be avoided.

Developments in statistics since the appearance of the first edition are reflected in most sections and every chapter of the revision. The determination of sample sizes is brought up to date in Section 3.2; the corresponding table in the Appendix (Table A.3) has been revised accordingly. Some recently proposed alternatives to simple randomization in clinical studies are discussed in two new sections, 4.3 and 7.3. The presentation of ridit analysis in Section 9.4 has been revised in the light of recent research. The effects and control of misclassification in both variables in a fourfold table are considered in Sections 11.3 and 12.2. The new Chapter 13, which is an expansion and updating of the old Section 12.2, presents recent results on the measurement of interrater agreement for categorical data. Some recent insights into indirect standardization are cited in Sections 14.3 and 14.5.

The emphasis continues to be on, and the examples continue to be from, the health sciences. The selection of illustrative material was determined by the field I know best, not by the field I necessarily consider the most important.

The revision is again aimed at research workers and students who have had at least a year's course in applied statistics, including chi square and correlation. Many of the problems that conclude the chapters have been revised. Several new problems have been added.

Several of my colleagues and a few reviewers urged me to include the solutions to at least some of the numerical problems. I have decided to provide the solutions to all of them. Teachers who wish to assign these problems for homework or on examinations may do so simply by changing some of the numerical values.

The mathematical prerequisites continue to be a knowledge of high school algebra and an ability to take logarithms and extract square roots. All methods presented can be applied using only a desktop or pocket calculator. As a consequence, the book does not present the powerful but mathematically complicated methods of log-linear or logistic regression analysis for high order cross-classification tables. The texts by D. R. Cox (*The analysis of binary data*, Methuen, London, 1970) and by Y. M. M. Bishop, S. E. Fienberg, and P. W. Holland (*Discrete multivariate analysis: Theory and practice*, M.I.T. Press, Cambridge, Mass., 1975) are excellent references at a somewhat advanced mathematical level. Two more recent short monographs (B. S. Everitt, *The analysis of contingency tables*, Halsted Press, New York, 1977 and S. E. Fienberg, *The analysis of cross-classified categorical data*, M.I.T. Press, Cambridge, Mass., 1977) provide less mathematically advanced reviews of these topics.

Professors Agnes Berger, John Fertig, Bruce Levin, and Patrick Shrout of Columbia University and Professor Gary Simon of the State University of

New York at Stony Brook reviewed draft copies of the revision and made many helpful suggestions. Professor Berger, Fertig, and Simon were especially critical, and offered advice that I took seriously but did not always follow.

Most helpful of all were the students who took my course on the analysis of categorical data the last couple of years at the Columbia University School of Public Health, and the students who took my course on advanced statistical methods in epidemiology in the 1978 Graduate Summer Session in Epidemiology at the University of Minnesota School of Public Health. They served as experimental subjects without informed consent as I tried out various approaches to the presentation of the new (and old) material. Students who took my course in the 1980 Graduate Summer Session in Epidemiology saw draft copies of the revision and pointed out several typographical errors I had made. I thank them all.

Ms. Blanche Agdern patiently and carefully typed the several drafts of the revision. Ms. Beatrice Shube, my editor at Wiley, was always supportive and a ready source of advice and encouragement. My wife Isabel was a constant source of inspiration and reinforcement when the going got tough.

The new table of sample sizes was generated by a program run at the computer center of the New York State Psychiatric Institute. The publishers of the *American Journal of Epidemiology, Biometrics*, and the *Journal of Chronic Disease* kindly gave me permission to use published data.

JOSEPH L. FLEISS

New York
December 1980

Preface to the First Edition

This book is concerned solely with comparisons of qualitative or categorical data. The case of quantitative data is treated in the many books devoted to the analysis of variance. Other books have restricted attention to categorical data (such as A. E. Maxwell, *Analysing qualitative data*. Methuen, London, 1961, and R. G. Francis, *The rhetoric of science: A methodological discussion of the two-by-two table*, University of Minnesota Press, Minneapolis, 1961), but an updated monograph seemed overdue. A recent text (D. R. Cox, *The analysis of binary data*, Methuen, London, 1970) is at once more general than the present book in that it treats categorical data arising from more complicated study designs and more restricted in that it does not treat such topics as errors of misclassification and standardization of rates.

Although the ideas and methods presented here should be useful to anyone concerned with the analysis of categorical data, the emphasis and examples are from the disciplines of clinical medicine, epidemiology, psychiatry and psychopathology, and public health. The book is aimed at research workers and students who have had at least a year's course in applied statistics, including a thorough grounding in chi square and correlation. Most chapters conclude with one or more problems. Some call for the proof of an algebraic identity. Others are numerical, designed either to have the reader apply what he has learned or to present ideas mentioned only in passing in the text.

No more complicated mathematical techniques than the taking of logarithms and the extraction of square roots are required to apply the methods described. This means that anyone with only high school algebra, and with only a desktop calculator, can apply the methods presented. It also means, however, that analysis requiring matrix inversion or other complicated mathematical techniques (e.g., the analysis of multiple contingency tables) are not described. Instead, the reader is referred to appropriate sources.

The estimation of the degree of association or difference assumes equal importance with the assessment of statistical significance. Except where the formulas are excessively complicated, I present the standard error of almost every measure of association or difference given in the text. The standard errors are used to test hypotheses about the corresponding parameters, to compare the precision of different methods of estimation, and to obtain a weighted average of a number of independent estimates of the same parameter.

I have tried to be careful in giving both sides of various arguments that are still unresolved about the proper design of studies and analysis of data. Examples are the use of matched samples and the measurement of association. Inevitably, my own biases have probably affected how I present the opposing arguments.

In two instances, however, my bias is so strong that I do not even permit the other side to be heard. I do not find confidence intervals to be useful, and therefore do not discuss interval estimation at all. The reader who finds a need for confidence intervals will have to refer to some of the cited references for details. He will find, by the way, that the proper interval is almost always more complicated than simply the point estimate plus or minus a multiple of its standard error.

The second instance is my bias against the Bayesian approach to statistical inference. See W. Edwards, H. Lindman, and L. J. Savage. Bayesian statistical inference for psychological research, *Psychol. Rec.*, **70**, 193–242, 1963, for a description of the Bayesian approach to data in psychology; and J. Cornfield, A Bayesian test of some classical hypotheses—with applications to sequential clinical trials, *J. Am. Stat. Assoc.*, **61**, 577–594, 1966, for a description of that approach to data in medicine. I believe that the kind of thinking described in Chapter 3, especially in Section 3.1, provides an adequate alternative to the Bayesian approach.

It is with gratitude that I acknowledge the advice, criticism, and encouragement of Professors John Fertig, Mervyn Susser, and Andre Varma of Columbia University and of Dr. Joseph Zubin of the Biometrics Research unit of the New York State Department of Mental Hygiene. Dr. Gary Simon of Princeton University and Professor W. Edwards Deming of New York University reviewed the manuscript and pointed out a number of errors I had made in an earlier draft. Needless to say, I take full responsibility for any and all errors that remain.

My wife Isabel was a constant source of inspiration as well as an invaluable editorial assistant.

The major portion of the typing was admirably performed by Vilma Rivieccio. Additional typing, collating, and keypunching were ably carried out by Blanche Agdern, Rosalind Fruchtman, Cheryl Keller, Sarah Lichtenstaedter, and Edith Pons.

My work was supported in part by grant DR 00793 from the National Institute of Dental Research (John W. Fertig, Ph.D., Principal Investigator) and in part by grant MH 08534 from the National Institute of Mental Health (Robert L. Spitzer, M.D., Principal Investigator). Except when noted otherwise, the tables in the Appendix were generated by programs run on the computers of the New York State Psychiatric Institute and of Rockland State Hospital.

I thank Professor E. S. Pearson and the Biometrika Trustees for permission to quote from Tables 1, 4, and 8 of *Biometrika tables for statisticians, Vol. I*, edited by E. S. Pearson and H. O. Hartley; John Wiley & Sons for permission to use Tables A.1 to A.3 Of *Statistical inference under order restrictions* by R. E. Bartlow, D. J. Bartholomew, L. M. Bremner and H. D. Brunk; Van Nostrand Reinhold Co. for permission to quote data from *Smoking and Health*; the Institute of Psychiatry of the University of London for permission to quote data from *Psychiatry diagnosis in New York and London* by J. E. Cooper et al.; and Sir Austin Bradford Hill and Oxford University Press for permission to quote from *Statistical methods in clinical and preventive medicine*.

I also thank the editors of the following journals for permission to use published data: the *American Journal of Public Health*, the *American Statistician*, *Biometrics*, the *Journal of Laboratory and Clinical Medicine*, the *Journal of the National Cancer Institute*, the *Journal of Psychiatric Research*, and *Psychometrika*.

JOSEPH L. FLEISS

New York
June 1972

CHAPTER 1

An Introduction to Applied Probability

Some elements of applied probability theory are needed fully to appreciate and work with the different kinds of rates and proportions that arise in research. Thus the clearest and most suggestive interpretation of a proportion is as a probability—as a measure of the chance that a specified event happens to, or that a specified characteristic is possessed by, a typical member of a population. An important use of probabilities is in estimating the number of individuals, out of a sample of size n, who have the characteristic under consideration. If P is the probability that an individual possesses the characteristic, the expected number having the characteristic is simply nP.

Section 1.1 presents notation and some important definitions, and Section 1.2 presents the rule of total probability, along with an application. The theory in Sections 1.1 and 1.2 is applied in Section 1.3 to the evaluation of a screening test, and in Section 1.4 to the bias possible when making inferences from selected samples.

1.1. NOTATION AND DEFINITIONS

In this book, the terms *probability, relative frequency,* and *proportion* are used synonymously. If A denotes the event that a randomly selected person from a population has a defined characteristic (e.g., has arteriosclerotic heart disease), then $P(A)$ denotes the proportion of all people who have the characteristic. For the given example, $P(A)$ is the probability that a randomly selected individual has arteriosclerotic heart disease. The term *rate* has two

Statistical Methods for Rates and Proportions, Third Edition
By Joseph L. Fleiss, Bruce Levin, and Myunghee Cho Paik
ISBN 0-471-52629-0   Copyright © 2003 John Wiley & Sons, Inc.

meanings: one is as a simple synonym for probability, whereas the other attaches a notion of time to the expression of probability. The time setting may be over a given interval such as a year, or may refer to a particular point in time, and may or may not be stated explicitly. For convenience we use *rate* mostly in its first sense, but where the second sense is important we so indicate. For the given example, in the terminology of vital statistics, $P(A)$ is the case rate for arteriosclerotic heart disease (at a particular point in time).

One can go only so far with overall rates, however. Of greater usefulness usually are so-called *specific rates*: the rate of the defined characteristic specific for age, race, sex, occupation, and so on. What is known in epidemiology and vital statistics as a specific rate is known in probability theory as a *conditional probability*. The notation is

$P(A|B)$ = probability that a randomly selected individual has characteristic A, given that he has characteristic B, or *conditional* on his having characteristic B.

If, in our example, we denote by B the characteristic of being aged 65–74, then $P(A|B)$ is the conditional probability that a person has arteriosclerotic heart disease, given that he is aged 65–74. In the terminology of vital statistics, $P(A|B)$ is the rate of arteriosclerotic heart disease specific to people aged 65–74.

Let $P(B)$ represent the proportion of all people who possess characteristic B, and let $P(A$ and $B)$ represent the proportion of all people who possess both characteristic A and characteristic B. Then, by definition, provided $P(B) \neq 0$,

$$P(A|B) = \frac{P(A \text{ and } B)}{P(B)}. \tag{1.1}$$

Similarly, provided $P(A) \neq 0$,

$$P(B|A) = \frac{P(A \text{ and } B)}{P(A)}. \tag{1.2}$$

By the *association* of two characteristics we mean that when a person has one of the characteristics, say B, his chances of having the other are affected. By the *independence* or lack of association of two characteristics we mean that the fact that a person has one of the characteristics does not affect his chances of having the other. Thus, if A and B are independent, then the rate at which A is present specific to people who possess B, $P(A|B)$, is equal to the overall rate at which A is present, $P(A)$. By (1.1), this implies that

$$\frac{P(A \text{ and } B)}{P(B)} = P(A),$$

or

$$P(A \text{ and } B) = P(A)P(B). \tag{1.3}$$

Equation (1.3) is often taken as the definition of independence, instead of the equivalent statement

$$P(A|B) = P(A).$$

A heuristic justification of (1.1) is the following. Let N denote the total number of people in the population, N_A the number of people who have characteristic A, N_B the number of people who have characteristic B, and N_{AB} the number of people who have both characteristics. It is then clear that

$$P(A) = \frac{N_A}{N},$$

$$P(B) = \frac{N_B}{N},$$

and

$$P(A \text{ and } B) = \frac{N_{AB}}{N}.$$

By $P(A|B)$ we mean the proportion out of all people who have characteristic B who also have characteristic A, so that both the numerator and the denominator of $P(A|B)$ must be specific to B. Thus

$$P(A|B) = \frac{N_{AB}}{N_B}. \tag{1.4}$$

If we now divide the numerator and denominator of (1.4) by N, we find that

$$P(A|B) = \frac{N_{AB}/N}{N_B/N} = \frac{P(A \text{ and } B)}{P(B)}.$$

Equation (1.2) may be derived similarly:

$$P(B|A) = \frac{N_{AB}}{N_A} = \frac{N_{AB}/N}{N_A/N} = \frac{P(A \text{ and } B)}{P(A)}.$$

Equations (1.1) and (1.2) are connected by means of *Bayes' theorem*:

$$P(B|A) = \frac{P(A|B)P(B)}{P(A)}. \tag{1.5}$$

Equation (1.5) follows from the definition of (1.2) of $P(B|A)$ and from the fact, seen by multiplying both sides of (1.1) by $P(B)$, that $P(A \text{ and } B) = P(A|B)P(B)$.

It should be clear by comparing the denominators in (1.1) and (1.2) that $P(A|B)$ may be very different from $P(B|A)$. For example, suppose A is a disease with multiple causes and B is a risk factor that is exceedingly rare, but almost always causes A when a person is exposed to it. Then $P(A|B)$ is close to 1 by assumption, but $P(B|A)$ may be close to 0, as most cases of A will be caused by factors other than B. A similar phenomenon is studied in Section 1.3. The moral is that for a conditional probability, as for any rate or proportion, the denominator should always be clearly identified.

1.2. THE RULE OF TOTAL PROBABILITY

Let us consider the denominator of (1.5) in a bit more detail. It often happens that information about characteristic A is available in the form of a schedule of stratum-specific rates. Suppose there are k mutually exclusive and exhaustive strata, identified by $B_1, \ldots, B_k$, with specific rates $P(A|B_1), \ldots, P(A|B_k)$. In the example from the previous section, stratum B_i would represent a ten-year age interval, and $P(A|B_i)$ would be the corresponding age-specific rate of arteriosclerotic heart disease. Given the stratum proportions $P(B_1), \ldots, P(B_k)$, which sum to unity, we can obtain the overall rate $P(A)$ as

$$P(A) = P(A|B_1)P(B_1) + \cdots + P(A|B_k)P(B_k). \qquad (1.6)$$

Equation (1.6) expresses the familiar result that an overall rate is a weighted average of specific rates, where the weights are the proportions of people in the several strata. The result holds because if characteristic A occurs at all, it must occur along with one (and only one) of the k exhaustive categories of stratification $B_1, \ldots, B_k$. Because these are mutually exclusive, the corresponding probabilities simply add:

$$P(A) = P[(A \text{ and } B_1) \text{ or } (A \text{ and } B_2) \text{ or} \ldots \text{or } (A \text{ and } B_k)]$$
$$= P(A \text{ and } B_1) + \cdots + P(A \text{ and } B_k). \qquad (1.7)$$

For each term we have $P(A \text{ and } B_i) = P(A|B_i)P(B_i)$, from which (1.6) follows. Equation (1.6) is called the *rule of total probability*. In the special case of two stratum categories, say B and $\bar{B}$, the rule can be written

$$P(A) = P(A|B)P(B) + P(A|\bar{B})P(\bar{B}). \qquad (1.8)$$

There is an interesting application of (1.8) in survey method known as the *randomized response technique*. Originally introduced by Warner (1965), the method is designed to reduce bias due to evasive answers when interviewing respondents on sensitive matters. Respondents will often evade a truthful answer to a sensitive question for fear of stigmatization or incrimination, even with routine assurances of confidentiality. In order to encourage more accurate responses, in the randomized response technique an interviewer seeks a yes or no answer to a randomized question, such that the interviewer has no way of knowing what question the respondent is actually answering. If the respondent can be assured that there can be no penalties from truthful responses under such circumstances, the method can be successful in reducing bias. The following scheme described by Horvitz, Shah, and Simmons (1967) is one of several variations; another is given in Problem 1.4. The interviewer hands the respondent a coin and a card on which there are two questions: question H is the sensitive question, while question T is an innocuous question, such as "Is your mother's maiden name spelled with an even number of letters?" Respondent is instructed to toss the coin, and without revealing the outcome to the interviewer, answers yes or no to question H or T according as the coin comes up heads or tails. Thus the interviewer never knows whether the answer the respondent records is to question H or T.

Suppose a proportion p out of n respondents answer yes in the above fashion. Let A denote the event $A = $ [respondent answered yes], and let B denote the event $B = $ [coin came up heads]. Then p is an estimate of $P(A)$, the proportion of all people in the population surveyed who would answer yes. We seek $P(A|B)$, the proportion of such respondents who would answer yes to the sensitive question. The remaining terms in (1.8) are known: $P(B) = P(\bar{B}) = \frac{1}{2}$ by the coin toss, and $P(A|\bar{B}) = \frac{1}{2}$ by design of the innocuous question. Then solving for $P(A|B)$ yields the estimate $(p - \frac{1}{2} \cdot \frac{1}{2})/(\frac{1}{2}) = 2p - \frac{1}{2}$. Since $P(A)$ must lie between 0.25 and 0.75, in large samples p will also lie in this interval and will yield a reasonable estimate of $P(A|B)$.

1.3. THE EVALUATION OF A SCREENING TEST

A frequent application of Bayes' theorem is in evaluating the performance of a diagnostic test intended for use in a screening program. Let B denote the event that a person has the disease in question, $\bar{B}$ the event that he does not have the disease, A the event that he gives a positive response to the test, and $\bar{A}$ the event that he gives a negative response. Note that we distinguish between a test giving a positive (or negative) response and a person truly having (or not having) the disease, i.e., we acknowledge that the test can be in error. Suppose now that the test has been applied to a sample of B's, that is, to a sample of people with the disease, and to a sample of $\bar{B}$'s, that is, to a sample of people without the disease.

The results of this trial of the screening test may be represented by the two conditional probabilities $P(A|B)$ and $P(A|\overline{B})$. $P(A|B)$ is the conditional probability of a positive response given that the person has the disease; the larger $P(A|B)$ is, the more *sensitive* the test is. $P(A|\overline{B})$ is the conditional probability of a positive response given that the person is free of the disease; the smaller $P(A|\overline{B})$ is [equivalently, the larger $P(\overline{A}|\overline{B})$ is], the more *specific* the test is. These definitions of a test's sensitivity and specificity are due to Yerushalmy (1947).

Of greater concern than the test's sensitivity and specificity, however, are the probabilities of correctly identifying people as truly diseased or not if the test is actually used in a screening program. If a positive result is taken to indicate the presence of the disease, then the test's *positive predictive value*, or PPV, is the proportion of people, among those responding positive, who truly have the disease, or $P(B|A)$. By Bayes' theorem,

$$\text{PPV} = P(B|A) = \frac{P(A|B) \cdot P(B)}{P(A)}. \tag{1.9}$$

If a negative result is taken to indicate the absence of the disease, then the test's *negative predictive value*, or NPV, is the proportion of people, among those responding negative, who truly do not have the disease, or $P(\overline{B}|\overline{A})$. Again by Bayes' theorem,

$$\text{NPV} = P(\overline{B}|\overline{A}) = \frac{P(\overline{A}|\overline{B}) \cdot P(\overline{B})}{P(\overline{A})} = \frac{P(\overline{A}|\overline{B}) \cdot \{1 - P(B)\}}{1 - P(A)}. \tag{1.10}$$

Let Sens denote sensitivity, Sens $= P(A|B)$; let Spec denote specificity, Spec $= P(\overline{A}|\overline{B})$; and let Π denote the prevalence of the disease in the population being studied, $\Pi = P(B)$. Then (1.9) and (1.10) are expressible as

$$\text{PPV} = \frac{\text{Sens} \cdot \Pi}{\text{Sens} \cdot \Pi + (1 - \text{Spec})(1 - \Pi)}, \tag{1.11}$$

and

$$\text{NPV} = \frac{\text{Spec} \cdot (1 - \Pi)}{\text{Spec} \cdot (1 - \Pi) + (1 - \text{Sens})\Pi}. \tag{1.12}$$

[In the previous edition of the book, we analyzed the complements of (1.9) and (1.10), quantities we labeled the *false positive rate* and the *false negative rate*. Given the inconsistent meanings that attach to these two quantities—see Galen and Gambino (1975) and Rogan and Gladen (1978)—we decided to work exclusively with predictive values in the present edition.]

Cochrane and Holland (1971) and Galen and Gambino (1975) analyzed the performance of screening and diagnostic tests for a variety of medical

Table 1.1. *Results of a trial of a screening test*

Disease Status	Test Result		Total
	$+ (A)$	$- (\overline{A})$	
Present (B)	950	50	1,000
Absent $(\overline{B})$	10	990	1,000

disorders. We see from (1.11) and (1.12) that, in general, the two predictive values are functions of sensitivity and specificity, which may be estimated from the results of a trial of the screening test, and of the prevalence of the disease, for which an accurate estimate is rarely available. Nevertheless, a range of likely values for the error rates may be determined as in the following example.

Suppose that the test is applied to a sample of 1,000 people known to have the disease and to a sample of 1,000 people known not to have the disease. Suppose that this trial resulted in the frequencies shown in Table 1.1. We would then have the estimate of sensitivity,

$$\text{Sens} = P(A|B) = 950/1,000 = 0.95,$$

and the estimate of specificity,

$$\text{Spec} = P(\overline{A}|\overline{B}) = 990/1,000 = 0.99,$$

a pair of probabilities indicating a test that is both sensitive and specific to the disease being studied.

Substitution of these two probabilities in (1.11) gives, as the value for the positive predictive value,

$$\text{PPV} = \frac{0.95 \cdot \Pi}{0.95 \cdot \Pi + (1 - 0.99)(1 - \Pi)} = \frac{95\Pi}{94\Pi + 1}. \tag{1.13}$$

Substitution in (1.12) gives, as the value of the negative predictive value,

$$\text{NPV} = \frac{0.99 \cdot (1 - \Pi)}{0.99 \cdot (1 - \Pi) + 0.05 \cdot \Pi} = \frac{99 - 99 \cdot \Pi}{99 - 94 \cdot \Pi}. \tag{1.14}$$

Table 1.2 gives the predictive values associated with various values of the disease prevalence, Π. For few disorders will the prevalence exceed 1% of the population.

If the disease is not too prevalent—if it affects, say, less than 1% of the population—the negative predictive value will be quite high but the positive predictive value will be rather small. From one point of view, the test is a successful one: NPV is greater than 9,995/10,000; therefore, of every 10,000

Table 1.2. *Predictive values associated with a screening test*

Π	Positive Predictive Value (PPV)	Negative Predictive Value (NPV)
1/1,000,000	0.0001	1.0
1/100,000	0.0009	1.0
1/10,000	0.0094	0.99999
1/1,000	0.087	0.99995
1/500	0.160	0.99990
1/200	0.323	0.99975
1/100	0.490	0.99949

people who respond negative and are thus presumably given a clean bill of health, no more than 5 should actually have been informed they were ill. From another point of view, the test is a failure: PPV is less than $50/100$; therefore, of every 100 people who respond positive and thus presumably are told they have the disease or are at least advised to undergo further tests, more than 50 will actually be free of the disease.

Bayes' theorem illuminates what is going on here. Write (1.9) in *odds form*, which expresses probabilities in the form of a ratio of the probability to its complement:

$$\frac{\text{PPV}}{1-\text{PPV}} = \frac{P(B|A)}{P(\overline{B}|A)} = \frac{P(A|B)}{P(A|\overline{B})} \cdot \frac{P(B)/P(A)}{P(\overline{B})/P(A)}$$

$$= \frac{P(A|B)}{P(A|\overline{B})} \cdot \frac{P(B)}{P(\overline{B})}. \tag{1.15}$$

We see that the odds on true disease versus not, among those testing positive, is the product of two factors: the first is $P(A|B)/P(A|\overline{B}) = $ Sens$/(1-$Spec$)$, and is called the *likelihood ratio*; the second factor is the prevalence odds on disease in the population. In words, then, equation (1.15) states that the posterior odds on disease, given a positive test result, is the product of the likelihood ratio and the *a priori* prevalence odds on disease, that is, the odds we would quote before knowledge of any test result. The likelihood ratio depends only on the sensitivity and specificity of the test, and so is an empirically determinable measure of the evidentiary value of a positive test result. In the example, the likelihood ratio is Sens$/(1-$Spec$) = 0.95/0.01 = 95$. Thus a positive test result is 95 times more likely to occur in a person with disease than in one without. When the prevalence odds on disease are low, however, the term $P(B)/P(\overline{B})$ dominates the salutary effect of the likelihood ratio, and yields a soberingly low posterior odds on disease, as the results in Table 1.2 for PPV indicate.

The final decision whether or not to use the test will depend on the seriousness of the disease and on the cost of further tests or treatment.

Because the positive predictive value is so low, however, it would be hard to justify using this screening test for any but the most serious diseases. Since the proportions $P(A|B)$ and $P(\overline{A}|\overline{B})$ considered in this example are better than those associated with most existing screening tests, it is disquieting to realize that their positive predictive values are probably far below the 50 out of 100 that we found as an upper limit here.

One method for improving the positive or negative predictive value associated with a diagnostic screening procedure (but thereby increasing its cost) is to repeat the test a number of times and to declare the final result positive if the subject responds positive to each administration of the test or if he responds positive to a majority of the administrations. Parts (b) and (c) of Problem 1.2 illustrate the improved performance of a screening procedure when a test is administered twice. Sandifer, Fleiss, and Green (1968) have shown that, for some disorders, a better rule is to administer the test three times and to declare the final result positive if the subject responds positive to at least two of the three administrations. Only those subjects who respond to one of the first two administrations and negative to the other will have to be tested a third time. Those who respond positive to both of the first two administrations will be declared positive, and those who respond negative to both will be declared negative.

A more accurate but more complex assessment of the performance of a screening procedure than the above is possible when disease severity is assumed to vary and not, as here, merely to be present or absent. The appropriate analysis was originally proposed by Neyman (1947) and later extended by Greenhouse and Mantel (1950) and by Nissen-Meyer (1964). The reader is referred to these papers and to a review article by McNeil, Keeler, and Adelstein (1975) for details.

1.4. BIASES RESULTING FROM THE STUDY OF SELECTED SAMPLES

The first clues to the association between diseases and antecedent conditions frequently come from the study of such selected samples as hospitalized patients and autopsy cases. Because not all subjects are equally likely to end up in the study samples, bias may result when the associations found in the selected samples are presumed to apply in the population at large.

A classic example of this kind of bias occurs in a study by Pearl (1929). A large number of autopsy cases were cross-classified by the presence or absence of cancer and by the presence or absence of tuberculosis. A negative association between these two diseases was found, that is, tuberculosis was less frequent in autopsy cases with cancer than in cases without cancer. Pearl inferred that the same negative association should apply to live patients, and in fact acted on the basis of this inference by conceiving a study to treat terminal cancer patients with tuberculin (the protein of the tubercle bacillus) in the anticipation that the cancer would be arrested. What Pearl ignored is

Table 1.3. *Locomotor disease by respiratory disease in hospitalized subsample*

Respiratory Disease	Locomotor Disease		Total	Proportion with Locomotor Disease
	Present	Absent		
Present	5	15	20	$0.25 = p_1$
Absent	18	219	237	$0.08 = p_2$
Total	23	234	257	$0.09 = p$

that, unless all deaths are equally likely to be autopsied, it is improper to extrapolate to live patients an association found for autopsied cases. It is even possible that there would be no association for live patients but, due to the differential selection of patients for autopsy, a strong association for autopsied cases.

The same kind of bias, known as Berkson's fallacy after the person who first studied it in detail (Berkson, 1946, 1955), is possible whenever a subject's chances of being included in the study sample vary. Berkson's fallacy has also been studied by Mainland (1953; 1963, pp. 117–124), White (1953), Mantel and Haenszel (1959), and Brown (1976). Curiously, the actual existence of the fallacy was not demonstrated empirically until a report by Roberts et al. (1978). It is illustrated below in data from Sackett (1979).

Of a random sample of 2,784 individuals interviewed in the community, 257 had been hospitalized during the prior six months. Data on the presence or absence of respiratory disease and on the presence or absence of disease of bones and organs of movement (abbreviated locomotor disease) for the subsample that had been hospitalized are presented in Table 1.3.

There is clearly an association between whether a hospitalized patient had or did not have respiratory disease and whether he or she had or did not have locomotor disease: the proportion of patients with locomotor disease among those who had respiratory disease, $p_1 = 0.25$, was over three times the proportion of patients with locomotor disease among those who did not have respiratory disease, $p_2 = 0.08$. Would it, however, be correct to conclude that the two kinds of disease were associated in the community?

Not necessarily. In fact, these two characteristics—respiratory disease and locomotor disease—are essentially independent in the community. As shown in Table 1.4, the rates of locomotor disease are virtually the same in people with and without respiratory disease.

Table 1.4. *Locomotor disease by respiratory disease in general population*

Respiratory Disease	Locomotor Disease		Total	Proportion with Locomotor Disease
	Present	Absent		
Present	17	207	224	$0.08 = p_1$
Absent	184	2,376	2,560	$0.07 = p_2$
Total	201	2,583	2,784	$0.07 = p$

The source of the apparent paradox lies in variations across the four possible kinds of people (both diseases present, only respiratory disease present, only locomotor disease present, neither disease present) in the likelihood of being hospitalized. It may be checked by comparing corresponding cell frequencies in Tables 1.3 and 1.4 that the hospitalization rate for people with both diseases, 29%, was about three times each of the rates for the other kinds of people, which ranged from 7% to 10%.

Berkson's fallacy is always possible when admission rates for people with different combinations of factors vary; it can reasonably be ruled out only when the disease or diseases in question almost always require care (e.g., leukemia and some other cancers). The algebra underlying the phenomenon is as follows. Let B denote the event that a person has one of the two characteristics under study (in this case, respiratory disease), and $\bar{B}$ the event that he or she does not. Let $P(B)$ denote the proportion of all people in the community who have the characteristic and let $P(\bar{B}) = 1 - P(B)$ denote the proportion of all people who do not.

Let A denote the event that a person has the other characteristic under study (in this case, locomotor disease), and $\bar{A}$ the event that he or she does not, and let $P(A)$ and $P(\bar{A}) = 1 - P(A)$ denote the corresponding proportions. Let $P(A \text{ and } B)$ denote the proportion of all people in the community who have both characteristics, and assume that the two characteristics are independent in the community. Thus by (1.3), $P(A \text{ and } B) = P(A)\,P(B)$.

Let H denote the event that a person from the community is hospitalized for some reason or other. Define $P(H|A \text{ and } B)$ as the proportion, out of all people who have both characteristics, who are hospitalized; $P(H|\bar{A} \text{ and } B)$ as the proportion, out of all people who have one characteristic but not the other, who are hospitalized; and $P(H|A \text{ and } \bar{B})$ and $P(H|\bar{A} \text{ and } \bar{B})$ similarly. Our problem is to evaluate, in terms of these probabilities,

$$p_1 = P(A|B \text{ and } H),$$

that is, the proportion, out of all people who are characterized by B and are hospitalized, that turns out to have A; and

$$p_2 = P(A|\bar{B} \text{ and } H),$$

that is, the proportion, out of all people who are not characterized by B and are hospitalized, that turns out to have A.

We make use of the following version of the definition of a conditional probability:

$$p_1 = P(A|B \text{ and } H) = \frac{P(A \text{ and } B|H)}{P(B|H)}. \tag{1.16}$$

Equation (1.16) differs from (1.2) only in that, once specified, the second condition H (for hospitalization) remains a condition qualifying all probabilities.

A similar expression holds for the complement of p_1,

$$1 - p_1 = P(\bar{A}|B \text{ and } H) = \frac{P(\bar{A} \text{ and } B|H)}{P(B|H)}, \tag{1.17}$$

and because the denominators of (1.16) and (1.17) are the same, the ratio of p_1 to its complement is

$$\frac{p_1}{1 - p_1} = \frac{P(A|B \text{ and } H)}{P(\bar{A}|B \text{ and } H)} = \frac{P(A \text{ and } B|H)}{P(\bar{A} \text{ and } B|H)}. \tag{1.18}$$

By Bayes' theorem,

$$P(A \text{ and } B|H) = \frac{P(H|A \text{ and } B)P(A \text{ and } B)}{P(H)}$$

$$= \frac{P(H|A \text{ and } B)P(A)P(B)}{P(H)}$$

because of the assumed independence of A and B. Similarly,

$$P(\bar{A} \text{ and } B|H) = \frac{P(H|\bar{A} \text{ and } B)P(\bar{A} \text{ and } B)}{P(H)}$$

$$= \frac{P(H|\bar{A} \text{ and } B)P(\bar{A})P(B)}{P(H)}$$

and so

$$\frac{p_1}{1 - p_1} = \frac{P(A|B \text{ and } H)}{P(\bar{A}|B \text{ and } H)} = \frac{P(H|A \text{ and } B)P(A)}{P(H|\bar{A} \text{ and } B)P(\bar{A})},$$

from which it follows that

$$p_1 = \frac{P(H|A \text{ and } B)P(A)}{P(H|A \text{ and } B)P(A) + P(H|\bar{A} \text{ and } B)P(\bar{A})}. \tag{1.19}$$

Similarly,

$$\frac{p_2}{1 - p_2} = \frac{P(A|\bar{B} \text{ and } H)}{P(\bar{A}|\bar{B} \text{ and } H)} = \frac{P(H|A \text{ and } \bar{B})P(A)}{P(H|\bar{A} \text{ and } \bar{B})P(\bar{A})},$$

from which it follows that

$$p_2 = \frac{P(H|A \text{ and } \bar{B})P(A)}{P(H|A \text{ and } \bar{B})P(A) + P(H|\bar{A} \text{ and } \bar{B})P(\bar{A})}. \tag{1.20}$$

The two probabilities in (1.19) and (1.20) are not equal if the rates of hospitalization are not equal, even though the corresponding probabilities in the community, $P(A|B)$ and $P(A|\bar{B})$, are equal.

In our example, with A denoting locomotor disease, $P(A) = 7\%$. The various hospitalization rates were

$$P(H|A \text{ and } B) = 29\%,$$

$$P(H|\bar{A} \text{ and } B) = 7\%,$$

$$P(H|A \text{ and } \bar{B}) = 10\%,$$

$$P(H|\bar{A} \text{ and } \bar{B}) = 9\%.$$

Substituting these values into (1.19) and (1.20), we find that

$$p_1 = \frac{0.29 \times 0.07}{0.29 \times 0.07 + 0.07 \times 0.93} = \frac{0.020}{0.085} = 0.24$$

and that

$$p_2 = \frac{0.10 \times 0.07}{0.10 \times 0.07 + 0.09 \times 0.93} = \frac{0.007}{0.091} = 0.08,$$

close to the values we found in Table 1.3.

The moral of this exercise is clear. Unless something is known about differential hospitalization rates or differential autopsy rates, a good amount of skepticism should be applied to any generalization from associations found for hospitalized patients or for autopsy cases to associations for people at large. This caveat obviously applies also to associations obtained from reports by volunteers.

PROBLEMS

1.1. Characteristics A and B are independent if $P(A \text{ and } B) = P(A)P(B)$. Show that, if this is so, then $P(A \text{ and } \bar{B}) = P(A)P(\bar{B})$, $P(\bar{A} \text{ and } B) = P(\bar{A})P(B)$, and $P(\bar{A} \text{ and } \bar{B}) = P(\bar{A})P(\bar{B})$. [*Hint.* $P(A) = P(A \text{ and } B) + P(A \text{ and } \bar{B})$, so that $P(A \text{ and } \bar{B}) = P(A) - P(A \text{ and } B)$. Use the given relation, $P(A \text{ and } B) = P(A)P(B)$, and use the fact that $P(\bar{B}) = 1 - P(B)$.]

1.2. Assume that the case rate for a specified disease, $P(B)$, is one case per 1000 population and that a screening test for the disease is being studied.

    (a) Suppose that the test is administered a single time to a sample of people with the disease, of whom 99% respond positive. Suppose that it is also administered to a sample of people without the disease, of whom 1% respond positive. What are the positive and negative predictive values? Do you think the test is a good one?

(b) Suppose now that the test is administered twice, with a positive overall result declared only if both tests are positive. Suppose, according to this revised definition, that 98% of the diseased sample respond positive, but that only one out of 10,000 nondiseased people respond positive. What are the positive and negative predictive values now? Would you be willing to employ the test for screening under these revised conditions?

(c) Note that not all people have to be tested twice. Only if the first test result is positive must a second test be administered; the final result will be declared positive only if the second test is positive as well. It is important to estimate the proportion of all people who will have to be tested again, that is, the proportion who are positive on their first test. What is this proportion? Out of every 100,000 people tested once, how many will not need to be tested again?

1.3. The opposite kind of bias from that considered in Section 1.3 can occur. That is, two characteristics may be associated in the community but may be independent when hospitalized samples are studied. Let A represent living alone, $\bar{A}$ living with family, B having a neurosis, and $\bar{B}$ not having a neurosis. Suppose that $P(A|B) = 0.40$ and $P(A|\bar{B}) = 0.20$. Thus 40% of neurotics live alone and 20% of nonneurotics live alone. Suppose that, in the population at large, 100,000 people are neurotic and one million are not neurotic.

(a) Consider first the 100,000 neurotics. (1) How many of them live alone? (2) If the annual hospitalization rate for neurotics living alone is 5/1000, how many such people will be hospitalized? Note that this is the number of hospitalized neurotics one would find who lived alone, that is, the numerator of p_1. (3) How many of the 100,000 neurotics live with their families? (4) If the annual hospitalization rate for neurotics living with their families is 6/1000, how many such people will be hospitalized? Note that the sum of the numbers found in (2) and (4) is the total number of hospitalized neurotics, that is, the denominator of p_1. (5) What is the value of p_1, the proportion of hospitalized neurotics who lived alone? (6) How does p_1 compare with $P(A|B)$, the proportion of neurotics in the community who live alone?

(b) Consider now the one million nonneurotics. (1) How many of them live alone? (2) If the annual hospitalization rate for nonneurotics living alone is 5/1000, how many such people will be hospitalized? Note that this is the number of hospitalized nonneurotics one would find who lived alone, that is, the numerator of p_2. (3) How many of the one million nonneurotics live with their families? (4) If the annual hospitalization rate for nonneurotics living with their families is 225/100,000, how many such people will be hospitalized? Note that the sum of the numbers found in (b2) and (b4) is the total number of hospitalized nonneurotics, that is, the denominator of p_2. (5) What is the value of p_2, the proportion of hospitalized nonneurotics who lived alone? (6) How does p_2 compare with $P(A|\bar{B})$, the proportion of nonneurotics in the community who live alone?

(c) What inference would you draw from the comparison of p_1 and p_2? How does this inference compare with the inference drawn from the comparison of $P(A|B)$ and $P(A|\bar{B})$?

1.4. In a variation of the randomized response technique described by Kuk (1990), the interviewer hands the respondent two decks of cards. After shuffling each deck, the respondent selects a card at random from either deck 1 or deck 2, according as the true answer to the sensitive question would be yes or no. Respondent reports the color of the card selected (red or black), but does not reveal to the interviewer which deck was used. In this version, respondent does not have to answer any yes-no question, and may thus feel more at ease following the rules. Assuming the proportion of red cards in deck 1 is P_1 and the proportion of red cards in deck 2 is P_2, with P_1 not equal to P_2:

(a) Find an estimate of the proportion of people for whom the answer to the sensitive question is yes, given that proportion p of respondents selected a red card.

(b) What is the variance of the estimate found in (a)?

(c) Discuss the trade-off between bias due to an evasive answer and the variance of the estimate as a function of the magnitudes of P_1 and P_2.

REFERENCES

Berkson, J. (1946). Limitations of the application of fourfold table analysis to hospital data. *Biom. Bull.* (now *Biometrics*), **2**, 47–53.

Berkson, J. (1955). The statistical study of association between smoking and lung cancer. *Proc. Staff. Meet. Mayo Clin.*, **30**, 319–348

Brown, G. W. (1976). Berkson fallacy revisited: Spurious conclusions from patient surveys. *Am. J. Dis. Child.*, **130**, 56–60.

Cochrane, A. L. and Holland, W. W. (1971). Validation of screening procedures. *Br. Med. Bull.*, **27**, 3–8.

Galen, R. S. and Gambino, S. R. (1975). *Beyond normality: The predictive value and efficiency of medical diagnosis*. New York: Wiley.

Greenhouse, S. W. and Mantel, N. (1950). The evaluation of diagnostic tests. *Biometrics*, **6**, 399–412

Horvitz, D. G., Shah, B. V., and Simmons, W. R. (1967). The unrelated question randomized response model. *Proc. Social Statist. Sec., Am. Statist. Assoc.*, 65–72.

Kuk, A. Y. C. (1990). Asking sensitive questions indirectly. *Biometrika*, **77**, 436–438.

Mainland, D. (1953). The risk of fallacious conclusions from autopsy data on the incidence of diseases with applications to heart disease. *Am. Heart J.*, **45**, 644–654.

Mainland, D. (1963). *Elementary medical statistics*, 2nd ed. Philadelphia: W. W. Saunders.

Mantel, N. and Haenszel, W. (1959). Statistical aspects of the analysis of data from retrospective studies of disease. *J. Natl. Cancer Inst.*, **22**, 719–748.

McNeil, B. J., Keeler, E., and Adelstein, S. J. (1975). Primer on certain elements of medical decision making. *New Engl. J. Med.*, **293**, 211–215.

Neyman, J. (1947). Outline of statistical treatment of the problem of diagnosis. *Public Health Rep.*, **62**, 1449–1456.

Nissen-Meyer, S. (1964). Evaluation of screening tests in medical diagnosis. *Biometrics*, **20**, 730–755.

Pearl, R. (1929). Cancer and tuberculosis. *Am. J. Hyg.* (now *Am. J. Epidemiol.*), **9**, 97–159.

Roberts, R. S., Spitzer, W. O., Delmore, T., and Sackett, D. L. (1978). An empirical demonstration of Berkson's bias. *J. Chronic Dis.*, **31**, 119–128.

Rogan, W. J. and Gladen, B. (1978). Estimating prevalence from the results of a screening test. *Am. J. Epidemiol.*, **107**, 71–76.

Sackett, D. L. (1979). Bias in analytic research. *J. Chronic Dis.*, **32**, 51–63.

Sandifer, M. G., Fleiss, J. L., and Green, L. M. (1968). Sample selection by diagnosis in clinical drug evaluations. *Psychopharmacologia*, **13**, 118–128.

Warner, S. L. (1965). Randomized response: A survey technique for eliminating evasive answer bias. *J. Am. Statist. Assoc.*, **60**, 63–69.

White, C. (1953). Sampling in medical research. *Br. Med. J.*, **2**, 1284–1288.

Yerushalmy, J. (1947). Statistical problems in assessing methods of medical diagnosis, with special reference to X-ray techniques. *Public Health Rep.*, **62**, 1432–1449.

CHAPTER 2

Statistical Inference for a Single Proportion

Most frequently studies compare two or more proportions, but occasionally we need to draw statistical inferences about a single proportion. For example, a survey has collected data on the prevalence of a health condition. How do we assess whether or not the data support prior claims about the prevalence of the condition? What are the limits of uncertainty that accompany the estimated population prevalence? Here is another example. A "Phase II" clinical trial is being planned to investigate a new drug for the acute treatment of stroke victims, in advance of a large-scale, "Phase III" randomized clinical trial. How many patient participants are needed to confirm initial hopes that the new drug is superior to the standard treatment?

This chapter presents a brief survey of inferential methods for such problems and lays a formal groundwork for statistical ideas used throughout the book. Section 2.1 discusses methods of testing hypotheses about the parameter of a binomial distribution, using exact binomial calculations. Sections 2.2 and 2.3 continue with a discussion of confidence intervals. Section 2.4 presents methods that are approximate, being based on large-sample normal theory, and that require only pencil-and-paper calculations, or at most a hand-held calculator. Section 2.5 takes up the important question of sample size planning for a single-sample study. The reader who wants a quick introduction to the fundamental ideas can stop there and browse the rest later. Sections 2.6* and 2.7* may be skipped on first reading without loss of continuity. Section 2.6* discusses how to calculate approximate standard errors by the delta method. Section 2.7* discusses different ways of determining p-values and confidence intervals for discrete and asymmetrical

Statistical Methods for Rates and Proportions, Third Edition
By Joseph L. Fleiss, Bruce Levin, and Myunghee Cho Paik
ISBN 0-471-52629-0   Copyright © 2003 John Wiley & Sons, Inc.

distributions. Readers already familiar with basic binomial inference can turn straightaway to statistical methods for fourfold tables in Chapter 3.

2.1. EXACT INFERENCE FOR A SINGLE PROPORTION: HYPOTHESIS TESTS

Consider a study in which a random sample of n individuals is drawn from a large population, and the presence or absence of a specified condition or trait is ascertained for each person in the sample. Let X denote the number of persons who are found to have the condition. The *binomial probability distribution* gives the likelihoods of the $n + 1$ possible outcomes of the study —no person has the condition ($X = 0$), exactly one has the condition ($X = 1$),..., all n have the condition ($X = n$). If P is the proportion of members of the underlying population who have the condition, then the probability that exactly $X = x$ members of the sample have the condition is denoted by $\text{Bin}(x|n, P)$ and given by the formula

$$P(X = x) = \text{Bin}(x|n, P) = \binom{n}{x} P^x Q^{n-x} = \frac{n!}{x!(n-x)!} P^x (1-P)^{n-x}. \quad (2.1)$$

[In this expression, $Q = 1 - P$,

$$\binom{n}{x} = \frac{n!}{x!(n-x)!} \qquad (\text{read "}n \text{ choose } x\text{"})$$

is called the binomial coefficient, and $x!$ (read "x factorial") is equal to the product $x! = x \times (x-1) \times \cdots \times 3 \times 2 \times 1$. For example, $5! = 5 \times 4 \times 3 \times 2 \times 1 = 120$, and

$$\binom{25}{5} = \frac{25!}{5!20!} = \frac{25 \times 24 \times 23 \times 22 \times 21}{5 \times 4 \times 3 \times 2 \times 1} = 53,130.$$

By convention, $0! = 1$.] The probability that x or more members of the sample have the condition is equal to

$$P(X \geq x) = \sum_{i=x}^{n} \text{Bin}(i|n, P),$$

and the probability that x or fewer do is equal to

$$P(X \leq x) = \sum_{i=0}^{x} \text{Bin}(i|n, P).$$

Suppose that each member of a sample of $n = 25$ patients known to have a certain disorder is evaluated with a new diagnostic procedure, and that $x_0 = 23$ of them are classified by it as positive. Positivity with the new diagnostic procedure is the "condition" of the preceding paragraph, and the sensitivity P of the new procedure is estimated to be $23/25$, or 92%. If the standard laboratory procedure for the disorder has a sensitivity of $P_0 = 0.75$, the probability that exactly 23 of 25 patients would be classified as positive, assuming that the new procedure has the same underlying sensitivity as the standard, is

$$\text{Bin}(23\,|\,25, 0.75) = \frac{25!}{23!\,2!}0.75^{23}0.25^2 = \frac{25 \times 24}{2}0.75^{23}0.25^2$$

$$= 300 \times 0.001338 \times 0.0625 = 0.0251.$$

A scientific or substantive hypothesis explains and predicts certain outcomes obtained either experimentally or observationally. The traditional statistical approach to testing such a hypothesis calls for the following steps: (i) setting up a competing *null hypothesis* that predicts those outcomes based on ordinary causes and/or chance (the scientific hypothesis is then referred to as the *alternative hypothesis*); (ii) calculating the probability, assuming the null hypothesis holds, of obtaining the outcome that actually occurred, plus the probabilities of all other outcomes as extreme as, or more extreme than, the one that was observed; and (iii) rejecting the null hypothesis in favor of the alternative hypothesis if the sum of all these probabilities—the so-called *p-value*—is less than or equal to a predetermined level, denoted by α, called the *significance level*. If the p-value exceeds α, the null hypothesis is not rejected. In the biological and social sciences, where variability of observations is substantial, typical values for the significance level α are 0.10, 0.05, and 0.01. In the physical sciences, where the precision of observations can be quite high, typical values for α are 0.01, 0.001, or less.

Note that rejection of the null hypothesis does *not* constitute proof that the alternative hypothesis is true. The null hypothesis could be entirely true, and an event of low likelihood—α or less—might have occurred. An error, called the *Type I error* in the jargon of statistics, would then have been committed: rejecting the null hypothesis when it is true. It is impossible to avoid ever making such an error. What one does in the traditional "frequentist" mode of statistical inference is to make the chances of committing a Type I error tolerably small. On the other hand, failing to reject the null hypothesis does not constitute proof that it is true. The competing alternative hypothesis could be entirely true, yet the probability of the outcomes by chance alone might be sufficiently large (above α), resulting in the failure to reject the null hypothesis. Such an error is called a *Type II error*; it frequently occurs because the study's sample size is not large enough, an issue that will be taken up in Section 2.5. We note also that neither the statistical nor the alternative hypothesis need be true—explanations other than those two may be correct. Weighing of the statistical evidence of one hypothesis versus another is best accomplished by examination of the *likelihood ratio*, which we introduced in Section 1.3 and discuss again in Section 2.7.

Returning to our example, the investigators who developed the new diagnostic procedure would be interested in testing the alternative hypothesis that it has sensitivity superior to the standard procedure's sensitivity of 75%. The competing null hypothesis is that the new procedure's underlying sensitivity is no better than 75%. If the estimated sensitivity of the new procedure turned out to be less than 75%, there would obviously be no basis for asserting that the new procedure was better than the standard. If the new procedure's sensitivity turned out to exceed 75%, the question would remain whether the difference was trivially small (as would be the case if x_0 were equal to 19, yielding an estimated sensitivity of 76%) or was large enough to cast serious doubt on the tenability of the null hypothesis.

We already found that Bin(23|25, 0.75) = 0.0251. To carry out the hypothesis test as described above, we also need the values of Bin(24|25, 0.75) = 0.0063 and Bin(25|25, 0.75) = 0.0008. The sum of these probabilities is the p-value, 0.0321 (adjusted for round-off). If the prespecified significance level was $\alpha = 0.05$, we would reject the null hypothesis and conclude that the new procedure's underlying true sensitivity was greater than 75%. In repeated applications of this statistical procedure, our conclusion would be incorrect no more than 5% of the time when the null hypothesis holds.

The above test is an example of a *one-tailed test*, in which the alternative hypothesis is that the new procedure is *better*, in terms of sensitivity, than the standard. Ruled out as unimportant or uninteresting is the possibility that the new procedure is worse than the standard. Another way of stating the circumstances under which a one-tailed test is appropriate is that the consequences of the new procedure's sensitivity being the same as the standard's for how one acts or what one thinks or believes are the same as the consequences of the new procedure's sensitivity being poorer than the standard's. Suppose that, on the contrary, it is interesting or important to distinguish between these two possibilities. For example, the investigators might continue to conduct research on the new procedure if it is equal in sensitivity to the standard, but might decide to discontinue research if its sensitivity is substantially poorer. A *two-tailed test* would then be in order, wherein the null hypothesis is that there is no difference in sensitivity. This null hypothesis would be rejected if the new procedure's estimated sensitivity was either significantly larger or significantly smaller than 75%.

Different two-tailed tests are possible, depending on how one wishes to apportion the Type I error rate, α, between an outcome suggesting superiority of the new procedure and one suggesting inferiority. The simplest and most widely used two-tailed test apportions the overall error rate equally, as follows. One rejects the null hypothesis in favor of the alternative that the new procedure has greater sensitivity than 75% if $P(X \geq x_0) \leq \alpha/2$, and one rejects the null hypothesis in favor of the alternative that the new procedure's sensitivity is worse than 75% if $P(X \leq x_0) \leq \alpha/2$.

In the example, with $n = 25$, $x_0 = 23$, and $P_0 = 0.75$, the null hypothesis H_0: $P = P_0$ would not be rejected with a two-tailed test having a significance level of $\alpha = 0.05$ because

$$P(X \geq 23) = \sum_{x=23}^{25} \text{Bin}(x | 25, 0.75) = 0.0321,$$

which is greater than the critical probability $0.05/2 = 0.025$. With respect to the upper tail, only the values $x = 24$ or $x = 25$ permit rejection of the null hypothesis in favor of the alternative that the new procedure is better than the standard. With respect to the lower tail, values of x that are 13 or less lead to rejecting the null hypothesis in favor of the alternative that the new procedure's sensitivity is poorer than the standard's: $\sum_{x=0}^{13} \text{Bin}(x | 25, 0.75)$ $= 0.0107$, which is less than the critical probability 0.025, but $\sum_{x=0}^{14} \text{Bin}(x | 25, 0.75) = 0.0297$, which is not.

Suppose the investigators had decided, *in advance of the experiment*, that a Type I error in the direction of finding the new procedure inferior to the standard was consequential only if the new procedure performed extremely poorly. They might then have set up the test procedure using an asymmetric rule such as to reject the null hypothesis in favor of the alternative that the new procedure has better sensitivity than P_0 if the observed value of $X = x_0$ is such that

$$\sum_{x=x_0}^{n} \text{Bin}(x | n, P_0) \leq 0.04,$$

and reject in favor of the alternative that the new procedure has poorer sensitivity than P_0 if x_0 is such that

$$\sum_{x=0}^{x_0} \text{Bin}(x | n, P_0) \leq 0.01.$$

In the case of such a prespecified rule, the outcome $x_0 = 23$ would lead to rejecting the null hypothesis.

What is the definition of the p-value in the two-tailed case? With symmetrical allocation of $\alpha/2$ in each tail, the simplest procedure is to double the smaller of the two one-tailed p-values. In the example, we have $P(X \geq 23) = 0.0321$, which is smaller than $P(X \leq 23) = 0.9930$, so the two-tailed p-value is $2 \times 0.0321 = 0.0642$. This definition of two-tailed p-value *works assuredly* in the sense that a hypothesis test based on rejecting the null hypothesis whenever the two-tailed p-value is less than or equal to α will have a Type I error no greater than α (so it "works"), and this holds true for any value of P_0 (so it's "assured"). A proof of this assertion is given in Problem 2.7. We note that in some cases symmetrical allocation of Type I error may be arbitrary. In the illustration given in the previous paragraph of an unequal allocation of Type I error, we would define the two-tailed p-value to be the smaller of 5 times the lower tail probability and $5/4$ times the upper tail probability (see Problem 2.8). Ultimately, one might wish to deploy a data-driven allocation of Type I error to the two tails, so long as the corresponding two-tailed p-values work assuredly. Section 2.7* demonstrates how to do this in a variety of ways.

2.2. EXACT INFERENCE FOR A SINGLE PROPORTION: INTERVAL ESTIMATION

2.2.1. Definition of an Exact Confidence Interval

More informative, usually, than a test of the null hypothesis that the underlying binomial parameter P is equal to some specified value P_0 is a *confidence interval* for P. A confidence interval for a statistical parameter is a set of values that are, in a sense to be made explicit, reasonable candidates for being the true underlying value. A candidate value for the parameter is said to be *supported by the data* at the α level of significance, if, were that value hypothesized to be the true one and were the hypothesis put to the test, it would not be rejected with a test having a significance level of α. A $100(1 - \alpha)\%$ confidence interval for a parameter includes all values that are supported by the data, and excludes all values that are not supported by the data, at the α level of significance. Each value falling outside of the interval is such that, if it were hypothesized to be the value of the underlying probability, that null hypothesis would be rejected at the α level of significance.

Just as the investigators have to decide whether a one-tailed or two-tailed test is more appropriate, so must they decide between a one-sided confidence interval and a two-sided interval. An upper one-sided confidence interval for an underlying probability P is an interval of the form $P > P_L$, where P_L denotes the lower bound for the interval. Similarly, a lower one-sided confidence interval is of the form $P < P_U$, where P_U denotes the upper bound for the interval. A two-sided confidence interval is of the form $P_L < P < P_U$.

Consider finding the lower bound P_L for an upper $100(1 - \alpha)\%$ confidence interval for P. Except in special circumstances, no explicit formulas are available for P_L; it must be found by trial and error, by means of a formal iterative computation, or by special tables as shown in Section 2.3. In general, one knows one has the correct value for P_L when

$$\sum_{x=x_0}^{n} \text{Bin}(x|n, P_L) = \alpha, \tag{2.2}$$

where x_0, recall, is the number of observations out of n possessing the characteristic under study. In the numerical example in which $n = 25$ and

$x_0 = 23$ with sample proportion $p = 0.92$, the desired upper 95% one-sided confidence interval is

$$P > 0.7690. \tag{2.3}$$

The reader may confirm that the value $P_L = 0.7690$ satisfies equation (2.2) for $n = 25$, $x_0 = 23$, and $\alpha = 0.05$. This has been the first statistical problem posed in this text in which "you know you have the right answer when some (possibly complicated) equation is satisfied." It is not the last.

When $x_0 = n$, so that all subjects in the sample are positive, an explicit equation is available for P_L. Because we want P_L to satisfy $P_L^n = \alpha$, it follows that $P_L = \alpha^{1/n}$. An equivalent equation for P_L is

$$P_L = e^{(\ln \alpha)/n}, \tag{2.4}$$

where ln denotes the natural logarithm and e^x is the antilog of x. Had all 25 subjects in our example been classified as positive, the lower 95% confidence bound on P would have been

$$P_L = 0.05^{1/25} = e^{-2.9957/25} = e^{-0.1198} = 0.8871.$$

Problem 2.1 gives a common application for an upper confidence limit $P_U = 1 - \alpha^{1/n}$ based on the opposite extreme $x_0 = 0$.

Notice that the 95% confidence interval in (2.3) excludes the value 0.75, and recall that the null hypothesis H_0: $P = 0.75$ was rejected by a one-tailed test with a significance level of 0.05. Such concordance between the verdict for or against a null hypothesis from an α-level significance test and the inclusion or exclusion of the hypothesized parameter value from a $100(1 - \alpha)\%$ confidence interval always exists when the confidence interval is *test-based*, that is, constructed according to the principle of including values supported by the data at the α level of significance, and excluding all others. We shall see in Section 2.4 that other methods of constructing confidence intervals do not always give results concordant with those of significance tests, although agreement tends to be good in large samples.

Just as many two-tailed significance tests exist, so do many two-sided confidence intervals: if α_1 and α_2 are any two probabilities that sum to α, the value P_L that satisfies

$$\sum_{x=x_0}^{n} \text{Bin}(x|n, P_L) = \alpha_1 \tag{2.5}$$

and the value P_U that satisfies

$$\sum_{x=0}^{x_0} \text{Bin}(x|n, P_U) = \alpha_2 \tag{2.6}$$

are lower and upper $100(1 - \alpha)\%$ confidence limits for P. It is standard practice, and simplest, to take $\alpha_1 = \alpha_2 = \alpha/2$. The reader is asked in Problem 2.2 to prove that, in the numerical example,

$$0.74 < P < 0.99 \tag{2.7}$$

is a two-sided 95% confidence interval for the underlying sensitivity of the new procedure. Notice that the sensitivity value 0.75 for the standard diagnostic procedure lies within the interval. This is (necessarily) consistent with our not having rejected the hypothesis that the underlying sensitivity was equal to 0.75, with a two-tailed test having a significance level of 0.05 (with 0.025 in each tail).

2.2.2. A Fundamental Property of Confidence Intervals

Confidence intervals have a *fundamental property* that justifies use of the term "confidence." The property concerns the *coverage probability* for the parameter in question:

> A $100(1 - \alpha)\%$ confidence interval contains the true parameter value with probability at least $1 - \alpha$.

Note that in hypothetical repetitions of the experiment, the endpoints of the confidence interval would vary, since they depend on experimental outcomes that are subject to sampling fluctuations. The fundamental property asserts that the chance is at least $1 - \alpha$ that the (random) confidence interval covers the true (fixed) parameter value. We thus have 95% confidence that the true value is contained inside a 95% confidence interval in the same sense that we might have 95% confidence that a baseball player with a (phenomenal) .950 batting average will get a hit on any given time at bat.

There is a subtle but important distinction between the fundamental coverage property and the following statement, which refers to the numerical example in expression (2.7): "The probability is at least 95% that P lies between 0.74 and 0.99." Within the classical frequentist approach to inference, the true P is regarded as a fixed, if unknown, constant. In that case, P lies either inside or outside the interval from 0.74 to 0.99 without doubt. The statement only makes sense as a person's subjective degree of belief about where P is, or if one regards the true P not as a fixed constant but as a random variable itself. This is the Bayesian approach, which we revisit in Section 9.6. The key distinction between the two statements, then, is that the fundamental coverage property refers to a predictive operating characteristic of the confidence interval procedure in general, not to after-the-fact, degree-of-belief evaluations of coverage in specific applications of the procedure.

2.3. USING THE F DISTRIBUTION

Earlier we needed to solve equation (2.2) for P_L. Thanks to a lovely relation between sums of binomial probabilities and percentage points of the F distribution, familiar from the analysis of variance, one may solve for P_L using tables of the F distribution, which appear in most introductory statistics texts and are reproduced here as Table A.3. Let $F_{a, b; \alpha}$ denote the $100(1 - \alpha)$th percentile of the F distribution with a and b degrees of freedom; that is, $F_{a, b; \alpha}$ cuts off the proportion α in the upper tail of this distribution. The value of P_L is given explicitly by

$$P_L = \frac{x_0}{x_0 + (n - x_0 + 1) F_{2(n - x_0 + 1), 2x_0; \alpha}}, \tag{2.8}$$

where x_0 is the observed frequency. If $x_0 = 0$, the value of P_L is taken as 0.

Consider again the example with $n = 25$, $x_0 = 23$, and the requirement to determine the lower limit of an upper one-sided 95% confidence interval for P. As may be found in Table A.3, after a bit of interpolation, $F_{2 \times 3, \, 2 \times 23; \, 0.05} = F_{6, 46; 0.05} = 2.30$, so that

$$P_L = \frac{23}{23 + 3 \times 2.30} = 0.77,$$

equal to the lower limit found in expression (2.3).

The upper limit of a lower one-sided $100(1 - \alpha)\%$ confidence interval for P is

$$P_U = \frac{(x_0 + 1) F_{2(x_0 + 1), 2(n - x_0); \alpha}}{(n - x_0) + (x_0 + 1) F_{2(x_0 + 1), 2(n - x_0); \alpha}}, \tag{2.9}$$

(see Problem 2.3). If $x_0 = n$, the value of P_U is taken as 1. The equation that implicitly determines the value of P_U is

$$\sum_{x=0}^{x_0} \text{Bin}(x | n, P_U) = \alpha. \tag{2.10}$$

Suppose that $n = 25$ and $x_0 = 19$, and that a lower one-sided 95% confidence interval is desired for P of the form $P < P_U$. The critical F value is

$F_{2\times20,\ 2\times6;\ 0.05} = F_{40,\ 12;\ 0.05} = 2.43$, so that

$$P_U = \frac{20 \cdot 2.43}{6 + 20 \times 2.43} = 0.89.$$

The reader may confirm that

$$\sum_{x=0}^{19} \text{Bin}(x \mid 25, 0.89) = 0.05.$$

The limits of a two-sided $100(1 - \alpha)\%$ confidence interval with the overall Type I error rate evenly split between the two tails are

$$P_L = \frac{x_0}{x_0 + (n - x_0 + 1) F_{2(n-x_0+1),\ 2x_0;\ \alpha/2}}$$

and

$$P_U = \frac{(x_0 + 1) F_{2(x_0+1),\ 2(n-x_0);\ \alpha/2}}{(n - x_0) + (x_0 + 1) F_{2(x_0+1),\ 2(n-x_0);\ \alpha/2}}.$$

For $n = 25$, $x_0 = 23$, and $\alpha = 0.05$, we have $F_{48,\ 4;\ 0.025} = 8.39$ and $F_{6,\ 46;\ 0.025} = 2.70$. Thus,

$$P_L = \frac{23}{23 + 3 \times 2.70} = 0.74$$

and

$$P_U = \frac{24 \times 8.39}{2 + 24 \times 8.39} = 0.99,$$

identical to the limits reported in (2.7).

2.4. APPROXIMATE INFERENCE FOR A SINGLE PROPORTION

When n is large, in the sense that $nP \geq 5$ and $nQ \geq 5$, the following procedures based on the normal distribution provide excellent approximations to the corresponding exact binomial procedures. They work in large samples thanks to the *central limit theorem*, which implies that the sample proportion, $p = X/n$, is approximately normally distributed with mean P and standard error

$$\text{se}(p) = \sqrt{\frac{PQ}{n}}. \tag{2.11}$$

The sample proportion p is called a *point estimator* of the binomial parameter P, and the preceding assertion concerns properties of the distribution of the point estimator. In the sequel we will often be interested in the distribution of point estimators.

2.4.1. Hypothesis Tests

In order to test the null hypothesis that P is equal to a prespecified P_0 against the two-sided alternative hypothesis that $P \neq P_0$, one may calculate the critical ratio

$$z = \frac{|p - P_0| - 1/(2n)}{\sqrt{P_0 Q_0 / n}}, \tag{2.12}$$

where $Q_0 = 1 - P_0$, and reject the hypothesis if z exceeds $z_{\alpha/2}$, the critical value of the normal distribution for the desired two-tailed significance level α. The quantity $1/(2n)$ subtracted in the numerator is a correction for continuity, bringing normal-curve tail probabilities into closer agreement with binomial tail probabilities. It should be applied only when it is numerically smaller than $|p - P_0|$.

Consider again the study of $n = 25$ patients with a certain disorder of whom $x_0 = 23$ test positive on a new diagnostic procedure, with estimated sensitivity $p = 23/25 = 0.92$. The null hypothesis that the underlying sensitivity is equal to $P_0 = 0.75$ may be tested with a two-tailed 0.05 level test by determining the value of the critical ratio in (2.12),

$$z = \frac{|0.92 - 0.75| - 1/(2 \times 25)}{\sqrt{\dfrac{0.75 \times 0.25}{25}}} = 1.73, \tag{2.13}$$

and comparing it with the two-tailed 0.05-level critical value in Table A.1, $z_{0.025} = 1.96$. Because z is less than 1.96, the hypothesis that $P = 0.75$ cannot be rejected with the approximate two-tailed normal theory test. The same conclusion was drawn in Section 2.1 from the exact two-tailed binomial test.

Equivalently, the approximate two-sided p-value associated with a normal deviate of $z = 1.73$ may be determined and compared with 0.05. This p-value is the probability that a standard normal random variable exceeds 1.73 in absolute value. From Table A.1, this probability is equal to 0.084, which exceeds the specified significance level of 0.05. Again, the hypothesis that $P = 0.05$ cannot be rejected.

One-tailed critical ratio tests are easily carried out. If the alternative hypothesis is that the true proportion P is greater than P_0, the null hypothesis is rejected in favor of this alternative when $p > P_0$ and

$$z = \frac{(p - P_0) - 1/(2n)}{\sqrt{P_0 Q_0/n}} \geq z_\alpha, \qquad (2.14)$$

where z_α is the critical value of the normal distribution cutting off probability α in the upper tail. For example, $z_{0.05} = 1.645$ and $z_{0.01} = 2.326$. If the alternative hypothesis is that $P < P_0$, the null hypothesis is rejected in favor of this alternative when $p < P_0$ and

$$z = \frac{(p - P_0) + 1/(2n)}{\sqrt{P_0 Q_0/n}} \leq -z_\alpha, \qquad (2.15)$$

The continuity correction is applied in (2.14) and (2.15) only if $1/(2n) < |p - P_0|$.

Consider testing the one-sided alternative hypothesis that sensitivity exceeds 0.75 in the example. Because $p = 0.92$ is greater than 0.75, one may calculate the value of the statistic in (2.14). It is $z = 1.73$, which exceeds the critical value of $z_{0.05} = 1.645$ required for a one-sided test with a significance level of 0.05. The hypothesis that $P > 0.75$ is thus adopted, as it was with the exact binomial analysis. The exact binomial probability of $x_0 = 23$ or more positives on the test being studied, assuming $P = 0.75$, was found to be 0.032. The approximate p-value from the normal curve is 0.042, slightly greater.

2.4.2. Confidence Intervals

An approximate two-sided $100(1 - \alpha)\%$ confidence interval for the underlying proportion consists of all those values of P that would not be rejected by a two-tailed critical ratio test at the α level of significance. If the test is based on the statistic given in (2.12), and if $z_{\alpha/2}$ denotes the value cutting off probability $\alpha/2$ in the upper tail of the normal distribution, an approximate $100(1 - \alpha)\%$ confidence interval consists of all those values of P satisfying

$$z = \frac{|p - P| - 1/(2n)}{\sqrt{PQ/n}} < z_{\alpha/2}, \qquad (2.16)$$

The limits of this interval are given by the two roots of the quadratic equation obtained by setting the square of the left-hand side of (2.16) equal to $z_{\alpha/2}^2$. Define $q = 1 - p$. The lower limit is given explicitly by

$$P_L = \frac{\left(2np + z_{\alpha/2}^2 - 1\right) - z_{\alpha/2}\sqrt{z_{\alpha/2}^2 - \{2 + (1/n)\} + 4p(nq + 1)}}{2\left(n + z_{\alpha/2}^2\right)}, \qquad (2.17)$$

and the upper limit by

$$P_U = \frac{\left(2np + z_{\alpha/2}^2 + 1\right) + z_{\alpha/2}\sqrt{z_{\alpha/2}^2 + \{2 - (1/n)\} + 4p(nq-1)}}{2\left(n + z_{\alpha/2}^2\right)} \quad (2.18)$$

(see Problem 2.4).

For the data being analyzed, $n = 25$, $p = 0.92$, and $q = 0.08$. For a two-sided 95% confidence interval for P, we have $z_{\alpha/2} = z_{0.025} = 1.96$. It may be checked that (2.17) and (2.18) yield $P_L = 0.725$ and $P_U = 0.986$, so

$$0.73 < P < 0.99$$

is an approximate 95% confidence interval for P. The agreement is excellent with the exact interval given in (2.7). Further, the reader may check that if $P_0 = 0.725$ or $P_0 = 0.986$ is hypothesized as the value of P, the resulting value of z in (2.12) is exactly equal to 1.96.

The preceding somewhat complicated procedure for setting a confidence interval around P is preferred amongst approximate methods when p is near zero or near unity. When p is of moderate size (say, $0.3 \leq p \leq 0.7$), the following more familiar and simpler procedure may be employed when n is large (again, $nP \geq 5$ and $nQ \geq n$). Because $\sqrt{u(1-u)}$ remains fairly constant for $0.3 \leq u \leq 0.7$, $\sqrt{PQ}$ in the denominator of (2.16) may be replaced by $\sqrt{pq}$ without materially affecting the quality of the large-sample normal approximation. This yields the interval

$$p - z_{\alpha/2}\sqrt{\frac{pq}{n}} - \frac{1}{2n} < P < p + z_{\alpha/2}\sqrt{\frac{pq}{n}} + \frac{1}{2n} \quad (2.19)$$

as an approximate $100(1 - \alpha)\%$ confidence interval for P. For the data at hand, however, the resulting interval is

$$0.79 < P < 1.05.$$

The interval is shifted so strongly to the right relative to the technically more accurate one that its upper limit is absurd. Problem 2.5 illustrates related problems with the interval in (2.19) when p is close to 0 or 1, and Problem 2.6 asks the reader to prove that the interval given by (2.17) and (2.18) always lies between 0 and 1.

2.5. SAMPLE SIZE FOR A ONE-SAMPLE STUDY

One of the most important steps in designing a study is the determination of the number of participants. In this section we consider the sample size problem for hypothesis testing and interval estimation in the prototype case of a single binomial sample. Section 2.5.1 introduces the related problems of sample size, statistical power, and detectable effect size for testing hypotheses about the binomial parameter P. Section 2.5.2 determines the sample size required to construct a confidence interval for P with maximum predetermined width.

2.5.1. Sample Size for Hypothesis Tests

The problem stated at the beginning of the chapter is typical of sample size determination problems. Here is a version in a bit more detail:

> A Phase II clinical trial is being planned to investigate a new drug for the acute treatment of stroke victims, in advance of a large-scale, Phase III randomized clinical trial. The new drug is actually a modified form of the tissue plasminogen activator (tPA) molecule that has been shown to be effective in helping stroke patients recover. In the Phase II trial the investigators want to determine whether the new preparation can substantially reduce the rate of intracerebral hemorrhage (ICH), a serious adverse side effect that occurs with a known frequency of 6% within three days of treatment by tPA . Stroke patients who consent will be given the new treatment in a single treatment arm. If the new drug is successful in reducing the rate of ICH substantially below 6%, the drug will be taken to the Phase III randomized controlled trial to test its efficacy and safety definitively in comparison with tPA. The investigators decide to conduct a one-sided test, on the following grounds. No further development of the drug will occur unless the ICH rate with the new drug is lower than 6%; so a Type I error in the direction of stating that the new drug is significantly worse than the standard with respect to ICH, when in fact it has the same rate, will have the same consequences as lackluster performance in the positive direction: further development will stop. The investigators want to control the Type I error rate in the direction of stating that the new drug has a significantly better rate of ICH than 6%, when in fact it does not, and they choose the significance level $\alpha = 0.05$. Finally, the investigators also consider a Type II error serious: failure to reject the null hypothesis that the ICH rate is no better than 6%, when in fact the new drug has a lower ICH rate, would represent an unfortunate loss of a treatment with better properties than the standard. The investigators want their study to have statistical power of 90% if, as they hope, the new drug can reduce the ICH rate to 2%. The main statistical question for planning the Phase II trial is: how many participants should be enrolled?

Let X denote the number of intracerebral hemorrhages to be observed among the n stroke patients treated with the new drug, let P denote the true ICH rate, and assume X has a binomial distribution with sample size n and parameter P, which we write as $X \sim \text{Bin}(n, P)$. The null hypothesis is that the ICH rate with the new drug is no better than 6%, that is, $H_0: P \geq P_0 = 0.06$. The alternative hypothesis is that the new drug improves over this rate: $H_1: P < P_0$. The statistical power is the probability of correctly rejecting H_0 when it is false. Because that probability depends on the true P, the statistical power is not a single number but a function of values as P varies. It is also the complement of the Type II error rate, β, for given values of P. In succinct form, the problem is to find n such that $P(\text{Reject } H_0|H_0 \text{ true}$ with any $P \geq P_0) \leq \alpha$ and $P(\text{Reject } H_0|H_0 \text{ false with any } P \leq 0.02) \geq 1 - \beta$, where $\alpha = 0.05$ is the level of significance and $1 - \beta = 0.90$ is the statistical power.

The required sample size will be large, so let us begin with the normal approximation to the binomial distribution, which states that if we *standardize* the random variable X by subtracting off its expected value nP and dividing by the square root of the variance, $nP(1 - P)$, so that

$$X^* = \frac{X - EX}{\sqrt{\text{Var } X}} = \frac{X - nP}{\sqrt{nP(1 - P)}},$$

then the standardized variable X^* has an approximately normal distribution with zero mean and unit variance, that is, X^* is approximately standard normal. The probability of rejection under H_0 will be greatest when $P = P_0$, so it suffices to consider this case to represent the null hypothesis. For an approximate one-tailed test of the hypothesis H_0: $P = P_0$, then, we reject H_0 when the observed value of X^* is less than or equal to $-z_\alpha$, where z_α is the critical value cutting off probability α in the upper tail of the standard normal distribution; in this case, $z_\alpha = 1.645$ from Table A.1. This is the same test as presented in (2.15), except we have postponed introducing the correction for continuity $1/(2n)$. In symbols, we reject H_0 when we observe the event

$$R = \left[X^* \leq -z_\alpha \right] = \left[X \leq nP_0 - z_\alpha\sqrt{nP_0(1 - P_0)} \right], \tag{2.20}$$

Now suppose that H_1 is true with $P = P_1 = 0.02$. The next step is to standardize the random variable X again, this time at the alternative parameter value. The power is then

$$\text{Power (at } P_1) = P\left(R = \text{Reject } H_0|P = P_1 \right)$$

$$= P\left[\frac{X - E_1X}{\sqrt{\text{Var}_1 X}} \leq \frac{nP_0 - z_\alpha\sqrt{nP_0(1 - P_0)} - nP_1}{\sqrt{nP_1(1 - P_1)}} \right]$$

$$\approx P\left[Z \leq \frac{n(P_0 - P_1) - z_\alpha\sqrt{nP_0(1 - P_0)}}{\sqrt{nP_1(1 - P_1)}} \right], \tag{2.21}$$

where Z denotes a standard normal random variable. In order for the expression on the right-hand side of (2.21) to be at least $1 - \beta$, the expression inside the square bracket has to be at least as large as z_β, the critical value cutting off probability β in the upper tail of the standard normal distribution. From Table A.1, $z_\beta = 1.282$. Cancelling $\sqrt{n}$ from numerator and denominator and solving for n establishes the sample size requirement:

$$n \geq \left[\frac{z_\alpha \sqrt{P_0(1-P_0)} + z_\beta \sqrt{P_1(1-P_1)}}{P_1 - P_0} \right]^2 . \tag{2.22}$$

Substituting the design constants in (2.22) yields a sample size of $n \geq 203.2$, so we take as minimum sample size $n = 204$.

How well does (2.22) perform? The rejection region R in (2.20) for $n = 204$ is $R = [X \leq 6.66]$, so the actual rejection region is the set of integers $\{0, 1, \ldots, 6\}$, and the exact binomial probability of rejection when $P = P_0$ is $\sum_{x=0}^{6} \text{Bin}(x \mid 204, 0.06) = 0.0359$, and when $P = P_1$ the exact power is $\sum_{x=0}^{6} \text{Bin}(x \mid 204, 0.02) = 0.8829$. The Type I error is a bit conservative, and the power is not quite the desired 90%, so we can do better, but the normal approximation has given a reasonably good start.

The performance of (2.22) can be improved by use of the $\frac{1}{2}$ continuity correction, which modifies the critical ratio X^* toward zero in such a way that the accuracy of the normal approximation for the probability of the event $R = [X^* \leq -z_\alpha]$ is increased:

$$R = [X^* \leq -z_\alpha] = \left[\frac{X + \frac{1}{2} - nP_0}{\sqrt{nP_0(1-P_0)}} \leq -z_\alpha \right]$$

$$= \left[X \leq nP_0 - \tfrac{1}{2} - z_\alpha \sqrt{nP_0(1-P_0)} \right] . \tag{2.23}$$

Following through the same derivation leads now to the requirement that n be so large that

$$\sqrt{n}(P_0 - P_1) - \frac{1}{2\sqrt{n}} \geq z_\alpha \sqrt{P_0(1-P_0)} + z_\beta \sqrt{P_1(1-P_1)} .$$

This expression is a quadratic equation in $\sqrt{n}$ that can be solved by the usual quadratic formula. The required sample size is

$$n = \frac{n'}{4} \left(1 + \sqrt{1 + \frac{2}{n' |P_1 - P_0|}} \right)^2 , \tag{2.24}$$

where n' is from the right-hand side of (2.22). To an excellent approximation,

$$n = n' + 1/|P_1 - P_0| .$$

In our application, the smallest value to satisfy the inequality is $n = 228$, equation (2.24) yields $n = 227.5$, and the approximation $203.2 + 1/0.04 = 228.2$ agrees quite well.

How well does (2.24) perform? The rejection region R in (2.23) for $n = 228$ is now $R = [X \leq 7.28]$, so the actual rejection region is the set of integers $\{0, 1, \ldots, 7\}$, and the exact binomial probability of rejection when $P = P_0$ is now $\sum_{x=0}^{7} \text{Bin}(x \mid 228, 0.06) = 0.0336$, and when $P = P_1$ the exact power is $\sum_{x=0}^{7} \text{Bin}(x \mid 228, 0.02) = 0.9105$. The Type I error is even a bit more conservative, but the power is now greater than the desired 90%, so (2.24) was successful in meeting the goals of the trial.

Actually, the value $n = 228$ is a little larger than necessary. An exact test based on the critical region $\{0, 1, \ldots, 7\}$ with $n = 217$ has Type I error $\sum_{x=0}^{7} \text{Bin}(x \mid 217, 0.06) = 0.0484$ and power $\sum_{x=0}^{7} \text{Bin}(x \mid 217, 0.02) = 0.9280$. While conservative compared to the theoretically exact result, the additional sample size implied by (2.24) is not a detriment when one considers the complexities of actually conducting clinical trials. Withdrawal of patient consent, poor compliance, protocol violations, and other threats to validity are risks in conducting any trial, and tend to diminish the effective sample size. Thus building in a realistic cushion in the sample size calculation is a practical and prudent step to take. The conclusion is that (2.24) is a reasonable *initial* solution to the sample size problem. Problem 2.9 explores the consequences of inadequate sample sizes and underpowered studies.

Sample size calculations for hypothesis tests of the form H_0: $P \leq P_0$ versus H_1: $P > P_0$ are almost identical. The only change required is a reversal of the sign of $P_0 - P_1$, so that the general approximate sample size requirement for one-tailed tests is given by

$$\sqrt{n} \, |P_1 - P_0| - \frac{1}{2\sqrt{n}} \geq z_\alpha \sqrt{P_0(1 - P_0)} + z_\beta \sqrt{P_1(1 - P_1)} \,. \qquad (2.25)$$

For two-tailed tests of H_0: $P = P_0$ versus H_1: $P \neq P_0$, with equal allocation $\alpha/2$ in each tail of the rejection region, the only change required in (2.22) is to replace the critical value z_α with $z_{\alpha/2}$:

$$\sqrt{n} \, |P_1 - P_0| - \frac{1}{2\sqrt{n}} \geq z_{\alpha/2} \sqrt{P_0(1 - P_0)} + z_\beta \sqrt{P_1(1 - P_1)} \,. \qquad (2.26)$$

Expression (2.24) remains the same. The reader is asked to derive (2.26) in Problem 2.10.

The basic relationship between sample size, statistical power, and effect size in all these problems is the expression for power. This was given by (2.21) without continuity correction in the one-tailed case. For two-tailed testing with continuity correction, the basic relationship is

$$\text{Power at } P_1 \approx P\left[Z \leq \frac{\sqrt{n}\,|P_1 - P_0| - \dfrac{1}{2\sqrt{n}} - z_{\alpha/2}\sqrt{P_0(1 - P_0)}}{\sqrt{P_1(1 - P_1)}} \right]. \quad (2.27)$$

If sample size is fixed by an external consideration like cost, then (2.27) can be used to calculate the power of the test for given alternative values of $P = P_1$.

A related question is to determine the *detectable effect size* with specified power and sample sizes. That is, given a fixed sample size n, how large must the difference $|P_1 - P_0|$ be for the power to reach a prespecified level? In the stroke example, if $n = 100$ subjects are available and no more, how small must the ICH rate be in order for the one-sided level $\alpha = 0.05$ test to reject with power of 90%? The answer is contained implicitly in (2.27), with the one-tailed critical value $z_{0.05} = 1.645$, namely, that value of P_1 rendering the expression on the right side of the inequality equal to $z_{0.90} = 1.282$. This leads to another quadratic equation. A computation shows that the solution is less than 0.01, that is, the detectable effect size is nearly a 90% reduction in ICH rate. It would be an outstandingly safe drug that could achieve this effect size, which is another way of characterizing the inadequacy of the sample size $n = 100$.

2.5.2. Sample Size for Confidence Intervals

In planning a study to determine a confidence interval for a population proportion P, we need to know how large a sample to draw. In addition to the confidence level, $100(1 - \alpha)\%$, where α is most often taken to be 0.05, the investigator will often be able to specify in advance the desired width of the interval, say $d = 0.10$, between the upper and lower limits. Two cases may be considered: in the first, no information about P is known or assumed; in the second, the investigator has a rough idea of the magnitude of P.

The width of the confidence interval in (2.17) and (2.18) is no greater than the quantity

$$\frac{1 + z_{\alpha/2}\sqrt{z_{\alpha/2}^2 + 2 + nk}}{n + z_{\alpha/2}^2}, \quad (2.28)$$

where $k = 4pq$ and $p = 1 - q$ is the sample proportion. The requirement that (2.28) be no greater than of width d imposes a constraint on n which can be solved for by means of a quadratic equation. To an excellent approximation,

Table 2.1. *Sample size determination for a confidence interval of prespecified width*

If P satisfies	Then use
$0 \leq P < d/2$	$k = 4d(1 - d)$
$d/2 \leq P < 0.3$	$k = 4(P + d/2)(Q - d/2)$
$0.3 \leq P \leq 0.7$	$k = 1$
$0.7 < P \leq 1 - d/2$	$k = 4(P - d/2)(Q + d/2)$
$1 - d/2 < P \leq 1$	$k = 4d(1 - d)$

the solution is given by

$$n \geq \frac{kz_{\alpha/2}^2}{d^2} + \frac{2}{d} - 2z_{\alpha/2}^2 + \frac{z_{\alpha/2} + 2}{k}. \tag{2.29}$$

The first two terms in (2.29), $kz_{\alpha/2}^2/d^2 + 2/d$, give the required sample size for the approximate confidence interval in (2.19), while the first term alone gives the required sample size for interval (2.19) without the continuity correction.

Because for any p we have $k = 4pq \leq 1$, an upper bound is obtained in (2.28) by setting $4pq = 1$, with corresponding sample size being given in (2.29) using $k = 1$. This is an appropriate value to use when no information is available about P. If P is known or assumed to lie outside the interval $[0.3, 0.7]$, then a value of k that is less than 1 could be used to reduce the required sample size. The values of k in Table 2.1 are recommended, assuming a choice of width d no greater than 0.6 (d would rarely be set so high in practice).

For example, suppose a two-sided 95% confidence interval is desired of width $d \leq 0.2$, where P is believed to be about 0.10. Using the value $k = 4 \times 0.2 \times 0.8 = 0.64$ from Table 2.1 in (2.29) yields $n \geq 73$. With this sample size the confidence interval in (2.17) and (2.18) will be of width at most 20 percentage points for any observed value of $p \leq 0.20$. Such values of p will occur with high probability if P is near 0.10. Suppose in our example we observe $p = 14/73 = 0.192$. Then (2.17) and (2.18) produce the interval (0.112, 0.304), of width 0.19. The exact confidence interval from (2.5) and (2.6) with $\alpha_1 = \alpha_2 = \alpha/2$ is nearly identical, (0.109, 0.301). If p is close to the anticipated $P = 0.10$, say $p = 7/73 = 0.096$, then (2.17) and (2.18) yield the interval (0.043, 0.193), of width 0.15; the exact confidence interval is (0.039, 0.188).

Now compare these results with those obtained from (2.29) using $k = 1$. In that case the required sample size is $n \geq 105$, for which the interval from (2.17) and (2.18) has width ≤ 0.20 for any value of p. For example, with $p = 53/105 = 0.505$, equations (2.17)–(2.18) produce the interval (0.406, 0.603).

The exact confidence interval is nearly identical, $(0.405, 0.604)$. If p is close to the anticipated value 0.10, say $p = 10/105 = 0.095$, the approximate confidence interval is $(0.049, 0.172)$, of width 0.123, and the exact confidence interval is $(0.047, 0.168)$.

2.6.* STANDARD ERRORS BY THE DELTA METHOD

Occasions arise when the parameter of interest is not the binomial parameter P itself but some function of it, say $f(P)$. One important such function is $f(P) = \ln\{P/(1 - P)\}$, the natural logarithm of the odds associated with P, or simply the log odds of P. This function will play a central role in later chapters. The methods of Section 2.4 based on the large-sample normal approximation can be used to draw inferences about $f(P)$, but require a standard error for the estimate of $f(P)$. What shall we use as a standard error for the estimate $f(p)$ of $f(P)$ based on the sample proportion $p = X/n$ when n is large? If f is a differentiable function, the answer is contained in another consequence of the central limit theorem: $f(p)$ is approximately normally distributed with mean $f(P)$ and with a standard error (se) given by

$$\text{se}\{f(p)\} = \left| \frac{df}{dP}(P) \right| \sqrt{P(1 - P)/n},$$

where the derivative of f is evaluated at P. If P is not known, then $\text{se}\{f(p)\}$ may itself be estimated by

$$\widehat{\text{se}}\{f(p)\} = \left| \frac{df}{dP}(p) \right| \sqrt{p(1 - p)/n},$$

where the sample proportion has replaced the unknown P.

For example, with f being the log odds function given above,

$$\frac{df}{dP}(P) = \frac{1}{P} + \frac{1}{1 - P} = \frac{1}{P(1 - P)},$$

so that

$$\text{se}\{f(p)\} = \frac{1}{P(1 - P)} \sqrt{P(1 - P)/n} = \frac{1}{\sqrt{nP(1 - P)}},$$

which can be estimated by

$$\widehat{\text{se}}\{f(p)\} = \frac{1}{\sqrt{np(1 - p)}}.$$

Note that while p has a small estimated standard error when p is close to 0 or 1, the log odds has a large standard error. Problem 2.13 gives another example of this phenomenon. Problem 2.14 shows there is a *variance-stabilizing* transformation for P, yielding a transformed parameter whose estimated standard error depends only on the sample size but not on p.

2.7.* ALTERNATIVE DEFINITIONS OF TWO-SIDED P-VALUES AND CONFIDENCE INTERVALS

The definition of a two-sided confidence interval discussed above in Section 2.2.1 at (2.5) and (2.6) required specifying α_1 and α_2 (each usually taken to be $\alpha/2$) in advance. The symmetrical choice $\alpha_1 = \alpha_2 = \alpha/2$ can and should be motivated by substantive considerations related to the relative seriousness of a Type I error in the upper versus the lower tail. More often, though, this choice is made for convenience or convention. Symmetrical statistical procedures are familiar from work with the standard normal distribution, due to the symmetry of its bell-shaped probability density function, which, after all, is a large-sample approximation to the binomial distribution. However, when n is not large, or when p is close to 0 or 1, the symmetry of the large-sample normal approximation is no longer pertinent, given the discrete and asymmetrical shape of the binomial distribution with P different from $\frac{1}{2}$. Even with perfectly symmetrical distributions, asymmetrical allocation of Type I error may still make good sense. Ultimately, however, it just seems unrealistic to expect advance specification of separate tail probabilities in every application of a hypothesis test or confidence interval. In these circumstances there are alternative approaches to two-sided testing and interval estimation that require specification only of the total Type I error rate α. In a sense, the data determine their own allocation of Type I error in these methods, but the methods still maintain the overall two-tailed Type I error probability at a maximum of α. They are "exact" in the sense that they use exact binomial theory as opposed to approximate normal theory.

Below we present three such methods. In practical terms the differences among them are slight, and no one method dominates another, so that any of the three methods is acceptable for general usage and, in terms of statistical power and length of confidence intervals, will usually improve a bit on the method employing symmetrical allocation of Type I error presented in Section 2.1. The first method presented in Section 2.7.1 is the simplest of the three.

2.7.1. The Point Probability Method

In this approach we define the two-sided p-value, corresponding to a binomial observation x_0 under the hypothesis H_0: $P = P_0$, to be the sum of all binomial probabilities that are less than or equal to the probability of x_0.

If we denote the p-value for x_0 under H_0 by $\text{pval}(x_0, P_0)$, then

$$\text{pval}(x_0, P_0) = \sum_x \text{Bin}(x|n, P_0), \qquad (2.30)$$

where the sum is taken over all values of x with

$$\text{Bin}(x|n, P_0) \leq \text{Bin}(x_0|n, P_0). \qquad (2.31)$$

The set of x's satisfying (2.31) generally comprises two tails. One is the familiar tail of x values on the same side of the average value nP_0 as x_0 is, but farther away from it. The other tail consists of values of x that are on the opposite side of nP_0 from x_0, and with probabilities no larger than $\text{Bin}(x_0|n, P_0)$. We call this the two-tailed p-value by the *point probability method*.

Given a binomial observation $X = x_0$ with sample size n, a two-sided test of the hypothesis H_0: $P = P_0$ at level α may be conducted by evaluating the p-value and rejecting H_0 if and only if $\text{pval}(x_0, P_0) \leq \alpha$. Problem 2.15 asks the reader to verify that such a test procedure does indeed have Type I error rate $\leq \alpha$ for any value of P_0, that is, $\text{pval}(x_0, P_0)$ works assuredly.

In our standard example with $x_0 = 23$ and $n = 25$, the two-sided p-value by the point probability method equals $\text{pval}(23, 0.75) = 0.0618$, slightly smaller than the p-value of 0.0642 found in Section 2.1 with equal allocation of Type I error in each tail.

It is possible to invert the test procedure just described to obtain an exact two-sided $100(1 - \alpha)\%$ confidence region for P. The confidence region consists of all values P' for which $\text{pval}(x_0, P') > \alpha$, that is, values of the parameter that would not be rejected as hypotheses of the form H_0: $P = P'$. By construction, this method agrees exactly with hypothesis testing, such as, one rejects H_0: $P = P_0$ if and only if P_0 is not contained in the confidence region given $X = x_0$. Problem 2.16 demonstrates that the region so obtained has coverage probability at least $1 - \alpha$ for all values of P, that is, the confidence region works assuredly as well.

We have used the term "region" instead of "interval" because it is possible for the confidence region to consist of a union of disjoint intervals, due to a slight nonmonotonicity in the p-value function. Problem 2.20 explores this infrequently occurring phenomenon. While theoretically there is nothing wrong with a disconnected confidence region, for simplicity we will modify the definition and take as our confidence interval the smallest connected interval containing the confidence region. The limits of this confidence interval are obtained by finding the value P_L, equal to the smallest value of P' (technically, the greatest lower bound) such that $\text{pval}(x_0, P') > \alpha$, and P_U, equal to the largest value of P' (technically, the least upper bound) such that $\text{pval}(x_0, P') > \alpha$. Although extending the confidence interval occasionally to include interior values that just miss being supported by the data could break the strict correspondence between hypothesis testing and confidence intervals, usually no such parameter values are included in the confidence interval, that is, the confidence region is already a connected interval; when there are unsupported values, they are always contained in a tiny interval, and are surrounded by neighboring values of P that are supported by the data. Defining the confidence interval to include these unsupported parameter values merely increases slightly the interval's coverage probability. We shall adopt this modification without further mention on the grounds that an interval with good coverage is what is usually desired in a confidence procedure. Where perfect correspondence between hypothesis testing and interval estimation is important, the original confidence region can be used.

One advantage of the point probability method is that it usually produces intervals of shorter length than other methods, while still guaranteeing $100(1 - \alpha)\%$ coverage. A disadvantage is that finding P_L and P_U generally requires computer iteration, although efficient computing algorithms exist to do this. The binary search technique described in any textbook on numerical analysis is well suited to this task.

In the example with $x_0 = 23$ and $n = 25$, the two-sided p-value by the point probability method equals 0.05 at $P' = 0.9856$ and is less than 0.05 for values of P' larger than 0.9856, so that this value is the upper limit P_U. In Problem 2.17 the reader will verify that $P_L = 0.7441$. Note that the interval $(0.7441, 0.9856)$ is slightly shorter than that obtained from (2.5) and (2.6) with $\alpha_1 = \alpha_2 = 0.025$, which is $(0.7397, 0.9902)$ to four decimals.

2.7.2. The Tail Probability Method

Other definitions of two-tailed p-values are possible. For example, instead of defining $\mathrm{pval}(x_0, P_0)$ by (2.30) and (2.31), we can define the values of x to sum in (2.30) by those x which satisfy either

$$\sum_{i=0}^{x} \mathrm{Bin}(i|n, P_0) \le \sum_{i=0}^{x_0} \mathrm{Bin}(i|n, P_0) \quad \text{or} \quad \sum_{i=x}^{n} \mathrm{Bin}(i|n, P_0) \le \sum_{i=0}^{x_0} \mathrm{Bin}(i|n, P_0)$$

$$(2.32)$$

if the observed lower tail probability on the right-hand side of either expression is less than $\frac{1}{2}$, that is, if x_0 is in the lower tail. If, instead, x_0 is in the upper tail with $\sum_{i=x_0}^{n} \mathrm{Bin}(i|n, P_0) < \frac{1}{2}$, then the values of x to sum in (2.30) are those x which satisfy either

$$\sum_{i=0}^{x} \mathrm{Bin}(i|n, P_0) \le \sum_{i=x_0}^{n} \mathrm{Bin}(i|n, P_0) \quad \text{or} \quad \sum_{i=x}^{n} \mathrm{Bin}(i|n, P_0) \le \sum_{i=x_0}^{n} \mathrm{Bin}(i|n, P_0)$$

$$(2.33)$$

In words, the p-value is the probability associated with all values of x for which the opposite-tail probability is no greater than the observed-tail probability. We call this the two-tailed p-value by the *tail probability method*, and it too works assuredly. See Problem 2.18.

In our running example with $x_0 = 23$ and $n = 25$, the two-sided p-value by the tail probability method equals pval$(23, 0.75) = 0.0618$, identical to that of the point probability method, though this is not always the case. Inverting the p-value by the tail probability method to obtain a 95% confidence interval for P, we find the interval $(P_L, P_U) = (0.7485, 0.9856)$. In this example, the 95% confidence interval is slightly shorter than that based on the point probability method, although again, this is not always the case.

2.7.3. The Likelihood Ratio Method

The third definition of two-tailed p-value is based upon the likelihood ratio test, which is of special interest in its own right. If X has a binomial distribution with sample size n and parameter P, the *likelihood ratio statistic* for testing the null hypothesis $H_0: P = P_0$ against an alternative hypothesis of the form $H_1: P = P_1$ is defined as

$$\mathrm{LR}(P_1 : P_0 | x_0) = \frac{\mathrm{Bin}(x_0 | n, P_1)}{\mathrm{Bin}(x_0 | n, P_0)} = \frac{P_1^{x_0}(1 - P_1^{n - x_0})}{P_0^{x_0}(1 - P_0^{n - x_0})}, \qquad (2.34)$$

and the log likelihood ratio statistic is the natural logarithm of LR:

$$\mathrm{LLR}(P_1 : P_0 | x_0) = \ln \mathrm{LR}(P_1 : P_0 | x_0) = x_0 \ln\left(\frac{P_1}{P_0}\right) + (n - x_0)\ln\left(\frac{1 - P_1}{1 - P_0}\right).$$
$$(2.35)$$

These statistics are of key importance because the likelihood ratio is the fundamental way to define the weight of evidence in the data concerning the hypothesis H_0 versus the alternative H_1. The larger $\mathrm{LR}(P_1 : P_0 | x_0)$ or $\mathrm{LLR}(P_1 : P_0 | x_0)$ is, the greater the evidence contained in the data x_0 is in favor of H_1 and against H_0. We saw an illustration of this in Section 1.3 in the context of a screening test.

The *generalized likelihood ratio statistic* for testing the null hypothesis H_0: $P = P_0$ against the omnibus alternative hypothesis $H_1 : P \neq P_0$ is obtained by replacing P_1 by the sample estimate $p = x_0/n$ of P under H_1, which maximizes the binomial likelihood in the numerator of LR:

$$\mathrm{GLR}(P_0 | x_0) = \mathrm{LR}(p : P_0 | x_0) = \max_{P_1 \text{ in } H_1} \mathrm{LR}(P_1 : P_0 | x_0). \qquad (2.36)$$

The *generalized log likelihood ratio statistic* is defined similarly as

$$\text{GLLR}(P_0|x_0) = \ln \text{GLR}(P_0|x_0) = x_0 \ln\left(\frac{x_0}{nP_0}\right) + (n - x_0)\ln\left(\frac{n - x_0}{n(1 - P_0)}\right).$$

$$(2.37)$$

The larger $\text{GLR}(P_0|x_0)$ or $\text{GLLR}(P_0|x_0)$ is, the greater the evidence there is contained in the observation x_0 against the null hypothesis $H_0 : P = P_0$ (and in favor of some other value of P, the most likely of which is the sample proportion $p = x_0/n$). The generalized likelihood ratio statistic thus provides an ordering of possible x values: those values of x with generalized likelihood ratio statistic greater than $\text{GLR}(P_0|x_0)$ are "more extreme" than x_0 with respect to the binomial distribution with parameter P_0, and can serve to define a two-tailed rejection region. Thus, instead of (2.31), we define the values of x to sum in (2.30) by those x satisfying

$$\text{GLR}(P_0|x) \geq \text{GLR}(P_0|x_0) \quad \text{or} \quad \text{GLLR}(P_0|x) \geq \text{GLLR}(P_0|x_0). \quad (2.38)$$

In words, the p-value is the probability associated with all values of x with at least as much weight of evidence against H_0: $P = P_0$ as there is contained in x_0. We call this the two-tailed p-value by the *likelihood ratio method*, and it too works assuredly. See Problem 2.19.

In the example with $x_0 = 23$ and $n = 25$, the two-sided p-value by the likelihood ratio method equals pval(23, 0.75) = 0.0428, which is legitimately significant at the $\alpha = 0.05$ level. Inverting the p-value by the likelihood ratio method to obtain a 95% confidence interval for P, we find the interval $(P_L, P_U) = (0.7560, 0.9856)$. In this example, the 95% confidence interval is slightly shorter than those based on all of the previous methods, although, again, this is not always the case. In this case, the 95% confidence interval excludes the value 0.75, consistent with the rejection of H_0 by virtue of the two-sided p-value being $< \alpha$.

2.7.4. Some Concluding Remarks

Any one of the ways presented in this section to define a two-sided p-value for the binomial distribution, which is discrete and generally asymmetrical, yields a legitimate method for conducting an exact test of a hypothesis about the binomial parameter P and for constructing an exact confidence interval for P. Of course, in practice, the method should be prespecified, and not chosen after looking at each method to find the "most significant" result.

We have also emphasized that all of the above methods "work assuredly." This criterion sets these methods apart from approximate methods, for which the approximate p-value may not always produce a test with Type I error no greater than α, and for which approximate confidence intervals may not always have coverage probability at least $1 - \alpha$. It also sets them apart from another method called the *mid-p correction* (Lancaster, 1949, 1952, 1961). For a one-sided tail probability, instead of defining the p-value as

$$P(X \leq x_0) = \sum_{i=0}^{x_0} \text{Bin}(i|n, P) \quad \text{or} \quad P(X \geq x_0) = \sum_{i=x_0}^{n} \text{Bin}(i|n, P),$$

the mid-p correction defines the p-value to be, respectively,

$$P(X \leq x_0) - \text{Bin}(x_0|n, P)/2 = P(X < x_0) + \text{Bin}(x_0|n, P)/2 \quad (2.39)$$

or

$$P(X \geq x_0) - \text{Bin}(x_0|n, P)/2 = P(X > x_0) + \text{Bin}(x_0|n, P)/2. \quad (2.40)$$

The rationale for this correction is to make the distribution of the p-value in repeated samples more closely resemble that of a uniform random variable under H_0; for example, to render the mean of the p-value closer to $\frac{1}{2}$ under H_0 than would be the case without the correction, and to remove the bit of conservatism introduced into the actual Type I error rate by the discreteness of the binomial distribution. That is, because of the discreteness, when a p-value is less than or equal to α, it is almost always strictly less than α, so that the actual Type I error of the test is somewhat less than α. Levin (1982) discusses such inherent conservatism in the context of fourfold tables, and different authors have expressed different views about whether or not to take steps to remove the conservatism.

In this book we have adopted the somewhat conservative attitude that the above concerns are not of fundamental importance, whereas the construction of p-values and confidence intervals that achieve their claims of Type I error and coverage probabilities is of fundamental importance. Indeed, *the mid-p corrected p-value is not "assured"* in the sense that we have been using this term. To illustrate in our standard example, the mid-p corrected upper tail probabilities under the hypothesis H_0: $P = 0.75$ for the outcomes $x_0 = 23, 24,$ and 25 are, respectively, 0.01956, 0.0039, and 0.0004, whereas for the outcome $x_0 = 22$, the mid-p corrected upper tail probability is 0.064. (See Problem 2.21.) Therefore, if we were to reject H_0 whenever the mid-p corrected upper tail probability is less than 0.025 (for a one-sided test at level $\alpha = 0.025$), we would reject H_0 for $x_0 = 23, 24,$ or 25. But the probability that this occurs under H_0 is, as we have seen, 0.032, which is greater than 0.025. Therefore this test has Type I error greater than the nominal value of α. A similar phenomenon occurs for two-sided p-values with a mid-p correction. On these grounds we do not recommend use of the mid-p correction. The other methods presented in this section help to alleviate the conservatism of the Type I error rate found with the equal-allocation method, while maintaining the guaranteed error and coverage rates.

Two-sided confidence intervals for the binomial distribution, comparing different methods both exact and approximate, were discussed by Blyth and

Still (1983), Vollset (1993), and Newcombe (1998). The subject has its roots in Wilson (1927) and Clopper and Pearson (1934).

PROBLEMS

2.1. A common experiment to test for a chemical's tumorgenicity is to supplement the diet of $n = 100$ rats with high doses of the chemical. After six months the animals are sacrificed and examined for tumor formation. Let P denote the probability that a randomly selected rat will develop a tumor. Suppose none of the rats in the experiment are observed to develop tumors ($x_0 = 0$). Verify that the upper one-sided $100(1 - \alpha)\%$ confidence limit is $P_U = 1 - \alpha^{1/n}$, and evaluate this for $\alpha = 0.05$. If this chemical is found in a human diet, are you comfortable with the knowledge that values of P as large as P_U are supported by the data? How can we reduce the upper limit?

2.2. Prove that for $n = 25$, $x_0 = 23$, and $\alpha_1 = \alpha_2 = 0.025$, the value $P_L = 0.74$ satisfies equation (2.5) and $P_U = 0.99$ satisfies equation (2.6). [*Hint.* It is not necessary to calculate each term in the sum $\sum_{x=0}^{23} \text{Bin}(x \mid 25, 0.99)$. Prove that

$$\sum_{x=0}^{x_0} \text{Bin}(x \mid n, P) = 1 - \sum_{x=x_0+1}^{n} \text{Bin}(x \mid n, P).]$$

2.3. An explicit formula for P_L is given in (2.8). Derive, by interchanging P with Q and positive response with negative response, the expression in (2.9) for P_U.

2.4. Prove that (2.17) and (2.18) provide the two solutions to the equation

$$\frac{n\{|p - P| - 1/(2n)\}^2}{PQ} = z_{\alpha/2}^2.$$

[*Hint.* Bear in mind that the purpose of the continuity correction is to bring the difference between p and P closer to zero. In deriving the lower limit, therefore, work with $p - P - 1/(2n)$ in the numerator; in deriving the upper limit, work with $p - P + 1/(2n).]$

2.5. Suppose that out of a sample of $n = 100$ subjects a proportion $p = 0.05$ had a specified characteristic.
   (a) To two decimal places, find the lower and upper 99% confidence limits on P using (2.17) and (2.18). Use $z_{0.005} = 2.576$.
   (b) To two decimal places, find the lower and upper 99% confidence limits on P using (2.19).
   (c) How do the two intervals compare? Would matters be improved any in (b) if the continuity correction were ignored?

2.6. Prove that P_L in (2.17) is never less than zero and that P_U in (2.18) is never greater than unity. [*Hint.* Use the defining equation (2.16) rather than the explicit formulas in (2.17) and (2.18).]

2.7. Prove that the definition of the two-tailed *p*-value with equal allocation of Type I error to the two tails given in Section 2.1 works assuredly in the sense that for any P_0, the test based on rejecting $H_0: P = P_0$ versus $H_0: P \neq P_0$ whenever the two-tailed p-value is $\leq \alpha$ has Type I error no greater than α. [*Hint.* Among the possible values of x_0, those that lead to a rejection of H_0 by virtue of the rule "p-value $\leq \alpha$" are those with tail probabilities $\leq \alpha/2$, that is, with $\sum_{x=0}^{x_0} \text{Bin}(x|n, P_0) \leq \alpha/2$ or $\sum_{x=x_0}^{n} \text{Bin}(x|n, P_0) \leq \alpha/2$. This subset is called the *rejection region* for the test, and is of the form $\{0, 1, \ldots, c_L\} \cup \{c_U, c_U + 1, \ldots, n\}$, where c_L and c_U are, respectively, lower and upper critical values for rejecting H_0, defined as follows: c_L is the largest value of x_0 with lower tail probability $\leq \alpha/2$, and c_U is the smallest value of x_0 with upper tail probability $\leq \alpha/2$. Because c_L and c_U are themselves in the rejection region, conclude that the Type I error is $\sum_{x=0}^{c_L} \text{Bin}(x|n, P_0) + \sum_{x=c_U}^{n} \text{Bin}(x|n, P_0) \leq \alpha/2 + \alpha/2 = \alpha$.]

2.8. Demonstrate that the definition of two-tailed p-value in the case of asymmetrical allocation of Type I errors to the two tails given at the end of Section 2.1 works assuredly.

2.9. (An underpowered study.) The case-fatality rate for a certain illness under standard therapy is $P_0 = 0.10$. A new treatment has just passed phase I testing (safety and dosage), and now a single-sample, phase II trial for efficacy is being planned. The experiment will use current knowledge of the case-fatality rates for historical control; a full-scale phase III randomized controlled clinical trial will be conducted if the result of the phase II experiment is promising. A halving of the case-fatality rate to $P_1 = 0.05$ is considered clinically significant, and important to declare as statistically significant with 80% power, using a two-sided $\alpha = 0.05$ level of significance.

   (a) How many patients must be studied to achieve this goal?

   (b) Unfortunately, funds for this trial can only cover a study of at most $n = 100$ patients. What is the power to detect $P_1 = 0.05$ with this sample size at the above α level?

   (c) With a sample of $n = 100$, what is the value of P_1 that can be detected with 80% power?

   (d) Redo your calculations for the above questions if it is decided to use a one-sided test of the hypothesis $H_0: P = P_0$ versus $H_1: P < P_1$.

2.10. Derive the sample size requirement (2.26) for a two-sided test of the hypothesis $H_0: P = P_0$ versus $H_1: P \neq P_0$, with equal allocation $\alpha/2$ in each tail of the rejection region and use of the continuity correction, which achieves power $1 - \beta$ at $P = P_1 \neq P_0$. [*Hint.* Remember that the continuity correction is applied in a direction to reduce the critical ratio. Also, in your expression for the power of the test, you may ignore one of the two tails of the critical region, which has only negligible probability of occurrence under the alternative hypothesis.]

2.11. A randomized trial of two analgesics to relieve postoperative pain is being planned. On day 1 each subject will be given medication A or medication B, selected at random, and then switched to the other medication on day 2. On day 3 the subject is asked to state his or her preference for A or B (with a coin toss if the subject is indifferent). Because of the randomization, differences between postoperative pain on day 1 and on day 2, and other carry-over effects, will be balanced. Let X denote the number of preferences for A, and let P denote the proportion of patients in the population of similarly situated patients who would prefer A. Under the null hypothesis of no true difference between the analgesics in terms of preference, $P = \frac{1}{2}$. A two-tailed test is needed because the investigators wish to limit to 5% the probability of a Type I error in either direction. How many subjects are required to achieve statistical power of 90% or more if the population value of P is above 60% or below 40%?

2.12. The *New York Times* for October 22, 1996 on page C3 reported the following:

> Rockville, Md., Oct. 21 (AP)—An advisory panel to the Food and Drug Administration recommended today against approving a new contraceptive device that is similar to the cervical cap, saying it was unclear how effective it was.
>
> Womens advocacy groups had urged the agency to grant quick approval to the device, Lea's Shield, arguing that the millions of unplanned pregnancies every year showed how desperate women were for better contraceptive options.
>
> "The appropriate response to the public health needs of women in the 90's is to expedite barrier controls," said Lisa Cox of the National Women's Health Network.
>
> But the manufacturer, Yama Inc., managed to get only 55 women to complete a six-month study of the device. The study found a 9 percent pregnancy rate. The company argued that was acceptable quality, indicating that had the women used Lea's Shield for a year, the maximum pregnancy rate would have been 18 percent, which it said was equivalent to most diaphragms.

But the agency's scientific advisers said no other contraceptive had ever been approved on the basis of such a small study. They maintained that a test involving 55 women was not enough to determine the pregnancy rate reliably. ...

Comment on the sample size issue. Determine what sample size would be necessary for a 95% confidence interval for the six-month pregnancy rate to exclude 9% if the observed six-month pregnancy rate p were as high as 15%.

2.13. Referring to the delta method in Section 2.6, let $f(p) = \ln(p)$ be the natural logarithm transformation of p. Show that the standard error, $\text{se}[\ln(p)]$ is estimated to be $\{q/(np)\}^{1/2}$ in large samples, where $q = 1 - p$. Compare this with the standard error of the relative error $(p - P_0)/P_0$ for a given value of the underlying parameter $P = P_0$.

2.14.* Use the delta method to derive the approximate standard error of the so-called *arcsine–square-root* transformation of p: $f(p) = \arcsin \sqrt{p}$. Does the standard error depend on p? Why might this be of interest?

2.15.* Let X have a binomial distribution with sample size n and probability parameter P. Let $\text{pval}(x_0, P_0)$ be the p-value function by the point probability method defined in Section 2.7.1. Verify that rejecting H_0: $P = P_0$ in favor of H_1: $P \neq P_0$ if and only if $\text{pval}(x_0, P_0) \leq \alpha$ incurs a Type I error rate no larger than α. [*Hint.* Let $R = R(P_0)$ denote the rejection region for the test, $R(P_0) = \{x: \text{pval}(x, P_0) \leq \alpha\}$. We want to show that the probability that X falls in R is $\leq \alpha$. Let x^* be any point in R with maximum probability, so that $\text{Bin}(x|n, P_0) \leq \text{Bin}(x^*|n, P_0)$ for all x in R; thus R is contained in the set of x such that $\text{Bin}(x|n, P_0) \leq \text{Bin}(x^*|n, P_0)$. Conclude that the probability that X is in R is no greater than $\text{pval}(x^*, P_0)$.]

2.16.* The confidence interval based on the two-sided p-value defined in (2.30) and (2.31) is the set of parameter values $I(x_0) = \{P': \text{pval}(x_0, P') > \alpha\}$. If $X \sim \text{Bin}(n, P_0)$, then $I(X)$ is a random interval that either covers P_0 or does not. Show that the event $E = [P_0$ is not contained in $I(X)]$ is the same as the event $[X$ is contained in $R(P_0)]$, where $R(P_0)$ is defined in Problem 2.15. Conclude that $P(E) \leq \alpha$, and thus that for any underlying P_0 the coverage probability of $I(X)$ is at least $1 - \alpha$.

2.17.* The p-value function $\text{pval}(x_0, P')$ for the point probability, tail probability, or likelihood ratio method has jump discontinuities as P' varies, as certain values of x are included (or excluded) from the tail region because the binomial probability at these values is less than (or greater than) $\text{Bin}(x_0|n, P')$.

(a) Evaluate $\text{Bin}(x_0|n, P')$ at $x_0 = 23$, $n = 25$, and $P' = 0.7441$. Also evaluate $\text{Bin}(x|n, P')$ at $x = 14$ and the same P'. Verify that $x = 14$ satisfies (2.31) with $P_0 = P'$, so that $x = 14$ is included in the lower tail region at this value of P' by the point probability method. The p-value is $\text{pval}(23, 0.7441) = 0.0627$.

(b) Evaluate $\text{Bin}(x|n, P')$ at $x = x_0$ and $x = 14$ with $P' = 0.7440$. Verify that at this value of P', $x = 14$ fails to satisfy (2.21), so that $x = 14$ is excluded from the lower tail region. The p-value is now $\text{pval}(23, 0.7440) = 0.0408$.

(c) Conclude that the lower 95% confidence limit is $P_L = 0.7441$.

2.18.* Show that the two-tailed p-value by the tail probability method works assuredly. [*Hint.* Let $R = R(P_0)$ denote the rejection region for the test, $R(P_0) = \{x: \text{pval}(x, P_0) \le \alpha\}$. We want to show that the probability that X falls in R is $\le \alpha$. If there are any values of x in the lower tail contained in R, there exists a largest such x^* with $\text{pval}(x^*, P_0) \le \alpha$; show that $\text{pval}(x, P_0) \le \text{pval}(x^*, P_0)$ for all $x \le x^*$ in the lower tail. Similarly, if there are any values of x in the upper tail contained in R, there exists a smallest such x^{**} with $\text{pval}(x^{**}, P_0) \le \alpha$ and $\text{pval}(x, P_0) \le \text{pval}(x^{**}, P_0)$ for all $x \ge x^{**}$ in the upper tail. Thus R is of the form $R = \{0, \dots, x^*\} \cup \{x^{**}, \dots, n\}$, and

$$P(X \in R) = \sum_{x=0}^{x^*} \text{Bin}(x|n, P_0) + \sum_{x=x^{**}}^{n} \text{Bin}(x|n, P_0).$$

(If there is no x in the lower tail contained in R, just omit the term involving x^*; similarly if there is no x in the upper tail contained in R, just omit the term involving x^{**}.) Now either

$$\sum_{x=0}^{x^*} \text{Bin}(x|n, P_0) \le \sum_{x=x^{**}}^{n} \text{Bin}(x|n, P_0)$$

or

$$\sum_{x=x^{**}}^{n} \text{Bin}(x|n, P_0) \le \sum_{x=0}^{x^*} \text{Bin}(x|n, P_0).$$

Suppose it's the latter; then conclude that $P(X \in R) \le \text{pval}(x^*, P_0) \le \alpha$; if the former, then $P(X \in R) \le \text{pval}(x^{**}, P_0) \le \alpha$.]

2.19.* Show that the two-tailed p-value by the likelihood ratio method works assuredly. [*Hint:* Let $R = R(P_0)$ denote the rejection region for the test, $R(P_0) = \{x: \text{pval}(x, P_0) \le \alpha\}$, where $\text{pval}(x_0, P_0) = $

$\Sigma_x \text{Bin}(x|n, P_0)$, where the sum is over all x such that $\text{GLR}(P_0|x) \geq \text{GLR}(P_0|x_0)$. We want to show that the probability that X falls in R is $\leq \alpha$. Pick any x^* contained in R that minimizes the generalized likelihood ratio statistic in R, that is, $x^* \in R$ is such that $\text{GLR}(P_0|x) \geq \text{GLR}(P_0|x^*)$ for all $x \in R$. First show that R is identical to the subset $R^* = \{x: \text{GLR}(P_0|x) \geq \text{GLR}(P_0|x^*)\}$. To do this, note that if x is any point in R, then by definition of x^*, $\text{GLR}(P_0|x) \geq \text{GLR}(P_0|x^*)$, so x is contained in R^*, whence $R \subseteq R^*$. Conversely, if x' is any point in R^*, then $\{x: \text{GLR}(P_0|x) \geq \text{GLR}(P_0|x')\} \subseteq \{x: \text{GLR}(P_0|x) \geq \text{GLR}(P_0|x^*)\}$, because $\text{GLR}(P_0|x') \geq \text{GLR}(P_0|x^*)$. So $\text{pval}(x', P_0) \leq \text{pval}(x^*, P_0) \leq \alpha$, because x^* is in R. Thus x' is in R, whence $R^* \subseteq R$, whence $R = R^*$. Conclude that $P(X \in R) = P(X \in R^*) = \Sigma_x \text{Bin}(x|n, P_0)$, where the sum is over all x such that $\text{GLR}(P_0|x) \geq \text{GLR}(P_0|x^*)$, which, by definition, is $\text{pval}(x^*, P_0)$, which is $\leq \alpha$, because x* is in R.]

2.20.* The use of the greatest lower bound in the definition of P_L and least upper bound in the definition of P_U is to allow for the following technicality in the two-tailed p-value functions by the point probability, tail probability, and likelihood ratio methods: they need not be strictly monotonic in P. It is therefore possible for the set of all P satisfying $\text{pval}(x_0, P) > \alpha$ to be not a single interval but a union of disconnected intervals. This happens occasionally as values of P neighboring a jump discontinuity have p-values above and below α. To illustrate, consider $x_0 = 37$, $n = 42$, and consider the values of P supported by the data at the $\alpha = 0.05$ level, i.e., those values with $\text{pval}(37, P) > 0.05$, near the lower limit. (A similar phenomenon occurs near the upper confidence limit with observed data $x_0 = 5$, $n = 42$.) Show that $\text{pval}(37, P)$ jumps from 0.0354 to 0.0505 around $P = 0.7409$; *decreases* to 0.04993 as P increases to about 0.7457, crossing 0.05 around 0.7440; and then increases again as P further increases, exceeding 0.05 for the second time at around 0.7474. Thus the 95% confidence region for P consists of the interval (0.7409, 0.7440) together with the main interval (0.7474, 0.9519), and excludes the region of unsupported values (0.7440, 0.7474). The smallest interval containing the confidence region is (0.7409, 0.9519), and this is taken as the 95% confidence interval. Show that the general procedure produces confidence intervals that have coverage probability at least as large as the corresponding confidence regions, and thus have coverage probability no less than $100(1 - \alpha)\%$.

2.21. Confirm that the mid-p corrected upper tail probabilities for $x_0 = 23$, 24, and 25 are, respectively, 0.01956, 0.0039, and 0.0004, whereas for the outcome $x_0 = 22$, the mid-p corrected upper tail probability is 0.064.

REFERENCES

Blyth, C. R. and Still, H. A. (1983). Binomial confidence intervals. *J. Am. Statist. Assoc.*, **78**, 108–116.

Clopper, C. J. and Pearson, E. S. (1934). The use of confidence or fiducial limits illustrated in the case of the binomial. *Biometrika*, **26**, 404–413.

Lancaster, H. O. (1949). The combination of probabilities arising from data in discrete distributions. *Biometrika*, **36**, 370.

Lancaster, H. O. (1952). Statistical control of counting experiments. *Biometrika*, **39**, 419–422.

Lancaster, H. O. (1961). Significance tests in discrete distributions. *J. Amer. Statist. Assoc.*, **56**, 223–234.

Levin, B. (1982). On the accuracy of a normal approximation to the power of the Mantel-Haenszel procedure. *J. Statist. Comp. Simul.*, **14**, 210–218.

Newcombe, R. G. (1998). Two-sided confidence intervals for the single proportion: Comparison of seven methods. *Statist. in Med.*, **17**, 857–872.

Vollset, S. E. (1993). Confidence intervals for a binomial proportion. *Statist. in Med.*, **12**, 809–824.

Wilson, E. B. (1927). Probable inference, the law of succession, and statistical inference. *J. Amer. Statist. Assoc.*, **22**, 209–212.

CHAPTER 3

Assessing Significance in a Fourfold Table

The fourfold table (see Table 3.1) has been and probably still is the most frequently employed means of presenting statistical evidence. The simplest and most frequently applied statistical test of the significance of the association indicated by the data is the classic chi squared test. It is based on the magnitude of the statistic

$$\chi^2 = \frac{n_{..}\left(|n_{11}n_{22} - n_{12}n_{21}| - \frac{1}{2}n_{..}\right)^2}{n_{1.}n_{2.}n_{.1}n_{.2}}. \tag{3.1}$$

The value obtained for χ^2 is referred to tables of the chi squared distribution with one degree of freedom (see Table A.2). If the value exceeds the entry tabulated for a specified significance level, the inference is made that A and B are associated. An interesting graphic assessment of significance is due to Zubin (1939).

Table 3.2 presents some hypothetical frequencies. The value of χ^2 is, by (3.1),

$$\chi^2 = \frac{200(|15 \times 40 - 135 \times 10| - \frac{1}{2}200)^2}{150 \times 50 \times 25 \times 175} = 2.58. \tag{3.2}$$

Since χ^2 would have to exceed 3.84 in order for significance at the 0.05 level to be declared, the conclusion for these data would be that no significant association was demonstrated.

It is perhaps unfortunate that the chi squared statistic (3.1) takes such a simple form, both because its calculation does not require the investigator to

Statistical Methods for Rates and Proportions, Third Edition
By Joseph L. Fleiss, Bruce Levin, and Myunghee Cho Paik
ISBN 0-471-52629-0   Copyright © 2003 John Wiley & Sons, Inc.

50

Table 3.1. *Model fourfold table*

Characteristic A	Characteristic B		Total
	Present	Absent	
Present	n_{11}	n_{12}	$n_{1.}$
Absent	n_{21}	n_{22}	$n_{2.}$
Total	$n_{.1}$	$n_{.2}$	$n_{..}$

Table 3.2. *A hypothetical fourfold table*

Characteristic A	Characteristic B		Total
	Present	Absent	
Present	15	135	150
Absent	10	40	50
Total	25	175	200

determine explicitly the proportions being contrasted—these representing the association being studied, not the raw frequencies—and because it invites the investigator to ignore the fact that the proper inference to be drawn from the magnitude of χ^2 depends on how the data were generated, even though the formula for χ^2 does not. These ideas are developed in Section 3.1. There, three methods for generating the frequencies of a fourfold table are presented and the statistical hypothesis appropriate to each is specified.

The "exact" test due to Fisher and Irwin is presented in Section 3.2, and the need for incorporating Yates' correction for continuity into the chi squared and critical ratio statistics is considered in Section 3.3. Some criteria for choosing between a one-tailed and a two-tailed significance test are offered in Section 3.4. Section 3.5 is devoted to setting confidence limits around the difference between two independent proportions; Section 3.6, to a critical ratio test, different from the classic one, that is closely related to the construction of confidence intervals.

3.1. METHODS FOR GENERATING A FOURFOLD TABLE

There are, in practice, essentially three methods of sampling that can give rise to the frequencies set out in a fourfold table (see Barnard, 1947, for a more complete discussion).

Method I
The first method of sampling, termed cross-sectional, naturalistic, or multinomial sampling, calls for the selection of a total of $n_{..}$ subjects from a larger

Table 3.3. *Joint proportions of A and B in the population*

Characteristic A	Characteristic B		Total
	Present	Absent	
Present	P_{11}	P_{12}	$P_{1.}$
Absent	P_{21}	P_{22}	$P_{2.}$
Total	$P_{.1}$	$P_{.2}$	1

population followed by the determination for each subject of the presence or absence of characteristic A and the presence or absence of characteristic B. Only the total sample size, $n_{..}$, can be specified prior to the collection of the data.

Much of survey research is conducted along such a line. Examples of the use of method I sampling are the following. In a study of the quality of medical care delivered to patients, all new admissions to a specified service of a hospital might be cross-classified by sex and by whether or not each of a number of examinations was made. In a study of the variation of disease prevalence in a community, a random sample of subjects may be drawn and cross-classified by race and by the presence or absence of each of a number of symptoms. In a study of the association between birthweight and maternal age, all deliveries in a given maternity hospital might be cross-classified by the weight of the offspring and by the age of the mother.

With method I sampling, the issue is whether the presence or absence of characteristic A is associated with the presence or absence of characteristic B. In the population from which the sample was drawn, the proportions (of course unknown) are as in Table 3.3.

By the definition of independence (see Section 1.1), characteristics A and B are independent if and only if each joint proportion (e.g., P_{12}) is the product of the two corresponding total or marginal proportions (in this example, $P_{1.}P_{.2}$). Whether the proportions actually have this property can only be determined by how close the joint proportions in the sample are to the corresponding products of marginal proportions. The cross-classification table in the sample should therefore be the analog of Table 3.3 and is obtained by dividing each frequency in Table 3.1 by $n_{..}$. Table 3.4 results.

Table 3.4. *Joint proportions of A and B in the sample*

Characteristic A	Characteristic B		Total
	Present	Absent	
Present	p_{11}	p_{12}	$p_{1.}$
Absent	p_{21}	p_{22}	$p_{2.}$
Total	$p_{.1}$	$p_{.2}$	1

Table 3.5. *Joint proportions for hypothetical data of Table 3.2*

Characteristic A	Characteristic B		Total
	Present	Absent	
Present	0.075	0.675	0.75
Absent	0.050	0.200	0.25
Total	0.125	0.875	1

The tenability of the hypothesis that A and B are independent depends on the magnitudes of the four differences $p_{ij} - p_{i.}p_{.j}$, where i and j equal 1 or 2. The smaller these differences are, the closer the data come to the standard of independence. The larger these differences are, the more questionable the hypothesis of independence becomes. (Actually, only a single one of these four differences needs to be examined, the other three being equal to it except possibly for a change in sign—see Problem 3.1.)

Pearson (1900) suggested a criterion for assessing the significance of these differences. His statistic, incorporating the continuity correction, is

$$\chi^2 = n_{..} \sum_{i=1}^{2} \sum_{j=1}^{2} \frac{\left\{ |p_{ij} - p_{i.}p_{.j}| - 1/(2n_{..}) \right\}^2}{p_{i.}p_{.j}}. \tag{3.3}$$

Problem 3.2 is devoted to the proof that (3.1) and (3.3) are equal. If χ^2 is found by reference to the table of chi squared with one degree of freedom to be significantly large, the investigator would infer that A and B were associated and would proceed to describe their degree of association. Chapter 6 is devoted to methods of describing association following method I sampling.

Suppose that the data of Table 3.2 were obtained from a study employing method I sampling. The proper summarization of the data is illustrated by Table 3.5. Note, for example, that $p_{22} = 0.20$, whereas if A and B were independent, we would have expected the proportion to be $p_{2.}p_{.2} = 0.25 \times 0.875 = 0.21875$. Furthermore, note that each of the four differences entering into the formula in (3.3) is equal to $|\pm 0.01875| - 0.0025 = 0.01625$.

Applied to the data of Table 3.5, (3.3) yields the value

$$\chi^2 = 200 \left(\frac{0.01625^2}{0.09375} + \frac{0.01625^2}{0.65625} + \frac{0.01625^2}{0.03125} + \frac{0.01625^2}{0.21875} \right) = 2.58, \tag{3.4}$$

equal to the value in (3.2).

Method II

The second method of sampling, sometimes termed purposive sampling, calls for the selection and study of a predetermined number, $n_{1.}$, of subjects who

Table 3.6. *Proportions with a specified characteristic in two independent samples*

	Sample Size	Proportion
Sample 1	$n_{1.}$	$p_1(=n_{11}/n_{1.})$
Sample 2	$n_{2.}$	$p_2(=n_{21}/n_{2.})$
Combined	$n_{..}$	$\bar{p}(=n_{.1}/n_{..})$

possess characteristic A and for the selection and study of a predetermined number, $n_{2.}$, of subjects for whom characteristic A is absent. This method of sampling forms the basis of comparative prospective and of comparative retrospective studies. In the former, $n_{1.}$ subjects with and $n_{2.}$ subjects without a suspected antecedent factor are followed to determine how many develop disease. In the latter, $n_{1.}$ subjects with and $n_{2.}$ subjects without the disease are traced back to determine how many possessed the suspected antecedent factor.

Of interest in method II sampling is whether the proportions in the two populations from which we have samples, say P_1 and P_2, are equal. It is therefore indicated that the sample data be so presented that information about these two proportions is afforded. The appropriate means of presentation is given in Table 3.6.

The statistical significance of the difference between p_1 and p_2 is assessed by means of the *z-score* or *critical ratio* statistic

$$z = \frac{|p_2 - p_1| - \frac{1}{2}(1/n_{1.} + 1/n_{2.})}{\sqrt{\bar{p}\bar{q}(1/n_{1.} + 1/n_{2.})}}, \qquad (3.5)$$

where $\bar{q} = 1 - \bar{p}$. To test the hypothesis that P_1 and P_2 are equal, in large samples z may be referred to the standard normal distribution. If z exceeds the normal curve value for a prespecified significance level—see Table A.1—P_1 and P_2 are inferred to be unequal. Since, by definition, the square of a quantity that has the standard normal distribution will be distributed as chi squared with one degree of freedom, z^2 may be referred to tables of chi squared with one degree of freedom. Problem 3.3 is devoted to the proof that z^2 is equal to the quantity in (3.1).

The analysis subsequent to the finding of statistical significance with method II sampling is shown in Chapter 7 to be quite different from the analysis appropriate to method I sampling.

Suppose, for illustration, that the data of Table 3.2 had been generated by deliberately studying 150 subjects with characteristic A and 50 subjects without it. The appropriate presentation of the data is illustrated in Table 3.7.

Table 3.7. *Proportions with characteristic B for subjects with and subjects without characteristic A—from hypothetical data of Table 3.2*

	Sample	Proportion with B
A Present	150	$0.10 = p_1$
A Absent	50	$0.20 = p_2$
Total	200	$0.125 = \bar{p}$

The value of z (3.5) is

$$z = \frac{|0.20 - 0.10| - \frac{1}{2}\left(\frac{1}{150} + \frac{1}{50}\right)}{\sqrt{0.125 \times 0.875\left(\frac{1}{150} + \frac{1}{50}\right)}} = 1.60, \tag{3.6}$$

which fails to reach the value 1.96 needed for significance at the 0.05 level. The square of the obtained value of z is 2.56, equal except for rounding errors to the value of χ^2 in (3.2).

Method III
The third method of sampling is like method II in that two samples of predetermined size are contrasted. Unlike method II, however, method III calls for the two samples to be constituted at random. This method lies at the basis of the controlled comparative clinical trial: of a total of $n_{..}$ subjects, $n_{1.}$ are selected at random to be treated with the control treatment, and the remaining $n_{2.}$ to be treated with the test treatment.

Of importance are the proportions from the two groups experiencing the outcome under study (e.g., the remission of symptoms). The significance of their difference is assessed by the same statistic (3.5) appropriate to method II. The appropriate further description of the data, however, is shown in Chapter 8 to be different for the two methods.

3.2. "EXACT" ANALYSIS OF A FOURFOLD TABLE

A version of the χ^2 statistic almost as familiar as that given in (3.1) is

$$\chi^2 = \sum_{i=1}^{2} \sum_{j=1}^{2} \frac{\left(|n_{ij} - N_{ij}| - \frac{1}{2}\right)^2}{N_{ij}}, \tag{3.7}$$

where

$$N_{ij} = \frac{n_{i.}n_{.j}}{n_{..}} \tag{3.8}$$

is the frequency one would expect to find in the ith row and jth column under the hypothesis of independence (for sampling method I; see Problem 3.4) or under the hypothesis of equal underlying probabilities (for sampling methods II and III; see Problem 3.5). If the marginal frequencies are small, in the sense that one or more values of N_{ij} are less than 5, it may not be accurate to base the significance test on the chi squared (or equivalent normal curve) distribution.

An alternative procedure, due to Fisher (1934) and Irwin (1935), proceeds from restricting attention to fourfold tables in which the marginal frequencies $n_{1.}$, $n_{2.}$, $n_{.1}$, and $n_{.2}$ are fixed at the observed values. Under this restriction, exact probabilities associated with the cell frequencies n_{11}, n_{12}, n_{21}, and n_{22} may be derived from the hypergeometric probability distribution:

$$P\{n_{11}, n_{12}, n_{21}, n_{22}\} = \frac{\binom{n_{1.}}{n_{11}}\binom{n_{2.}}{n_{21}}}{\binom{n_{..}}{n_{.1}}} = \frac{\binom{n_{.1}}{n_{11}}\binom{n_{.2}}{n_{12}}}{\binom{n_{..}}{n_{1.}}} = \frac{n_{1.}!n_{2.}!n_{.1}!n_{.2}!}{n_{..}!n_{11}!n_{12}!n_{21}!n_{22}!},$$

(3.9)

where, as in Section 2.1, $n! = n(n-1)\ldots 3 \times 2 \times 1$ and $0! = 1$.

The Fisher-Irwin "exact" test consists of evaluating the probability in (3.9) for the fourfold table actually observed, say P_{obs}, as well as for all the other tables having the same marginal frequencies. Attention is restricted to those probabilities that are less than or equal to P_{obs}. If the sum of all these probabilities is less than or equal to the prespecified significance level, the hypothesis is rejected; otherwise, it is not. The sum is called the two-sided p-value by the point probability method (see Section 2.7).

Consider the hypothetical data in Table 3.8. The exact probability associated with the table is

$$P_{\text{obs}} = \frac{5!4!6!3!}{9!2!3!4!0!} = 0.1190.$$

(3.10)

**Table 3.8. *Hypothetical data representing
small marginal frequencies***

	B	$\bar{B}$	Total
A	2	3	5
$\bar{A}$	4	0	4
Total	6	3	9

Table 3.9. *Remaining possible fourfold tables consistent with the marginal frequencies of Table 3.8*

Table	Associated Probability
3 2	
3 1	0.4762
4 1	
2 2	0.3571
5 0	
1 3	0.0476

The three other possible tables consistent with the marginal frequencies of Table 3.8, together with their associated probabilities, are presented in Table 3.9.

Only the last of these tables has an associated probability less than or equal to $P_{obs} = 0.1190$, so the exact significance level associated with the observed table is $0.1190 + 0.0476 = 0.1666$. The value of χ^2 for the data of Table 3.8 is 1.41. The probability of finding a value this large or larger is 0.23, which is somewhat different from the exact value of 0.17.

Fairly extensive tables exist of the hypergeometric probability distribution. One of the more accessible ones is Table 38 of the Biometrika Tables (Pearson and Hartley, 1970). More extensive tabulations have been compiled by Lieberman and Owen (1961) and by Finney et al. (1963).

For most of the illustrative examples in the remainder of this text, the marginal frequencies will be sufficiently large for the chi squared or critical ratio tests to be valid.

3.3. YATES' CORRECTION FOR CONTINUITY

Yates (1934) suggested that the correction

$$C_1 = -\tfrac{1}{2}n_{..} \tag{3.11}$$

be incorporated into expression (3.1) for χ^2 and that the correction

$$C_2 = -\frac{1}{2}\left(\frac{1}{n_{1.}} + \frac{1}{n_{2.}}\right) \tag{3.12}$$

be incorporated into expression (3.5) for z. These corrections take account of the fact that a continuous distribution (the chi squared and normal, respectively) is being used to represent the discrete distribution of sample frequencies.

Studies of the effects of the continuity correction have been made by Pearson (1947), Mote, Pavate, and Anderson (1958), and Plackett (1964). On the basis of these and of their own analyses, Grizzle (1967) and Conover (1968, 1974) recommend that the correction for continuity not be applied. They give as their reason an apparent lowering of the actual significance level when the correction is used. A lowered significance level results in a reduction in *power*, that is, in a reduced probability of detecting a real association or real difference in rates.

Mantel and Greenhouse (1968) point out the inappropriateness of Grizzle's (and, by implication, of Conover's) analyses and refute their argument against the use of the correction. The details of Mantel and Greenhouse's refutation are beyond the scope of this book. An outline of their reasoning is provided instead.

In method I, the investigator hypothesizes no association between factors A and B, which means that all four cell probabilities are functions of the marginal proportions $P_{1.}$, $P_{2.}$, $P_{.1}$, and $P_{.2}$ (see Table 3.3). Because the investigator is almost never in the position to specify what the values of these proportions are, he or she must use the obtained marginal frequencies to estimate them.

In methods II and III, the investigator hypothesizes no difference between two independent proportions, P_1 and P_2. Because the investigator is almost never in the position to specify what the value of the hypothesized common proportion is, he or she must use the obtained marginal frequencies to estimate it.

For each of the three sampling methods, the investigator must therefore proceed to analyze the data with the restriction that his marginal proportions instead of the unknown population proportions characterize the factors under study. This restriction is equivalent to considering the four marginal frequencies $n_{1.}$, $n_{2.}$, $n_{.1}$, and $n_{.2}$ obtained (see Table 3.1) as fixed. As pointed out in Section 3.2, exact probabilities associated with the observed cell frequencies may, under the restriction of fixed marginal frequencies, be derived from the hypergeometric probability distribution. Because the incorporation of the correction for continuity brings probabilities associated with χ^2 and z into closer agreement with the exact probabilities than when it is not incorporated, the correction should always be used.

3.4. ONE-TAILED VERSUS TWO-TAILED TESTS

The chi squared test, z-score, and Fisher-Irwin exact test presented so far are examples of *two-tailed* tests. Specifically, a significant difference is declared either if p_2 is sufficiently *greater* than p_1 or if p_2 is sufficiently *less* than p_1. Analogously to the discussion begun in Section 2.1 for a single binomial sample, suppose now that the investigator is interested in an alternative hypothesis specifying a difference in one direction only, say in P_2, the underlying proportion in group 2, being greater than P_1, the underlying proportion in group 1. The power of the comparison can be increased by performing a *one-tailed* test. The investigator can make one of two inferences after a one-tailed test, either that p_2 is significantly greater than p_1 or that it is not; the possible inference that p_1 is significantly greater than p_2 is ruled out as unimportant, and no Type I error rate has been allocated to it.

The one-tailed test begins with an inspection of the data to see if they are in the direction specified by the alternative hypothesis. If they are not (e.g., if $p_1 > p_2$ but the investigator was only interested in a difference in the reverse direction), no further calculations are performed and the inference is made that P_2 might not be greater than P_1. If the data are consistent with the alternative hypothesis, the investigator proceeds to calculate either the χ^2 statistic (3.1) or the z-score statistic (3.5).

The magnitude of χ^2 is assessed for significance as follows. If the investigator desires to have a significance level of α, he enters Table A.2 in the column for 2α. If the calculated value of χ^2 exceeds the tabulated critical value, the investigator infers that the underlying proportions differ in the direction predicted by the alternative hypothesis (e.g., that $P_2 > P_1$). If not, he or she infers that the underlying proportions might not differ in that direction. The magnitude of z is assessed similarly. When the desired significance level is α, Table A.1 is entered with 2α.

It is seen from Tables A.1 and A.2 that critical values for a significance level of 2α are less than those for a significance level of α. An obtained value for the test statistic (either χ^2 or z) that fails to exceed the critical value for a significance level of α may nevertheless exceed the critical value for a significance level of 2α. Because it is easier to reject a hypothesis of no difference with a one-tailed than with a two-tailed test when the proportions differ in the direction specified by the alternative hypothesis, the former test is more powerful than the latter.

As presented here, a one-tailed test is called for only when the investigator is not interested in a difference in the reverse direction from that hypothe-sized. For example, if the hypothesis is that $P_2 > P_1$, then it will make no difference if either $P_2 = P_1$ or $P_2 < P_1$. Such an instance is assuredly rare. One example where a one-tailed test is called for is when an investigator is comparing the response rate for a new treatment (p_2) with the response rate for a standard treatment (p_1), and when the new treatment will be substi-tuted for the standard in practice only if p_2 is significantly greater than p_1. It will make no difference if the two treatments are equally effective or if the new treatment is actually worse than the standard; in either case, the investigator will stick with the standard.

If, however, the investigator intends to report the results to professional colleagues, he is ethically bound to perform a two-tailed test. For if the results indicate that the new treatment is actually worse than the standard—

an inference possible only with a two-tailed test—the investigator is obliged to report this as a warning to others who might plan to study the new treatment.

In the vast majority of comparative research undertakings, two-tailed tests are called for. Even if a theory or a large accumulation of published data suggests that the difference being studied should be in one direction and not the other, the investigator should nevertheless guard against the unexpected by performing a two-tailed test. Especially in such cases, the scientific importance of a difference in the unexpected direction may be greater than yet another confirmation of the difference being in the expected direction.

3.5. A SIMPLE CONFIDENCE INTERVAL FOR THE DIFFERENCE BETWEEN TWO INDEPENDENT PROPORTIONS

When the underlying proportions P_1 and P_2 are not hypothesized to be equal, a good estimate of the standard error of $p_2 - p_1$ is

$$\widehat{se}(p_2 - p_1) = \sqrt{\frac{p_1 q_1}{n_{1.}} + \frac{p_2 q_2}{n_{2.}}}, \tag{3.13}$$

where $q_1 = 1 - p_1$ and $q_2 = 1 - p_2$. Suppose that both $n_{1.}$ and $n_{2.}$ are large in the sense that $n_{i.} p_i \geq 5$ and $n_{i.} q_i \geq 5$ for $i = 1, 2$, and that a $100(1 - \alpha)\%$ confidence interval is desired for the difference $P_2 - P_1$. Let $z_{\alpha/2}$ denote the value cutting off the proportion $\alpha/2$ in the upper tail of the standard normal curve. The interval

$$(p_2 - p_1) - z_{\alpha/2} \sqrt{\frac{p_1 q_1}{n_{1.}} + \frac{p_2 q_2}{n_{2.}}} - \frac{1}{2}\left(\frac{1}{n_{1.}} + \frac{1}{n_{2.}}\right) \leq P_2 - P_1$$

$$\leq (p_2 - p_1) + z_{\alpha/2} \sqrt{\frac{p_1 q_1}{n_{1.}} + \frac{p_2 q_2}{n_{2.}}} + \frac{1}{2}\left(\frac{1}{n_{1.}} + \frac{1}{n_{2.}}\right) \tag{3.14}$$

is such that it will include the true difference approximately $100(1 - \alpha)\%$ of the time.

Consider, for example, the data of Table 3.7. The sample difference is $p_2 - p_1 = 0.10$, and its estimated standard error is

$$\widehat{se}(p_2 - p_1) = \sqrt{\frac{0.10 \times 0.90}{150} + \frac{0.20 \times 0.80}{50}} = 0.062.$$

An approximate 95% confidence interval for the true difference is

$$0.10 - 1.96 \times 0.062 - 0.013 \leq P_2 - P_1 \leq 0.10 + 1.96 \times 0.062 + 0.013,$$

or

$$-0.035 \leq P_2 - P_1 \leq 0.235.$$

The interval includes the value 0, which is consistent with the failure above [see equation (3.6)] to find a significant difference between p_1 and p_2.

3.6. AN ALTERNATIVE CRITICAL RATIO TEST

Occasionally, the consistency just found between the test for the significance of the difference between p_1 and p_2 and the confidence interval for $P_2 - P_1$ will not obtain. For example, the critical ratio test (3.5) may fail to reject the hypothesis that $P_1 = P_2$, but the confidence interval (3.14) may exclude the value zero. Partly in order to overcome such a possible inconsistency, Eberhardt and Fligner (1977) and Robbins (1977) considered an alternative critical ratio test in which the denominator of the statistic (3.5) is replaced by (3.13). The test statistic then becomes, say,

$$z' = \frac{|p_2 - p_1| - \frac{1}{2}(1/n_1 + 1/n_2)}{\sqrt{\dfrac{p_1 q_1}{n_1} + \dfrac{p_2 q_2}{n_2}}}. \tag{3.15}$$

Eberhardt and Fligner (1977) compared the performance of the test based on the critical ratio in (3.5) with that of the test based on the statistic in (3.15), although they did not include the continuity correction in their analysis. When $n_1 = n_2$, they found that the test based on z' is always more powerful than the test based on z, but that it also tends to reject the hypothesis, when the hypothesis is true, more frequently than the nominal proportion of times, α. When $n_1 \neq n_2$, there are some pairs of proportions P_1 and P_2 for which the test based on z' is more powerful, and other pairs for which the test based on z is more powerful.

Consider again the data of Table 3.7. The value of z' is

$$z' = \frac{|0.20 - 0.10| - \frac{1}{2}\left(\frac{1}{150} + \frac{1}{50}\right)}{\sqrt{\dfrac{0.10 \times 0.90}{150} + \dfrac{0.20 \times 0.80}{50}}} = 1.41,$$

which is less than the value of z in (3.6). For these data, it happens that the classic z-score test [see (3.5)] comes closer to rejecting the hypothesis than the test based on z' [see (3.15)].

Further analysis shows that when the test based on z' is more powerful than the one based on z, the increase in power is slight except when P_1 and P_2 are greatly different [measured by an odds ratio greater than 10; see equation (4.1) for a definition of the odds ratio]. There do not, therefore, seem to be any overwhelming reasons for replacing the familiar test based on z (and the equivalent classic chi squared test) with the test based on z'.

In situations where the choice of test statistic or confidence interval would make a difference to the inferences drawn, exact methods should be relied upon rather than normal approximations. In that way disagreements over "borderline significant" results can be minimized.

PROBLEMS

3.1. Consider the joint proportions of Table 3.4. Prove that $p_{12} - p_{1.}p_{.2} = -(p_{11} - p_{1.}p_{.1})$, that $p_{21} - p_{2.}p_{.1} = -(p_{11} - p_{1.}p_{.1})$, and that $p_{22} - p_{2.}p_{.2} = p_{11} - p_{1.}p_{.1}$. [*Hint.* Because $p_{11} + p_{12} = p_{1.}$, therefore $p_{12} = p_{1.} - p_{11}$. Use the fact that $1 - p_{.2} = p_{.1}$.]

3.2. Prove that formulas (3.3) and (3.1) for χ^2 are equal. [*Hint.* Begin by using the result of Problem 3.1 to factor $\{|p_{11} - p_{1.}p_{.1}| - 1/(2n_{..})\}^2$ out of the summation in formula (3.3). Bring the four remaining terms, $1/(p_{i.}p_{.j})$, over a common denominator and show, using the facts that $p_{1.} + p_{2.} = p_{.1} + p_{.2} = 1$, that the numerator of the resulting expression is unity. Finally, replace each proportion by its corresponding ratio of frequencies.]

3.3. Prove that the square of z—see (3.5)—is equal to the expression for χ^2 given in (3.1).

3.4. Show that the estimated expected entry in the ith row and jth column of a fourfold table generated by sampling method I is given by expression (3.8) under the hypothesis of independence. [*Hint.* The expected entry is equal to $n_{..}P_{ij}$. What is the estimate of P_{ij} under the hypothesis of independence?]

3.5. Show that the estimated expected entry in the ith row and jth column of a fourfold table generated by sampling method II or III is given by expression (3.8) under the hypothesis of equal underlying probabilities. [*Hint.* Under the hypothesis, $P_1 = P_2 = P$, say. The expected entries are equal to $N_{i1} = n_{i.}P$ and $N_{i2} = n_{i.}Q$, where $Q = 1 - P$. What are the estimates of P and Q under the hypothesis?]

3.6. When the two sample sizes are equal, the denominator of (3.5) involves $2\bar{p}\bar{q}$, whereas the denominator of (3.15) involves $p_1q_1 + p_2q_2$. Prove that $p_1q_1 + p_2q_2 \leq 2\bar{p}\bar{q}$ when $n_{1.} = n_{2.}$, with equality if and only if $p_1 = p_2$.

REFERENCES

Barnard, G. A. (1947). Significance tests for 2×2 tables. *Biometrika*, **34**, 123–138.

Conover, W. J. (1968). Uses and abuses of the continuity correction. *Biometrics*, **24**, 1028.

Conover, W. J. (1974). Some reasons for not using the Yates continuity correction on 2×2 contingency tables. (With comments.) *J. Am. Statist. Assoc.*, **69**, 374–382.

Eberhardt, K. R. and Fligner, M. A. (1977). A comparison of two tests for equality of two proportions. *Am. Statist.*, **31**, 151–155.

Finney, D. J., Latscha, R., Bennett, B. M., and Hsu, P. (1963). *Tables for testing significance in a 2×2 contingency table.* Cambridge, England: Cambridge University Press.

Fisher, R. A. (1934). *Statistical methods for research workers*, 5th ed. Edinburgh: Oliver and Boyd.

Grizzle, J. E. (1967). Continuity correction in the χ^2-test for 2×2 tables. *Am. Statist.*, **21** (October), 28–32.

Irwin, J. O. (1935). Tests of significance for differences between percentages based on small numbers. *Metron*, **12**, 83–94.

Lieberman, G. J. and Owen, D. B. (1961). *Tables of the hypergeometric probability distribution.* Stanford: Stanford University Press.

Mantel, N. and Greenhouse, S. W. (1968). What is the continuity correction? *Am. Statist.*, **22**, 27–30.

Mote, V. L., Pavate, M. V., and Anderson, R. L. (1958). Some studies in the analysis of categorical data. *Biometrics*, **14**, 572–573.

Pearson, E. S. (1947). The choice of statistical tests illustrated on the interpretation of data classed in a 2×2 table. *Biometrika*, **34**, 139–167.

Pearson, E. S. and Hartley, H. O. (Eds.) (1970). *Biometrika tables for statisticians*, Vol. 1, 3rd ed. Cambridge, England: Cambridge University Press.

Pearson, K. (1900). On the criterion that a given system of deviations from the probable in the case of a correlated system of variables is such that it can be reasonably supposed to have arisen from random sampling. *Philos. Mag.*, **50**(5), 157–175.

Plackett, R. L. (1964). The continuity correction in 2×2 tables. *Biometrika*, **51**, 327–337.

Robbins, H. (1977). A fundamental question of practical statistics. *Am. Statist.*, **31**, 97.

Yates, F. (1934). Contingency tables involving small numbers and the χ^2 test. *J. R. Statist. Soc. Suppl.*, **1**, 217–235.

Zubin, J. (1939). Nomographs for determining the significance of the differences between the frequencies of events in two contrasted series or groups, *J. Am. Statist. Assoc.*, **34**, 539–544.

CHAPTER 4

Determining Sample Sizes Needed to Detect a Difference between Two Proportions

There are two kinds of errors one must guard against in designing a comparative study. Even though these errors can occur in any statistical evaluation, such as in the single sample study of Section 2.1, their discussion here is restricted to the case where proportions from two independent samples are compared, that is, to sampling methods II and III. The reader is referred to Cohen (1988, Chapter 7) for a discussion of the two kinds of errors in sampling method I.

The first, called the Type I error, consists in declaring that the difference in proportions being studied is real when in fact the difference is zero. This kind of error has been given the greater amount of attention in elementary statistics books, and hence in practice. It is typically guarded against simply by setting the significance level for the chosen statistical test, denoted α, at a suitably small probability such as 0.01 or 0.05.

This kind of control is not totally adequate, because a literal Type I error probably never occurs in practice. The reason is that the two populations giving rise to the observed samples will inevitably differ to some extent, albeit possibly by a trivially small amount. This is as true in the case of the improvement rates associated with any two treatments as in the case of the disease rates for people possessing and for people not possessing any suspected antecedent factor. It is shown in Problem 4.2 that no matter how small the difference is between the two underlying proportions—provided it is nonzero—samples of sufficiently large size can virtually guarantee statistical significance. Assuming that an investigator desires to declare significant

Statistical Methods for Rates and Proportions, Third Edition
By Joseph L. Fleiss, Bruce Levin, and Myunghee Cho Paik
ISBN 0-471-52629-0   Copyright © 2003 John Wiley & Sons, Inc.

64

only differences that are of practical importance, and not merely differences of any magnitude, he should impose the added safeguard of not employing sample sizes that are larger than he needs to guard against the second kind of error.

The second kind of error, called the Type II error, consists in failing to declare the two proportions significantly different when in fact they are different. As just pointed out, such an error is not serious when the proportions are only trivially different. It becomes serious only when the proportions differ to an important extent. The practical control over the Type II error must therefore begin with the investigator's specifying just what difference is of sufficient importance to be detected, and must continue with the investigator's specifying the desired probability of actually detecting it. This probability, denoted $1 - \beta$, is called the *power* of the test; the quantity β is the probability of failing to find the specified difference to be statistically significant.

Some means of specifying an important difference between proportions are given in Section 4.1. Having specified the quantities α, $1 - \beta$, and the minimum difference in proportions considered important, the investigator may use the mathematical results of Section 4.2 or the values in Table A.4 (described in Section 4.3) to find the sample sizes necessary to assure that (1) any smaller sample sizes will reduce the chances below $1 - \beta$ of detecting the specified difference and (2) any appreciably larger sample sizes may increase the chances well above α of declaring a trivially small difference to be significant.

Frequently an investigator is restricted to working with sample sizes dictated by a prescribed budget or by a set time limit. He or she will still find the values in Table A.4 useful, for they can be used to find those differences that the investigator has a reasonable probability of detecting and thus to obtain a realistic appraisal of the chances for success of the study.

Section 4.4 is devoted to the case where unequal sample sizes are planned for beforehand. Section 4.5 discusses some additional uses of the tables, including detectable effect sizes. Some final comments are made in Section 4.6.

4.1. SPECIFYING A DIFFERENCE WORTH DETECTING

An investigator will often have some idea of the order of magnitude of the proportions he or she is studying. This knowledge may come from previous research, from an accumulation of clinical experience, from small-scale pilot work, or from vital-statistics reports. Given at least some information, the investigator can, using his or her imagination and expertise, come up with an estimate of a difference between two proportions that is scientifically or clinically important. Given no information, the investigator has no basis for designing the study intelligently and would be hard put to justify designing it at all.

In this section only two of the many approaches to the specification of a difference are illustrated, each with two examples. Let P_1 denote the proportion of members of the first group who possess the attribute or experience the outcome being studied. In general, the designation of one of the groups as the first and the other as the second is arbitrary. Here, however, we designate the first group to be the one that might be viewed as a standard, typically because more information may be available for it than for the other group. Our problem is to determine that value of P_2, the proportion in the second group, which, if actually found, would be deemed on practical grounds to differ sufficiently from P_1 to warrant the conclusion that the two groups are different.

Example 4.1.1. In a comparative clinical trial, the first group might represent patients treated by a standard form of therapy. The proportion P_1 might then refer to their observed response (e.g., remission) within a specified period of time following the beginning of treatment. The second group might represent patients treated with an as yet untested alternative form of therapy. A clinically important proportion P_2 associated with the alternative treatment might be determined as follows.

Suppose that it can be assumed that all patients responding to the standard treatment would also respond to the new therapy. Suppose further that if at least an added fraction f, specified by the investigator, of nonresponders to the standard treatment respond to the new one, then the investigator would wish to identify the new treatment as superior to the old. Since the proportion of nonresponders to the standard treatment is $1 - P_1$, a clinically important value of P_2 is therefore $P_1 + f(1 - P_1)$.

For example, the remission rate associated with the standard treatment might be $P_1 = 0.60$. If the investigator will view the alternative treatment as superior to the standard only if it succeeds in remitting the symptoms of at least one quarter of those patients who would not otherwise show remission, so that $f = 0.25$, then he is in effect specifying a value $P_2 = 0.60 + 0.25 \times (1 - 0.60) = 0.70$ as one that is different to a practically important extent from $P_1 = 0.60$.

In this example, the proportions P_1 and P_2 refer to a favorable outcome, namely, a remission of symptoms. Similar reasoning can be applied to studies in which an untoward event (e.g., morbidity or mortality) is of especial interest.

Example 4.1.2. Suppose that the rate of premature births is P_1 among women of a certain age and race who attend the prenatal clinic in their community hospital. An intensive education program aimed at nonattenders is to be undertaken only if P_2, the rate of premature births among prospective mothers not attending the clinic but otherwise similar to the clinic attenders, is sufficiently greater than P_1.

It is reasonable to assume that a mother who delivered a premature offspring even after having attended the clinic would also have done so if she had not attended the clinic. The added risk of prematurity associated with nonattendance can thus only operate on mothers who do not deliver premature offspring after attending the clinic. If f denotes an added risk that is of practical importance, the hypothesized value of P_2 is then $P_1 + f(1 - P_1)$.

Suppose, for example, that the prematurity rate for clinic attenders is $P_1 = 0.25$. Suppose further that an education program is to be undertaken only if, of women who attend the clinic and who do not deliver a premature offspring, at least 20% would have delivered a premature offspring by not attending the clinic. The value of f is then 0.20, and the hypothesized value of P_2 is $0.25 + 0.20 \times (1 - 0.25) = 0.40$.

The approach to the comparison of two proportions exemplified by these two examples has been recommended and applied by Sheps (1958, 1959, 1961). It is considered again in Chapter 8, where the *relative difference* $f = (P_2 - P_1)/(1 - P_1)$ is studied in greater detail.

Example 4.1.3. One often undertakes a study in order to replicate (or refute) another's research findings, or to see if one's own previous findings hold up in a new setting. One must be careful, however, to control for the possibility that the rates in the groups being compared are at levels in the new setting different from those in the old. This possibility effectively rules out attempting to recapture the simple difference between rates found previously.

For example, suppose that the rate of depression among women aged 20–49 was found in the mental hospitals of one community to be 40 percentage points higher than the rate among men aged 20–49. It will be impossible to find the same difference in the mental hospitals of a new community if, there, the rate of depression among males aged 20–49 is 70%, since a difference of 40 percentage points implies an impossible rate of 110% for women similarly aged.

A measure of the degree of inequality between two rates is therefore needed that may be expected to remain constant if the levels at which the rates apply vary across settings. A measure frequently found to have this property is the *odds ratio*, denoted ω. The odds ratio is discussed in greater detail in Chapters 6 and 7. Here we give only its definition.

If P_1 is the rate at which an event occurs in the first population, then the odds associated with that event in the first population are, say, $\Omega_1 = P_1/Q_1$, where $Q_1 = 1 - P_1$. Similarly, the odds associated with the event in the second population are $\Omega_2 = P_2/Q_2$. The odds ratio is simply the ratio of these two odds,

$$\omega = \frac{\Omega_2}{\Omega_1} = \frac{P_2 Q_1}{P_1 Q_2}. \tag{4.1}$$

The odds ratio is also termed the cross-product ratio (Fisher, 1962) and the approximate relative risk (Cornfield, 1951). If $P_2 = P_1$, then $\omega = 1$. If $P_2 < P_1$, then $\omega < 1$. If $P_2 > P_1$, then $\omega > 1$.

Suppose that a study is to be carried out in attempt to replicate the results of a previous study in which the odds ratio was found to be ω. If, in the community in which the new study is to be conducted, the rate of occurrence of the event in the first group is P_1, and if the same value ω for the odds ratio is hypothesized to apply in the new community, then the value hypothesized for P_2 is

$$P_2 = \frac{\omega P_1}{\omega P_1 + Q_1}. \tag{4.2}$$

For example, suppose that the value $\omega = 2.5$ had previously been found as the ratio of the odds for depression among female mental hospital patients aged 20–49 to the odds for male mental hospital patients similarly aged. If the same value for the odds ratio is hypothesized to obtain in the mental hospitals of a new community, and if in that community's mental hospitals the rate of depression among male patients aged 20–49 is approximately $P_1 = 0.70$, then the rate among female patients aged 20–49 is hypothesized to be approximately

$$P_2 = \frac{2.5 \times 0.70}{2.5 \times 0.70 + 0.30} = 0.85.$$

An important property of the odds ratio to be demonstrated in Chapters 6 and 7 is that the same value should be obtained whether the study is a prospective or retrospective one. This fact may be taken advantage of if an investigator wishes to replicate a previous study but alters the research design from, say, a retrospective to a prospective study.

Example 4.1.4. Suppose that a case-control (retrospective) study was conducted in a certain school district. School children with emotional disturbances requiring psychological care were compared with presumably normal children on a number of antecedent characteristics. Suppose it was found that one-quarter of the emotionally disturbed children versus one-tenth of the normal controls had lost (by death, divorce, or separation) at least one parent before age 5. The odds ratio is then, from (4.1),

$$\omega = \frac{0.25 \times 0.90}{0.10 \times 0.75} = 3.0.$$

Suppose that a study of this association is to be conducted prospectively in a new community by following through their school year a sample of children who begin school with both parents alive and at home (group 1) and a sample who begin with at least one parent absent from the home (group 2), with the proportions developing emotional problems being compared. From a survey of available school records, the investigator in the new school district is able to estimate that P_1, the proportion of children beginning school with both parents at home who ultimately develop emotional problems, is $P_1 = 0.05$. If the value $\omega = 3.0$ found in the retrospective study is hypothesized to apply in the new school district, the investigator is effectively hypothesizing a value (see equation 4.2)

$$P_2 = \frac{3.0 \times 0.05}{3.0 \times 0.05 + 0.95} = 0.136,$$

or approximately 15%, as the rate of emotional disturbance during school years among children who have lost at least one parent before age 5.

The methods just illustrated may be of use in generating hypotheses for studies to be carried out within a short time, but are likely to prove inadequate for long-term comparative studies. Halperin et al. (1968) give a model and some numerical results when two long-term therapies are to be compared and when few or no dropouts are expected. When droputs are likely to occur, the model of Schork and Remington (1967) may be useful for generating hypotheses. If the study calls for the comparison of more than two treatments, or if outcome is measured on a scale with more than two categories, the results of Lachin (1977) should be useful.

4.2. THE MATHEMATICS OF SAMPLE SIZE DETERMINATION

We assume in this section and the next that the sample sizes from the two populations being compared, n_1 and n_2, are equal to a common n. We find the value for the common sample size n so that (1) if in fact there is no difference between the two underlying proportions, then the chance is approximately α of falsely declaring the two proportions to differ, and (2) if in fact the proportions are P_1 and $P_2 \neq P_1$, then the chance is approximately $1 - \beta$ of correctly declaring the two proportions to differ. Since this section only derives the mathematical results on which the values in Table A.4 (described in Section 4.3) are based, it is not essential to the sections that follow.

We begin by deriving the sample size, say n', required in both the groups if we ignore the continuity correction. With n' as a first approximation, we then obtain a formula for the desired sample size per group, n, that is appropriate when the test statistic incorporates the continuity correction.

Suppose that the proportions found in the two samples are p_1 and p_2. The statistic used for testing the significance of their difference is, temporarily ignoring the continuity correction,

$$z = \frac{p_2 - p_1}{\sqrt{2\bar{p}\bar{q}/n'}}, \tag{4.3}$$

where

$$\bar{p} = \tfrac{1}{2}(p_1 + p_2)$$

and

$$\bar{q} = 1 - \bar{p}.$$

To assure that the probability of a Type I error is α, the difference between p_1 and p_2 will be declared significant only if

$$|z| > z_{\alpha/2}, \tag{4.4}$$

where $z_{\alpha/2}$ denotes the value cutting off the proportion $\alpha/2$ in the upper tail of the standard normal curve and $|z|$ is the absolute value of z, always a nonnegative quantity. For example, if $\alpha = 0.05$, then $z_{0.05/2} = z_{0.025} = 1.96$, and the difference is declared significant if either $z > 1.96$ or $z < -1.96$.

If the difference between the underlying proportions is actually $P_2 - P_1$, we wish the chances to be $1 - \beta$ of rejecting the hypothesis, that is, of having the outcome represented in (4.4) actually occur. Thus we must find the value of n' such that, when $P_2 - P_1$ is the difference between the proportions,

$$P\left\{\frac{|p_2 - p_1|}{\sqrt{2\bar{p}\bar{q}/n'}} > z_{\alpha/2}\right\} = 1 - \beta. \tag{4.5}$$

The probability in (4.5) is the sum of two probabilities,

$$1 - \beta = P\left\{\frac{p_2 - p_1}{\sqrt{2\bar{p}\bar{q}/n'}} > z_{\alpha/2}\right\} + P\left\{\frac{p_2 - p_1}{\sqrt{2\bar{p}\bar{q}/n'}} < -z_{\alpha/2}\right\}. \tag{4.6}$$

If P_2 is hypothesized to be greater than P_1, then the second probability on the right-hand side of (4.6)—representing the event that p_2 is appreciably less than p_1—is near zero (see Problem 4.1). Thus we need only find the value of n' such that, when $P_2 - P_1$ is the actual difference,

$$1 - \beta = P\left\{\frac{p_2 - p_1}{\sqrt{2\bar{p}\bar{q}/n'}} > z_{\alpha/2}\right\}. \tag{4.7}$$

The probability in (4.7) cannot yet be evaluated, because the mean and the standard error of $p_2 - p_1$ appropriate when $P_2 - P_1$ is the actual difference have not yet been taken into account. The mean of $p_2 - p_1$ is $P_2 - P_1$, and its standard error is

$$\text{se}(p_2 - p_1) = \sqrt{(P_1 Q_1 + P_2 Q_2)/n'}, \tag{4.8}$$

where $Q_1 = 1 - P_1$ and $Q_2 = 1 - P_2$.

The following development of (4.7) can be traced using only simple algebra:

$$1 - \beta = P\left\{(p_2 - p_1) > z_{\alpha/2}\sqrt{2\bar{p}\bar{q}/n'}\right\}$$

$$= P\left\{(p_2 - p_1) - (P_2 - P_1) > z_{\alpha/2}\sqrt{2\bar{p}\bar{q}/n'} - (P_2 - P_1)\right\}$$

$$= P\left\{\frac{(p_2 - p_1) - (P_2 - P_1)}{\sqrt{(P_1 Q_1 + P_2 Q_2)/n'}} > \frac{z_{\alpha/2}\sqrt{2\bar{p}\bar{q}/n'} - (P_2 - P_1)}{\sqrt{(P_1 Q_1 + P_2 Q_2)/n'}}\right\}. \quad (4.9)$$

The final probability in (4.9) can be evaluated using tables of the normal distribution, because, when the underlying proportions are P_2 and P_1, the quantity

$$Z = \frac{(p_2 - p_1) - (P_2 - P_1)}{\sqrt{(P_1 Q_1 + P_2 Q_2)/n'}} \quad (4.10)$$

has, to a good approximation if n' is large, the standard normal distribution.

Let z_β denote the value cutting off the proportion β in the upper tail of the standard normal curve. Then, by the symmetry of the normal curve

$$1 - \beta = P(Z > -z_\beta) \quad (4.11)$$

By matching (4.11) with the last probability of (4.9), we find that the value of n' we seek is the one that satisfies

$$z_\beta = \frac{(P_2 - P_1) - z_{\alpha/2}\sqrt{2\bar{p}\bar{q}/n'}}{\sqrt{(P_1 Q_1 + P_2 Q_2)/n'}}$$

$$= \frac{(P_2 - P_1)\sqrt{n'} - z_{\alpha/2}\sqrt{2\bar{p}\bar{q}}}{\sqrt{P_1 Q_1 + P_2 Q_2}}. \quad (4.12)$$

Before presenting the final expression for n', we note that (4.12) is a function not only of P_1 and P_2, which may be hypothesized by the investigator, but also of $\bar{p}\bar{q}$, which is observable only after the study is complete. If n' is fairly large, however, $\bar{p}$ will be close to

$$\bar{P} = \frac{P_1 + P_2}{2}, \quad (4.13)$$

and, more importantly, $\bar{p}\bar{q}$ will be close to $\bar{P}\bar{Q}$, where $\bar{Q} = 1 - \bar{P}$. Therefore, replacing $\sqrt{2\bar{p}\bar{q}}$ in (4.12) by $\sqrt{2\bar{P}\bar{Q}}$ and solving for n', we find

$$n' = \frac{\left(z_{\alpha/2}\sqrt{2\bar{P}\bar{Q}} + z_{\beta}\sqrt{P_1 Q_1 + P_2 Q_2}\right)^2}{(P_2 - P_1)^2} \tag{4.14}$$

to be the required sample size from *each* of the two populations being compared when the continuity correction is not employed.

Haseman (1978) found that equation (4.14) gives values that are too low, in the sense that the power of the test based on sample size $n_1 = n_2 = n'$ is less than $1 - \beta$ when P_1 and P_2 are the underlying probabilities. Kramer and Greenhouse (1959) proposed an adjustment to (4.14) based on a double use of the continuity correction, once in the statistic (4.3) and again in the statistic (4.10). Their adjustment, which was tabulated in the first edition of this book, was found by Casagrande, Pike, and Smith (1978b) to result in an overcorrection.

By incorporating the continuity correction only in the test statistic (4.3), the latter authors derived

$$n = \frac{n'}{4}\left(1 + \sqrt{1 + \frac{4}{n'|P_2 - P_1|}}\right)^2 \tag{4.15}$$

as the sample size required in each group to provide, to an excellent degree of approximation, the desired significance level and power. The sample sizes tabulated in Table A.4 (which is different from Table A.3 of the first edition) are based on this formula. The values there agree very well with those tabulated by Casagrande, Pike, and Smith (1978a) and Haseman (1978). Ury and Fleiss (1980) present comparisons with some other formulas.

Levin and Chen (1999) show how the continuity correction can be used, in a logically consistent manner, both in the test statistic (4.3) and again in the statistic (4.10) to obtain (4.14) and (4.15). By a careful analysis of the round-off error created in the normal approximation by discreteness in the exact distribution of the test, they demonstrate that while it may appear that (4.14) and (4.15) result from only one use of the $\frac{1}{2}$ continuity correction, two uses are actually required logically. When the second continuity correction is properly employed in the Z statistic (4.10) used for approximating power, it effectively cancels out the round-off error, and leaves only one correction apparent in the formula. Curiously, when Kramer and Greenhouse (1959) considered use of two continuity corrections, they applied the second correction in the wrong direction, which explains the inaccuracy of their sample sizes. Thus Levin and Chen (1999) settle three puzzles from the first two editions of this book: why the sample size table from the first edition had to be replaced (because of an improper use of the second continuity correction); why the Casagrande, Pike, and Smith (1978b) formula is so accurate (because it is a valid approximation to the exact hypergeometric test procedure); and why it is so though it uses only one (logically inconsistent) application of the continuity correction (because it actually uses two logically consistent corrections when properly derived).

To a remarkable degree of accuracy (especially when n' and $|P_2 - P_1|$ are such that $n'|P_2 - P_1| \geq 4$),

$$n = n' + \frac{2}{|P_2 - P_1|}. \tag{4.16}$$

This result, due to Fleiss, Tytun, and Ury (1980), is useful both in arriving quickly at an estimate of required sample sizes and in estimating the power associated with a study involving prespecified sample sizes. Suppose that one can study no more than a total of $2n$ subjects. If the significance level is α and if the two underlying proportions one is seeking to distinguish are P_1 and P_2, one can invert (4.16) and (4.14) to obtain

$$z_\beta = \frac{|P_2 - P_1|\sqrt{n - \dfrac{2}{|P_2 - P_1|}} - z_{\alpha/2}\sqrt{2\overline{PQ}}}{\sqrt{P_1 Q_1 + P_2 Q_2}} \tag{4.17}$$

as the equation defining the normal curve deviate corresponding to the power $1 - \beta$ associated with the proposed sample sizes. Table A.1 may then be used to find the power itself.

4.3. USING THE SAMPLE SIZE TABLES

Table A.4 gives the equal sample sizes necessary in each of the two groups being compared for varying values of the hypothesized proportions P_1 and P_2, for varying significance levels ($\alpha = 0.01, 0.02, 0.05, 0.10$, and 0.20), and for varying powers [$1 - \beta = 0.50, 0.65(0.05)0.95$, and 0.99]. The value $1 - \beta = 0.50$ is included not so much because an investigator will intentionally embark on a study for which the chances of success are only 50:50, but rather to help provide a baseline for the minimum sample sizes necessary.

The probability of a Type I error, α, is frequently specified first. If, on the basis of declaring the two proportions to differ significantly, the decision is made to conduct further (possibly expensive) research or to replace a standard form of treatment with a new one, the Type I error is serious and α should be kept small (say, 0.01 or 0.02). If the study is aimed only at adding to the body of published knowledge concerning some theory, then the Type I error is less serious, and α may be increased to 0.05 or 0.10 (the more the published evidence points to a difference, the higher may α safely be set).

Having specified α, the investigator needs next to specify the chances $1 - \beta$ of detecting the proportions as different if, in the underlying populations, the proportions are P_1 and P_2. The criterion suggested by Cohen (1988, p. 56) seems reasonable. He supposes it to be the typical case that a Type I error is some four or five times as serious as a Type II error. This implies that one should set β, the probability of a Type II error, approximately equal to 4α, so that the power becomes, approximately, $1 - \beta = 1 - 4\alpha$. Thus when $\alpha = 0.01$, $1 - \beta$ may be set at 0.95; for $\alpha = 0.02$, at 0.90; and for $\alpha = 0.05$, at 0.80. When α is larger than 0.05, it seems safe to take $1 - \beta = 0.75$.

The use of Table A.4 will be illustrated for each of the examples of Section 4.1.

Example 4.3.1. The investigator hypothesizes a remission rate of $P_1 = 0.60$ for the standard treatment and one of $P_2 = 0.70$ for the new treatment. The significance level α is set at 0.01, and the power $1 - \beta = 0.95$. It is necessary to study 827 patients under the standard treatment and 827 under the new one, the assignment of patients to treatment groups being at random, in order to guarantee the desired significance level and power.

To reduce the chances of detecting a difference to $1 - \beta = 0.75$ without increasing the significance level, it is necessary to study 499 patients with each treatment. If the investigator can afford to study no more than a total of 600 patients, so that each treatment would be applied to no more than 300 subjects, the chances of detecting the hypothesized difference become less than 50:50.

Example 4.3.2. The investigator hypothesizes a prematurity rate of $P_1 = 0.25$ for clinic attenders and one of $P_2 = 0.40$ for nonattenders. The significance level α is set at 0.01 and the power $1 - \beta$ at 0.95. It is necessary to study 357 mothers from each group, all women being within a specified age range. If the significance level is increased to $\alpha = 0.02$ and the power lowered to $1 - \beta = 0.90$, then 65 mothers from each group are needed.

Example 4.3.3. The investigator hypothesizes the rate of depression among male mental hospital patients aged 20–49 to be $P_1 = 0.70$, and the rate among similarly aged female patients to be $P_2 = 0.85$. The significance level α is set at 0.05, and the power $1 - \beta$ at 0.80. It is necessary to study 134 patients of each sex. If the investigator had planned to study 200 patients of each sex, the chances of picking up the hypothesized difference would be nearly 95%, a value that might be larger than necessary. The value of z_β from (4.17) is

$$z_\beta = \frac{0.15\sqrt{200 - \dfrac{2}{0.15}} - 1.96\sqrt{2 \times 0.775 \times 0.225}}{\sqrt{0.70 \times 0.30 + 0.85 \times 0.15}} = 1.535.$$

Example 4.3.4. The investigator hypothesizes that the proportion developing emotional problems among children beginning school with both parents at home is $P_1 = 0.05$, and that the proportion among children beginning school with at least one parent absent is approximately $P_2 = 0.15$. The significance level α is set at 0.05, and the power $1 - \beta$ at 0.80. It is necessary to follow up 160 of each kind of child, making certain that the two cohorts are similar with respect to sex and race. If the investigator can afford to study no more than 120 of each kind of child, and if he or she is willing to increase the chance of making a Type I error to $\alpha = 0.10$, there will still be over a 75% chance of finding the groups to be different if the hypothesized values of P_1 and P_2 are correct. The value of z_β from (4.17) is 0.722.

The reader will note in each of these examples that the required sample size is *substantially larger* than that required for a comparable single sample problem. For instance, in Example 4.3.4, if the proportion among children beginning school with both parents at home were known to be $P_0 = 0.05$ and a single sample among children with at least one parent absent were to be used to test H_0: $P = P_0$ with a two-tailed test at level $\alpha = 0.05$ and power $1 - \beta = 0.80$ at $P = 0.15$, then (2.24) would yield $n = 62.6$, about 5 times smaller than $N = 320$ for the two-sample study. Comparing an observed proportion against a hypothesized one is obviously a great deal more efficient than comparing one observed proportion against another, but the comparison is valid only if the hypothesized proportion actually pertains to the study population. In the example, if P_0 pertains to a population of children with fewer emotional problems than the one to be studied, then the one-sample test is invalid, and an erroneous conclusion would likely follow that children with one or both parents absent are at higher risk for emotional problems, even if this were not true in the study population. For such reasons single-sample studies with *historical controls* are generally unpersuasive. Only in fields with a good understanding and control of sources of variation, or with a high degree of certainty in outcomes with standard treatments, are historical-controlled studies accepted. For example, in the care of patients with terminal illness where standard therapies are known to be hopeless, compassionate treatment with experimental therapies may be considered without concurrent controls. Animal carcinogenesis studies commonly incorporate information from historical controls (see Section 9.3), although the logic here is less compelling.

4.4. UNEQUAL SAMPLE SIZES

Suppose that considerations of relative cost, the desire for more precise estimates for one group than for the other, or other factors (Walter, 1977) lead to the selection of samples of unequal size from the two populations. Let the required sample size from the first population be denoted by m and that from the second by rm $(0 < r < \infty)$, with r specified in advance. The total sample size is, say, $N = (r + 1)m$.

If p_1 and p_2 are the two resulting sample proportions, the test statistic incorporating the continuity correction is

$$
z = \frac{|p_2 - p_1| - \dfrac{1}{2m}\left(\dfrac{r + 1}{r}\right)}{\sqrt{\dfrac{\bar{p}\bar{q}(r + 1)}{mr}}},
$$

where $\bar{p} = (p_1 + rp_2)/(r + 1)$ and $\bar{q} = 1 - \bar{p}$. If the desired significance level is α, and if a power of $1 - \beta$ is desired against the alternative hypothesis that $P_1 \neq P_2$, with P_1 and P_2 specified, the same kind of development as in Section 4.2 leads to the value

$$
m = \frac{m'}{4}\left(1 + \sqrt{1 + \frac{2(r + 1)}{m'r|P_2 - P_2|}}\right)^2
\tag{4.18}
$$

for the required sample size from the first population, and rm for that from the second. In (4.18),

$$
m' = \frac{\left\{z_{\alpha/2}\sqrt{(r + 1)\overline{PQ}} + z_\beta\sqrt{rP_1Q_1 + P_2Q_2}\right\}^2}{r(P_2 - P_1)^2},
\tag{4.19}
$$

where $\overline{P} = (P_1 + rP_2)/(r + 1)$ and $\overline{Q} = 1 - \overline{P}$. Expression (4.19) would be the required sample size if the continuity correction $-\{1/(2m)\}\{(r + 1)/r\}$ were omitted from the z-score.

As found by Fleiss, Tytun, and Ury (1980), m is approximately equal to

$$
m = m' + \frac{r + 1}{r|P_2 - P_1|}.
\tag{4.20}
$$

Note that equations (4.14)–(4.16) are special cases of those presented above when the two sample sizes are equal (i.e., when $r = 1$).

Consider again the example of comparing the rates of prematurity in the offspring of clinic attenders (P_1 is hypothesized to be 0.25) and in the offspring of nonattenders (P_2 is hypothesized to be 0.40). The significance level is again set at $\alpha = 0.01$, and the power at $1 - \beta = 0.95$. Suppose that recruitment of clinic attenders is easier than recruitment of nonattenders and that the investigator decides to study half as many nonattenders as attenders, so that $r = 0.5$. The value of m' in (4.19) is

$$m' = \frac{\left(2.576\sqrt{1.5 \times 0.30 \times 0.70} + 1.645\sqrt{0.5 \times 0.25 \times 0.75 + 0.40 \times 0.60}\,\right)^2}{0.5(0.15)^2}$$

$$= 510.34,$$

so that, by (4.18), the required sample size from the population of clinic attenders is

$$m = \frac{510.34}{4}\left(1 + \sqrt{1 + \frac{2(1.5)}{510.34 \times 0.5 \times 0.15}}\,\right)^2 = 530.$$

Equation (4.20) yields the same value to the nearest integer.

The two required sample sizes are therefore $n_1 = m = 530$ and $n_2 = 0.5m = 265$. The total number of women required is $N = 795$, some 80 more than were required for the case of equal sample sizes (see Example 2 of Section 4.3).

It is generally true that N is minimized, for given α, β, P_1, and P_2, when sample sizes are equal, $r = 1$.

Problem 4.5 is devoted to further applications of the results of this section.

4.5. SOME ADDITIONAL USES OF THE TABLES

One-Tailed Tests
It has so far been assumed that a two-tailed test (see Section 3.4) would be used in comparing the two proportions. If the investigator chooses to perform a one-tailed test, he can still use Table A.4, but should enter it with twice the significance level. Thus for a one-tailed significance level of 0.01, one uses $\alpha = 0.02$; for a one-tailed significance level of 0.05, one uses $\alpha = 0.10$. No change in the value of $1 - \beta$ is necessary.

Unequal Sample Sizes
As discussed by Mantel (1983) and Lee (1984), sample size tables for equal group sizes can be used for unequal sample sizes by the following reasonable approximation (see Problem 4.6). If n is the tabulated value per group from Table A.4 for the given values of α, β, P_1, and P_2, then, approximately,

$$m = \frac{n(r + 1)}{2r} \qquad (4.21)$$

In the example of the previous section comparing rates of prematurity in the offspring of clinic attenders (with $P_1 = 0.25$) and nonattenders (with $P_2 = 0.40$), where $\alpha = 0.01$, and $1 - \beta = 0.95$, use of Table A.4 and (4.21) yields

$m = 357(0.5 + 1)/(2 \times 0.5) = 536$, reasonably close to the result using (4.18) and (4.19) of 530.

One Sample Size Given

Suppose that one of the two sample sizes, say m ($= n_1$) is given. For example, m may represent the fixed number of cases available for a case-control study. There may or may not then be a value of r such that, with the second sample size, $n_2 = rm$, the study will have the desired power. If n denotes the common sample size from Table A.4 for the given parameters and the specified values of α and β, then the required value of r is approximately

$$r = \frac{n}{2m - n} \tag{4.22}$$

If $m \leq n/2$, no positive value for r exists and the study as planned must be abandoned. (The power might have to be reduced; the values of P_1 and P_2 might have to be moved further apart; etc.)

Suppose, for example, that the population from which controls will be selected is characterized by a probability of $P_1 = 0.15$ for the characteristic under study, and suppose that a probability of $P_2 = 0.30$ is sufficiently different from P_1 that, if it were the underlying probability in the population of cases, the power should be equal to 0.80. Let the two-tailed significance level be $\alpha = 0.05$, and suppose that only $m = 100$ cases will be available for the study.

If the study could be carried out with equal numbers of cases and controls, the required sample size per group would be $n = 134$ from Table A.4. The required ratio of sample sizes given that $m = 100$ is therefore $r = 134/(2 \times 100 - 134) = 2.03$, and the required number of controls is $2.03 \times 100 = 203$.

Interpolation

Suppose the investigator hypothesizes a pair of probabilities P_1 and P_2, with $P_2 > P_1$, one or both of which are not tabulated in Table A.4. If $P_1^* \leq P_1$ and $P_2^* \geq P_2$ and if n^* is the required sample size for P_1^* and P_2^* and the specified values of α and β, then the required sample size n for P_1 and P_2 is approximately equal to

$$n = \frac{n^*(P_2^* - P_1^*)^2}{(P_2 - P_1)^2}. \tag{4.23}$$

Assume, for example, that $P_1 = 0.33$, $P_2 = 0.40$, $\alpha = 0.05$, and $1 - \beta = 0.80$. The value of P_1^* is then 0.30, the value of n^* from the table is 376, and, from (4.23), the required sample size for $P_1 = 0.33$ versus $P_2 = 0.40$ is $n = \{376(0.40 - 0.30)^2\}/(0.40 - 0.33)^2 = 767.3$. This value is within 1% of the sample size produced by the formulas in (4.14) and (4.15) for $P_1 = 0.33$ and $P_2 = 0.40$, $n = 769.6$.

The example highlights a disturbing feature of sample size determination, the possibly inordinate sensitivity of the sample sizes to the values of P_1 and P_2. The sample size required for the hypothesized difference between 0.33 and 0.40, $n = 770$ per group, is more than twice the sample size required for the hypothesized difference between 0.30 and 0.40, $n = 376$ per group. Investigators will often be tempted to round off their hypothesized values of P_1 or P_2 so that they become multiples of 0.05, but they should be aware that, if the resulting values of P_1^* and P_2^* are farther apart than the original values, the sample sizes they determine may be much too low.

Detectable Effect Size

The key expression for power with equal sample sizes is (4.17). For unequal sample sizes, m in group 1 and rm in group 2, the corresponding expression using the continuity correction is

$$z_\beta = \frac{|P_2 - P_1|\sqrt{rm - \dfrac{r+1}{|P_2 - P_1|}} - z_{\alpha/2}\sqrt{(r+1)\overline{PQ}}}{\sqrt{rP_1Q_1 + P_2Q_2}}. \qquad (4.24)$$

Expression (4.24) may be used to approximate the power of the test of H_0: $P_1 = P_2$ at alternative values of P_1 and P_2.

Given α and the sample sizes, how does one invert (4.17) or (4.24) to find the magnitudes of P_1 and P_2 at which the test of H_0 has prespecified power $1 - \beta$? Such a pair is called *detectable* (with power $1 - \beta$ at the α level of significance). Usually, one of the probabilities will be known, at least approximately; say it's P_1. Then (4.24) could in principle be solved for the desired P_2, but the solution generally will require an iterative computation.

Table A.4 may be used to locate approximate values of P_2 for given P_1, α, and power by bracketing the sample size at hand between two tabled values. For example, with equal sample sizes of $n = 100$ per group and $P_1 = 0.30$, $\alpha = 0.05$, and $1 - \beta = 0.80$, a value of P_2 slightly above 0.50 can be *detected* (i.e., allows testing with 80% power at $\alpha = 0.05$ two-tailed).

For unequal sample sizes, one finds the values of P_2 that bracket the *harmonic mean* of m and rm, i.e., $n = 2rm/(r+1)$. (See Problem 4.6.) Thus for $m = 75$ and $r = 2$, we bracket $n = 2 \times 2 \times 75/(2+1) = 100$ to find the detectable $P_2 = 0.50$ again. For $m = 75$ and $r = \frac{2}{3}$, the harmonic mean of 75 and 50 is $n = 60$, and bracketing this sample size in Table A.4 we find P_2 between 0.55 and 0.60. Checking in (4.24) shows that the detectable P_2 is 0.57. More precise solutions require an iterative computation to solve (4.24) for P_2. The values from Table A.4 are useful as starting values for the iteration.

4.6. SOME ADDITIONAL COMMENTS

Cohen (1988, Chapter 6) gives a set of tables and Feigl (1978) gives a set of graphs for determining sample sizes when the same parameters as those preceding are specified. Since the significance test they consider is different from the standard one, their sample sizes are slightly different from those in Table A.4. In general, Cohen's tables and Feigl's charts have to be used if the investigator can hypothesize the order of magnitude of the difference between P_1 and P_2, but not their separate magnitudes. If the investigator can hypothesize the separate values of P_1 and P_2, the current table is preferable.

A number of authors have considered the problem of determining the required sample sizes for a two-group study when a confidence interval is desired for some parameter (Greenland, 1988; Satten and Kupper, 1990). Greenland (1988) shows how the power approach may be adopted when one's interest is in an interval that has a high probability of excluding one or the other of two competing values for a parameter. Satten and Kupper (1990) present a method for deriving sample sizes, and present tables of results, when one desires a confidence interval for the odds ratio that has a high probability of having a maximum prespecified length. McHugh and Le (1984) and O'Neill (1984) present simple sample size formulas for interval estimation of the difference between two probabilities or of their odds ratio. The resulting sample sizes will be adequate when the underlying probabilities are close to $\frac{1}{2}$, but otherwise will be too small.

PROBLEMS

4.1. Suppose that $P_2 > P_1$ and that n' is the sample size studied in each group. Let Z represent a random variable having the standard normal distribution.

(a) Show that the probability that p_2 is significantly *less* than p_1,

$$P\left(\frac{p_2 - p_1}{\sqrt{2\,\overline{p}\overline{q}/n'}} < -z_{\alpha/2} \right),$$

is approximately equal to

$$\Pi = P\left(Z < \frac{-z_{\alpha/2}\sqrt{2\,\overline{PQ}} - (P_2 - P_1)\sqrt{n'}}{\sqrt{P_1 Q_1 + P_2 Q_2}} \right).$$

(b) If $P_2 = P_1$, then $\Pi = \alpha/2$. Thus if $P_2 > P_1$, show why $\Pi < \alpha/2$. [*Hint.* Prove that $\sqrt{P_1 Q_1 + P_2 Q_2} < \sqrt{2\,\overline{PQ}}$ whenever $P_2 \neq P_1$.

Therefore, if $P_2 > P_1$,

$$\frac{-z_{\alpha/2}\sqrt{2\overline{PQ}} - (P_2 - P_1)\sqrt{n'}}{\sqrt{P_1Q_1 + P_2Q_2}} < -z_{\alpha/2} - \frac{(P_2 - P_1)\sqrt{n'}}{\sqrt{P_1Q_1 + P_2Q_2}} < -z_{\alpha/2}.]$$

(c) Π is small even if P_2 is only slightly larger than P_1 and even if n' is small. Find the value of Π when $P_1 = 0.10$, $P_2 = 0.11$, $n' = 9$, and $\alpha = 0.05$. Note that the probability found in Table A.1 must be *halved*.

4.2. Let the notation and assumptions of Problem 4.1 be used again. The power of the test for comparing p_1 and p_2 is approximately

$$1 - \beta = P\left\{Z > \frac{z_{\alpha/2}\sqrt{2\overline{PQ}} - (P_2 - P_1)\sqrt{n'}}{\sqrt{P_1Q_1 + P_2Q_2}}\right\},$$

(a) Show that $1 - \beta$ approaches unity as n' becomes large but α remains fixed. [*Hint.* What is the probability that a standard normal random variable exceeds -1? -2? -3? What value does the expression to the right of the inequality sign above approach as n' increases?]

(b) Show that $1 - \beta$ decreases as α becomes small but n' remains fixed.

4.3. Show that, when the test statistic incorporates the continuity correction, equation (4.15) gives the sample size needed in each group to achieve a power of $1 - \beta$ when the underlying probabilities are P_1 and P_2. [*Hint.* The hypothesis that $P_1 = P_2$ is rejected if

$$\frac{|p_2 - p_1| - \dfrac{1}{n}}{\sqrt{2\overline{pq}/n}} > z_{\alpha/2}.$$

Assume that $P_2 > P_1$, and apply the same algebraic development as in Section 4.2 to arrive at

$$\sqrt{n} - \frac{1}{\sqrt{n}\,(P_2 - P_1)} = \sqrt{n'}$$

as the equation defining n, where n' is defined in (4.14). Finally, solve the above quadratic equation for $\sqrt{n}$ and then for n, noting that one of the two roots is negative and therefore inadmissible.]

4.4. An investigator hypothesizes that the improvement rate associated with a placebo is $P_1 = 0.45$, and that the improvement rate associated with an active drug is $P_2 = 0.65$. The plan is to perform a *one-tailed* test.

(a) If a significance level of $\alpha = 0.01$ and a power of $1 - \beta = 0.95$ are desired, how large a sample per treatment must he study?

(b) How large must the sample sizes be if the significance level is relaxed to $\alpha = 0.05$ and the power to $1 - \beta = 0.80$?

(c) What is the power of his one-tailed test if he can study only 52 patients per group, and if his significance level is $\alpha = 0.05$? [*Hint.* Because we are considering a one-tailed test, be sure to replace $z_{\alpha/2}$ in equation (4.17) by 1.645.]

4.5. The comparison of two populations with hypothesized probabilities $P_1 = 0.25$ and $P_2 = 0.40$ was considered several times in the text.

(a) Continuing to take $\alpha = 0.01$ and $1 - \beta = 0.95$, fill in the remaining values in the second, third, and fourth columns of the following table:

Ratio of Sample Sizes $(n_2/n_1 = r)$	n_1	n_2	Required Total Sample Size	Total Cost
0.5	530	265	795	$8,480
0.6	—	—	—	—
0.7	—	—	—	—
0.8	—	—	—	—
0.9	—	—	—	—
1	357	357	714	$7,854

(b) Suppose that the average cost of studying a member of group 1 is $10, and that the average cost for group 2 is $12. Find the total cost associated with each tabulated value of r. For which of these ratios of sample sizes is the total cost minimized?

(c) Suppose that the investigator can afford to spend only $6,240 on the study and decides to employ the value of r found in part (b). What is the value of m? What is the corresponding value of m' when $P_1 = 0.25$ and $P_2 = 0.40$? [Solve equation (4.20) for m'.] What is the corresponding value of z_β when $\alpha = 0.01$? What, finally, is the power of the test?

4.6. Suppose that n is the required sample size per group for specified values of α, β, P_1, and P_2. Another study with sample sizes $n_1 = m$ and $n_2 = rm$ has, approximately, the same power as the first if the harmonic mean of n_1 and n_2 is equal to n. Prove that the required value of m is given by (4.21). [*Hint.* The harmonic mean of two positive numbers x and y is $2/(x^{-1} + y^{-1})$.]

4.7. In a discussion of the landmark studies defining the role of elevated oxygen concentration in causing retrolental fibroplasia (RLF), a condition that causes blindness in premature infants, a commentary by Day et al. (1979) provided the following data from one of the original studies by Lanman et al. (1954). The clinical dilemma at the time was that the higher oxygen concentration given to the premature infants to improve their chances of survival (with risk of death due to insufficient lung function) caused the RLF condition, leading to blindness. The study by Lanman et al. (1954) prospectively compared two groups of premies, those given low O_2 concentration ($n_1 = 40$) and those given high O_2 concentration ($n_2 = 45$). Two fourfold tables of interest can be derived from the reports:

Group	Died	Lived	Total	Blind	Not Blind	Survived
Low O_2	12	28	40	0	28	28
High O_2	9	36	45	6	30	36

The fourfold table on the left indicates higher mortality (30%) for the low-O_2-concentration group than for the high-O_2-concentration group (20%). The fourfold table on the the right indicates no blindness among those infants who survived the perinatal period in the low-O_2-concentration group, and a higher incidence of blindness among those who survived in the high-O_2-concentration group.

(a) Test the hypothesis of no effect of O_2 concentration on mortality against the one-sided alternative hypothesis that lowered O_2 concentration increases mortality. What is the p-value?

(b) Assuming a true mortality of $P_1 = 0.30$ versus $P_2 = 0.20$, what is the power of the hypothesis test conducted in part (a)? What would be the equal sample sizes required to test the above hypothesis at the 0.05 level of significance and 80% power at the specified alternative mortalities? Assuming the high-O_2-concentration group had a true mortality of 20%, what mortality for the low-O_2-concentration group P_1 can be detected at 80% power with the given sample sizes?

(c) How do you interpret the finding of part (a) in light of the findings of part (b)?

(d) Use Fisher's exact test to test the hypothesis of no effect of O_2 concentration on blindness among the surviving premies versus the two-sided alternative. What is the exact two-tailed p-value by the point probability method?

REFERENCES

Casagrande, J. T., Pike, M. C., and Smith, P. G. (1978a). The power function of the "exact" test for comparing two binomial distributions. *Appl. Statist.*, **27**, 176–180.

Casagrande, J. T., Pike, M. C., and Smith, P. G. (1978b). An improved approximate formula for calculating sample sizes for comparing two binomial distributions, *Biometrics*, **34**, 483–486.

Cohen, J. (1988). *Statistical power analysis for the behavioral sciences*, 2nd ed. New York: Academic Press.

Cornfield, J. (1951). A method of estimating comparative rates from clinical data. Applications to cancer of the lung, breast, and cervix. *J. Natl. Cancer Inst.*, **11**, 1269–1275.

Day, R. L., Dell, R. B., Darlington, R. B., and Fleiss, J. L. (1979). Interpretation of statistical nonsignificance and retrolental fibroplasia. *Pediatrics*, **63**, 342–344.

Feigl, P. (1978). A graphical aid for determining sample size when comparing two independent proportions. *Biometrics*, **34**, 111–122.

Fisher, R. A. (1962). Confidence limits for a cross-product ratio. *Aust. J. Statist.*, **4**, 41.

Fleiss, J. L., Tytun, A., and Ury, H. K. (1980). A simple approximation for calculating sample sizes for comparing independent proportions. *Biometrics*, **36**, 343–346.

Greenland, S. (1988). On sample-size and power calculations for studies using confidence intervals. *Amer. J. Epidemiol.*, **128**, 231–237.

Halperin, M., Rogot, E., Gurian, J., and Ederer, F. (1968). Sample sizes for medical trials with special reference to long-term therapy. *J. Chronic Dis.*, **21**, 13–24.

Haseman, J. K. (1978). Exact sample sizes for use with the Fisher-Irwin test for 2×2 tables. *Biometrics*, **34**, 106–109.

Kramer, M. and Greenhouse, S. W. (1959). Determination of sample size and selection of cases. Pp. 356–371 in National Academy of Sciences—National Research Council Publication 583, *Psychopharmacology: Problems in evaluation*. Washington, D.C.

Lachin, J. M. (1977). Sample size determinations for $r \times c$ comparative trials. *Biometrics*, **33**, 315–324.

Lanman, J. T., Guy, L. P., and Dancis, J. (1954). Retrolental fibroplasia and oxygen therapy. *J. Am. Med. Assoc.*, **155**, 223.

Lee, Y. J. (1984). Quick and simple approximation of sample sizes for comparing two independent binomial distributions: Different sample size case. *Biometrics*, **40**, 239–241.

Levin, B. and Chen, X. (1999). Is the one-half continuity correction used once or twice to derive a well known approximate sample size formula to compare two independent binomial distributions? *Am. Statist.*, **53**, 62–66.

Mantel, N. (1983). Extended use of binomial sample size tables. *Biometrics*, **39**, 777–779.

McHugh, R. B. and Le, C. T. (1984). Confidence estimation and the size of a clinical trial. *Controlled Clinical Trials*, **5**, 157–163.

O'Neill, R. T. (1984). Sample sizes for estimation of the odds ratio in unmatched case-control studies. *Am. J. Epidemiol.*, **120**, 145–153.

Satten, G. A. and Kupper, L. L. (1990). Sample size requirements for interval estimation of the odds ratio. *Am. J. Epidemiol.*, **131**, 177–184. (See also **131**, 578.)

Schork, M. A. and Remington, R. D. (1967). The determination of sample size in treatment-control comparisons for chronic disease studies in which drop-out or non-adherence is a problem. *J. Chronic Dis.*, **20**, 233–239.

Sheps, M. C. (1958). Shall we count the living or the dead? *New Engl. J. Med.*, **259**, 1210–1214.

Sheps, M. C. (1959). An examination of some methods of comparing several rates or proportions. *Biometrics*, **15**, 87–97.

Sheps, M. C. (1961). Marriage and mortality. *Am. J. Public Health*, **51**, 547–555.

Ury, H. K. and Fleiss, J. L. (1980). On approximate sample sizes for comparing two independent proportions with the use of Yates' correction. *Biometrics*, **36**, 347–351.

Walter, S. D. (1977). Determination of significant relative risks and optimal sampling procedures in prospective and retrospective comparative studies of various sizes. *Am. J. Epidemiol.*, **105**, 387–397.

CHAPTER 5

How to Randomize

A number of references have been made so far to randomization. Subjects were described as being "randomly selected" from a larger group of subjects, as being "randomly assigned" to one or another treatment group, and so on. This chapter gives some methods for achieving randomness of selection (needed in sampling methods I and II; see Section 5.1) or of assignment (needed in sampling method III; see Sections 5.2 and 5.3).

It is important to bear in mind that randomness inheres not in the samples one ends up with, but in the method used to generate those samples. When we say that a group of a given size is a *simple random sample* from a larger group, we mean that each possible sample of that size has the same chance of being selected. When we say that treatments are assigned to subjects *at random*, we mean that each subject is equally likely to receive each of the treatments.

The necessity for randomization in controlled experiments was first pointed out by Fisher (1935). In the context of comparative trials, Hill (1962) describes what is accomplished by the random assignment of treatments to subjects:

> [Randomization] ensures three things: it ensures that neither our personal idiosyncrasies ... nor our lack of balanced judgement has entered into the construction of the different treatment groups ...; it removes the danger, inherent in an allocation based upon personal judgement, that believing we may be biased in our judgements we endeavor to allow for that bias, to exclude it, and that in so doing we may overcompensate and by thus "leaning over backward" introduce a lack of balance from the other direction; and, having used a random allocation, the sternest critic is unable to say when we eventually dash into print that quite probably the groups were differentially biased through our predilections or through our stupidity [p. 35].

Statistical Methods for Rates and Proportions, Third Edition
By Joseph L. Fleiss, Bruce Levin, and Myunghee Cho Paik
ISBN 0-471-52629-0   Copyright © 2003 John Wiley & Sons, Inc.

In spite of the widespread use of randomization in comparative trials, debate continues as to its universal appropriateness. This issue will be addressed in Section 8.3.

Table A.5 presents 20,000 random digits, arrayed on each page in ten columns of 50 numbers, with five digits to each number. Some illustrations of the use of the table follow. Modern computers generate lists like those in A.5 with ease, and most readers will have no trouble producing their own lists of random digits by computer. Still, the manual method presented below has a certain charm, and is instructive on a number of points.

5.1. SELECTING A SIMPLE RANDOM SAMPLE

Suppose that a firm has 250 employees, of whom 100 are to be selected for a thorough physical examination and an interview to determine health habits. A simple random sample of 100 out of the larger group of 250 may be selected as follows.

Examine consecutive three-digit numbers, ignoring any that are 000 or between 251 and 999. Of the numbers between 001 and 250, list the first 100 distinct ones that are encountered. When a column is completed, proceed to the next one. The 100 numbers listed designate the employees to be selected. If a file exists containing the names of all employees—the order in which the names appear is immaterial—the employees may be numbered from 1 to 250 and those whose numbers appear on the list of random numbers would be selected.

To illustrate, let us begin in the second column of the second page of Table A.5. Each number in the column contains five digits, of which only the first three will be examined. The first five numbers in the column, after deleting their last two digits, are 670, 716, 367, 988, and 283—all greater than 250. The sixth number, 142, is between 001 and 250 and thus designates one of the employees to be selected. The other numbers selected from the second column are seen to be 021, 166, 127, 060, 098, 219, 161, 042, 043, 157, 113, 234, 024, 028, and 128.

Having exhausted the second column, and still requiring 84 additional numbers, we proceed to examine the third column of the second page. At the end of the third column, 29 distinct numbers between 001 and 250 are available. In numerical order, they are:

001	028	052	107	142	166
014	034	059	113	146	219
021	042	060	121	157	234
024	043	080	127	160	244
026	047	098	128	161	

Subsequent columns are examined similarly until an additional 71 distinct numbers between 001 and 250 are found. If a previously selected number is encountered (e.g., 244 is encountered again in column 4), it is ignored.

The above method has the virtue of being *self-documenting*, in the sense that, considering Table A.5 as a fixed, public record, any random sample drawn using it can be reconstructed by revealing the starting location and selection rules. This is useful for auditing purposes. The reader may wonder how a sequence of numbers can be both "random" and yet completely reproducible. That is the secret of *pseudorandom* sequences, like those modern computers use universally. A pseudorandom number generator is a deterministic algorithm whose output exhibits certain properties of theoretical random sequences: the numbers tend to be *uniformly* distributed and *chaotic*, in the sense of extreme sensitivity to initial conditions, and thus they are *difficult to predict*. These features help assure that a documentable and replicable (pseudo)random number generator is beyond suspicion of manipulation.

To illustrate the chaotic nature of pseudorandom number generators, if one had used columns 2, 3, and 4 instead of 1, 2, and 3 in the preceding paragraph, a radically different set of numbers would have resulted. As another illustration, consider the following example of a pseudorandom number generator known as a *multiplicative congruential generator*. With a prespecified *multiplier a*, a fixed *modulus m*, and a given *seed X_0*, generate the next number as follows: multiply X_0 by a, divide the result by m, throw away the whole number quotient, and set X_1 equal to the remainder. The next number is generated similarly starting with X_1, and so on. The numbers generated will fall in the interval from 1 to $m - 1$, and with suitably chosen a and m, the sequence will not repeat until all $m - 1$ integers have been exhausted. For example, if $a = 7$, $m = 101$, and we choose seed $X_0 = 1$, the generator produces the sequence $(X_1, X_2, X_3, \ldots) = (7, 49, 40, 78, 41, 85, 90, 24, 67, 65, \ldots)$. The third number generated is 40 because $7 \times 49 = 343$, and 343 has a remainder of 40 upon division by 101. Although the first two numbers generated, 7, 49, are easily predictable, the sequence soon loses that property. Furthermore, if instead of choosing seed 1 we choose seed $X_0 = 2$, the generator produces $(14, 98, 80, 55, 82, 69, 79, 48, 33, 29, \ldots)$, which, as a sequence of numbers from 1 to 100, bears little resemblance to the first sequence after the first few numbers, even though each number in the second sequence is equal to twice that in the first modulo 101.

The above pseudorandom number generator will start repeating after 101 numbers have been generated. In modern computers the multiplier and modulus are chosen to be huge numbers, so that the sequence does not start repeating except after an immensely long time. A popular multiplicative congruential generator is given by $a = 2 \times 7^2 \times 4{,}053{,}103 = 397{,}204{,}094$ and $m^{31} - 1 = 2{,}147{,}483{,}647$. The modulus m is related to the length of a computer word, 31 bits, when this congruential generator was developed. The multiplier a is chosen carefully to assure the sequence of numbers appears as uniformly distributed as possible in several dimensions. Some computer installations select the seed X_0 by reading the time of day down to hundredths of a second when the random number generator is invoked. The chaotic nature of the process insures that if one wanted to manipulate the system in order to predict the outcome of the selection process, one would have to know the time the algorithm was executed down to the hundredth of a second; otherwise a completely unrelated selection would result. At the same time, if the seed is recorded at the moment of execution, the deterministic nature of the procedure guarantees replicability of the selection for auditing.

5.2. RANDOMIZATION IN A CLINICAL TRIAL

Suppose that a clinical trial is to be carried out to compare the effectiveness of a drug with that of an inert placebo, and suppose that 50 patients are to be studied under each drug, requiring a total of 100 patients. Suppose, finally, that patients enter the study serially over time, and so are not all available at once.

Two randomization methods exist. The first calls for selecting 50 distinct numbers between 001 and 100, as described in Section 5.1, and for letting these numbers designate the patients who will receive the active drug. The remaining 50 numbers designate the patients who will receive the placebo.

This method has two drawbacks. First, if the study must be terminated prematurely, there exists a strong likelihood that the total number of patients who had been assigned the active drug up to the termination date will not equal the total number who had been assigned the placebo. Statistical comparisons lose sensitivity if the sample sizes differ. This can be especially annoying in multicenter studies or highly stratified studies (see Section 5.3) where many individual stratum sizes may be small. Second, if the clinical characteristics of the patients entering the trial during one interval of time differ from those of patients entering during another, or if the standards of assessment change over time, then the two treatment groups might well end up being different, in spite of randomization, either in the kinds of patients they contain or in the standards of assessment applied to them (see Cutler et al., 1966, p. 865).

The second possible method of randomization guards against these potential weaknesses in the first method. It calls for independently randomizing, to one treatment group or the other, patients who enter the trial within each successive short interval of time.

Suppose, for example, that ten patients are expected to enter the trial each month. A reasonable strategy is to assign at random five of the first ten patients to one treatment group and the other five to the second treatment group, and to repeat the random assignment of five patients to one group and five to the other for each successive group of ten.

The procedure is implemented as follows, beginning at the top of the fifth column of the first page of Table A.5. Because selection is from ten subjects, only single digits need be examined, with 0 designating the tenth subject. The first five distinct digits are found to be 2, 5, 4, 8, and 6. Therefore, the second, fourth, fifth, sixth, and eighth patients out of the first ten will be assigned the active drug, and the others—the first, third, seventh, ninth, and tenth—will be assigned the placebo.

Examination of the column continues for the second series of ten patients. The next five distinct digits are found to be 3, 1, 8, 0, and 5, implying that, of the second group of ten patients, the first, third, fifth, eighth, and tenth are assigned the active drug and the second, fourth, sixth, seventh, and ninth are assigned the placebo. As soon as the leading digits in a column are exhausted, the second digits may be examined.

It is important that a new set of random numbers be selected for each successive group, lest an unsuspected periodicity in the kind of patient entering the trial, or a pattern soon apparent to personnel who should be kept ignorant of which drugs the patients are receiving, introduce a bias.

A special case of the method just illustrated is the pairing of subjects, with one member of the pair randomly assigned the active drug and the other assigned the placebo. Random assignment becomes especially simple when subjects are paired. To begin with, one member of the pair must be designated the first, and the other, the second. The designation might be on the basis of time of entry into the study, of alphabetical order of the surname, or of any other criterion, provided that the designation is made before the randomization is performed.

Table A.5 is entered at any convenient point, and successive single digits are examined, one digit for each pair. If the digit is odd—1, 3, 5, 7, or 9—the first member of the pair is assigned the active drug and the second member, the placebo. If the digit is even—2, 4, 6, 8, or 0—the second member of the pair is assigned the active drug and the first member the placebo.

To illustrate, let us begin at the top of the first column on the third page of Table A.5. The first digit encountered, 2, is even, indicating that, in the first pair, the active drug is given to the second member and the placebo to the first. The second digit encountered, 8, is also even, so that, in the second pair, too, the active drug is given to the second member and the placebo to the first. The sixth, seventh, and eighth digits—3, 9, and 1—are all odd. Therefore, in the sixth through eighth pairs, the active drug is given to the first member and the placebo to the second.

The methods just described for balanced assignment in blocks of size ten or two are special cases of *randomly permuted blocks* (Zelen, 1974; see also Fleiss, 1986, from which we freely paraphrase). To simplify matters, let us reformulate the method as follows. First, exhaustively enumerate all possible permuted blocks of size $2k$ for a given choice of k. Each block contains equal numbers of treatment assignments to treatments, say, A and B. Table 5.1

Table 5.1. *Permuted blocks of length 2, 4, 6, and 8*

	Length 2		
1. AB		2. BA	

	Length 4		
1. AABB		4. BAAB	
2. ABAB		5. BABA	
3. ABBA		6. BBAA	

Length 6

1. AAABBB	6. ABABAB	11. BAAABB	16. BABBAA
2. AABABB	7. ABABBA	12. BAABAB	17. BBAAAB
3. AABBAB	8. ABBAAB	13. BAABBA	18. BBAABA
4. AABBBA	9. ABBABA	14. BABAAB	19. BBABAA
5. ABAABB	10. ABBBAA	15. BABABA	20. BBBAAA

Length 8

1. AAAABBBB	15. AABBBBAA	29. ABBABAAB	43. BAABBAAB	57. BBAAABAB
2. AAABABBB	16. ABAAABBB	30. ABBABABA	44. BAABBABA	58. BBAAABBA
3. AAABBABB	17. ABAABABB	31. ABBABBAA	45. BAABBBAA	59. BBAABAAB
4. AAABBBAB	18. ABAABBAB	32. ABBBAAAB	46. BABAAABB	60. BBAABABA
5. AAABBBBA	19. ABAABBBA	33. ABBBAABA	47. BABAABAB	61. BBAABBAA
6. AABAABBB	20. ABABAABB	34. ABBBABAA	48. BABAABBA	62. BBABAAAB
7. AABABABB	21. ABABABAB	35. ABBBBAAA	49. BABABAAB	63. BBABAABA
8. AABABBAB	22. ABABABBA	36. BAAAABBB	50. BABABABA	64. BBABABAA
9. AABABBBA	23. ABABBAAB	37. BAAABABB	51. BABABBAA	65. BBABBAAA
10. AABBAABB	24. ABABBABA	38. BAAABBAB	52. BABBAAAB	66. BBBAAAAB
11. AABBABAB	25. ABABBBAA	39. BAAABBBA	53. BABBAABA	67. BBBAAABA
12. AABBABBA	26. ABBAAABB	40. BAABAABB	54. BABBABAA	68. BBBAABAA
13. AABBBAAB	27. ABBAABAB	41. BAABABAB	55. BABBBAAA	69. BBBABAAA
14. AABBBABA	28. ABBAABBA	42. BAABABBA	56. BBAAAABB	70. BBBBAAAA

gives the enumerations for $k = 1, 2, 3,$ and 4. The length of each enumeration is the binomial coefficient $\binom{2k}{k} = \{(2k)!\}/(k!)^2$, equal to 2, 6, 20, and 70 for $k = 1, 2, 3,$ and 4 for blocks of length 2, 4, 6, and 8.

Second, from Table A.5 generate a sequence of random numbers from 1 to the length of the enumeration. Treatment assignment for the first $2k$ subjects begins in the permuted block with the index number specified by the first number in the sequence. When these have been assigned, the second number in the sequence specifies which permuted block to use for treatment assignment, and so on.

To illustrate the use of permuted blocks of length 6 ($k = 3$), let us begin (arbitrarily) at the top of the sixth column of the sixth page of Table A.5. We need a sequence of numbers from 1 to 20, and use the method of Section 5.1: looking at only the first two digits in each row, we obtain the sequence 14, 7, 11, 3, 13, 13, 1, 10, 11, 10, 16, and 8 before exhausting the column. Notice that repetitions are allowed in the sequence. Then the first six subjects to be randomized are assigned treatments B, A, B, A, A, B; the next six subjects are assigned treatments, A, B, A, B, B, A; the next six B, A, A, A, B, B; and so on.

If the two treatments are sufficiently similar in their side effects and in other characteristics to assure that the investigator can be kept ignorant (i.e., *masked* or *blinded* to) which treatment a patient is receiving, then randomly permuted blocks of size two should suffice. It is unlikely that the person responsible for recruiting patients into the study will catch on to the fact that randomization occurs within consecutive pairs. Even if the investigator does catch on, he or she may not know which treatment was assigned to the first patient in a pair and will therefore not be in a position to know with certainty which treatment will be assigned to the next patient. Such knowledge could easily cause the investigator to delay enrolling the next patient until, in his or her clinical judgement, the "right" one came along for that treatment.

In studies comparing different methods of surgery or any kinds of treatments for which maintenance of the investigator's masking is unlikely or impossible, the use of blocks of size two is risky. Randomly permuted blocks of size four, six, or perhaps even eight ought to be used, and one may even randomly change the block size over the course of the study as an added control over the investigator's "catching on."

For example, suppose the trial protocol calls for randomly permuted blocks of sizes four, six, and eight. First, generate three sequences of numbers from 1 to 6, 1 to 20, and 1 to 70, calling them, say, F, S, and E, respectively. Thus, using the first digit of the fourth column of the fourth page of Table A.5, we generate for the F list the sequence beginning 6, 6, 5, 1, 4, 4, 1, 6, 6, 5, ... For the S list we can use the sequence illustrated above, 14, 7, 11, 3, 13, 13, 1, 10, 11, 10, ... For the E list, using the first two digits of the eighth column of the eighth page of Table A.5, we generate the sequence beginning 61, 66, 22, 28, 65, 8, 32, 19, 70, 19, ... Second, generate an auxiliary list to randomize between the F, S, or E sequences. Use digits 1, 2, or 3 for F; 4, 5, or 6 for S; 7, 8, or 9 for E; and ignore digit 0. The first digit of the first column on the first page of Table A.5 gives the sequence E, E, S, F, E, E, F, F, F, S, ... Then the first block of subjects to be randomized is of length eight, and we use the permuted block corresponding to the first number on the E list, 61. This gives the treatment assignment B, B, A, A, B, B, A, A. The second block is also of length eight, and using the second number on the E list, 66, gives the treatment assignment B, B, B, A, A, A, A, B for the next eight subjects. The third block is of length six, and we can use, for example, the third number on the S list, 11, to assign treatments B, A, A, A, B, B to the next six subjects. The fourth block is of length four, and the fourth number on the F list, 1, assigns treatments A, A, B, B to the next four subjects; and so on. (Instead of using the *n*th number on the F, S, or E list for the *n*th permuted block, one could use the sequences consecutively, making sure to cross off sequence numbers as they are used.)

As emphasized in Fleiss (1986, p. 51), the lists of treatment assignments must be kept under lock and key and not made known to the investigator or anyone else who must remain blinded to treatment assignment until the study is over. During the course of a study, the investigator opens an envelope, calls the statistician or an automated randomization telephone number set up for the trial, or does any of a number of other things to learn what treatment to assign after each new eligible patient has been enrolled.

Investigators who require more than the 20,000 random digits of Table A.5 are referred to the Rand Corporation's extensive table (1955). Those whose research designs call for applying each of a number (more than two) of treatments to each of a sample of subjects will find Moses and Oakford's tables of random permutations (1963) indispensable. Their tables also facilitate each of the uses of randomization illustrated above.

5.3. VARIATIONS ON SIMPLE RANDOMIZATION

The randomization procedures discussed in the preceding section are all such that each new patient has a 50:50 chance of being assigned one or the other of the two treatments being compared. With the exception of studies in which patients are matched on characteristics associated with the outcome variable, these procedures run the risk of producing a lack of balance between the treatment groups in the distributions of age, sex, initial severity, or other prognostic factors. A solution other than matching on these characteristics is to stratify patients into predetermined strata (e.g., males aged 20–29, females aged 20–29, males aged 30–39, etc.), and to apply one of the simple randomization methods described above separately and independently within each stratum.

The risk of imbalance is reduced but not totally removed by simple stratified randomization, especially if patients enter the trial serially over time so that the total number of patients ending up in each stratum is not known until the recruitment of patients is completed. As a means of reducing even further the risk of imbalance, Efron (1971) introduced and Pocock and Simon (1975) elaborated on the concept of the *biased coin*. Suppose that a new patient is in a stratum for which, to date, more patients have been assigned one treatment than the other. Biased coin allocation calls for this new patient to be assigned, with prespecified probability $p > 0.5$, the treatment that is currently underrepresented in his stratum. His chances of being assigned the currently overrepresented treatment are $1 - p < 0.5$. If the two treatments have so far been assigned to equal numbers of patients in his stratum, the new patient is assigned to one or the other with probability 0.5.

We illustrate Efron's biased coin scheme with the value of p he proposed as generally being good, that is, $p = \frac{2}{3}$. Suppose a new patient is in a stratum where unequal numbers of patients have so far been assigned the two treatments. A single digit from Table A.5 is examined for this patient, with the digit 0 ignored. If the selected digit is not divisible by 3 (1, 2, 4, 5, 7, or 8), the patient is assigned the currently underrepresented treatment. If the selected digit is divisible by 3 (3, 6, or 9), he or she is assigned the currently overrepresented treatment.

Probabilities of assignment other than 50:50 are also called for in so-called adaptive clinical trials, where the intent is to have, by the time the trial is concluded, more patients treated with the superior than with the inferior treatment (see Chapter 8 for discussion and references). Let $p > 0.5$ be the prespecified probability that a new patient is assigned the treatment that, to date, seems to be superior (if the two treatments appear to be equally effective, the new patient is assigned one or the other treatment with probability 0.5). Two-digit numbers in Table A.5 may be examined. If the selected number for a new patient lies between 01 and $100p$, inclusive, he or she is assigned the currently superior treatment; if it exceeds $100p$ (00 is taken to be 100), he or she is assigned the currently inferior treatment. For example, $p = 0.60$ leads to any number in the interval from 01 to 60 assigning the patient the currently superior treatment, and any number in the interval from 61 to 00 the currently inferior treatment.

REFERENCES

Cutler, S. J., Greenhouse, S. W., Cornfield, J., and Schneiderman, M. A. (1966). The role of hypothesis testing in clinical trials: Biometrics seminar. *J. Chronic Dis.*, **19**, 857–882.

Efron, B. (1971). Forcing a sequential experiment to be balanced. *Biometrika*, **58**, 403–417.

Fisher, R. A. (1935). *The design of experiments*. Edinburgh: Oliver and Boyd.

Fleiss, J. L. (1986). *The design and analysis of clinical experiments*. New York: Wiley.

Hill, A. B. (1962). *Statistical methods in clinical and preventive medicine*. New York: Oxford University Press.

Moses, L. E. and Oakford, R. V. (1963). *Tables of random permutations*. Stanford: Stanford University Press.

Pocock, S. J. and Simon, R. (1975). Sequential treatment assignment with balancing for prognostic factors in the controlled clinical trial. *Biometrics*, **31**, 103–115.

Rand Corporation (1955). *A million random digits with 100,000 normal deviates*. New York: The Free Press.

Zelen, M. (1974). The randomization and stratification of patients to clinical trials. *J. Chron. Dis.*, **27**, 365–375.

CHAPTER 6

Comparative Studies: Cross-sectional, Naturalistic, or Multinomial Sampling

In this chapter we study what was identified in Section 3.1 as method I sampling. This method of sampling, referred to as *cross-sectional, naturalistic,* or *multinomial* sampling, does not attempt to prespecify any frequencies except the overall total.

We consider only the case where the resulting data are arrayed in a 2×2 table. Most statistics texts describe the chi squared test for association when there are more than two rows or more than two columns in the resulting cross-classification table (e.g., Dixon and Massey, 1969, Section 13.3; Everitt, 1977, Chapter 3). The accuracy of the chi squared test for general contingency tables when the total sample size is small has been studied by Craddock and Flood (1970). Methods for estimating association in such tables are given by Goodman (1964), Goodman and Kruskal (1979), and Altham (1970a, 1970b).

In Section 6.1 we present some hypothetical data that are referred to repeatedly in this and the next chapter. In Section 6.2 we examine estimation by means of measures based on χ^2 of the degree of association between the two characteristics studied. Some properties of the odds ratio and its logarithm are presented in Section 6.3.

Exact methods for testing hypotheses about the odds ratio are discussed in Section 6.4, and exact methods for constructing confidence intervals for the odds ratio in Section 6.5. Section 6.6 discusses approximate methods for hypothesis tests and confidence intervals. Section 6.7 presents some criticisms of the odds ratio by Berkson, Sheps, Feinstein, and others, and some

Statistical Methods for Rates and Proportions, Third Edition
By Joseph L. Fleiss, Bruce Levin, and Myunghee Cho Paik
ISBN 0-471-52629-0   Copyright © 2003 John Wiley & Sons, Inc.

alternative measures of association that better serve their needs. Section 6.8 defines and presents methods for making inferences about the attributable risk. Section 6.9 concludes the chapter with some formulas for the standard errors of the measures of association presented earlier.

6.1. SOME HYPOTHETICAL DATA

Suppose that we are studying the association, if any, between the age of the mother (A represents a maternal age less than or equal to 20 years; $\overline{A}$, a maternal age over 20 years) and the birthweight of her offspring (B represents a birthweight less than or equal to 2500 grams; $\overline{B}$, a birthweight over 2500 grams). Since the association might vary as a function of social and demographic factors, let us agree to study only women of a given level of education, race, and type of insurance coverage, who deliver in a single large urban hospital. For example, we might specify the study population to be high school graduates who are black and covered by Medicaid delivering at New York Presbyterian Hospital. Such information is available from birth certificates and/or the hospital's records.

Suppose that all the data we need are on file in the hospital's record system and that, for each delivery, an entry is created recording the birthweight of the infant and the age, education, race, and type of insurance coverage of the mother. After filtering out records from the mothers who do not fit the study criteria, we are left with a file for deliveries of the desired study population. Suppose that the number of records remaining is quite large. The decision might then be made to examine only a sample, say 200, of all the records.

The sample should ideally be a simple random sample (see Chapter 5), but alternatives exist that may be more practical for noncomputerized files, especially those without a record locator index. Suppose that there are a total of 1,000 records. A *systematic random sample* of 200 may be selected by drawing every fifth record, with the starting record (the first, second, third, fourth, or fifth) chosen at random. Another alternative is to base the selection on the last digit of the identification number, choosing only those records whose last digit is, for example, a 3 or a 7. These methods are not truly random, and one needs to assume there are no hidden periodicities in the filing system that might cause every fifth record to be more or less likely to represent certain characteristics. Imagine, for example, a file ordered by day of week, and choosing every seventh record.

Let us suppose that the sample of 200 records has been selected, and that the data are as in Table 6.1. As pointed out in Chapter 3, a more appropriate means of presenting the data resulting from method I sampling is as in Table 6.2.

A consequence of multinomial sampling is that all probabilities may be estimated. Thus the proportion of all deliveries in which the mother was aged

Table 6.1. *Association between birthweight and maternal age: cross-sectional study*

	Birthweight		
Maternal Age	B	$\overline{B}$	Total
A	10	40	50
$\overline{A}$	15	135	150
Total	25	175	200

Table 6.2. *Joint proportions derived from Table 6.1*

	Birthweight		
Maternal Age	B	$\overline{B}$	Total
A	$0.050\ (=p_{11})$	$0.200\ (=p_{12})$	$0.25\ (=p_{1.})$
$\overline{A}$	$0.075\ (=p_{21})$	$0.675\ (=p_{22})$	$0.75\ (=p_{2.})$
Total	$0.125\ (=p_{.1})$	$0.875\ (=p_{.2})$	1.

20 years or less and in which the offspring weighed 2500 grams or less is estimated as $p(A$ and $B) = p_{11} = 0.05$. The proportion of all deliveries in which the mother was aged 20 years or less is estimated as $p(A) = p_{1.} = 0.25$, and the proportion of all deliveries in which the offspring weighed 2500 grams or less is $p(B) = p_{.1} = 0.125$.

The significance of the association between maternal age and birth weight (the first, but by no means the most important, issue) may be assessed by means of the standard chi squared test. The value of the test statistic is

$$\chi^2 = \frac{200(|10 \times 135 - 40 \times 15| - \frac{1}{2}200)^2}{50 \times 150 \times 25 \times 175} = 2.58, \tag{6.1}$$

indicating an association that is not statistically significant.

6.2. MEASURES OF ASSOCIATION DERIVED FROM χ^2

The failure to find statistical significance would presumably signal the completion of the analysis. For later comparative purposes, however, we proceed to consider the estimation of the *degree* of association between the two characteristics, beginning with estimates based on the magnitude of χ^2.

A common mistake is to use the value of χ^2 itself as the measure of association. Even though χ^2 is excellent as a measure of the *significance* of the association, it is not at all useful as a measure of the *degree* of association. Generally, a test statistic makes a poor measure of association.

Table 6.3. *Association between birthweight and maternal sge: Sampling method I with 400 births*

| | Birthweight | | |
Maternal Age	B	$\overline{B}$	Total
A	20	80	100
$\overline{A}$	30	270	300
Total	50	350	400

Most importantly, a test statistic is constructed under a null hypothesis, and is thus not designed to estimate a nonnull association. In addition, the number of subjects studied plays a role in the chances of finding significance if association exists, but should play no role in determining the extent of association (see, e.g., Fisher, 1954, pp. 89–90).

Suppose, for example, that another investigator studied the characteristics of 400 births from the same hospital, and suppose that the resulting data were as in Table 6.3. The value of χ^2 for these data is

$$\chi^2 = \frac{400\left(|20 \times 270 - 80 \times 30| - \frac{1}{2}400\right)^2}{100 \times 300 \times 50 \times 350} = 5.97,$$

which indicates an association significant at the 0.05 level.

The inferences are different for the data of Tables 6.1 and 6.3: nonsignificance for the first but significance for the second. The only reason for the difference, however, is that twice as many births were used in Table 6.3 as in Table 6.1. The joint proportions (see Table 6.2) are obviously identical for Tables 6.1 and 6.3, so that the associations between maternal age and birthweight implied by both are also identical. The larger value of χ^2 for the data of Table 6.3 is thus a reflection of the larger total sample size (the doubling of all frequencies has in fact more than doubled the value of chi squared), and not of a greater degree of association.

A measure of the degree of association between characteristics A and B which is related to χ^2 but is free of the influence of the total sample size, $n_{..}$, is the *phi coefficient*:

$$\varphi = \sqrt{\frac{\chi_u^2}{n_{..}}}, \tag{6.2}$$

where χ_u^2 is the uncorrected chi squared statistic,

$$\chi_u^2 = \frac{n_{..}\left(n_{11}n_{22} - n_{12}n_{21}\right)^2}{n_{1.}n_{2.}n_{.1}n_{.2}}. \tag{6.3}$$

The phi coefficient is especially popular as a measure of association in the behavioral sciences, and is interpretable as a correlation coefficient (which is the actual reason that phi is a measure of association—not the fact that it is derived from the χ^2 test statistic). In fact, φ may be computed by assigning any two distinct numbers (0 and 1, for simplicity) to A and $\overline{A}$, assigning any two to B and $\overline{B}$, and calculating the usual product-moment correlation coefficient between the resulting values.

Values of φ close to zero indicate little if any association, whereas values close to unity indicate almost perfect predictability: if φ is near 1, then knowing whether the subject is A or $\overline{A}$ permits an accurate prediction of whether the subject is B or $\overline{B}$. The maximum value of φ is unity (if the marginal distributions are not equal, the maximum is less than unity), and, as a rule of thumb, any value less than 0.30 or 0.35 may be taken to indicate no more than trivial association.

For the data of Table 6.1,

$$\chi_u^2 = \frac{200(10 \times 135 - 40 \times 15)^2}{50 \times 150 \times 25 \times 175} = 3.43,$$

so that

$$\varphi = \sqrt{\frac{3.43}{200}} = 0.13 \tag{6.4}$$

hardly of appreciable magnitude. The value of φ for the data of Table 6.3 is obviously also equal to 0.13.

The phi coefficient finds its greatest usefulness in the study of items contributing to psychological and educational tests (Lord and Novick, 1968) and in the *factor analysis* of a number of yes-no items. See Harman (1960) and Nunnally (1978) for a general description of factor analysis, and Nunnally (1978) and Lord and Novick (1968) for the validity of factor analysis when applied to phi coefficients. Berger (1961) has presented a method for comparing phi coefficients from two independent studies.

The phi coefficient has a number of serious deficiencies, however. As shown in Chapter 7, the values of φ obtained when the association between characteristics A and B is studied prospectively and retrospectively are not comparable, nor is either value comparable with that obtained when the association is studied naturalistically. Carroll (1961) has shown that if either or both characteristics are dichotomized by cutting a continuous distribution into two parts, then the value of φ depends strongly on where the cutting point is set.

This lack of invariance of the phi coefficient and of other measures derived from χ^2 (see Goodman and Kruskal, 1954, pp. 739–740), plus presumably other reasons, led Goodman and Kruskal to assert that they "have been unable to find any convincing published defense of χ^2-like statistics as measures of association" (1954, p. 740). Whereas this assertion ignores the usefulness of φ in psychometrics, it does point to the avoidance of φ and of other statistics based on χ^2 as measures of association in those areas of research where comparability of findings is essential.

Goodman and Kruskal (1954, 1959) present a great many measures of association for 2×2 tables that are not functions of χ^2 and give their statistical properties in two later papers (1963, 1972), which also appear in a collection (1979).

6.3. THE ODDS RATIO AND ITS LOGARITHM

Frequently, one of the two characteristics being studied is antecedent to the other. In the example we have been considering, maternal age is antecedent to birthweight. A measure of the risk of experiencing the outcome under study when the antecedent factor is present is

$$\Omega_A = \frac{P(B|A)}{P(\overline{B}|A)} \tag{6.5}$$

(see Section 1.1 for a definition of conditional probabilities). Ω_A is the *odds* that B will occur when A is present. Now $P(B|A)$ may be estimated by

$$p(B|A) = \frac{p_{11}}{p_{1.}},$$

and $P(\overline{B}|A)$ by

$$p(\overline{B}|A) = \frac{p_{12}}{p_{1.}};$$

therefore Ω_A may be estimated by

$$O_A = \frac{p_{11}/p_{1.}}{p_{12}/p_{1.}} = \frac{p_{11}}{p_{12}}. \tag{6.6}$$

For our example, the estimated odds that a mother aged 20 years or less will deliver an offspring weighing 2500 grams or less are, from Table 6.2,

$$O_A = \frac{0.05}{0.20} = \frac{1}{4} = 0.25 \tag{6.7}$$

Thus, for every four births weighing over 2500 grams to mothers aged 20 years or less, there is one birth weighing 2500 grams or less.

The information conveyed by these odds is exactly the same as that conveyed by the rate of low birthweight specific to young mothers,

$$p(B|A) = \frac{0.05}{0.25} = \frac{1}{5} = 0.20$$

but the emphases differ. One can imagine attempting to educate prospective mothers aged 20 years or less. The impact of the statement, "One out of every five of you is expected to deliver an infant with a low birthweight," may well be different from the impact of "For every four of you who deliver infants of fairly high weight, one is expected to deliver an infant of low birthweight."

When A is absent, the odds of B's occurrence are defined as

$$\Omega_{\bar{A}} = \frac{P(B|\bar{A})}{P(\bar{B}|\bar{A})},\qquad(6.8)$$

which may be estimated as

$$O_{\bar{A}} = \frac{p_{21}/p_{2.}}{p_{22}/p_{2.}} = \frac{p_{21}}{p_{22}}.\qquad(6.9)$$

For our example, the estimated odds that a mother aged more than 20 years will deliver an offspring weighing 2500 grams or less are

$$O_{\bar{A}} = \frac{0.075}{0.675} = \frac{1}{9} = 0.11.\qquad(6.10)$$

Thus for every nine births weighing over 2500 grams to mothers aged more than 20 years (as opposed to every four to younger mothers), there is one birth weighing 2500 grams or less.

The two odds, Ω_A (6.5) and $\Omega_{\bar{A}}$ (6.8), may be contrasted in a number of ways in order to provide a measure of association. One such measure, due to Yule (1900), is

$$Q = \frac{\Omega_A - \Omega_{\bar{A}}}{\Omega_A + \Omega_{\bar{A}}}.\qquad(6.11)$$

Another, also due to Yule (1912), is

$$Y = \frac{\sqrt{\Omega_A} - \sqrt{\Omega_{\bar{A}}}}{\sqrt{\Omega_A} + \sqrt{\Omega_{\bar{A}}}}.\qquad(6.12)$$

the measure of association based on Ω_A and $\Omega_{\bar{A}}$ that is currently in greatest use is simply their ratio,

$$\omega = \frac{\Omega_A}{\Omega_{\bar{A}}},\qquad(6.13)$$

which may be estimated by the sample odds ratio,

$$o = \frac{O_A}{O_{\overline{A}}} = \frac{p_{11}/p_{12}}{p_{21}/p_{22}} = \frac{p_{11}p_{22}}{p_{12}p_{21}}. \tag{6.14}$$

If the two rates $P(B|A)$ and $P(B|\overline{A})$ are equal, indicating the independence or lack of association between the two characteristics, then the two odds Ω_A and $\Omega_{\overline{A}}$ are also equal (see Problem 6.1), so that the odds ratio $\omega = 1$. If $P(B|A) > P(B|\overline{A})$, then $\Omega_A > \Omega_{\overline{A}}$ and $\omega > 1$ (see Problem 6.2). If $P(B|A) < P(B|\overline{A})$, then $\Omega_A < \Omega_{\overline{A}}$ and $\omega < 1$.

For our data, the estimated odds ratio is

$$o = \frac{0.05 \times 0.675}{0.20 \times 0.075} = 2.25, \tag{6.15}$$

indicating that the odds of a young mother's delivering an offspring with low birthweight are $2\frac{1}{4}$ times those for an older mother. Because the odds ratio may also be estimated as

$$o = \frac{n_{11}n_{22}}{n_{12}n_{21}}, \tag{6.16}$$

it is sometimes also referred to as the *cross-product ratio*.

The standard error of the estimated odds ratio is estimated in large samples by

$$\widehat{se}(o) = \frac{o}{\sqrt{n_{..}}} \sqrt{\frac{1}{p_{11}} + \frac{1}{p_{12}} + \frac{1}{p_{21}} + \frac{1}{p_{22}}}. \tag{6.17}$$

For the data of Table 6.2, the standard error is found to be

$$\widehat{se}(o) = \frac{2.25}{\sqrt{200}} \sqrt{\frac{1}{0.05} + \frac{1}{0.20} + \frac{1}{0.075} + \frac{1}{0.675}} = 1.00 \tag{6.18}$$

An equivalent formula in terms of the original frequencies is

$$\widehat{se}(o) = o\sqrt{\frac{1}{n_{11}} + \frac{1}{n_{12}} + \frac{1}{n_{21}} + \frac{1}{n_{22}}}. \tag{6.19}$$

The standard error is useful in gauging the precision of the estimated odds ratio, but not in testing its significance or in constructing confidence intervals. The classic chi squared test should be used as a test of the hypothesis that the odds ratio in the population is equal to 1; the methods of Section 6.6 should be used for constructing confidence intervals.

Anscombe (1956), Gart (1966), and Gart and Zweifel (1967) have studied the sampling properties of o and its standard error. Note that if either n_{12} or

n_{21} is equal to zero, then o in (6.16) is undefined. If any one of the four cell frequencies is equal to zero, then se(o) in (6.19) is undefined. Suggested improved estimates are

$$o' = \frac{(n_{11} + 0.5)(n_{22} + 0.5)}{(n_{12} + 0.5)(n_{21} + 0.5)} \tag{6.20}$$

for the odds ratio and

$$\widehat{se}(o') = o' \sqrt{\frac{1}{(n_{11} + 0.5)} + \frac{1}{(n_{12} + 0.5)} + \frac{1}{(n_{21} + 0.5)} + \frac{1}{(n_{22} + 0.5)}} \tag{6.21}$$

for its standard error. The addition of $\frac{1}{2}$ to each frequency is *not* a continuity correction, but a bias reduction device. See the discussion at the end of this section.

A number of important properties of the odds ratio as measure of association will be demonstrated in the sequel. Advantages of using the odds ratio instead of other measures have been illustrated by Mosteller (1968). Edwards (1963) considered the advantages to be so great that he recommended that only the odds ratio or functions of it be used to measure association in 2×2 tables. We indicate further reasons for the importance of the odds ratio in Section 11.2.

The odds ratio was originally proposed by Cornfield (1951) as a measure of the degree of association between an antecedent factor and an outcome event such as morbidity or mortality, but only because it provided a good approximation to another measure he proposed, the *relative risk*, also called the *rate ratio*. If the risk of the occurrence of event B when A is present is taken simply as the rate of B's occurrence specific to the presence of A, $P(B|A)$, and similarly for the risk of B when A is absent, then the relative risk is simply the ratio of the two risks,

$$R = \frac{P(B|A)}{P(B|\bar{A})}. \tag{6.22}$$

R may be estimated by

$$r = \frac{p_{11}/p_{1.}}{p_{21}/p_{2.}} = \frac{p_{11} p_{2.}}{p_{21} p_{1.}}. \tag{6.23}$$

If the occurrence of event B is unlikely whether or not characteristic A is present, then, as shown in Problem 6.3, r is approximately equal to o [see

(6.14)]. For the data of Table 6.2,

$$r = \frac{0.05 \times 0.75}{0.075 \times 0.25} = 2.0, \tag{6.24}$$

only slightly less than the value found for the odds ratio, $o = 2.25$ [see (6.15)].

There is more to the odds ratio, however, than merely an approximation to the relative risk. There exists a mathematical model, the so-called *logistic model*, that naturally gives rise to the odds ratio as a measure of association. Consider, for specificity, the association between cigarette smoking and lung cancer. Mortality from lung cancer is a function not only of whether one smokes, but also, as but one example, of the amount of air pollution in the environment of the community where one works or lives.

Let us agree to study the association between smoking and lung cancer in one community only, and let x represent the mean amount of a specified pollutant in the atmosphere surrounding that community. A possible representation of the mortality rate from lung cancer for cigarette smokers is

$$P_S = \frac{1}{1 + e^{-(ax+b_S)}}, \tag{6.25}$$

and of the mortality rate for nonsmokers,

$$P_N = \frac{1}{1 + e^{-(ax+b_N)}}, \tag{6.26}$$

where $e = 2.718$, the base of natural logarithms. The parameter a measures the dependence of mortality on the specified air pollutant. The use of the same parameter, a, in (6.25) and (6.26) is equivalent to the assumption of no synergistic effect of smoking and air pollution on mortality. If a is positive, then both P_S and P_N approach unity as x, the mean amount of the pollutant, becomes large.

According to the model represented by (6.25) and (6.26), the effect of smoking on mortality is reflected only in the possible difference between the parameters b_S and b_N. When $x = 0$, that is, when a community is completely free of the specified pollutant, then b_S is directly related to the mortality rate for smokers and b_N is directly related to the mortality rate for nonsmokers.

Consider, now, the odds that a smoker from the selected community will die of lung cancer. These odds are

$$\Omega_S = \frac{P_S}{1 - P_S}.$$

Since

$$1 - P_S = \frac{e^{-(ax+b_S)}}{1 + e^{-(ax+b_S)}},$$

therefore

$$\Omega_S = \frac{1}{e^{-(ax+b_S)}} = e^{ax+b_S}. \tag{6.27}$$

Similarly, the odds that a nonsmoker from that community will die of lung cancer are

$$\Omega_N = e^{ax+b_N}. \tag{6.28}$$

Thus, if the logistic model is correct, the odds ratio, that is, the ratio of the odds in (6.27) to the odds in (6.28), becomes simply

$$\omega = \frac{\Omega_S}{\Omega_N} = \frac{e^{ax+b_S}}{e^{ax+b_N}} = e^{b_S-b_N}, \tag{6.29}$$

independent of x. The natural logarithm of the odds ratio is then simply

$$\ln \omega = b_S - b_N, \tag{6.30}$$

which is also independent of x, and, moreover is the simple difference between the two parameters assumed to distinguish smokers from non-smokers.

The importance of this result is that, if the odds ratio or its logarithm is found to be stable across many different kinds of populations, then one may reasonably infer that the logistic model is a fair representation of the phenomenon under study. Given this inference, one may predict the value of the odds ratio in a new population and test the difference between the observed and predicted values; one may predict the effects on mortality of controlling the factor represented by x (in our example, an air pollutant); and one may of course predict the effects on mortality of controlling smoking habits.

The representation of (6.30) of the logarithm of ω suggests that the logarithm of the sample odds ratio,

$$L = \ln o, \tag{6.31}$$

is an important measure of association. Natural logarithms are tabulated in Table A.6. The standard error of L has been studied by Woolf (1955), Haldane (1956), and Gart (1966). A better estimate of $\ln(\omega)$ was found to be

$$L' = \ln o', \tag{6.32}$$

where o' is defined in (6.20), and a good estimate of its standard error was found to be

$$\widehat{\text{se}}(L') = \sqrt{\frac{1}{(n_{11}+0.5)} + \frac{1}{(n_{12}+0.5)} + \frac{1}{(n_{21}+0.5)} + \frac{1}{(n_{22}+0.5)}}.$$

(6.33)

The addition of $\frac{1}{2}$ is not arbitrary. Haldane (1956) showed that of all estimators of a log odds parameter of the form $\ln\{(p+a/n)/(q+a/n)\}$ for different values of a, the choice $a = \frac{1}{2}$ removes the leading term in the expression for bias in large samples. See Problem 6.5.

When the logistic model of (6.25) and (6.26) obtains, $\ln \omega$ is seen by (6.30) to be completely independent of x. Even if, instead, a model specified by a cumulative normal distribution is assumed, $\ln \omega$ is nearly independent of x (Edwards, 1966; Fleiss, 1970). The logistic model is far more manageable for representing rates and proportions than the cumulative normal model, however, and has been so used by Bartlett (1935), Winsor (1948), Dyke and Patterson (1952), Cox (1958, 1970), Grizzle (1961, 1963), Maxwell and Everitt (1970), and Fienberg (1977). We devote Chapter 11 to its study.

6.4. EXACT INFERENCE FOR AN ODDS RATIO: HYPOTHESIS TESTS

In this section we present exact methods of testing hypotheses for an odds ratio from a fourfold table collected under cross-sectional sampling. Readers who wish to use approximate methods only may proceed directly to Section 6.6.

The Noncentral Hypergeometric Distribution.
We restrict attention to fourfold tables as in Table 3.1 with marginal frequencies $n_{1.}$, $n_{2.}$, $n_{.1}$, and $n_{.2}$ fixed at the values actually observed, and suppose that the value of the underlying odds ratio is equal to

$$\omega = \frac{P_{11}/P_{12}}{P_{21}/P_{22}} = \frac{P_{11}/P_{21}}{P_{12}/P_{22}} = \frac{P_{11}P_{22}}{P_{12}P_{21}},$$

(6.34)

where the P_{ij}'s are the true or population cell frequencies as in Table 3.3. Because the margins are being held fixed, any one cell in the table will determine all the other cells by subtraction, so we will choose n_{11} and denote it by X. The reference cell frequency X, given all four margins fixed, has the conditional distribution known as the *noncentral hypergeometric distri-bution*. It's probability function $P(X=x|n_{..}, n_{1.}, n_{.1})$ will be denoted by

$H(x|n_{..}, n_{1.}, n_{.1}, \omega)$ and is given by

$$
H(x|n_{..}, n_{1.}, n_{.1}, \omega) = \frac{\binom{n_{1.}}{x}\binom{n_{2.}}{n_{.1}-x}\omega^x}{\displaystyle\sum_{i=\max(0, n_{1.}+n_{.1}-n_{..})}^{\min(n_{1.}, n_{.1})}\binom{n_{1.}}{i}\binom{n_{2.}}{n_{.1}-i}\omega^i}
$$

$$
= \frac{\binom{n_{.1}}{x}\binom{n_{.2}}{n_{1.}-x}\omega^x}{\displaystyle\sum_{i=\max(0, n_{1.}+n_{.1}-n_{..})}^{\min(n_{1.}, n_{.1})}\binom{n_{.1}}{i}\binom{n_{.2}}{n_{1.}-i}\omega^i}. \qquad (6.35)
$$

The summation in the denominator of (6.35) is a normalizing constant that insures the point probabilities sum to 1. The terms in the summation extend over all possible cell frequencies for the reference cell. The maximum possible reference cell frequency is the smaller of $n_{1.}$ and $n_{.1}$, denoted by $\min(n_{1.}, n_{.1})$, and the minimum possible cell frequency is the quantity $l = n_{1.} + n_{.1} - n_{..}$, or 0 if $l < 0$, denoted by $\max(0, l)$; (6.35) gives the probability of finding $X = x$ for all values of $x = \max(0, l), \dots, \min(n_{1.}, n_{.1})$. In Problem 6.6 the reader is asked to derive (6.35) and to prove that the two expressions in (6.35) are identical. Thus it does not matter which factors are used for the rows or columns of the table. The Fisher-Irwin exact probability function in (3.9) is the special case of (6.35) when the odds ratio $\omega = 1$.

The most remarkable property of (6.35) is that it depends on the four underlying cell probabilities P_{11}, P_{12}, P_{21}, and P_{22} *only through the odds ratio* ω in (6.34). This reduces what would otherwise be a more complicated, three-dimensional inference problem about an odds ratio in the presence of two other nuisance parameters into a simpler, one-dimensional problem of inference about the odds ratio alone. Thanks to the conditioning on the observed margins of the fourfold table (i.e., regarding them as fixed), we can proceed with methods of inference in analogy to those presented in Chapter 2.

The general method for exact testing of a hypothesis about ω is the same as that for exact testing of a hypothesis about P in the binomial distribution presented in Section 2.1; in principle, one merely substitutes the noncentral hypergeometric distribution (6.35) for the binomial distribution (2.1). Given the observed value of $X = n_{11} = x_0$, say, the upper tail probability for testing the null hypothesis H_0: $\omega = \omega_0$ against the one-sided alternative hypothesis H_1: $\omega > \omega_0$ is

$$
P(X \geq x_0) = \sum_{x=x_0}^{\min(n_{1.}, n_{.1})} H(x|n_{..}, n_{1.}, n_{.1}, \omega_0), \qquad (6.36)
$$

and the lower tail probability for testing the same null hypothesis against the one-sided alternative H_1: $\omega < \omega_0$ is

$$P(X \leq x_0) = \sum_{x=\max(0,l)}^{x_0} H(x|n_{..}, n_{1.}, n_{.1}, \omega_0), \qquad (6.37)$$

where $l = n_{1.} + n_{.1} - n_{..}$.

Two-tailed p-values for testing the null hypothesis H_0: $\omega = \omega_0$ against the alternative H_1: $\omega \neq \omega_0$ are defined analogously to those in Section 2.1 and 2.7. In particular, a two-tailed p-value with equal allocation of Type I error in each tail is defined as twice the observed one-tailed p-value (or 1, whichever is smaller). A two-tailed p-value by the point probability method of Section 2.7.1 is defined as

$$\text{pval}(x_0, \omega_0) = \sum_x H(x|n_{..}, n_{1.}, n_{.1}, \omega_0) \qquad (6.38)$$

where the sum is taken over all values of x with

$$H(x|n_{..}, n_{1.}, n_{.1}, \omega_0) \leq H(x_0|n_{..}, n_{1.}, n_{.1}, \omega_0) \qquad (6.39)$$

as we did in Section 3.2 for the special case of the Fisher-Irwin exact test, $\omega_0 = 1$. All four definitions of two-tailed p-values discussed in Section 2.7 (equal allocation, point probability, tail probability, and likelihood ratio) carry over analogously to the case of the noncentral hypergeometric distribution, and provide hypothesis tests for odds ratios that work assuredly.

Consider testing the hypothesis that the value of the odds ratio ω underlying the data of Table 6.1 equals $\omega_0 = 5$ against the two-sided alternative $\omega \neq 5$. The noncentral hypergeometric distribution with total sample size $n_{..} = 200$, margins $n_{1.} = 50$ and $n_{.1} = 25$, and parameter $\omega_0 = 5$ is given in Table 6.4.

Table 6.4. Values of the noncentral hypergeometric distribution
$H(x|200, 50, 25, \omega_0 = 5)$

x	$P(X=x)$	x	$P(X=x)$	x	$P(X=x)$
0	0.0000	10	0.0335	20	0.0055
1	0.0000	11	0.0671	21	0.0013
2	0.0000	12	0.1114	22	0.0002
3	0.0000	13	0.1534	23	0.0000
4	0.0000	14	0.1750	24	0.0000
5	0.0000	15	0.1650	25	0.0000
6	0.0003	16	0.1280		
7	0.0013	17	0.0811		
8	0.0047	18	0.0416		
9	0.0138	19	0.0170		

The reference cell has observed frequency $x_0 = 10$, with point probability 0.0335. The lower tail probability is the sum of the probabilities for $x = 0, \ldots, 10$, which is 0.0535 (corrected for round-off). The two-tailed p-value by the equal allocation method is thus twice this value, or 0.1070. The two-tailed p-value by the point probability method is the lower tail probability, 0.0535, plus the sum of the probabilities in the upper tail with values no greater than 0.0335, corresponding to $x = 19, 20, \ldots, 25$. The resulting p-value, corrected for roundoff, is 0.0776.

Mean and Variance of the Noncentral Hypergeometric Distribution
Unlike the binomial distribution, there are no general closed-form formulas for the mean and variance of the noncentral hypergeometric distribution, except for certain special cases. One special case is $\omega = 1$, for which $EX = n_{1.}n_{.1}/n_{..}$ as in (3.8). The variance is given by

$$\text{Var } X = \frac{n_{1.}n_{2.}n_{.1}n_{.2}}{n_{..}^2(n_{..} - 1)}. \tag{6.40}$$

Another important special case arises in the context of matched samples (see Chapter 13) which correspond to a collection of fourfold tables in which $n_{1.} = 1$ for each table. In that case the reference cell frequency is a binary variable taking on values 0 or 1. The reader is asked to show in Problem 6.7 that when $n_{1.} = 1$ and $n_{..} = 1 + n_{2.}$, the mean and variance of the noncentral hypergeometric distribution are

$$E\left(X | n_{..}, 1, n_{.1}, \omega\right) = \frac{n_{.1}\omega}{n_{.1}(\omega - 1) + n_{..}} = \frac{n_{.1}\omega}{n_{.1}\omega + n_{..} - n_{.1}} \tag{6.41}$$

and

$$\text{Var}\left(X | n_{..}, 1, n_{.1}, \omega\right) = \frac{n_{.1}(n_{..} - n_{.1})\omega}{\left\{n_{.1}(\omega - 1) + n_{..}\right\}^2}. \tag{6.42}$$

Of course, for exact computation of a p-value, one does not need formulas for the mean and variance, only terms of (6.35) for tail probabilities. If needed for other applications, the exact mean may be calculated directly from the definition,

$$E_{11} = E\left(X | n_{..}, n_{1.}, n_{.1}, \omega\right) = \frac{\displaystyle\sum_{i=\max(0, n_{1.}+n_{.1}-n_{..})}^{\min(n_{1.}, n_{.1})} i \binom{n_{.1}}{i}\binom{n_{.2}}{n_{1.} - i}\omega^i}{\displaystyle\sum_{i=\max(0, n_{1.}+n_{.1}-n_{..})}^{\min(n_{1.}, n_{.1})} \binom{n_{.1}}{i}\binom{n_{.2}}{n_{1.} - i}\omega^i}; \tag{6.43}$$

the other cell expectations are obtained by subtraction from the margins:

$$E_{12} = E(n_{12}|n_{1.}, n_{.1}, n_{..}, \omega) = n_{1.} - E_{11},$$

$$E_{21} = E(n_{21}|n_{1.}, n_{.1}, n_{..}, \omega) = n_{.1} - E_{11},$$

$$E_{22} = E(n_{22}|n_{1.}, n_{.1}, n_{..}, \omega) = E_{11} - l,$$

where $l = n_{1.} + n_{.1} - n_{..}$. The variance is, by definition,

$$\text{Var}(X|n_{..}, n_{1.}, n_{.1}, \omega)$$

$$= \frac{\sum\limits_{i=\max(0, n_{1.}+n_{.1}-n_{..})}^{\min(n_{1.}, n_{.1})} \{i - E(X|n_{..}, n_{1.}, n_{.1}, \omega)\}^2 \cdot \binom{n_{.1}}{i}\binom{n_{.2}}{n_{1.}-i}\omega^i}{\sum\limits_{i=\max(0, n_{1.}+n_{.1}-n_{..})}^{\min(n_{1.}, n_{.1})} \binom{n_{.1}}{i}\binom{n_{.2}}{n_{1.}-i}\omega^i};$$

$$(6.44)$$

The variances of the other cells are identical to (6.44), because they differ from the reference cell only by constants, conditional on fixed margins.

For future reference, the exact expected values of the cells in Table 6.1 when $\omega = 5$ are $E_{11} = 14.140$, $E_{12} = 50 - 14.140 = 35.860$, $E_{21} = 25 - 14.140 = 10.860$, and $E_{22} = 14.140 - (50 + 25 - 200) = 139.140$. The variance of each cell frequency is $\text{Var}(X|200, 50, 25, \omega = 5) = 5.093$, and the standard deviation is the square root, 2.257.

We note here that the cross-product ratio calculated from the expected cell frequencies E_{ij} is close, but not exactly equal, to the underlying odds ratio of 5: $(E_{11}E_{22})/(E_{12}E_{21}) = 5.052$. Mantel and Hankey (1975) explore this oddity, and show that for the noncentral hypergeometric distribution, it is not the cross-product ratio of expected cell frequencies that equals ω, but rather the ratio of expected cross-products:

$$\frac{E\{X(X-l)\}}{E\{(n_{1.}-X)(n_{.1}-X)\}} = \omega = \frac{E_{11}E_{22} + \text{Var}(X|n_{..}, n_{1.}, n_{.1}, \omega)}{E_{12}E_{21} + \text{Var}(X|n_{..}, n_{1.}, n_{.1}, \omega)}.$$

Levin (1984, 1990) exploits these relations to offer simple but highly accurate approximations to the mean of a noncentral hypergeometric random variable. When the margins of the table are large, the cross-product ratio of the expected cell frequencies is approximately equal to the underlying odds ratio, and this forms the basis for a simple approximation for the mean and variance in large samples, which is taken up in Section 6.6. For matched samples and other situations with one or more small margins, the exact formulas (6.41) and (6.42) or the more general (6.43) and (6.44) should be used.

Another point estimator for the odds ratio, in addition to (6.14) and (6.20), is given by the *conditional maximum likelihood estimate* (cmle), denoted by $\hat{\omega}_c$. It is defined as that value of ω which maximizes (6.35) for the observed value $x = x_0$ of X, and it satisfies the so-called *likelihood equation* (see Appendix B)

$$E\left(X | n_{..}, n_{1.}, n_{.1}, \hat{\omega}_c\right) = x_0, \qquad (6.45)$$

where the left-hand side is given by (6.43). Solving this equation for $\hat{\omega}_c$ generally requires an iterative computation. In large samples the cmle is close to $(p_{11} p_{22})/(p_{12} p_{21})$. The standard error of $\hat{\omega}_c$ is estimated in large samples by

$$\widehat{se}(\hat{\omega}_c) = \hat{\omega}_c / \sqrt{\mathrm{Var}\left(X | n_{..}, n_{1.}, n_{.1}, \hat{\omega}_c\right)},$$

with the conditional variance of X given by (6.44) evaluated at the cmle. The standard error for ln(cmle) is estimated by

$$\widehat{se}(\ln \hat{\omega}_c) = 1 / \sqrt{\mathrm{Var}\left(X | n_{..}, n_{1.}, n_{.1}, \hat{\omega}_c\right)},$$

analogous to the relation between (6.21) and (6.33). Further approximations for $\mathrm{Var}(X | n_{..}, n_{1.}, n_{.1}, \omega)$ are given in Section 6.6.

For the data in Table 6.1, the cmle is $\hat{\omega}_c = 2.24$, essentially the same as the value in (6.15). The variance of X at $\omega = \hat{\omega}_c$ is 5.056, and so the standard error of $\hat{\omega}_c$ is estimated to be $2.24/5.056^{1/2} = 0.996$, very close to (6.18). The cmle of ln ω is ln $2.24 = 0.806$, with estimated standard error $1/5.056^{1/2} = 0.445$.

6.5. EXACT INFERENCE FOR AN ODDS RATIO: CONFIDENCE INTERVALS

An exact confidence interval for the odds ratio underlying the data in a fourfold table observed under cross-sectional sampling can be obtained by the same methods used in Section 2.2 for a binomial proportion: the $100(1 - \alpha)\%$ confidence interval contains all those odds ratios which, if considered as null hypotheses and put to the test with all margins regarded as fixed, would have p-value strictly greater than α.

More precisely, consider finding the upper limit ω_U of a one-sided lower $100(1 - \alpha)\%$ confidence interval for ω of the form $(0, \omega_U)$. One knows one has the correct value for ω_U when

$$\sum_{x=\max(0, l)}^{x_0} H\left(x | n_{..}, n_{1.}, n_{.1}, \omega_U\right) = \alpha, \qquad (6.46)$$

where x_0, recall, is the observed value of the reference cell, n_{11}, and $l = n_{1.} + n_{.1} - n_{..}$. Similarly, the lower limit ω_L of a one-sided upper $100(1 - \alpha)\%$ confidence interval for ω of the form (ω_L, ∞) satisfies

$$\sum_{x=x_0}^{\min(n_{1.}, n_{.1})} H(x|n_{..}, n_{1.}, n_{.1}, \omega_L) = \alpha, \qquad (6.47)$$

For two-sided intervals of the form (ω_L, ω_U) using the equal allocation method, the upper limit sets the left-hand side of (6.46) equal to $\alpha/2$, and the lower limit sets the left-hand side of (6.47) equal to $\alpha/2$. For two-sided intervals using the point probability method, the lower limit ω_L is the greatest lower bound of all ω for which the p-value in (6.38) and (6.39) satisfies pval$(x_0, \omega) > \alpha$, and the upper limit ω_U is the least upper bound of all ω for which the p-value satisfies pval$(x_0, \omega) > \alpha$. (The use of the greatest lower bound and least upper bound in the definition was explained in Section 2.7 and Problem 2.20 for the binomial distribution. Similar remarks apply in the present context.)

For the data of Table 6.1, the one-sided upper 95% confidence limit is just larger than $\omega = 5$, because Table 6.4 shows the lower tail probability, 0.0535, to be just larger than 0.05. Iterative methods provide the desired upper 95% confidence limit of $\omega_U = 5.072$ satisfying (6.46). For the lower confidence limit, iterative methods yield the value $\omega_L = 0.9650$ for (6.47). For the two-sided 95% confidence interval using the equal allocation method, the confidence interval is (0.831, 5.820). The two-sided 95% confidence interval using the point probability method is (0.926, 5.390), narrower than the interval by the equal allocation method. In neither case would the method reject the null hypothesis of no association between maternal age and low birthweight, as the confidence intervals contain $\omega = 1$.

Agresti (1992) gives a good review of exact methods for fourfold and larger tables.

6.6. APPROXIMATE INFERENCE FOR AN ODDS RATIO

When the margins of the fourfold table are large, such that the expected cell frequencies inside the table are all five or more, the approximate methods presented in this section are accurate enough for general use. Indeed, the second edition of this book used the first-order approximations N_{ij} presented below in expressions (6.52) through (6.55) as if they were the exact expected cell frequencies E_{ij} defined at (6.43). Although this was not perfectly accurate, and the exact expressions should be used when the table violates the "rule of five," the approximation is perfectly adequate for the large-sample case illustrated in this section.

Table 6.5. *Expected frequencies in a fourfold table*

	Factor B		
Factor A	Present	Absent	Total
Present	N_{11}	N_{12}	$n_{1.}$
Absent	N_{21}	N_{22}	$n_{2.}$
Total	$n_{.1}$	$n_{.2}$	$n_{..}$

6.6.1. Hypothesis Tests

We continue to restrict attention to fourfold tables with marginal frequencies $n_{1.}$, $n_{2.}$, $n_{.1}$, and $n_{.2}$ fixed at the values actually observed, and suppose that the value of the underlying odds ratio is equal to ω. A first-order approximation N_{ij} to the expected cell frequencies E_{ij} associated with ω is such that (a) they are consistent with the original data in the sense that they reproduce the marginal frequencies (see Table 6.5), and (b) they are consistent with the value ω in the sense that

$$\frac{N_{11} N_{22}}{N_{12} N_{21}} = \omega. \tag{6.48}$$

The hypothesis that the value of the underlying odds ratio is equal to ω may be tested by referring the value of

$$\chi^2 = \sum_{i=1}^{2} \sum_{j=1}^{2} \frac{\left(|n_{ij} - N_{ij}| - \frac{1}{2} \right)^2}{N_{ij}} \tag{6.49}$$

to the chi squared distribution with one degree of freedom. The form of the test statistic in (6.49) is identical to the form of the classic statistic presented in (3.7), and the interpretation of the N_{ij}'s as expected cell frequencies associated with hypothesized values of the odds ratio [$\omega = 1$ in (3.7), ω arbitrary in (6.49)] are also identical.

When ω is the hypothesized value of the odds ratio, and when $\omega \neq 1$, the approximate expected cell frequency N_{11} may be found as a solution of

$$\frac{N_{11}\{N_{11} - (n_{1.} + n_{.1} - n_{..})\}}{(n_{1.} - N_{11})(n_{.1} - N_{11})} = \omega,$$

as follows. Define

$$A = \omega(n_{1.} + n_{.1}) + (n_{2.} - n_{.1}) \tag{6.50}$$

and

$$B = \sqrt{A^2 - 4n_{1.}n_{.1}\omega(\omega - 1)} \; ; \qquad (6.51)$$

then

$$N_{11} = \frac{A - B}{2(\omega - 1)}, \qquad (6.52)$$

$$N_{12} = n_{1.} - N_{11}, \qquad (6.53)$$

$$N_{21} = n_{.1} - N_{11}, \qquad (6.54)$$

and

$$N_{22} = N_{11} - l = N_{11} - n_{1.} - n_{.1} + n_{..} . \qquad (6.55)$$

Levin (1984) gave an improved approximation to the expected cell frequency:

$$E_{11} \approx N_{11} + \frac{(\omega - 1)n_{..}/(n_{..} - 1)}{BW},$$

where B is (6.51) and W is given in (6.56) below.

The following result was proved by Stevens (1951) and by Cornfield (1956). When the marginal frequencies are held fixed and when ω is the value of the odds ratio, n_{ij} (for any one of the four cells) is approximately normally distributed with mean N_{ij} and standard error $1/\sqrt{W}$, where

$$W = \sum_{i=1}^{2} \sum_{j=1}^{2} \frac{1}{N_{ij}} \qquad (6.56)$$

and the N_{ij}'s are defined by (6.52)–(6.55).

Again consider testing the hypothesis that the value of the odds ratio underlying the data of Table 6.1 is $\omega = 5$. The value of A in (6.57) is

$$A = 5(50 + 25) + (150 - 25) = 500, \qquad (6.57)$$

and that of B in (6.51) is

$$B = \sqrt{500^2 - 4 \times 50 \times 25 \times 5 \times 4} = 387.30. \qquad (6.58)$$

The four expected cell frequencies are presented in Table 6.6. Note that the odds ratio for the expected frequencies is

$$\frac{14.1 \times 139.1}{35.9 \times 10.9} = 5.0. \qquad (6.59)$$

Table 6.6. *Expected frequencies for data in Table 6.1 when the odds ratio is 5*

| Maternal Age | Birthweight | | Total |
	B	$\bar{B}$	
A	14.1	35.9	50
$\bar{A}$	10.9	139.1	150
Total	25	175	200

The value of chi squared in (6.49) is

$$\chi^2 = \frac{(|10 - 14.1| - 0.5)^2}{14.1} + \frac{(|40 - 35.9| - 0.5)^2}{35.9}$$

$$+ \frac{(|15 - 10.9| - 0.5)^2}{10.9} + \frac{(|135 - 139.1| - 0.5)^2}{139.1}$$

$$= 2.56, \tag{6.60}$$

and so the hypothesis that $\omega = 5$ is not rejected.

Another test of this hypothesis may be based on results given in the preceding section at (6.32) and (6.33). If $\lambda = \ln \omega$, the quantity

$$\chi^2 = \frac{(L' - \lambda)^2}{\{se(L')\}^2} \tag{6.61}$$

may be referred to the chi squared distribution with one degree of freedom. For the data at hand,

$$\lambda = \ln 5 = 1.61, \tag{6.62}$$

$$L' = \ln \frac{10.5 \times 135.5}{40.5 \times 15.5} = 0.82, \tag{6.63}$$

and

$$\widehat{se}(L') = \sqrt{\frac{1}{10.5} + \frac{1}{40.5} + \frac{1}{15.5} + \frac{1}{135.5}} = 0.438. \tag{6.64}$$

The value of the chi squared statistic in (6.61) is then

$$\chi^2 = \frac{(0.82 - 1.61)^2}{0.438^2} = 3.25, \tag{6.65}$$

which is larger than the value of the statistic in (6.60) but still indicates a nonsignificant difference from $\omega = 5$.

The value of the chi squared statistic in (6.61) based on the log odds ratio usually exceeds that of the statistic in (6.49) based on a comparison of the n_{ij}'s with the N_{ij}'s but the difference is small when the marginal frequencies are large. If the statistic in (6.49) were defined without the continuity correction, its value would be close to that of the statistic in (6.61) even for moderate sample sizes (see Problem 6.9).

The procedure described in this section is more complicated than the one based on the log odds ratio, but is more accurate. It should be used whenever a hypothesized value of ω is tested.

6.6.2. Confidence Intervals

An approximate $100(1 - \alpha)\%$ confidence interval for ω may be constructed as follows. The interval consists of all those values of ω for which, when the N_{ij}'s are the associated expected cell frequencies from (6.52)–(6.55),

$$\chi^2 = \sum_{i=1}^{2} \sum_{j=1}^{2} \frac{\left(|n_{ij} - N_{ij}| - \frac{1}{2}\right)^2}{N_{ij}} \leq z_{\alpha/2}^2. \tag{6.66}$$

The upper and lower limits are those for which the value of χ^2 equals $z_{\alpha/2}^2$.

The statistic in (6.66) depends on ω not explicitly but only implicitly through (6.50)–(6.55). The criterion for finding the upper and lower limits is therefore not simple. However, it is not overly complicated and can be implemented as follows.

The lower confidence limit, say ω_L, is associated with values of N_{11} and N_{22} smaller than n_{11} and n_{22} and with values of N_{12} and N_{21} larger than n_{12} and n_{21}. The continuity correction in (6.66) is then such that the χ^2 criterion simplifies to, say,

$$\chi_L^2 = \left(n_{11} - N_{11} - \tfrac{1}{2}\right)^2 W = z_{\alpha/2}^2, \tag{6.67}$$

where W is defined in (6.56). The lower limit, ω_L, will have been found when

$$F = \left(n_{11} - N_{11} - \tfrac{1}{2}\right)^2 W - z_{\alpha/2}^2 = 0. \tag{6.68}$$

The following describes Newton's method for iteratively solving (6.68). Define

$$T = \frac{1}{2(\omega - 1)^2} \left[B - n_{..} - \frac{\omega - 1}{B} \{A(n_{1.} + n_{.1}) - 2n_{1.}n_{.1}(2\omega - 1)\} \right], \tag{6.69}$$

$$U = \frac{1}{N_{12}^2} + \frac{1}{N_{21}^2} - \frac{1}{N_{11}^2} - \frac{1}{N_{22}^2}, \tag{6.70}$$

and

$$V = T\left\{\left(n_{11} - N_{11} - \tfrac{1}{2}\right)^2 U - 2W\left(n_{11} - N_{11} - \tfrac{1}{2}\right)\right\} \tag{6.71}$$

Let $\omega_L^{(1)}$ be a first approximation to ω_L, let A and B be the corresponding values of (6.50) and (6.51), and let N_{11}, N_{12}, N_{21}, and N_{22} be the corresponding values of (6.52)–(6.55). If the value of F in (6.68) is not equal to zero, a second, better approximation to ω_L is

$$\omega_L^{(2)} = \omega_L^{(1)} - \frac{F}{V}. \tag{6.72}$$

If the value of F associated with the second approximation is still not zero (say, if its absolute value exceeds 0.05), the process has to be repeated.

Convergence to ω_U, the upper confidence limit, proceeds by exactly the same process, except that the continuity correction is taken as $+\tfrac{1}{2}$ in (6.67), (6.68), and (6.71). Good first approximations to ω_L and ω_U are provided by the limits of the interval based on the log odds ratio,

$$\omega_L^{(1)} = \text{antilog}\left[L' - z_{\alpha/2}\,\text{se}(L')\right] \tag{6.73}$$

and

$$\omega_U^{(1)} = \text{antilog}\left[L' + z_{\alpha/2}\,\text{se}(L')\right]. \tag{6.74}$$

Consider again the data of Table 6.1, and suppose that a 95% confidence interval is desired for ω. From (6.63) and (6.64),

$$\omega_L^{(1)} = \text{antilog}(0.82 - 1.96 \times 0.438)$$
$$= \text{antilog}(-0.04) = 0.96 \tag{6.75}$$

and

$$\omega_U^{(1)} = \text{antilog}(0.82 - 1.96 \times 0.438)$$
$$= \text{antilog}(1.68) = 5.37. \tag{6.76}$$

Consider first the lower confidence limit. The value of A in (6.50) associated with $\omega_L^{(1)} = 0.96$ is

$$A = 0.96(50 + 25) + (150 - 25) = 197.00, \tag{6.77}$$

and that of B in (6.51) is

$$B = \sqrt{197^2 - 4 \times 50 \times 25 \times 0.96 \times (-0.04)} = 197.49. \tag{6.78}$$

The value of N_{11} in (6.52) is therefore

$$N_{11} = \frac{197.00 - 197.49}{2(-0.04)} = 6.13, \tag{6.79}$$

and the values of the other cell frequencies to be expected if the odds ratio is 0.96 are $N_{12} = 43.87$, $N_{21} = 18.87$, and $N_{22} = 131.13$. The value of W in (6.56) is

$$W = \frac{1}{6.13} + \frac{1}{43.87} + \frac{1}{18.87} + \frac{1}{131.13} = 0.2465, \tag{6.80}$$

and that of F in (6.68) is

$$F = (10 - 6.13 - 0.5)^2 \times 0.2465 - 3.84 = -1.04. \tag{6.81}$$

The value of the chi squared criterion is 1.04 units below the desired value of 3.84, and the iterative process therefore has to be initiated.

The required values of the quantities in (6.69)–(6.71) are

$$T = \frac{1}{2(-0.04)^2} \left(197.49 - 200 \right.$$

$$\left. - \frac{-0.04}{197.49} [197(50 + 25) - 2 \times 50 \times 25 \times (1.92 - 1)] \right)$$

$$= 5.22, \tag{6.82}$$

$$U = \frac{1}{43.87^2} + \frac{1}{18.87^2} - \frac{1}{6.13^2} - \frac{1}{131.13^2} = -0.0233, \tag{6.83}$$

and

$$V = 5.22 \left[(10 - 6.13 - 0.5)^2 \times (-0.0233) - 2 \times 0.2465 \times (10 - 6.13 - 0.5) \right]$$

$$= -10.05. \tag{6.84}$$

The second approximation to ω_L is then, from (6.72),

$$\omega_L^{(2)} = 0.96 - \frac{-1.04}{-10.05} = 0.86. \tag{6.85}$$

This turns out to be, to two decimal places, the lower 95% confidence limit on ω. The table of expected cell frequencies is given in Table 6.7, and the value of the chi squared criterion in (6.67) is

$$\chi_L^2 = (10 - 5.66 - 0.5)^2 \times 0.2586 = 3.81, \tag{6.86}$$

which is close to the desired value 3.84.

Table 6.7. *Expected frequencies for data in Table 6.1 when the odds ratio is 0.86*

| | Birthweight | | |
Maternal Age	B	$\bar{B}$	Total
A	5.66	44.34	50
$\bar{A}$	19.34	130.66	150
Total	25	175	200

Problem 6.10 is devoted to applying the same kind of iterative procedure to the upper 95% confidence limit, which turns out to be 5.84. The desired 95% confidence interval for the odds ratio underlying the data of Table 6.1 is therefore

$$0.86 \leq \omega \leq 5.84. \tag{6.87}$$

Note that it is somewhat wider than the interval based on the log odds ratio, (0.96, 5.37). This phenomenon has been found in other analyses by Gart (1962), Gart and Thomas (1972), and Fleiss (1979a); that is, the interval defined by endpoints satisfying equality in (6.66) is wider (but more accurate) than the interval defined by (6.73) and (6.74), and in fact wider (but more accurate) than a number of other suggested approximate confidence intervals.

For a limited number of tables, exact upper and lower confidence bounds on the odds ratio have been tabulated by Thomas and Gart (1977). For general fourfold tables, among approximate procedures, the one just described is the method of choice. It is more complicated than its competitors, but it is more accurate and is easily programmed for analysis on a programmable calculator or desktop computer.

Although presented in the context of a fourfold table generated by sampling method I, the procedures described in this section are also applicable to tables generated by sampling methods II and III. The reason is that, once attention is restricted to fourfold tables having a specified set of marginal frequencies, the probability structure of the internal cell frequencies is independent of the way the data were generated.

6.6.3.* A Confidence Interval Method to Be Avoided

The second edition of this book stated that the values of *any function* of the expected frequencies (e.g., the phi coefficient or the relative risk) evaluated for the entries in the tables associated with the lower and upper confidence limits on the odds ratio would provide lower and upper confidence limits for the corresponding parameter. This assertion was unfortunately ambiguous, and while true in a limited sense to be made precise in this section, the method does not work assuredly in the wider context in which it would ordinarily be interpreted. This section explains the difficulty with the method, which is that the procedure does not guarantee the desired probability of coverage for the given parametric function of the underlying cell probabilities. Due to this failure, general use of this method is not recommended.

Let θ be a scale-invariant function of the cells of the fourfold table, that is, a function $\theta = \theta(u_{11}, u_{12}, u_{21}, u_{22})$ taking the same value for any constant multiple of the arguments, such as $(n_{..}u_{11}, n_{..}u_{12}, n_{..}u_{21}, n_{..}u_{22})$. Assume further that θ increases in u_{11} for fixed values of $u_{1.}, u_{2.}, u_{.1}, u_{.2}$. For example, the relative risk, $\theta = (u_{11}/u_{1.})/(u_{21}/u_{2.}) = (u_{11}/u_{1.})/\{(u_{.1} - u_{11})/u_{2.}\}$, is such a function, as are all of the measures of association discussed in this chapter. We call such a function simply an *association function*.

> *Correct statement:* Any association function θ evaluated for the entries in the tables of *conditional expected frequencies* associated with the lower and upper confidence limits on the odds ratio provides lower and upper confidence limits for the corresponding parametric function of the *conditional expected frequencies* given the true odds ratio, i.e., $\theta(E_{11}, E_{12}, E_{21}, E_{22})$, where $E_{ij} = E(n_{ij}|n_{..}, n_{1.}, n_{.1}, \omega)$ and $\omega = (P_{11}P_{22})/(P_{12}P_{21})$.

> *Incorrect statement:* The above procedure provides lower and upper confidence limits for the corresponding parametric function of the *cell probabilities* underlying the cross-sectional sampling, that is, $\theta(P_{11}, P_{12}, P_{21}, P_{22})$.

To clarify the distinction between these two statements, consider the coverage property for an exact, two-sided confidence interval for the odds ratio. When based on the conditional distribution of X given fixed margins, the coverage property guarantees that for all values of the true odds ratio, ω, we have

$$P[\omega_L(X) < \omega < \omega_U(X)|n_{..}, n_{1.}, n_{.1}, \omega] \geq 1 - \alpha, \qquad (6.88)$$

where we have written the lower and upper confidence limits as $\omega_L(X)$ and $\omega_U(X)$ to remind us that these limits depend on the random variable $X = n_{11}$ in the reference cell. Now, in sampling method I, the margins are all random variables before conditioning, so we first inquire if the coverage property holds unconditionally as well. That is, we want to confirm that under sampling method I, for any set of underlying cell probabilities $P_{11}, P_{12}, P_{21}, P_{22}$, the assertion

$$P[\omega_L(\{n_{ij}\}) < \omega < \omega_U(\{n_{ij}\})|n_{..}, P_{11}, P_{12}, P_{21}, P_{22}] \geq 1 - \alpha \quad (6.89)$$

holds, where $\{n_{ij}\}$ represents all the frequencies inside the table (without fixed margins, X alone no longer suffices to represent all the cells), and

$\omega_L(\{n_{ij}\})$ and $\omega_U(\{n_{ij}\})$ are the confidence limits based on them. The unconditional coverage probability in (6.89) is obtained by averaging (6.88) over all values of the margins, the joint distribution of which is determined by the multinomial cell probabilities P_{11}, P_{12}, P_{21}, P_{22}. Because the inequality in (6.88) holds for all margins, for any P_{11}, P_{12}, P_{21}, P_{22},

$$P\left[\omega_L(\{n_{ij}\}) < \omega < \omega_U(\{n_{ij}\})|n_{..}, P_{11}, P_{12}, P_{21}, P_{22}\right]$$
$$= E\{P[\omega_L(X) < \omega < \omega_U(X)|n_{..}, n_{1.}, n_{.1}, \omega]|n_{..}, P_{11}, P_{12}, P_{21}, P_{22}\}$$
$$\geq 1 - \alpha.$$

Thus the coverage property in (6.89) holds, and the confidence interval for the odds ratio works assuredly, unconditionally as well as conditionally.

Now let θ_L and θ_U denote the association function evaluated at the conditional expected frequencies corresponding to the lower and upper confidence limits for ω:

$$\begin{aligned}
\theta_L &= \theta\left(E_{11}^{(L)}, E_{12}^{(L)}, E_{21}^{(L)}, E_{22}^{(L)}\right) \\
\theta_U &= \theta\left(E_{11}^{(U)}, E_{12}^{(U)}, E_{21}^{(U)}, E_{22}^{(U)}\right),
\end{aligned} \tag{6.90}$$

where the expected cell frequencies corresponding to the upper and lower confidence limits are denoted by $E_{ij}^{(L)}$ and $E_{ij}^{(U)}$, respectively, and depend on $\{n_{ij}\}$. Expression (6.88) implies that $(E_{11}^{(L)}, E_{11}^{(U)})$ is an exact conditional confidence interval for $E_{11} = E(X|n_{..}, n_{1.}, n_{.1}, \omega)$, because the expectation in (6.43) is a monotonic increasing function of ω. Thus for every ω and every set of fixed margins $n_{1.}, n_{2.}, n_{.1}, n_{.2}$,

$$P\left[E_{11}^{(L)} < E_{11} < E_{11}^{(U)}|n_{..}, n_{1.}, n_{.1}, \omega\right] \geq 1 - \alpha,$$

whence by the monotonicity of θ in E_{11} for fixed margins,

$$P\left[\theta_L < \theta(E_{11}, E_{12}, E_{21}, E_{22}) < \theta_U|n_{..}, n_{1.}, n_{.1}, \omega\right] \geq 1 - \alpha.$$

This demonstrates the correct, conditional statement. The problem is that the quantity inside the limits, $\theta(E_{11}, E_{12}, E_{21}, E_{22})$, based on the conditional expected frequencies given fixed margins and evaluated at the true odds ratio ω, is generally *not* equal to the population parameter, $\theta = \theta(P_{11}, P_{12}, P_{21}, P_{22})$. Therefore one cannot conclude that (θ_L, θ_U) is a valid confidence interval for θ, either conditionally or unconditionally.

To illustrate, consider the fourfold table with cell frequencies $(n_{11}, n_{12}, n_{21}, n_{22}) = (3, 1, 6, 0)$ based on a sample of size 10 collected cross-sectionally from a population with true cell probabilities $(0.25, 0.25, 0.375, 0.125)$. In the population, the relative risk parameter is $\theta = (0.25/0.50)/(0.375/0.50) = 0.50/0.75 = \frac{2}{3}$. The exact two-tailed lower conditional confidence limit $\omega_L(3)$ is zero, and the corresponding expected frequency $E_{11}^{(L)}$ is 3, so that the relative risk at the lower limit is 0.75. (See Problem 6.8.) No matter how small the odds ratio, for the given margins the relative risk based on the conditional expected frequencies at the lower limit cannot take values smaller than the population relative risk. This is just one extreme case, but other, less extreme tables similarly exclude the population relative risk of $\theta = \frac{2}{3}$, and similar coverage failures occur as well for row margins other than the $(5,5)$ margins in the illustration. Together these cases occur with nonnegligible probability, and an exhaustive computation shows that as a result, the unconditional coverage probability of (6.90) is only 0.916.

The computation referred to above used the point probability method for setting two-sided 95% confidence intervals for the odds ratio. It also credited (6.90) with coverage of θ for indeterminate fourfold tables that occur in sampling method I when there is a zero frequency in one or both sets of margins. The coverage probability would have been worse if those cases had been excluded from consideration.

The difficulty with (6.90) is not just a small-sample aberration. For example, with sample size $n_{..} = 40$, and population probabilities $(P_{11}, P_{12}, P_{21}, P_{22}) = (0.125, 0.375, 0.375, 0.125)$, such that the expected cell frequencies (unconditionally) are all 5 or more, the coverage probability for the population relative risk of $\frac{1}{3}$ is only 0.929 using exact 95% confidence intervals for the odds ratio.

We emphasize that the exact confidence intervals for the odds ratio have coverage probability at least 95%. The fundamental difficulty with exact procedures for other association functions is that fixing the margins does not produce a conditional distribution that depends only on that association parameter, as it does for the odds ratio, and so one is forced to deal with an additional nuisance parameter. Santner and Snell (1980) discuss methods for setting exact confidence intervals in small samples for the difference of two rates and the relative risk. These are either complicated or conservative, and will not be discussed here. Methods for constructing approximate confidence intervals in large samples for measures of association other than the odds ratio are discussed in Section 6.9.

6.7. CRITICISMS OF THE ODDS RATIO

The multiplicative comparison of risks confers useful properties on the odds ratio and the rate ratio, which we examine in the next chapter. However, Berkson (1958) and Feinstein (1973) strongly criticized taking the ratio of rates as a measure of association, pointing out that the level of the rates is lost. Thus a tenfold increase over a rate of one per million would be considered equivalent to a tenfold increase over a rate of one per thousand,

Table 6.8. *Mortality rates per 100,000 person-years from lung cancer and coronary artery disease for smokers and nonsmokers of cigarettes*

Disease	Smokers	Nonsmokers	o	Difference
Cancer of the lung	48.33	4.49	10.8	43.84
Coronary artery disease	294.67	169.54	1.7	125.13

even though the latter increase is far more serious than the former. Berkson and Feinstein maintain that the simple difference between two rates is the proper measure of the practical magnitude, in terms of public health importance, of an association.

Data from Table 26 of *Smoking and Health* (1964, p. 110) illustrate their point. Table 6.8 gives the approximate death rates per 100,000 person-years for smokers and for nonsmokers of cigarettes.

If we compared only the odds ratios o, we would conclude that cigarette smoking has a greater effect on lung cancer than on coronary artery disease. It was this conclusion, from a number of studies, that Berkson felt was unwarranted. He contended, quite correctly, that the odds ratio throws away all information on the number of deaths due to either cause. Berkson went farther, however, and maintained that it is *only* the excess in mortality that permits a valid assessment of the effect of smoking on a cause of death: "...of course, from a strictly practical viewpoint, it is only the total number of increased deaths that matters" [1958, p. 30].

He maintained that the effect of smoking is greater on that cause of death with the greater number of excess deaths. Thus, since smoking is associated with an excess mortality of over 120 per 100,000 person-years from coronary artery disease and with an excess mortality of under 50 per 100,000 person-years from lung cancer, Berkson concluded that the association is stronger for coronary artery disease than for lung cancer.

Sheps (1958, 1961) proposed a simple and elegent modification of Berkson's index. Let p_c denote the mortality rate (in general, the rate at which an untoward event occurs) in a control sample, and p_s the corresponding rate in a study sample presumed to be at higher risk. Thus by assumption, $p_s > p_c$.

Sheps contends that the excess risk associated with being in the study group, say p_e, can operate only on those individuals who would not have had the event occurring to them otherwise. Thus she postulates the model

$$p_s = p_c + p_e(1 - p_c); \qquad (6.91)$$

that is, the rate in the study group, p_s, is the sum of the rate in the control group, p_c, and of the excess risk, p_e, applied to those who would not otherwise have had the event, $1 - p_c$. Sheps suggests that p_e be used as a measure of added or excess risk. Because, clearly,

$$p_e = \frac{p_s - p_c}{1 - p_c},$$ (6.92)

p_e may also be called the *relative difference*.

This differs from Berkson's index, $p_s - p_c$, only in that the difference is divided by $1 - p_c$, the proportion of the people actually at added risk. If p_c is small, then Sheps' and Berkson's indexes are close. Thus for the data of Table 6.8, the excess mortality due to cancer of the lung is $p_e = 43.84/(100,000 - 4.49) = 43.84$ additional deaths attributable to cigarette smoking per 100,000 person-years saved by not having smoked. For coronary artery disease, the excess mortality is $p_e = 125.13/(100,000 - 169.54) = 125.34$ deaths per 100,000 person-years saved by not having smoked.

If research into the etiology of disease were concerned *solely* with public health issues, then Berkson's simple difference or Sheps' relative difference would be the only valid measures of the association between the antecedent factor and the outcome event. Because retrospective studies are incapable of providing estimates of either measure, such studies are necessarily useless from the point of view of public health. As Cornfield et al. (1959) and Greenberg (1969) have pointed out, however, etiological research is also concerned with the search for regularities in many sets of data, with the development of models of disease causation and distribution, and with the generation of hypotheses by one set of data that can be tested on other sets.

Given these concerns, that measure of association is best which is suggested by a mathematical model, which is capable of assuming predicted values for certain kinds of populations and can thus serve as the basis of a test of a hypothesis, and which is invariant under different methods of studying association. Because the odds ratio, or its logarithm, comes closest to providing such a measure (Cox and Snell, 1989, pp. 20–21), and because the odds ratio is estimable from a retrospective study (as we shall see in the next chapter), retrospective studies are eminently valid from the more general point of view of the advancement of knowledge. Peacock (1971) warns, however, against the uncritical assumption that the odds ratio should be constant across different kinds of populations.

That Sheps' measure, like Berkson's, lacks the regularity so often observed with the odds ratio is seen from the data of Table 6.9. It gives overall death rates for smokers and nonsmokers of varying ages, taken from the graph on p. 88 of *Smoking and Health* (1964). In that graph two rates appear for the nonsmokers aged 75–79. The value that seemed the more reasonable was used.

As is so often the case, one comes to different conclusions depending on which measure is chosen. Looking at p_e, the conclusion is that the effect of smoking steadily increases with increasing age. In terms of lives lost among

Table 6.9. *Death rates from all causes by age and smoking*

Age Interval	Death Rate (per 100,000) Smokers	Nonsmokers	o	p_e (per 100,000)
45–49	580	270	2.2	310
50–54	1050	440	2.4	610
55–59	1600	850	1.9	750
60–64	2500	1500	1.7	1000
65–69	3700	2000	1.9	1700
70–74	5300	3000	1.8	2400
75–79	9200	4800	2.0	4600

those not otherwise expected to die, this conclusion is correct. The increase in p_e, however, is so erratic that no precise mathematical extrapolation or even interpolation seems possible.

Looking at o, on the other hand, the conclusion is that the effect of smoking on overall mortality is essentially constant across all the tabulated ages. The epidemiological importance of this conclusion is that one may validly predict that the odds ratio would be approximately 2.0 for specific ages between 45 and 79, for ages below 45, and for ages above 79. If the observed odds ratio for any such interpolated or extrapolated age departed appreciably from 2.0, further research would clearly be indicated.

We turn next to a measure of association that combines elements of both multiplicative and additive comparisons of risk.

6.8. ATTRIBUTABLE RISK

Let A denote the presence of the risk factor under study, and B the presence of the outcome condition. The overall rate of occurrence of the condition is $P(B) = P(B|A)P(A) + P(B|\overline{A})P(\overline{A})$. Unfortunately, there are several definitions available for the *attributable risk*; of these, the one due to Levin (1953) [no relation to the author] makes the most substantive sense. It is that fraction of $P(B)$ that can uniquely be attributed to the presence of the risk factor.

Exposure to the risk factor is not necessary for the occurrence of the outcome condition; a proportion, $P(B|\overline{A})$, of people without the risk factor will develop it. If the risk factor were without any effect, we would expect this same proportion to apply to the exposed group, so that its contribution to $P(B)$ would be $P(B|\overline{A})P(A)$. Its actual contribution is $P(B|A)P(A)$, and the difference between these two quantities, relative to $P(B)$, is Levin's attributable risk, say,

$$
\begin{aligned}
R_A &= \frac{P(B|A)P(A) - P(B|\overline{A})P(A)}{P(B)} \\
&= \frac{P(A)\left[P(B|A) - P(B|\overline{A})\right]}{P(B|A)P(A) + P(B|\overline{A})[1 - P(A)]} \\
&= \frac{P(A)\left[P(B|A) - P(B|\overline{A})\right]}{P(B|\overline{A}) + P(A)\left[P(B|A) - P(B|\overline{A})\right]} \\
&= \frac{P(A)(R-1)}{1 + P(A)(R-1)},
\end{aligned}
\tag{6.93}
$$

where R is the relative risk,

$$
R = \frac{P(B|A)}{P(B|\overline{A})}.
\tag{6.94}
$$

The attributable risk, also known as the *population attributable risk fraction* or the *etiologic fraction*, is interpreted as follows. If the risk factor could be eliminated, R_A is the proportion by which $P(B)$, the rate of occurrence of the outcome characteristic in the population, would be reduced. Therefore it has important uses in educational programs and in health planning, but its dependence on $P(A)$, the rate of exposure to the risk factor, limits its use in making comparisons between populations in which this rate varies. (There are some striking exceptions, however; see Problem 6.12.)

The population attributable risk as just defined should not be confused with the so-called *attributable risk among the exposed*, defined as

$$
R_E = \frac{P(B|A) - P(B|\overline{A})}{P(B|A)} = 1 - \frac{1}{R}.
\tag{6.95}
$$

This measure expresses the excess risk as a fraction of the risk among those *exposed to the antecedent factor*. It finds its widest applicability in the law, where issues of causation in civil toxic tort cases require a determination of whether it was more likely than not that plaintiffs who were exposed to risk factor A and suffered disease B did so because of their exposure (Finkelstein and Levin, 2001). Thus if the relative risk $R = P(B|A)/P(B|\overline{A})$ exceeds 2, (6.95) shows that more than half of the exposed plaintiffs might not have been expected to have suffered the disease but for their exposure, suggesting the more-likely-than-not standard is met. Because the attributable risk among the exposed, R_E, does not depend at all on the prevalence of the exposure A, it does not indicate the impact of the exposure among the wider group of all those who have the disease in the population, as does the attributable risk, R_A. Thus R_A is the more useful measure for etiologic research.

The population attributable risk can be expressed equivalently in two other ways of interest. From the first equality in (6.93) defining R_A, we can write

$$R_A = \frac{P(B|A)P(A) - P(B|\bar{A})\{1 - P(\bar{A})\}}{P(B)}$$

$$= \frac{P(B|A)P(A) + P(B|\bar{A})P(\bar{A}) - P(B|\bar{A})}{P(B)}$$

$$= \frac{P(B) - P(B|\bar{A})}{P(B)} = 1 - \frac{1}{P(B)/P(B|\bar{A})}. \qquad (6.96)$$

Thus R_A can be expressed in a manner similar to (6.95), where the relative risk R is replaced by the ratio of the *population* risk of disease irrespective of exposure, to that among the unexposed. This ratio is not generally of interest other than to express (6.93) in a form similar to (6.95), and the relative risk should be used as the standard rate ratio comparison.

A more informative expression for R_A is the following, which starts from the first equality of (6.93), factors out the product $P(B|A)P(A)$, and applies Bayes' theorem:

$$R_A = \frac{P(B|A)P(A)\left\{1 - \frac{1}{P(B|A)/P(B|\bar{A})}\right\}}{P(B)} = R_E \cdot P(A|B). \quad (6.97)$$

Expression (6.97) shows that the population attributable risk is equal to the attributable risk among the exposed, reduced by the prevalence of the antecedent factor among those with the disease. In method I sampling, each of the required rates or conditional probabilities can be estimated. Moreover, the use of $P(A|B)$ makes expression (6.97) useful in the context of a retrospective study, in which antecedent exposures are estimated amongst those with and without disease. We return to this point in Section 7.3.

Expression (6.97) has another important advantage. The interpretation of attributable risk as the proportion by which $P(B)$ would be reduced if the risk factor A could be eliminated is an oversimplification and idealization of actual experience in public health practice. There are usually confounding factors that correlate with both exposure and disease, and would not disappear even if the exposure were eliminated. For example, smokers may have habits other than smoking, like sedentary lifestyles, that contribute to their higher rates of heart disease. Interventions to eliminate risk factors are only modestly successful in most cases, and exposed persons may substitute other risk-elevating factors if compelled to give up the original exposure. These realities often produce much smaller reductions in disease than the attributable risk would predict, unless adjustments are made. The adjustment takes the form of replacing the rate of disease given no exposure (only) in the denominator of the relative risk R by the rate of disease among those unexposed if the exposure alone were eliminated, but assuming all other characteristics of exposed persons remain the same. Such adjustments can be made by conditioning on covariate information, by stratification in the cross-sectional sampling method, or by regression methods. The advantage of (6.97) is that if such adjustments to the relative risk are made, the adjusted relative risk can be used in R_E and then in R_A to produce a valid adjusted attributable risk estimate. Other expressions do not lend themselves to this kind of adjustment. Expression (6.97) also generalizes easily to the case of more than two exposure categories. Rockhill, Newman, and Weinberg (1998) review these and other properties of the population attributable risk.

When, as pointed out by Markush (1977), data are collected in cross-sectional surveys (such as those conducted by the National Center for Health Statistics) or as part of routine registration (such as the recording of vital events by local health departments), the attributable risk may be estimated by, say,

$$r_A = \frac{p_{11} p_{22} - p_{12} p_{21}}{p_{.1} p_{2.}} \tag{6.98}$$

(see Problem 6.11). Walter (1976) derived a complicated expression for the standard error of r_A. A related but much simpler expression was derived by Fleiss (1979b) for the standard error of $\ln(1 - r_A)$,

$$\widehat{\text{se}}\{\ln(1 - r_A)\} = \sqrt{\frac{p_{12} + r_A(p_{11} + p_{22})}{n_{..} p_{21}}} . \tag{6.99}$$

Its use is illustrated on the data in Table 6.10, which cross-classifies birthweight and infant mortality among whites in 1974 in New York City. The

Table 6.10. *Infant mortality by birthweight for 72,730 live white births in 1974 in New York City*

Birthweight (g)	Outcomes at One Year		Total
	Dead	Alive	
≤ 2500	0.0085	0.0632	0.0717
> 2500	0.0058	0.9225	0.9283
Total	0.0143	0.9857	1

estimated risk of infant death attributable to low birthweight is

$$r_A = \frac{0.0085 \times 0.9225 - 0.0632 \times 0.0058}{0.0143 \times 0.9283} = 0.563, \qquad (6.100)$$

with an estimated standard error of $\ln(1 - r_A)$ given by

$$\widehat{se}\{\ln(1 - r_A)\} = \sqrt{\frac{0.0632 + 0.563(0.0085 + 0.9225)}{72,730 \times 0.0058}} = 0.037. \quad (6.101)$$

The natural logarithm of $1 - r_A$ is

$$\ln(1 - r_A) = \ln(1 - 0.563) = -0.828, \qquad (6.102)$$

and an approximate 95% confidence interval for $\ln(1 - R_A)$ is

$$-0.828 - 1.96 \times 0.037 \le \ln(1 - R_A) \le -0.828 + 1.96 \times 0.037, \quad (6.103)$$

or

$$-0.901 \le \ln(1 - R_A) \le -0.755. \qquad (6.104)$$

By taking antilogarithms of these limits, and then complements from unity, we obtain

$$0.530 \le R_A \le 0.594 \qquad (6.105)$$

as an approximate 95% confidence interval for the attributable risk itself. With 95% confidence, therefore, between 53% and 59% of all white infant deaths in New York City in 1974 could have been prevented if low (birthweights less than or equal to 2500 grams) had been eliminated

6.9.* STANDARD ERRORS FOR MEASURES OF ASSOCIATION

In this chapter we have seen several formulas for the standard error of measures of association: the odds ratio [see (6.17), (6.19), or (6.21)], the log odds ratio [(6.33)], and the log complementary attributable risk [(6.99)]. Standard error formulas for many other measures of association may be derived using the delta method of Section 2.6. Here we record the results for some other measures mentioned in this chapter, viz., the risk difference, the relative risk, the phi coefficient, and Sheps' relative difference, each estimated in a cross-sectional sample. Because the most important use of the standard error of an estimate of association is to set approximate confidence intervals for the corresponding population parameter, we state the standard error formula for whichever transformation of the measure is best approximated by the normal distribution in large samples, typically the logarithmic transformation.

Sampling method I involves the multinomial distribution, so we state an appropriate multivariable version of the delta method. In large samples, the sample proportions p_{ij} estimated from the fourfold table are jointly distributed approximately with a multivariate normal distribution with mean $(P_{11}, P_{12}, P_{21}, P_{22})$ and covariance matrix

$$\text{Cov}(p_{11}, p_{12}, p_{21}, p_{22})$$

$$= \frac{1}{n} \begin{bmatrix} P_{11}(1 - P_{11}) & -P_{11}P_{12} & -P_{11}P_{21} & -P_{11}P_{22} \\ -P_{11}P_{12} & P_{12}(1 - P_{12}) & -P_{12}P_{21} & -P_{12}P_{22} \\ -P_{11}P_{21} & -P_{12}P_{21} & P_{21}(1 - P_{21}) & -P_{21}P_{22} \\ -P_{11}P_{22} & -P_{12}P_{22} & -P_{21}P_{22} & P_{22}(1 - P_{22}) \end{bmatrix}.$$

$$(6.106)$$

The variances of the sample proportions lie on the main diagonal of (6.106), and the covariance of the ith and jth sample proportions lies in the ith row and jth column. The assertion about the large-sample joint distribution of the sample proportions follows from the multivariate version of the central limit theorem. Expression (6.106) can be written in the equivalent matrix form

$$\text{Cov}(p_{11}, p_{12}, p_{21}, p_{22})$$

$$= \frac{1}{n} \left(\text{Diag}(P_{11}, P_{12}, P_{21}, P_{22}) - \begin{bmatrix} P_{11} \\ P_{12} \\ P_{21} \\ P_{22} \end{bmatrix} \begin{bmatrix} P_{11} & P_{12} & P_{21} & P_{22} \end{bmatrix} \right)$$

$$(6.107)$$

where $\text{Diag}(P_{11}, P_{12}, P_{21}, P_{22})$ is a 4×4 matrix with $P_{11}, P_{12}, P_{21}, P_{22}$ on the main diagonal and 0 for the off-diagonal entries, and matrix multiplication is used to multiply the column vector of cell probabilities by the row vector of cell probabilities.

Now let $\theta = f(P_{11}, P_{12}, P_{21}, P_{22})$ be a differentiable function of the cell probabilities in the fourfold table. θ represents a population parameter we want to estimate by substituting the sample proportions for the P_{ij}, i.e., $\hat{\theta} = f(p_{11}, p_{12}, p_{21}, p_{22})$. The estimate $\hat{\theta}$ is then a maximum likelihood estimate of θ. What is the distribution of $\hat{\theta}$ in large samples, and what is its standard error? The answer is normal with mean $\theta = f(P_{11}, P_{12}, P_{21}, P_{22})$ and standard error given by the square root of the following expression:

$$
\begin{aligned}
\text{Var}\{\hat{\theta}\} &= \text{Var}\{f(p_{11}, p_{12}, p_{21}, p_{22})\} \\
&\approx \nabla f(P_{11}, P_{12}, P_{21}, P_{22}) \cdot \text{Cov}(p_{11}, p_{12}, p_{21}, p_{22}) \\
&\quad \cdot \nabla f(P_{11}, P_{12}, P_{21}, P_{22})'
\end{aligned}
\tag{6.108}
$$

The quantity $\nabla f(P_{11}, P_{12}, P_{21}, P_{22})$ is called the *gradient vector* and is defined as the row vector of partial derivatives of f with respect to the P_{ij}'s:

$$
\nabla f(P_{11}, P_{12}, P_{21}, P_{22}) = \left(\frac{\partial f}{\partial P_{11}}, \frac{\partial f}{\partial P_{12}}, \frac{\partial f}{\partial P_{21}}, \frac{\partial f}{\partial P_{22}} \right).
\tag{6.109}
$$

Matrix multiplication is used in (6.108), and the prime on $\nabla f'$ refers to the transpose of the gradient vector. As usual, the variance of $\hat{\theta}$ is estimated by substituting the sample proportions p_{ij} for the population proportions P_{ij} wherever they appear in (6.106)–(6.109).

For example, consider Berkson's risk difference, $p_s - p_c$, which in the current notation is an estimate of $\theta = f(P_{11}, P_{12}, P_{21}, P_{22}) = (P_{11}/P_{1.}) - (P_{21}/P_{2.})$. The gradient of f is the vector

$$
\nabla f(P_{11}, P_{12}, P_{21}, P_{22}) = \left(\frac{P_{12}}{P_{1.}^2}, -\frac{P_{11}}{P_{1.}^2}, -\frac{P_{22}}{P_{2.}^2}, \frac{P_{21}}{P_{2.}^2} \right);
$$

the term in (6.108) equal to $\nabla f\{\text{Diag}(P_{11}, P_{12}, P_{21}, P_{22})\}\nabla f'$ is

$$
\frac{P_{11}P_{12}^2}{P_{1.}^4} + \frac{P_{12}P_{11}^2}{P_{1.}^4} + \frac{P_{21}P_{22}^2}{P_{2.}^4} + \frac{P_{22}P_{21}^2}{P_{2.}^4}
$$

$$
= \frac{P_{11}P_{12}}{P_{1.}^3} + \frac{P_{21}P_{22}}{P_{2.}^3} = \frac{P_{11}}{P_{1.}}\left(1 - \frac{P_{11}}{P_{1.}}\right)\Big/P_{1.} + \frac{P_{21}}{P_{2.}}\left(1 - \frac{P_{21}}{P_{2.}}\right)\Big/P_{2.},
$$

and the other term in (6.108) involving the product of $(P_{11}, P_{12}, P_{21}, P_{22})\nabla f'$ with itself is equal to 0 (do you see why?). Thus the standard error of the risk difference is

$$
\text{se}(p_s - p_c) = \frac{1}{\sqrt{n_{..}}} \sqrt{\frac{P_{11}P_{12}}{P_{1.}^3} + \frac{P_{21}P_{22}}{P_{2.}^3}},
\tag{6.110}
$$

which is estimated by

$$\widehat{se}(p_s - p_c) = \sqrt{\frac{n_{11}n_{12}}{n_{1.}^3} + \frac{n_{21}n_{22}}{n_{2.}^3}} \ . \tag{6.111}$$

For the data in Table 6.1, the risk difference is estimated as $0.20 - 0.10 = 0.10$, the standard error of the risk difference is estimated from (6.111) to be 0.0616, and an approximate 95% confidence interval is given by $0.10 \pm 1.96 \times 0.0616 = (0.021, 0.221)$.

Next consider the log relative risk, $\theta = \ln R = \ln\{(P_{11}/P_{1.})/(P_{21}/P_{2.})\}$. Problem 6.13 asks the reader to demonstrate that the standard error of the sample log relative risk is estimated by

$$\widehat{se}[\ln r] = \widehat{se}\left[\ln\left\{\left(\frac{P_{11}}{P_{1.}}\right)\middle/\left(\frac{P_{21}}{P_{2.}}\right)\right\}\right] = \sqrt{\frac{n_{12}}{n_{11}n_{1.}} + \frac{n_{22}}{n_{11}n_{2.}}} \ . \tag{6.112}$$

Another application of the delta method shows that in large samples, the standard error of the relative risk itself is estimated by

$$\widehat{se}[r] = \widehat{se}\left[\left(\frac{P_{11}}{P_{1.}}\right)\middle/\left(\frac{P_{21}}{P_{2.}}\right)\right] = r\sqrt{\frac{n_{12}}{n_{11}n_{1.}} + \frac{n_{22}}{n_{21}n_{2.}}} \ . \tag{6.113}$$

As for the odds ratio, the preferred method for setting an approximate confidence interval for the relative risk is *not* to take the sample estimate plus or minus a critical value times (6.113), but rather to construct a confidence interval for the log relative risk and then to exponentiate the lower and upper limits. Thus an approximate $100(1 - \alpha)\%$ confidence interval for the log relative risk $\lambda = \ln R$ in large samples is given by $\ln r \pm z_{\alpha/2} se\{\ln r\}$, obtaining, say, λ_L and λ_U, and then taking as the confidence limits for R itself $R_L = \exp(\lambda_L)$ and $R_U = \exp(\lambda_U)$.

For the data of Table 6.1, the estimated log relative risk is $\ln 2 = 0.693$, and the standard error is estimated to be $[\{40/(10 \times 50) + 135/(15 \times 150)\}^{1/2} = 0.374$. Thus an approximate 95% confidence interval for the log relative risk is $0.693 \pm 1.96 \times 0.374 = (-0.040, 1.426)$, and thus an approximate 95% confidence interval for the relative risk is $(\exp(-0.040), \exp(1.426)) = (0.961, 4.16)$. A comparison of (6.75)–(6.76) with (6.87) for the odds ratio suggests that the confidence interval just obtained for the relative risk may be overoptimistic in its width.

For the attributable risk among the exposed, $R_E = 1 - 1/R$, we do not need a separate standard error formula. Confidence limits for R_E, say $R_{E,L}$ and $R_{E,U}$, are obtained by using the corresponding confidence limits for the relative risk, such that, $R_{E,L} = 1 - 1/R_L$ and $R_{E,U} = 1 - 1/R_U$.

For Sheps' relative difference p_e in (6.92) it is simplest to work with the logarithm of the complement of the relative difference, $1 - p_e = (1 - p_{11}/p_{1.})/(1 - p_{21}/p_{2.}) = (p_{12}/p_{1.})/(p_{22}/p_{2.})$. Then the standard error of the sample log complementary relative difference is given by

$$\text{se}\left[\ln(1 - p_e)\right] = \frac{1}{\sqrt{n_{..}}} \sqrt{\frac{P_{11}}{P_{12}P_{1.}} + \frac{P_{21}}{P_{22}P_{2.}}}$$

$$= \frac{1}{\sqrt{n_{..}}} \sqrt{\frac{1}{P_{12}} - \frac{1}{P_{1.}} + \frac{1}{P_{22}} - \frac{1}{P_{2.}}}$$

and is estimated by

$$\widehat{\text{se}}\left[\ln(1 - p_e)\right] = \sqrt{\frac{n_{11}}{n_{12}n_{1.}} + \frac{n_{21}}{n_{22}n_{2.}}} = \sqrt{\frac{1}{n_{12}} - \frac{1}{n_{1.}} + \frac{1}{n_{22}} - \frac{1}{n_{2.}}}. \quad (6.114)$$

The reader is asked to derive (6.114) in Problem 6.14.

For the data of Table 6.1, Sheps' relative difference is $p_e = (0.2 - 0.1)/(1 - 0.1) = 0.111$. The estimated log complementary relative difference is $\ln\{(1 - 0.2)/(1 - 0.1)\} = \ln(\frac{8}{9}) = -0.118$, and the standard error is estimated at $(\frac{1}{40} - \frac{1}{50} + \frac{1}{135} - \frac{1}{150})^{1/2} = 0.0758$. Thus an approximate 95% confidence interval for the log complementary relative difference is $-0.118 \pm 1.96 \times 0.0758 = (-0.267, 0.0306)$. Taking antilogs and then complements, an approximate 95% confidence interval for Sheps' relative difference is $(1 - \exp(0.0306), 1 - \exp(-0.267)) = (-0.031, 0.234)$.

For the phi coefficient, in order to preserve the sign or direction of the association, write the measure as

$$\varphi = \frac{n_{11}n_{22} - n_{12}n_{21}}{\sqrt{n_{1.}n_{2.}n_{.1}n_{.2}}} \quad (6.115)$$

First consider the case in which the population phi coefficient,

$$\Phi = \frac{P_{11}P_{12} - P_{12}P_{21}}{\sqrt{P_{1.}P_{2.}P_{.1}P_{.2}}}, \quad (6.116)$$

is zero. We demonstrate in this case that the standard error of the sample phi coefficient is $1/(n-1)^{1/2}$. To see this, write the sample version as

$$\phi = \frac{n_{11}n_{22} - n_{12}n_{21}}{\sqrt{n_{1.}n_{2.}n_{.1}n_{.2}}} = \frac{n_{11} - n_{1.}n_{.1}/n_{..}}{\sqrt{n_{1.}n_{2.}n_{.1}n_{.2}/n_{..}^2}}$$

$$= \frac{n_{11} - n_{1.}n_{.1}/n_{..}}{\sqrt{n_{1.}n_{2.}n_{.1}n_{.2}/\{n_{..}^2(n_{..} - 1)\}}} \cdot \frac{1}{\sqrt{n_{..} - 1}}, \quad (6.117)$$

where the first equality follows from the identity

$$n_{11}n_{22} - n_{12}n_{21} = n_{11}(n_{..} - n_{11} - n_{12} - n_{21}) - n_{12}n_{21}$$
$$= n_{..}n_{11} - (n_{11} + n_{12})(n_{11} + n_{21}) = n_{..}(n_{11} - n_{1.}n_{.1}/n_{..}).$$
$$\tag{6.118}$$

Referring to (6.40), we recognize (6.117) as $(n_{..} - 1)^{1/2}$ times a standardized central hypergeometric random variable, given fixed margins. Thus we have, conditionally, that φ is approximately normal in large samples, with

$$E(\phi|n_{..}, n_{1.}, n_{.1}, \Phi = 0) = 0 \quad \text{and} \quad \text{Var}\{\phi|n_{..}, n_{1.}, n_{.1}, \Phi = 0\} = \frac{1}{n_{..} - 1}.$$
$$\tag{6.119}$$

The unconditional variance of phi is then also $1/(n_{..} - 1)$, because of the general identity for any two random variables, X and Y, with finite means and variances,

$$\text{Var}(Y) = E\{\text{Var}(Y|X)\} + \text{Var}\{E(Y|X)\}. \tag{6.120}$$

Thus $\text{Var}(\phi) = E\{1/(n_{..} - 1)\} + \text{Var}\{0\} = 1/(n_{..} - 1)$, so that the exact standard error of ϕ is

$$\text{se}(\phi|n_{..}, \Phi = 0) = \frac{1}{\sqrt{n_{..} - 1}}. \tag{6.121}$$

This simple result provides a good approximation to the standard error of the phi coefficient when the population value is small but nonzero, although it slightly underestimates se$\{\phi\}$.

For the data in Table 6.1, the approximate standard error is $1/\sqrt{199} = 0.071$. A simulation experiment shows that for cross-sectional sampling with underlying cell probabilities equal to those shown for the sample in Table 6.2, the standard error of ϕ is 0.079. An approximate 95% confidence interval for ϕ using (6.121) is then $0.13 \pm 1.96 \times 0.071 = (-0.01, 0.27)$.

When the population phi coefficient is not close to zero, the situation is more complicated. We shall assume in this case that all of the true marginal cell probabilities are positive, and that the sample size is sufficiently large that the sample phi coefficient will be bounded away from zero with high probability, in order that we may work with the logarithm of phi:

$$\theta = \ln \Phi = \ln|P_{11}P_{22} - P_{12}P_{21}| - \tfrac{1}{2}\{\ln(P_{11} + P_{12}) + \ln(P_{21} + P_{22})$$
$$+ \ln(P_{11} + P_{21}) + \ln(P_{12} + P_{22})\}.$$

Define $\Delta = |P_{11}P_{22} - P_{12}P_{21}|$ and $a_{ij} = P_{i.}^{-1} + P_{.j}^{-1}$. Then a calculation shows that the standard error of $\ln \varphi$ is given by

$$\mathrm{se}(\ln \phi) = \frac{1}{\sqrt{n_{..}}} \sqrt{B_1 + B_2 + B_3 - B_4 - B_5 - B_6}, \qquad (6.122)$$

where

$$B_1 = \frac{1}{\Delta^2}\{P_{11}P_{22}(P_{11} + P_{22}) + P_{12}P_{21}(P_{12} + P_{21})\},$$

$$B_2 = \tfrac{1}{4}\{a_{11}^2 P_{11}(1 - P_{11}) + a_{12}^2 P_{12}(1 - P_{12})$$

$$+ a_{21}^2 P_{21}(1 - P_{21}) + a_{22}^2 P_{22}(1 - P_{22})\},$$

$$B_3 = 2(a_{11}P_{11} + a_{12}P_{12} + a_{21}P_{21} + a_{22}P_{22}),$$

$$B_4 = 4,$$

$$B_5 = \left(\frac{1}{P_{1.}} + \frac{1}{P_{2.}} + \frac{1}{P_{.1}} + \frac{1}{P_{.2}}\right),$$

$$B_6 = \tfrac{1}{2}(a_{11}a_{12}P_{11}P_{12} + a_{11}a_{21}P_{11}P_{21} + a_{11}a_{22}P_{11}P_{22}$$

$$+ a_{12}a_{21}P_{12}P_{21} + a_{12}a_{22}P_{12}P_{22} + a_{21}a_{22}P_{21}P_{22}).$$

As usual, the standard error may be estimated by substituting the sample proportions for the P_{ij}.

For a cross-sectional sample of size 1,000 with sample proportions as in Table 6.2, (6.122) yields an estimated standard error of 0.270 for $\ln \phi$. Thus an approximate 95% confidence interval for $\ln \phi$ is $\ln 0.13 \pm 1.96 \times 0.270 = (-2.56, -1.50)$, and taking antilogs, a 95% confidence interval for ϕ is $(0.08, 0.22)$. This is close to the interval $(0.07, 0.19)$ based on the simpler standard error formula (6.121) for ϕ with a sample of size $n_{..} = 1,000$.

PROBLEMS

6.1. The odds Ω_A and $\Omega_{\bar{A}}$ are defined by (6.5) and (6.8). Prove that $\Omega_A = \Omega_{\bar{A}}$ if and only if $P(B|A) = P(B|\bar{A})$.

6.2. The odds ratio ω is defined by (6.13). Prove that $\omega > 1$ if and only if $P(B|A) > P(B|\bar{A})$.

6.3. The relative risk r is defined by (6.23), and the odds ratio o by (6.14). Prove that r is approximately equal to o if p_{21} is small relative to p_{22} and if p_{11} is small relative to p_{12}. [*Hint.* $p_{2.} = p_{22}(1 + p_{21}/p_{22})$ and $p_{1.} = p_{12}(1 + p_{11}/p_{12}).$]

6.4. It had long been known that, among first admissions to American public mental hospitals, schizophrenia as diagnosed by the hospital psychiatrists was more prevalent than the affective disorders, whereas the reverse was true for British public mental hospitals. A cooperative study between New York and London psychiatrists was designed to determine the extent to which the difference was a result of differences in diagnostic habits. The following data are from a study reported by Cooper et al. (1972).

(a) **(1)** One hundred and forty-five patients in a New York hospital and 145 in a London hospital were selected for study. The New York hospital diagnosed 82 patients as schizophrenic and 24 as affectively ill, whereas the London hospital diagnosed 51 as schizophrenic and 67 as affectively ill. Ignoring the patients given other diagnosis, set up the resulting fourfold table.

(2) The project psychiatrists made diagnoses using a standard set of criteria after conducting standardized interviews with the patients. In New York, the project diagnosed 43 patients as schizophrenic and 53 as affectively ill. In London, the project diagnosed 33 patients as schizophrenic and 85 as affectively ill. Ignoring the patients given other diagnoses, set up the resulting fourfold table.

(3) The results of the standardized interview served as input to a computer program that yields psychiatric diagnoses. In New York, the computer diagnosed 67 patients as schizophrenic and 27 as affectively ill. In London, the computer diagnosed 56 patients as schizophrenic and 37 as affectively ill. Ignoring the patients given other diagnoses, set up the resulting fourfold table.

(b) Three diagnostic contrasts between New York and London are possible: by the hospitals' diagnoses, by the project's diagnoses, and by the computer's diagnoses. Compute, for each of the three sources of diagnoses, the ratio of the odds that a New York patient will be diagnosed schizophrenic rather than affective to the corresponding odds for London. How do the odds ratios for the project's and computer's diagnoses compare? How do these two compare with the odds ratio for the hospital's diagnoses?

(c) For each source of diagnosis, all four cell frequencies are large, indicating that the improved estimate (6.20) may not be necessary. Check that, for each source of diagnosis, the estimate of the odds ratio given by (6.20) is only slightly less than the estimate given by (6.14).

6.5. * Prove Haldane's (1956) result that among all estimators of $\ln(P/Q)$ of the form $\ln\{(p + a/n)/(q + a/n)\}$, the choice $a = \frac{1}{2}$ removes the term of order $1/n$ in the asymptotic expansion of the bias of the estimator. [*Hint*. Write the estimator in the following form:

$$\ln\left(\frac{p+a/n}{q+a/n}\right) = \ln\left(\frac{P}{Q}\right) + \ln\left(1 + \frac{p-P+a/n}{P}\right) - \ln\left(1 + \frac{q-Q+a/n}{Q}\right).$$

Use the approximation $\ln(1+x) \approx x - x^2/2$ for small x to write the estimator approximately as

$$\ln\left(\frac{p+a/n}{q+a/n}\right) \approx \ln\left(\frac{P}{Q}\right) + \frac{p-P+a/n}{P} - \frac{1}{2}\left(\frac{p-P+a/n}{P}\right)^2$$

$$- \frac{q-Q+a/n}{Q} + \frac{1}{2}\left(\frac{q-Q+a/n}{Q}\right)^2$$

$$= \ln\left(\frac{P}{Q}\right) + \frac{p-P+a/n}{P} - \frac{q-Q+a/n}{Q}$$

$$- \frac{1}{2P^2}(p-P)^2 - \frac{a}{nP^2}(p-P) + \frac{1}{2Q^2}(q-Q)^2 + \frac{a}{nQ^2}(q-Q),$$

ignoring terms of order $1/n^2$ and higher. Now take expectations, and use the fact that $E(p-P) = 0$ and $E(p-P)^2 = PQ/n$ to express the bias of the estimator, ignoring terms of order $1/n^2$ and higher, as

$$\text{bias} = E\left[\ln\left(\frac{p+a/n}{q+a/n}\right)\right] - \ln\left(\frac{P}{Q}\right)$$

$$\approx \frac{a}{n}\left(\frac{1}{P} - \frac{1}{Q}\right) - \frac{1}{2n}\left(\frac{Q}{P} - \frac{P}{Q}\right) = \frac{Q-P}{nPQ}\left(a - \frac{1}{2}\right).]$$

6.6. The *joint multinomial probability function* for cross-sectional sampling is given by

$$P(n_{11}, n_{12}, n_{21}, n_{22}) = \frac{N!}{n_{11}!n_{12}!n_{21}!n_{22}!} P_{11}^{n_{11}} P_{12}^{n_{12}} P_{21}^{n_{21}} P_{22}^{n_{22}}$$

for all quadruplets of nonnegative integers $n_{11}, n_{12}, n_{21}, n_{22}$ that sum to $n_{..}$. Show that the conditional distribution of n_{11} given the two conditions $n_{11} + n_{12} = n_{1.}$ and $n_{11} + n_{21} = n_{.1}$ is given by either expression in (6.35). [*Hint*. Write the conditional probability as the joint multinomial probability for $n_{11}, n_{12}, n_{21}, n_{22}$ divided by the joint multinomial probability for the conditioning events. Write $n_{12} = n_{1.} - n_{11}$, $n_{21} = n_{.1} - n_{11}$, and $n_{22} = n_{11} - n_{1.} - n_{.1} + n_{..}$ and substitute these into the expression. Cancel terms that involve only $n_{1.}, n_{.1}$, and $n_{..}$ and that appear in both numerator and denominator.]

6.7. Show that when $n_{1.} = 1$, the reference cell in the noncentral hypergeometric distribution (6.35) is a binary outcome with $P(X = 1)$ given by (6.41). Deduce the mean and variance formulas (6.41) and (6.42).

6.8. For the fourfold table with cell frequencies $(n_{11}, n_{12}, n_{21}, n_{22}) = (3, 1, 6, 0)$, show that the upper conditional tail probability above $x_0 = 3$ is 1 for any odds ratio, and hence the lower confidence limit is $\omega_L = 0$. Confirm the same by the approximate method of Section 6.6.2. Conclude that the corresponding expected frequency is 3, and that the corresponding relative risk is 0.75.

6.9. When the continuity correction is not incorporated into the test statistic in (6.49), the resulting value usually agrees very well with that of the statistic in (6.61). Find the value of

$$\chi^2 = \sum_{i=1}^{2} \sum_{j=1}^{2} \frac{(n_{ij} - N_{ij})^2}{N_{ij}}$$

for the data in Tables 6.1 and 6.6, and compare with the value found in (6.65).

6.10. Apply the iterative procedure of Section 6.6.2 to find the upper 95% confidence limit on the odds ratio underlying the data of Table 6.1. Use as the initial approximation the value $\omega_U^{(1)} = 5.37$ from (6.76).

6.11. Show that, when the components of the population attributable risk defined in (6.93) are replaced by their sample estimators [$P(A)$ by $p_{1.}$ and R by the expression in (6.23)], and when the resulting expression is simplified, equation (6.95) results.

6.12. Data on infant mortality by birthweight for whites were presented in Table 6.10. Data for 37,840 nonwhite live births in New York City in 1974 are

Birthweight	Outcome at One Year		
(g)	Dead	Alive	Total
≤ 2500	0.0140	0.1147	0.1287
> 2500	0.0088	0.8625	0.8713
Total	0.0228	0.9772	1

(a) What is the estimated attributable risk for nonwhite live births? How does this compare with the value found in (6.100) for white live births?

(b) What is the estimated standard error of $\ln(1 - r_A)$ for the estimate found in (a)? What is an approximate 95% confidence interval for R_A in nonwhite live births? How does this compare with the interval found in (6.105) for white live births?

6.13.* Show that for the log relative risk function $\ln R$ with $f(P_{11}, P_{12}, P_{21}, P_{22}) = \ln\{(P_{11}/P_{1.})/(P_{21}/P_{2.})\}$, the gradient is given by

$$\left[\frac{P_{12}}{P_{11}P_{1.}}, -\frac{1}{P_{1.}}, -\frac{P_{22}}{P_{21}P_{2.}}, \frac{1}{P_{2.}} \right]$$

and that the matrix multiplication of the gradient on the left by the covariance matrix (6.107) on the right yields the vector

$$\left[\frac{P_{12}}{P_{1.}}, -\frac{P_{12}}{P_{1.}}, -\frac{P_{22}}{P_{2.}}, \frac{P_{22}}{P_{2.}} \right],$$

so that multiplying the result on the right by the transpose of the gradient vector yields

$$\mathrm{Var}(\ln r) = \frac{P_{12}}{P_{11}P_{1.}} + \frac{P_{22}}{P_{21}P_{2.}}.$$

Deduce that when sample estimates of the cell and marginal probabilities are substituted, expression (6.112) results as the estimated standard error of the log relative risk.

6.14.* Consider the log complementary relative difference function $f(P_{11}, P_{12}, P_{21}, P_{22}) = \ln\{(P_{12}/P_{1.})/(P_{22}/P_{2.})\}$. Derive the standard error formula (6.114). [*Hint.* Use Problem 6.13.]

6.15. Referring to Problem 4.7, consider the right-hand data set for blindness outcomes among premature infants who survived the perinatal period, comparing low versus high O_2 concentration.

(a) Find the exact two-sided 95% confidence interval for the odds ratio relating blindness to oxygen concentration, using the point probability method. Confirm that the value for the odds ratio $\omega = 1$ is excluded from the confidence interval. This is consistent with the exact two-tailed p-value 0.031 by the point probability method for Fisher's exact test.

(b) An approximate confidence interval for the log odds ratio appears in expressions (6.73) and (6.74) using the definitions in (6.20), (6.32), and (6.33). Construct the approximate 95% confidence for the same data as in part (a). Exponentiate the endpoints of this interval to arrive at a commonly used confidence interval for the odds ratio. Compare the results with the exact interval in part (a). What are your conclusions in this small-sample case?

(c) Repeat part (b) for the mortality data in the left-hand table of Problem 4.7. Compare the results with the exact interval for the odds ratio (two-sided, using the point probability method) of (0.615, 4.730). What are your conclusions in this larger sample size case?

REFERENCES

Agresti, A. (1992). A survey of exact inference for contingency tables. *Statist. Sci.*, **7**, 131–153, with discussion, 154–177.

Altham, P. M. E. (1970a). The measurement of association of rows and columns for an $r \times s$ contingency table. *J. R. Statist. Soc., Ser. B*, **32**, 63–73.

Altham, P. M. E. (1970b). The measurement of association in a contingency table: Three extensions of the cross-ratios and metric methods. *J. R. Statist. Soc., Ser. B.*, **32**, 395–407.

Anscombe, F. J. (1956). On estimating binomial response relations. *Biometrika*, **43**, 461–464.

Bartlett, M. S. (1935). Contingency table interactions. *J. R. Statist. Soc. Suppl.*, **2**, 248–252.

Berger, A. (1961). On comparing intensities of association between two binary characteristics in two different populations. *J. Am. Statist. Assoc.*, **56**, 889–908.

Berkson, J. (1958). Smoking and lung cancer: Some observations on two recent reports. *J. Am. Statist. Assoc.*, **53**, 28–38.

Carroll, J. B. (1961). The nature of the data, or how to choose a correlation coefficient. *Psychometrika*, **26**, 347–372.

Cooper, J. E., Kendell, R. E., Gurland, B. J., Sharpe, L., Copeland, J. R. M., and Simon, R. (1972). *Psychiatric diagnosis in New York and London*. London: Oxford University Press.

Cornfield, J. (1951). A method of estimating comparative rates from clinical data. Applications to cancer of the lung, breast, and cervix. *J. Natl. Cancer Inst.*, **11**, 1269–1275.

Cornfield, J. (1956). A statistical problem arising from retrospective studies. Pp. 135–148 in J. Neyman (Ed.). *Proceedings of the third Berkeley symposium on mathematical statistics and probability*, Vol. 4. Berkeley: University of California Press.

Cornfield, J., Haenszel, W., Hammond, E. C., Lilienfeld, A. M., Shimkin, M. B., and Wynder, E. L. (1959). Smoking and lung cancer: Recent evidence and a discussion of some questions. *J. Natl. Cancer Inst.*, **22**, 173–203.

Cox, D. R. (1958). The regression analysis of binary sequences. *J. R. Statist. Soc., Ser. B*, **20**, 215–242.

Cox, D. R. (1970). *Analysis of binary data*. London: Methuen.

Cox, D. R. and Snell, E. J. (1989). *Analysis of binary data*, 2nd ed. Boca Raton: Chapman & Hall/CRC Press.

Craddock, J. M. and Flood, C. R. (1970). The distribution of the χ^2 statistic in small contingency tables. *Appl. Statist.*, **19**, 173–181.

Dixon, W. J. and Massey, F. J. (1969). *Introduction to statistical analysis*, 3rd ed. New York: McGraw-Hill.

Dyke, G. V. and Patterson, H. D. (1962). Analysis of factorial arrangements when the data are proportions. *Biometrics*, **8**, 1–12.

Edwards, A. W. F. (1963). The measure of association in a 2×2 table. *J. R. Statist. Soc., Ser. A*, **126**, 109–114.

Edwards, J. H. (1966). Some taxonomic implications of a curious feature of the bivariate normal surface. *Brit. J. Prev. Soc. Med.*, **20**, 42–43.

Everitt, B. S. (1977). *The analysis of contingency tables*. London: Chapman and Hall.

Feinstein, A. R. (1973). Clinical biostatistics XX. The epidemiologic trohoc, the ablative risk ratio, and retrospective research. *Clinical Pharmacol. Ther.*, **14**, 291–307.

Fienberg, S. E. (1977). *The analysis of cross-classified categorical data*. Cambridge, Mass.: MIT Press.

Finkelstein, M. O. and Levin, B. (2001). *Statistics for lawyers*, 2nd ed. New York: Springer-Verlag.

Fisher, R. A. (1954). *Statistical methods for research workers*, 12th ed. Edinburgh: Oliver and Boyd.

Fleiss, J. L. (1970). On the asserted invariance of the odds ratio. *Brit. J. Prev. Soc. Med.*, **24**, 45–46.

Fleiss, J. L. (1979a). Confidence intervals for the odds ratio in case-control studies: The state of the art. *J. Chronic Dis.*, **32**, 69–77.

Fleiss, J. L. (1979b). Inference about population attributable risk from cross-sectional studies. *Am. J. Epidemiol.*, **110**, 103–104.

Gart, J. J. (1962). Approximate confidence limits for the relative risk. *J. R. Statist. Soc., Ser. B*, **24**, 454–463.

Gart, J. J. (1966). Alternative analysis of contingency tables. *J. R. Statist. Soc., Ser. B*, **28**, 164–179.

Gart, J. J. and Thomas, D. G. (1972). Numerical results on approximate confidence limits for the odds ratio. *J. R. Statist. Soc., Ser. B*, **34**, 441–447.

Gart, J. J. and Zweifel, J. R. (1967). On the bias of various estimators of the logit and its variance, with applications to quantal bioassay. *Biometrika*, **54**, 181–187.

Goodman, L. A. (1964). Simultaneous confidence limits for cross-product ratios in contingency tables. *J. R. Statist. Soc., Ser. B*, **26**, 86–102.

Goodman, L. A. and Kruskal, W. H. (1954). Measures of association for cross classifications. *J. Am. Statist. Assoc.*, **49**, 732–764.

Goodman, L. A. and Kruskal, W. H. (1959). Measures of association for cross classifications II: Further discussion and references. *J. Am. Statist. Assoc.*, **54**, 123–163.

Goodman, L. A. and Kruskal, W. H. (1963). Measures of association for cross classifications III: Approximate sampling theory. *J. Am. Statist. Assoc.*, **58**, 310–364.

Goodman, L. A. and Kruskal, W. H. (1972). Measures of association for cross classifications IV: Simplification of asymptotic variances. *J. Am. Statist. Assoc.*, **67**, 415–421.

Goodman, L. A. and Kruskal, W. H. (1979). *Measures of association for cross classifications*. New York: Springer-Verlag.

Greenberg, B. G. (1969). Problems of statistical inference in health with special reference to the cigarette smoking and lung cancer controversy. *J. Am. Statist. Assoc.*, **64**, 739–758.

Grizzle, J. E. (1961). A new method of testing hypotheses and estimating parameters for the logistic model. *Biometrics*, **17**, 372–385.

Grizzle, J. E. (1963). Tests of linear hypotheses when the data are proportions. *Am. J. Public Health*, **53**, 970–976.

Haldane, J. B. S. (1956). The estimation and significance of the logarithm of a ratio of frequencies. *Ann. Hum. Genet.*, **20**, 309–311.

Harman, H. H. (1960). *Modern factor analysis*. Chicago: University of Chicago Press.

Levin, B. (1984). Simple improvements on Cornfield's approximation to the mean of a noncentral hypergeometric random variable. *Biometrika*, **71**, 630–632.

Levin, B. (1990). The saddlepoint correction in conditional logistic likelihood analysis. *Biometrika*, **77**, 275–285.

Levin, M. L. (1953). The occurrence of lung cancer in man. *Acta Unio Int. contra Cancrum*, **19**, 531–541.

Lord, F. M. and Novick, M. R. (1968). *Statistical theories of mental test scores*. Reading, Mass. Addison-Wesley.

Mantel, N., and Hankey, B. (1975). The odds ratio of a 2×2 contingency table. *Am. Statistician*, **29**, 143–145.

Markush, R. E. (1977). Levin's attributable risk statistic for analytic studies and vital statistics. *Am. J. Epidemiol.*, **105**, 401–406.

Maxwell, A. E. and Everitt, B. S. (1970). The analysis of categorical data using a transformation. *Brit. J. Math. Statist. Psychol.*, **23**, 177–187.

Mosteller, F. (1968). Association and estimation in contingency tables. *J. Am. Statist. Assoc.*, **63**, 1–28.

Nunnally, J. (1978). *Psychometric theory*, 2nd ed. New York: McGraw-Hill.

Peacock, P. B. (1971). The noncomparability of relative risks from different studies. *Biometrics*, **27**, 903–907.

Rockhill, B., Newman, B., and Weinberg, C. (1998). Use and misuse of population attributable fractions. *Am. J. Public Health*, **88**, 15–19.

Santner, T. J. and Snell, M. K. (1980). Small-sample confidence intervals for $p_1 - p_2$ and p_1/p_2 in 2×2 contingency tables. *J. Am. Statist. Assoc.*, **75**, 386–394.

Sheps, M. C. (1958). Shall we count the living or the dead? *New Engl. J. Med.*, **259**, 1210–1214.

Sheps, M. C. (1961). Marriage and mortality. *Am. J. Public Health*, **51**, 547–555.

Smoking and Health (1964). Report of the Advisory Committee to the Surgeon General of the Public Health Service. Princeton: Van Nostrand.

Stevens, W. L. (1951). Mean and variance of an entry in a contingency table. *Biometrika*, **38**, 468–470.

Thomas, D. G. and Gart, J. J. (1977). A table of exact confidence limits for differences and ratios of two proportions and their odds ratio. *J. Am. Statist. Assoc.*, **72**, 73–76.

Walter, S. D. (1976). The estimation and interpretation of attributable risk in health research. *Biometrics*, **32**, 829–849.

Winsor, C. P. (1948). Factorial analysis of a multiple dichotomy. *Hum. Biol.*, **20**, 195–204.

Woolf, B. (1955). On estimating the relation between blood group and disease. *Ann. Hum. Genet.*, **19**, 251–253.

Yule, G. U. (1900). On the association of attributes in statistics. *Philos. Trans. R. Soc. Ser. A*, **194**, 257–319.

Yule, G. U. (1912). On the methods of measuring the association between two attributes. *J. R. Statist. Soc.*, **75**, 579–642.

CHAPTER 7

Comparative Studies: Prospective and Retrospective Sampling

Section 3.1 introduced sampling method II as the selection of a sample from each of two populations, a predetermined number n_1 from the first and a predetermined number n_2 from the second. Method II sampling is used in comparative prospective studies [in which one of the two populations is defined by the presence and the second by the absence of a suspected antecedent factor (MacMahon and Pugh, 1970, Chapter 11)], and is also used in comparative retrospective studies [in which one of the two populations is defined by the presence and the second by the absence of the outcome under study (MacMahon and Pugh, 1970, Chapter 12)].

The analysis of data from a comparative prospective study is discussed in Section 7.1, and the analysis of data from a comparative retrospective study in Section 7.2. Inferences about the attributable risk when the data are from retrospective studies are considered in Section 7.3. Section 7.4 compares the prospective and retrospective approaches.

7.1. PROSPECTIVE STUDIES

The comparative prospective study (also termed the *cohort*, or *forward-going*, or *follow-up* study) is characterized by the identification of the two study samples on the basis of the presence or absence of the antecedent factor and by the estimation for both samples of the proportions developing the disease or condition under study.

Consider again the hypothetical association between maternal age (the antecedent factor) and birthweight (the outcome) introduced in Chapter 6.

Statistical Methods for Rates and Proportions, Third Edition
By Joseph L. Fleiss, Bruce Levin, and Myunghee Cho Paik
ISBN 0-471-52629-0   Copyright © 2003 John Wiley & Sons, Inc.

A design fitting the paradigm of a comparative prospective study would be indicated if, for example, the file containing records for mothers aged 20 years or less were kept separate from the file containing records for mothers aged more than 20 years. Suppose that 100 mothers of each kind are sampled from the respective lists, and the weights of their offspring ascertained.

The precise outcome is of course subject to chance variation, but let us suppose that the data turn out to be perfectly consistent with those obtained with sampling method I (see Section 6.1). From Table 6.2, the rate of low birthweight specific to mothers aged 20 years or less is estimated to be

$$p(B|A) = \frac{p_{11}}{p_{1.}} = \frac{0.05}{0.25} = 0.20. \tag{7.1}$$

Thus we would expect to have 20% of the offspring of mothers aged 20 years or less, or 20 infants, weighing 2500 grams or less, and the remaining 80 weighing over 2500 grams.

The rate of low birthweight specific to mothers aged over 20 years is estimated from Table 6.2 to be

$$p(B|\overline{A}) = \frac{p_{21}}{p_{2.}} = \frac{0.075}{0.75} = 0.10. \tag{7.2}$$

We would therefore expect to have ten of the offspring of mothers aged over 20 years weighing 2500 grams or less, and the remaining 90 weighing over 2500 grams. The expected table is therefore as shown in Table 7.1.

The value of χ^2 for these data is

$$\chi^2 = 3.18, \tag{7.3}$$

so that the association fails to reach significance at the 0.05 level. What is noteworthy is that the total sample sizes of Tables 6.1 and 7.1 are equal and that the frequencies of the two tables are consistent. Nevertheless, the chi squared value for the latter table is greater than that for the former. The inference from this comparison holds in general: a prospective study with equal sample sizes yields a more *powerful* chi squared test than a cross sectional study with the same total sample size (see Lehmann, 1997, p. 158).

Table 7.1. *Association between birthweight and maternal age: Prospective study*

Maternal Age	Birthweight		Total	Proportion with Low Birthweight
	B	$\overline{B}$		
A	20	80	$100\,(=N_A)$	$0.20\,[=p(B|A)]$
$\overline{A}$	10	90	$100\,(=N_{\overline{A}})$	$0.10\,[=p(B|\overline{A})]$
Total	30	170	200	

The odds ratio ω was introduced in Section 6.3 as a measure of associa-tion between characteristics A and B. Because of the way the separate odds Ω_A in (6.5) and $\Omega_{\bar{A}}$ in (6.8) were defined, it is clear that the odds ratio may be estimated from a comparative prospective study as well as from a cross-sectional study. The estimate is

$$o = \frac{p(B|A)p(\bar{B}|\bar{A})}{p(\bar{B}|A)p(B|\bar{A})}. \tag{7.4}$$

For the data of Table 7.1, the estimated odds ratio is

$$o = \frac{0.20 \times 0.90}{0.80 \times 0.10} = 2.25, \tag{7.5}$$

which is precisely equal to the value found in (6.15) for the data from the cross-sectional study.

Formula 6.16 for o as a function of the cross-products of cell frequencies applies to the data from comparative prospective studies as well. For the data of Table 7.1, obviously,

$$o = \frac{20 \times 90}{80 \times 10} = 2.25.$$

The standard error of the odds ratio estimated from a comparative prospective study is estimated as

$$\widehat{se}(o) = o\sqrt{\frac{1}{N_A p(B|A)p(\bar{B}|A)} + \frac{1}{N_{\bar{A}} p(B|\bar{A})p(\bar{B}|\bar{A})}}. \tag{7.6}$$

For the data of Table 7.1, the estimated standard error is

$$\widehat{se}(o) = 2.25\sqrt{\frac{1}{100 \times 0.20 \times 0.80} + \frac{1}{100 \times 0.10 \times 0.90}}$$

$$= 0.94. \tag{7.7}$$

An equivalent expression for the standard error in terms of the original frequencies (see Problem 7.1) is

$$\widehat{se}(o) = o\sqrt{\frac{1}{n_{11}} + \frac{1}{n_{12}} + \frac{1}{n_{21}} + \frac{1}{n_{22}}}, \tag{7.8}$$

which is identical to expression (6.19).

We found above that the chi squared test applied to data from a compara-tive prospective study with equal sample sizes is more powerful than the chi squared test applied to data from a cross-sectional study. A similar phenomenon holds for the *precision* of the estimated odds ratio. Even though the total sample sizes in Tables 6.1 and 7.1 are equal, and even though the association between the two characteristics is the same, the odds ratio from the latter table is estimated more precisely [$\widehat{se}(o) = 0.94$, from (7.7)] than the odds ratio from the former [$\widehat{se}(o) = 1.00$, from (6.18)]. A prospective study with equal sample sizes is thus superior in both power and precision to a cross-sectional study with the same total sample size.

Using the methods described in Section 6.6, an approximate 95% confidence interval for the odds ratio based on the data of Table 7.1 may be shown to be

$$0.93 \leq \omega \leq 5.51, \tag{7.9}$$

which is narrower than (and thus superior to) the interval found in (6.87) for data from the corresponding cross-sectional study.

The value of the uncorrected chi squared statistic (see equation 6.3) for the data of Table 7.1 is

$$\chi_u^2 = \frac{200(20 \times 90 - 80 \times 10)^2}{100 \times 100 \times 30 \times 170} = 3.92.$$

It yields a phi coefficient (see equation 6.2) of

$$\phi = \sqrt{\frac{3.92}{200}} = 0.14, \tag{7.10}$$

which is only slightly greater than the value 0.13 found in (6.4) for the data of Table 6.1. Recall, however, that the data of Tables 6.1 and 7.1 are perfectly consistent.

7.2. RETROSPECTIVE STUDIES

The comparative retrospective study (also termed the *case-control* study) is characterized by the identification of the two study samples on the basis of the presence or absence of the outcome factor and by the estimation for both samples of the proportions possessing the antecedent factor under study.

This method might be easily applied to the study of the association between maternal age and birthweight if, for example, the file containing records for infants of low birthweight (less than or equal to 2500 grams) were kept separate from the file containing records for infants of higher birthweight. Suppose that 100 infants of both kinds are sampled from the respective lists and that the ages of their mothers are ascertained.

Let us suppose, as we did in Section 7.1, that the data turn out to be perfectly consistent with those already given. We need the rates $p(A|B)$ and

$p(A|\bar{B})$, that is, the proportions of mothers aged 20 years or less among infants to low and among infants of high birthweight. From Table 6.2 we find that

$$p(A|B) = \frac{p_{11}}{p_{.1}} = \frac{0.05}{0.125} = 0.40, \qquad (7.11)$$

implying that 40% of the mothers of the 100 low-birthweight infants, or 40, should be aged 20 years or less, and the remaining 60, over 20 years. We also find that

$$p(A|\bar{B}) = \frac{p_{12}}{p_{.2}} = \frac{0.20}{0.875} = 0.23, \qquad (7.12)$$

implying that 23% of the mothers of the 100 higher-birthweight infants, or 23, should be aged 20 years or less, and the remaining 77, over 20 years.

Standard practice is to set out the data resulting from sampling method II as in Table 3.6, so that the two study samples appear one above the other and the characteristic determined for each subject is located across the top. This causes something of an anomaly when applied to data from a comparative retrospective study, because the characteristic determined for each subject is the suspected antecedent factor and not the outcome characteristic that is hypothesized to follow from it. Miettinen (1970) stressed the necessary shift in thinking required for analyzing data from a comparative retrospective study: that the outcome characteristic follows the antecedent factor in a logical sequence, but precedes it in a retrospective study.

Following, then, the format of Table 3.6, we present the expected data as shown in Table 7.2. The value of χ^2 for these data is

$$\chi^2 = 5.93, \qquad (7.13)$$

which indicates that the association is significant at the 0.05 level.

The gradient in the magnitude of χ^2 from the cross-sectional study ($\chi^2 = 2.58$) to the prospective study ($\chi^2 = 3.18$) to the retrospective study ($\chi^2 = 5.93$) is noteworthy because the three sets of data were all generated according to the same set of underlying rates and because the three total

Table 7.2. *Association between birthweight and maternal age: Retrospective study*

Birthweight	Maternal Age		Total	Proportion with Low Age
	A	$\bar{A}$		
B	40	60	$100 \, (= N_B)$	$0.40 \, [= p(A|B)]$
$\bar{B}$	23	77	$100 \, (= N_{\bar{B}})$	$0.23 \, [= p(A|\bar{B})]$
Total	63	137	200	

sample sizes were equal. It is true in general that a retrospective study with equal sample sizes yields a more powerful chi squared test than a cross sectional study with the same total sample size. If, in addition, the outcome characteristic is rarer than the antecedent factor—more precisely, if

$$|P(B) - 0.5| > |P(A) - 0.5|, \tag{7.14}$$

then the chi squared test on the data of a retrospective study with equal sample sizes is more powerful than the chi squared test on the data of a prospective study with equal sample sizes (Lehmann, 1997, p. 158).

For the data of Table 7.2, the value of the uncorrected chi squared statistic is

$$\chi_u^2 = \frac{200(40 \times 77 - 60 \times 23)^2}{100 \times 100 \times 63 \times 137} = 6.70.$$

The value of the associated phi coefficient is

$$\phi = \sqrt{\frac{6.70}{200}} = 0.18, \tag{7.15}$$

nearly 40% higher than the value, $\phi = 0.13$, associated with the data of Table 6.1, and nearly 30% higher than the value, $\phi = 0.14$, associated with the data of Table 7.1. Now, if a given measure is to be more than a mere uninterpretable index, it should have the property that different investigators studying the same phenomenon should emerge with at least similar estimates even though they studied the phenomenon differently. Since the phi coefficient obviously lacks the property of *invariance*, it should not be used as a measure of association for data from comparative prospective or retrospective studies.

The odds ratio ω, on the other hand, is invariant across the three kinds of studies we are considering. It is defined by

$$\omega = \frac{P(B|A)P(\bar{B}|\bar{A})}{P(\bar{B}|A)P(B|\bar{A})}. \tag{7.16}$$

When expressed in this form, ω seems to be estimable only from cross-sectional and comparative prospective studies, because only these two kinds of studies provide estimates of the rates $P(B|A)$ and $P(B|\bar{A})$. An equivalent expression for ω (see Problem 7.2), however, is

$$\omega = \frac{P(A|B)P(\bar{A}|\bar{B})}{P(\bar{A}|B)P(A|\bar{B})}, \tag{7.17}$$

and, when expressed in this form, ω is clearly estimable from comparative retrospective studies, too (see Cornfield, 1956).

The estimate is

$$o = \frac{p(A|B)p(\bar{A}|\bar{B})}{p(\bar{A}|B)p(A|\bar{B})}. \tag{7.18}$$

For the data of Table 7.2, the estimated odds ratio is

$$o = \frac{0.40 \times 0.77}{0.60 \times 0.23} = 2.23, \tag{7.19}$$

equal except for rounding errors to the value $o = 2.25$ found previously. Formula (6.16), which involves the cell frequencies, continues to apply as well.

The standard error of the odds ratio estimated from a comparative retrospective study is estimated as

$$\widehat{se}(o) = o\sqrt{\frac{1}{N_B\, p(A|B)p(\bar{A}|B)} + \frac{1}{N_{\bar{B}}\, p(A|\bar{B})p(\bar{A}|\bar{B})}}. \tag{7.20}$$

Expressions (6.19) and (7.8) for the standard error as a function of the original frequencies are also valid for the data of a comparative retrospective study.

For the data of Table 7.2,

$$\widehat{se}(o) = 2.23\sqrt{\frac{1}{100 \times 0.40 \times 0.60} + \frac{1}{100 \times 0.23 \times 0.77}}$$

$$= 2.23\sqrt{\frac{1}{40} + \frac{1}{60} + \frac{1}{23} + \frac{1}{77}}$$

$$= 0.70. \tag{7.21}$$

The gradient noted above in the magnitude of χ^2 is matched by a gradient in the precision with which the odds ratio is estimated. For the cross-sectional study, $\widehat{se}(o) = 1.00$ [see (6.18)]; for the comparative prospective study, $\widehat{se}(o) = 0.94$ [see (7.7)]; and for the comparative retrospective study, $\widehat{se}(o) = 0.70$ [see (7.21)].

An approximate 95% confidence interval for the odds ratio based on the data of Table 7.2, using the methods described in Section 6.6, is

$$1.16 \leq \omega \leq 4.33. \tag{7.22}$$

Exactly the same gradient across the three kinds of studies is therefore found for the length of the 95% confidence interval for the odds ratio. The length of the interval for the cross-sectional study [see (6.87)] is largest; that for the prospective study [see (7.9)], smaller; and that for the retrospective study [see (7.22)], smallest of all.

According to the criteria of precision, power, and length of confidence interval, therefore, when the total sample sizes are equal and (7.14) holds, a comparative retrospective study with equal sample sizes is superior to both a cross-sectional study and a comparative prospective study with equal sample sizes.

7.3. ESTIMATING ATTRIBUTABLE RISK FROM RETROSPECTIVE STUDIES

Levin's (1953) attributable risk, R_A, was presented in Section 6.8 as the fraction of all occurrences of a condition due to exposure to a specified risk factor. As motivated there, and as defined in (6.93), R_A appears to be estimable only from a cross-sectional study, which simultaneously permits the estimation of $P(A)$, the proportion of the population exposed to the risk factor, and of R, the relative risk. As pointed out by Levin (1953), Walter (1975, 1976), and Taylor (1977), however, R_A can be approximated from a retrospective study under certain assumptions. If $P(B)$, the rate of occurrence of the outcome characteristic in the population, is low, then the odds ratio ω approximates R. If, in addition, the control group $(\bar{B})$ in the study is a random sample of the corresponding group in the population, then $P(A|\bar{B})$ approximates $P(A)$.

Under these assumptions,

$$\tilde{r}_A = \frac{p(A|B) - p(A|\bar{B})}{1 - p(A|\bar{B})} \qquad (7.23)$$

is a good estimate of the population attributable risk (Levin and Bertell, 1978). (See Problem 7.5.) For the hypothetical data of Table 7.2, the estimated risk for low birthweight attributable to low maternal age is

$$\tilde{r}_A = \frac{0.40 - 0.23}{1 - 0.23} = 0.22. \qquad (7.24)$$

For the corresponding data from a cross-sectional study (Table 6.2), $p(A) = 0.25$ and the relative risk is $r = 2.0$; thus from (6.93),

$$r_A = \frac{0.25(2.0 - 1)}{1 + 0.25(2.0 - 1)} = 0.20, \qquad (7.25)$$

which is reasonably close to the estimate in (7.24) from a retrospective study. In either case, the hypothetical data suggest that the rate of low birthweight could be reduced about a fifth if pregnancy among women aged 20 years or less could be avoided.

Walter (1975) showed that when the attributable risk is estimated from a retrospective study using formula (7.23), the estimated standard error of the natural logarithm of its complement, $1 - \tilde{r}_A$, is given by

$$\widehat{se}\{\ln(1 - \tilde{r}_A)\} = \sqrt{\frac{p(A|B)}{N_B p(\bar{A}|B)} + \frac{p(A|\bar{B})}{N_{\bar{B}} p(\bar{A}|\bar{B})}}, \qquad (7.26)$$

where N_B is the number of cases and $N_{\bar{B}}$ the number of controls. This formula is the same as one would use upon recognizing that (7.23) is formally identical to Sheps' relative difference—applied, however, to the retrospective probabilities $p(A|B)$ and $p(A|\bar{B})$—and then applying the result of Problem 2.13. See Problem 7.6. The formula is also identical to (6.114).

For the data of Table 7.2,

$$\ln(1 - \tilde{r}_A) = \ln(1 - 0.22) = -0.25 \qquad (7.27)$$

and

$$\widehat{se}\{\ln(1 - \tilde{r}_A)\} = \sqrt{\frac{0.40}{100 \times 0.60} + \frac{0.23}{100 \times 0.77}} = 0.10. \qquad (7.28)$$

An approximate 95% confidence interval for $\ln(1 - R_A)$ is

$$-0.25 - 1.96 \times 0.10 \le \ln(1 - R_A) \le -0.25 + 1.96 \times 0.10, \qquad (7.29)$$

or

$$-0.45 \le \ln(1 - R_A) \le -0.05. \qquad (7.30)$$

By taking antilogarithms of these limits, and then complements from unity, we obtain an approximate 95% confidence interval for the attributable risk itself:

$$0.05 \le R_A \le 0.36. \qquad (7.31)$$

Problem 7.5 shows that only the approximation $P(A|\bar{B}) \approx P(A)$ is required to show that $\tilde{r}_A$ is a good estimate of R_A when $P(B)$ is small, but not the other approximate equality, $\omega \approx R$, which is also true under the rare-disease assumption. The latter approximate equality can be used in expression (6.97) for the attributable risk to provide an equivalent estimate of R_A in retrospective studies:

$$\tilde{r}_A = \left(1 - \frac{1}{o}\right) p(A|B). \qquad (7.32)$$

For the data in Table 7.2,

$$\tilde{r}_A = \left(1 - \frac{1}{2.23}\right) \times 0.40 = 0.22, \tag{7.33}$$

which is identical to (7.24), apart from roundoff. Problem 7.7 demonstrates that (7.23) is identical to (7.32) in general.

7.4. THE RETROSPECTIVE APPROACH VERSUS THE PROSPECTIVE APPROACH

If a scientist accepts the argument of Section 6.7 that the odds ratio and thus the retrospective study are inherently valid, he or she must still bear in mind that retrospective studies are subject to more sources of error than prospective studies. Hammond (1958), for example, has cited the bias that may arise because historical data are obtained only after subjects become ill, and frequently only after they are diagnosed. A patient's knowledge that he has a certain disease might easily affect his recollection, intentionally or unintentionally, of which factors preceded his illness.

Another difficulty pointed out by Hammond is in finding an adequate control series for the sample of patients: one must, after all, find groups of subjects who are like the cases in all respects save for having the disease. Mantel and Haenszel (1959) cite these and other deficiencies in the retrospective approach. When, for example, the subjects having the disease are found in hospitals or clinics, inferences from retrospective studies may be subject to the kind of bias illustrated in Section 1.4. Specifically, the antecedent factors may appear to be associated with the disease, but in reality be more associated with admission to a treatment facility. Feinstein (1973) describes the closely related bias due to differential surveillance of individuals with and individuals without the suspected risk factor.

This does not imply that only the retrospective approach, and not the prospective, is open to bias. Similar biases have been shown to operate in prospective studies as well (Mainland and Herrera, 1956; Yerushalmy and Palmer, 1959; Mantel and Haenszel, 1959; Greenland, 1977; Joffres et al., 1990). For example, the bias possible in those retrospective studies that require hospitalized patients to be evaluated is matched by the potential bias in those prospective studies that require volunteers to be followed up. Errors of diagnosis and insufficiently frequent screening are also problems associated with prospective studies (Schlesselman, 1977).

What does seem to be true, however, is that a greater degree of ingenuity is needed for the proper design of a retrospective study than for the design of a prospective study. Thus Levin (1954) controlled for the first bias cited above—that due to a patient's report possibly being influenced by his knowledge that he has the disease being studied—by questioning all subjects prior to the final diagnosis. By this means, the possible bias due to the examiner's applying different standards to the responses of cases and controls is also controlled. Rimmer and Chambers (1969) suggested another means of control. They found greater accuracy in the recollections of relatives than in those of the patients themselves.

Improper identification or sampling of a control group can cause such selection biases. Analytic methods to adjust for selection bias have been proposed (Kleinbaum, Morgenstern, and Kupper, 1981; Weinberg and Wacholder, 1990; Maclure and Hankinson, 1990; Lin and Paik, 2001).

As a means of reducing the bias possible in contrasting cases with only one control series, Doll and Hill (1952) studied two control groups. One was a sample of hospitalized patients with other diseases than the one studied, and the second was a sample from the community. Matching (see Chapter 13) is another device for reducing bias. The validity of the retrospective approach can only increase as investigators learn which kinds of information can be accurately recalled by a subject and which cannot. For example, Gray (1955) and Klemetti and Saxén (1967) have shown that the occurrence or nonoccurrence of a past event can be recalled accurately, but not the precise time when the event occurred.

Jick and Vessey (1978) have reviewed the major sources of error in those retrospective studies in particular that seek to elucidate the role of prescribed drug use in the development of illness, and they indicate methods for their control. The January 1979 issue of the *Journal of Chronic Diseases* (Ibrahim, 1979) is devoted to the art of designing retrospective studies; the contribution by Sackett (1979) is especially useful for its cataloguing of several sources of bias and for its prescriptions for their control or measurement.

The reduction of bias is discussed again in Chapter 17. To the extent that bias can be controlled, the following points made by Mantel and Haenszel argue strongly for the retrospective approach:

> Among the desirable attributes of the retrospective study is the ability to yield results from presently collectible data.... The retrospective approach is also adapted to the limited resources of an individual investigator.... For especially rare diseases a retrospective study may be the only feasible approach.... In the absence of important biases in the study setting, the retrospective method could be regarded, according to sound statistical theory, as the study method of choice [1959, p. 720].

PROBLEMS

7.1. Prove the equality of expressions (7.6) and (7.8) for the standard error of the odds ratio. [*Hint.* $p(B|A) = n_{11}/N_A$; $p(\overline{B}|A) = n_{12}/N_A$; $p(B|\overline{A}) = n_{21}/N_{\overline{A}}$; and $p(\overline{B}|\overline{A}) = n_{22}/N_{\overline{A}}$. Also, $N_A = n_{11} + n_{12}$ and $N_{\overline{A}} = n_{21} + n_{22}$.]

7.2. Prove the equality of expressions (7.16) and (7.17) for the odds ratio. [*Hint*. Use the definitions of Section 1.1 to replace all conditional probabilities in (7.16) by joint probabilities. The probabilities $P(A)$ and $P(\overline{A})$ are seen to cancel out. Multiply and divide by $P(B)$ and by $P(\overline{B})$, and use the definition of conditional probabilities to arrive at (7.17).]

7.3. The phi coefficient [see (6.2)] is a valid measure of association only for method I (naturalistic or cross-sectional) sampling. Phi coefficients applied to data from method II (prospective or retrospective) studies are not at all comparable to those applied to data from method I studies. Even more is true. When two studies are both conducted according to either the prospective or retrospective approaches, but with proportionately different allocations of the total sample, the phi coefficient for one will not in general be comparable to that for the other.

    (a) In a retrospective study of factors associated with cancer of the oral cavity, Wynder et al. (1958) studied 34 women with cancer of the oral cavity and 214 women, matched by age, with nonmalignant conditions. Twenty-four percent of the cancer cases, as opposed to 66% of the controls, were nonsmokers. Set up the resulting fourfold table, and calculate uncorrected chi squared and the associated phi coefficient.

    (b) Suppose that Wynder et al. had studied, instead, 214 cancer cases and 34 controls. Assuming the same proportions of nonsmokers as above, set up the expected fourfold table, and calculate uncorrected chi squared and the associated phi. How do the phi coefficients compare?

    (c) Suppose, now, that 124 of both kinds of women had been studied, and assume the same proportions of nonsmokers as above. Set up the resulting expected fourfold table and calculate uncorrected chi squared and the associated phi. How does this phi coefficient compare with those in (a) and (b)? What is the percentage difference between the phi coefficient of (a) and that of (c)? What would you conclude about the comparability of phi coefficients in retrospective studies with varying allocations of a total sample?

7.4. Three criteria were suggested in this chapter for comparing the cross-sectional, prospective, and retrospective approaches. Another criterion is the total sample size necessary for the standard error of the odds ratio to assume some specified value. The data for the following questions are those employed throughout Chapters 6 and 7. Suppose that the correct values of $o = 2.25$ and of all the necessary proportions are known.

    (a) The approximate standard error of o with cross-sectional sampling is given by (6.17). What value of $n_{..}$ is needed to give a standard error of 0.50?

(b) The approximate standard error of o with prospective sampling is given by (7.6). Let $N_A + N_{\bar{A}}$, the total sample size, be denoted N_P, and suppose for simplicity that $N_A = N_{\bar{A}} = N_P/2$. What value of N_P is needed to give a standard error of 0.50? What is the percentage reduction from $n_{..}$ to N_P?

(c) The approximate standard error of o with retrospective sampling is given by (7.20). Let $N_B + N_{\bar{B}}$, the total sample size, be denoted N_R, and suppose for simplicity that $N_B = N_{\bar{B}} = N_R/2$. What value of N_R is needed to give a standard error of 0.50? What is the percentage reduction from $n_{..}$ to N_R? From N_P to N_R?

(d) Is the reduction in (b) of much practical (e.g., monetary) importance? How about the reductions in (c)?

7.5. Starting from expression (6.97), show that another formula for R_A is

$$R_A = \frac{P(A|B) - P(A)}{1 - P(A)}.$$

Deduce that (7.23) is an estimator in retrospective sampling that approximates R_A, assuming $P(A|\bar{B}) \approx P(A)$, which would obtain with small $P(B)$. [*Hint.* Use Bayes' theorem to write all probabilities in retrospective form, and put all terms over a common denominator $P(\bar{A}) = 1 - P(A)$.]

7.6. Show that (7.26) results when (7.23) is recognized as Sheps' relative difference applied to the retrospective probabilities $p(A|B)$ and $p(A|\bar{B})$, rather than the prospective probabilities $p(B|A)$ and $p(B|\bar{A})$ as originally proposed by Sheps (1958, 1961). [*Hint.* Write $1 - \tilde{r}_A = p(\bar{A}|B)/p(\bar{A}|\bar{B})$, and notice that in retrospective sampling, $\ln(1 - \tilde{r}_A)$ is the difference of two independent random variables. Then apply the result of Problem 2.13.]

7.7. Show that (7.23) and (7.32) are identical.

7.8. An article in the February 8, 2002 issue of the *New York Times* (p. A18) excitedly discusses a new blood test currently being developed for detecting ovarian cancer. Some initial results regarding the sensitivity and specificity of this test have been published. In a preliminary study, 50 women known to have ovarian cancer and 66 women known to be free of ovarian cancer were tested. Of the 50 women with ovarian cancer, all 50 tested positive. Of the 66 women without ovarian cancer, 3 tested positive and 63 tested negative.

(a) Assume the prevalence of ovarian cancer is 40 per 100,000 women. What then is the positive predictive value (PPV) of this test?

(b) Find an approximate two-sided 95% confidence interval for the PPV. [*Hint.* Write the PPV odds as $\text{PPV}/(1 - \text{PPV}) = R \cdot (\text{prevalence odds})$, where R is the rate ratio $R = P(+\mid D)/P(+\mid \text{no } D)$, and the prevalence odds, $4/9{,}996$, is a given constant. Take logs, and note that the log PPV odds is the sum of $\ln R$ plus a constant. Find the standard error for the estimate of $\ln R$, and use that to find an approximate 95% confidence interval for the log PPV odds. Back-transform the endpoints of this interval to find an approximate 95% confidence interval for PPV.]

REFERENCES

Cornfield, J. (1956). A statistical problem arising from retrospective studies. Pp. 135–148 in J. Newman (Ed.). *Proceedings of the third Berkeley symposium on mathematical statistics and probability*, Vol. 4, Berkeley: University of California Press.

Doll, R. and Hill, A. B. (1952). A study of the etiology of carcinoma of the lung. *Brit. Med. J.*, **2**, 1271–1286.

Feinstein, A. R. (1973). Clinical biostatistics XX. The epidemiologic trohoc, the ablative risk ratio, and retrospective research. *Clin. Pharmacol. Ther.*, **14**, 291–307.

Gray, P. G. (1955). The memory factor in social surveys. *J. Am. Stat. Assoc.*, **50**, 344–363.

Greenland, S. (1977). Response and follow-up bias in cohort studies. *Am. J. Epidemiol.*, **106**, 184–187.

Hammond, E. C. (1958). Smoking and death rates: A riddle in cause and effect. *Am. Sci.*, **46**, 331–354.

Ibrahim, M. A. (Ed.) (1979). The case-control study: Consensus and controversy. *J. Chronic Dis.*, **32**, 1–144.

Jick, H. and Vessey, M. P. (1978). Case-control studies in the evaluation of drug-induced illness. *Am. J. Epidemiol.*, **107**, 1–7.

Joffres, M. R., MacLean, C. J., Reed, D. M., Yano, K., and Benfante, R. (1990). Potential bias due to prevalent diseases in prospective studies, *Int. J. Epidemiol.*, **19**, 459–465.

Kleinbaum, D. G., Morgenstern, H., and Kupper, L. L. (1981). Selection bias in epidemiologic studies. *Am. J. Epidemiol.*, **113**, 452–463.

Klemetti, A. and Saxén, L. (1967). Prospective versus retrospective approach in the search for environmental causes of malformations. *Am. J. Public Health*, **57**, 2071–2075.

Lehmann, E. L. (1997). *Testing statistical hypotheses*, 2nd ed. New York: Springer.

Levin, M. L. (1953). The occurrence of lung cancer in man. *Acta Unio Int. contra Cancrum*, **19**, 531–541.

Levin, M. L. (1954). Etiology of lung cancer: Present status. *N. Y. State J. Med.*, **54**, 769–777.

Levin, M. L. and Bertell, R. (1978). Re: "Simple estimation of population attributable risk from case-control studies." *Am. J. Epidemiol.*, **108**, 78–79.

Lin, I.-F. and Paik, M. C. (2001). Matched case-control data analysis with selection bias. *Biometrics*, **57**, 1106–1112.

Maclure, M. and Hankinson, S. (1990). Analysis of selection bias in a case-control study of renal adenocarcinoma. *Epidemiology*, **1**, 441–447.

MacMahon, B. and Pugh, T. F. (1970). *Epidemiology: Principles and methods*, Boston: Little, Brown.

Mainland, D. and Herrera, L. (1956). The risk of biased selection in forward-going surveys with nonprofessional interviewers. *J. Chronic Dis.*, **4**, 240–244.

Mantel, N. and Haenszel, W. (1959). Statistical aspects of the analysis of data from retrospective studies of disease. *J. Natl. Cancer Inst.*, **22**, 719–748.

Miettinen, O. S. (1970). Matching and design efficiency in retrospective studies. *Am. J. Epidemiol.*, **91**, 111–118.

Rimmer, J. and Chambers, D. S. (1969). Alcoholism: Methodological considerations in the study of family illness. *Am. J. Orthopsychiatry*, **39**, 760–768.

Sackett, D. L. (1979). Bias in analytic research. *J. Chronic Dis.*, **32**, 51–63.

Schlesselman, J. J. (1977). The effect of errors of diagnosis and frequency of examination on reported rates of disease. *Biometrics*, **33**, 635–642.

Sheps, M. C. (1958). Shall we count the living or the dead? *New Engl. J. Med.*, **259**, 1210–1214.

Sheps, M. C. (1961). Marriage and mortality. *Am. J. Public Health*, **51**, 547–555.

Taylor, J. W. (1977). Simple estimation of population attributable risk from case-control studies. *Am. J. Epidemiol.*, **106**, 260.

Walter, S. D. (1975). The distribution of Levin's measure of attributable risk. *Biometrika*, **62**, 371–374.

Walter, S. D. (1976). The estimation and interpretation of attributable risk in health research. *Biometrics*, **32**, 829–849.

Weinberg, C. R. and Wacholder, S. (1990). The design and analysis of case-control studies with biased sampling. *Biometrics*, **46**, 953–975.

Wynder, E. L., Navarrette, A., Arostegui, G. E., and Llambes, J. L. (1958). Study of environmental factors in cancer of the respiratory tract in Cuba. *J. Natl. Cancer Inst.*, **20**, 665–673.

Yerushalmy, J. and Palmer, C. E. (1959). On the methodology of investigations of etiologic factors in chronic diseases. *J. Chronic Dis.*, **10**, 27–40.

CHAPTER 8

Randomized Controlled Trials

Sampling method III is exemplified by the comparative clinical trial in which treatments are assigned to subjects at random. The philosophy of the controlled clinical trial is discussed by Hill (1962, Chapters 1–3), and solutions to some practical problems arising in the execution of a clinical trial are offered by Mainland (1960) and in an entire issue of *Clinical Pharmacology and Therapeutics* (Roth and Gordon, 1979). Ethical issues are discussed by Fox (1959), Meier (1975), and Royall (1991). Considerations needed in deciding how many patients to study and some unfortunate consequences of studying too few are discussed by Friedman et al. (1978).

In the twenty years since publication of the second edition of this book, there has been an explosion in the literature both of the methods and of the ethics of controlled clinical trials. An entire journal dedicated to the field (*Controlled Clinical Trials*) had its inaugural publication in 1981, as the official journal of the Society for Clinical Trials. A theme issue of the *British Medical Journal* recently celebrated the fiftieth anniversary of its publication of a randomized controlled trial of streptomycin in pulmonary tuberculosis, arguably the first such publication of a trial to describe explicitly the method of randomization (Smith, 1998). The volume also contains several articles on the deficiencies of randomized trials, and the "huge scope for doing better" (Smith, 1998). Of several textbooks on the design and conduct of clinical trials, four of note are (in their current editions) by Pocock (1984), Piantadosi (1997), Friedman, Furberg, and DeMets (1998), and Everitt and Pickles (2000). Levine (1999) gives an excellent review of current thinking about ethical issues in randomized clinical trials.

A distinctive feature of clinical trials is the opportunity to terminate the study prematurely if one of the groups being compared is found to be experiencing an alarmingly high rate of serious adverse reactions or if the

Statistical Methods for Rates and Proportions, Third Edition
By Joseph L. Fleiss, Bruce Levin, and Myunghee Cho Paik
ISBN 0-471-52629-0   Copyright © 2003 John Wiley & Sons, Inc.

therapeutic difference between the treatments is so overwhelming that to withhold the superior treatment from all future eligible patients is deemed unethical. The University Group Diabetes Program (Report of the Committee for the Assessment of Biometric Aspects of Controlled Trials of Hypoglycemic Agents, 1975) provides a noteworthy example of the former reason to terminate a trial, and the Anturane Trial (Anturane Reinfarction Trial Research Group, 1978) provides a noteworthy example of the latter. Meier (1979) suggests a framework for deciding whether to continue or to terminate a trial. The development of sequential and group sequential methods for interim monitoring and early stopping of clinical trials has also been remarkable. The textbook by Friedman, Furberg, and DeMets (1998) contains useful guidance in these areas. An early monograph on the application of sequential methods to clinical trials is Armitage (1975), and the monograph by Siegmund (1985) gives the advanced mathematical theory underpinning the field. Modern treatments are given by Whitehead (1997) and Jennison and Turnbull (1999).

Friedman and DeMets (1981) and Ellenberg, Fleming, and DeMets (2002) discuss the role of monitoring committees, variously called Data and Safety Monitoring Committees (DSMCs), Performance and Safety Monitoring Boards (PSMBs), or variations on these names. See also Levin (2003). As the names suggest, a PSMB has responsibility as an independent, deliberative body to review data and consider issues related to the safety of the participants and the performance and integrity of the trial. These issues include: accumulating data concerning serious adverse events; interim analyses showing evidence strongly favoring efficacy of one treatment arm relative to another earlier in the trial, or the lack of any efficacy differences later in the trial; late-breaking developments from other studies suggesting an alteration of the clinical equipoise under which the trial began; poor subject accrual and other performance matters directly affecting statistical power and/or the ability of the study to achieve its primary goals; protocol violations or proposals to alter the protocol after the trial is underway. The PSMB must weigh these and other matters, and, ultimately, advise on whether a trial should be allowed to continue or stopped. Current guidelines by federal funding and regulatory agencies call for increasing deployment of such independent monitoring committees whenever there are potential risks to the participants above a minimal level.

The scope of randomized controlled trials has become so broad that we must limit consideration in this chapter just to salient statistical points related to the comparison of two treatments. Section 8.1 describes the analysis of data from a simple comparative trial, and Section 8.2 discusses the crossover design—both for the case where the outcome is a yes-no variable, such as recovery–no-recovery. Section 8.3 discusses some issues that affect the power of the primary statistical analysis of a randomized trial. One is the intent-to-treat principle. A second is the design of a trial for goals other than the classical test of the null hypothesis of no treatment effect. Some proposed

Table 8.1. *Hypothetical data from a comparative clinical trial*

	Number of Patients	Proportion Improved
Treatment 1	$80 \; (= n_1)$	$0.60 \; (= p_1)$
Treatment 2	$70 \; (= n_2)$	$0.80 \; (= p_2)$
Overall	$150 \; (= n)$	$0.69 \; (= \bar{p})$

alternatives to simple randomization in comparative trials are discussed in Section 8.4.

8.1.   THE SIMPLE COMPARATIVE TRIAL

Suppose that the data of Table 8.1 resulted from a trial in which one treatment was applied to a sample of $n_1 = 80$ subjects randomly selected from a total of $n = 150$ and the other treatment was applied to the remaining $n_2 = 70$ subjects.

The statistical significance of the difference between the two improvement rates is tested using the statistic given in (3.5). For the data of Table 8.1, the value is

$$z = \frac{|0.80 - 0.60| - \frac{1}{2}\left(\frac{1}{80} + \frac{1}{70}\right)}{\sqrt{0.69 \times 0.31 \left(\frac{1}{80} + \frac{1}{70}\right)}} = 2.47, \tag{8.1}$$

indicating that the difference is significant at the 0.05 level.

The simple difference between the two improvement rates,

$$d = p_2 - p_1, \tag{8.2}$$

is the measure most frequently used to describe the differential effectiveness of the second treatment over the first. The standard error of d is estimated by

$$\widehat{se}(d) = \sqrt{\frac{p_1 q_1}{n_1} + \frac{p_2 q_2}{n_2}}. \tag{8.3}$$

For the data of Table 8.1, the simple difference is

$$d = 0.80 - 0.60 = 0.20, \tag{8.4}$$

implying that among every 100 patients given the first treatment an additional 20 would have been expected to improve had they been given the second treatment. The estimated standard error of d is

$$\widehat{se}(d) = \sqrt{\frac{0.60 \times 0.40}{80} + \frac{0.80 \times 0.20}{70}} = 0.07. \tag{8.5}$$

An approximate 95% confidence interval for the difference between the two underlying rates of improvement is

$$0.20 - 1.96 \times 0.07 \leq P_2 - P_1 \leq 0.20 + 1.96 \times 0.07, \tag{8.6}$$

or

$$0.06 \leq P_2 - P_1 \leq 0.34. \tag{8.7}$$

Occasionally one can assume that the two treatments are such that any patient who responds to the first treatment is also expected to respond to the second. This assumption may be tenable if the first treatment is an inert placebo, or if the first treatment is an active drug and the second is that drug plus another compound or that drug at a greater dosage level. A consequence of the assumption is that any greater effectiveness of the second treatment can only be manifested on subjects who were refractory to the first (see Sheps, 1958, for further examples and discussion).

Let P_1 denote the proportion improving in the population of patients given the first treatment and P_2 the proportion improving in the population given the second. Let f denote the proportion of patients, among those failing to respond to the first treatment, who would be expected to respond to the second. It is then assumed that

$$P_2 = P_1 + f(1 - P_1), \tag{8.8}$$

that is, the improvement rate under the second treatment is equal to that under the first plus an added improvement rate which applies only to patients who fail to improve under the first treatment. The value of f is clearly

$$f = \frac{P_2 - P_1}{1 - P_1}, \tag{8.9}$$

which was introduced in Section 6.7 as *Sheps' relative difference.*

Because the sample proportions p_1 and p_2 are estimates of the corresponding population proportions, an estimate of the relative difference is

$$p_e = \frac{p_2 - p_1}{1 - p_1}. \tag{8.10}$$

Its standard error (see Sheps, 1959) is approximately

$$\widehat{se}(p_e) = \frac{1}{q_1} \sqrt{\frac{p_2 q_2}{n_2} + (1 - p_e)^2 \frac{p_1 q_1}{n_1}}. \tag{8.11}$$

Walter (1975) showed, however, that more accurate inferences about f could be made by taking $\ln(1 - p_e)$ as normally distributed with a mean of $\ln(1 - f)$ and an estimated standard error of [see also (6.114)]

$$\widehat{se}\left[\ln(1 - p_e)\right] = \sqrt{\frac{p_2}{n_2 q_2} + \frac{p_1}{n_1 q_1}} \,. \tag{8.12}$$

For the data of Table 8.1, the relative difference is

$$p_e = \frac{0.80 - 0.60}{1 - 0.60} = 0.50, \tag{8.13}$$

implying that, of every 100 patients who fail to improve under the first treatment, 50 would be expected to improve under the second. The value of $\ln(1 - p_e)$ is -0.69, and an estimate of its standard error is

$$\widehat{se}\left[\ln(1 - p_e)\right] = \sqrt{\frac{0.80}{70 \times 0.20} + \frac{0.60}{80 \times 0.40}} = 0.28. \tag{8.14}$$

An approximate 95% confidence interval for $\ln(1 - f)$ is

$$-0.69 - 1.96 \times 0.28 \le \ln(1 - f) \le -0.69 + 1.96 \times 0.28,$$

or

$$-1.24 \le \ln(1 - f) \le -0.14. \tag{8.15}$$

By taking antilogarithms of the limits of this interval and then their complements from unity, one obtains an approximate 95% confidence interval for the relative difference itself:

$$0.13 \le f \le 0.71. \tag{8.16}$$

A perspective different from the usual one is required when the aim of the study is to demonstrate that two treatments are therapeutically equivalent or, at least, that they differ by an amount that is clinically unimportant. Examples of such studies and a method of analysis are given by Dunnett and Gent (1977), and considered further in Section 8.5.

8.2. THE TWO-PERIOD CROSSOVER DESIGN

Chapter 13 presents means for analyzing data from, *inter alia*, a controlled trial in which patients are first matched on characteristics associated with the outcome and then randomly assigned the treatments. An extreme example of matching is when, as in a *crossover design*, each patient serves as his own control, that is, when each patient receives each treatment.

Table 8.2. *Layout of data from a two-period crossover design*

	Order AB			Order BA	
Response to A	Response to B		Response to A	Response to B	
	Good	Poor		Good	Poor
Good	n_{11}	n_{12}	Good	m_{11}	m_{12}
Poor	n_{21}	n_{22}	Poor	m_{21}	m_{22}

Half of the sample of patients is randomly selected to be given the two treatments in one order, and the other half to be given the treatments in the reverse order. A number of factors must be guarded against in analyzing the data from such studies, however.

Meier, Free, and Jackson (1958) have shown that the order in which the treatments are given may affect the response. The following test, due to Gart (1969), is valid when order effects are present and when the outcome is measured as good or poor.

Let the data be arrayed as in Table 8.2, where, for example, n_{12} denotes the number of patients, among those receiving the treatments in the order AB, who had a good response to treatment A but a poor response to treatment B. For the sample of patients receiving the two treatments in the order AB, those with a good response to both treatments (n_{11} in number) and those with a poor response to both (n_{22} in number) provide no information about a difference between the two treatments and may be ignored in the analysis. Similarly, the $m_{11} + m_{22}$ patients with similar responses to the two treatments, among those receiving them in the order BA, are uninformative about a difference between A and B and may also be ignored.

The resulting data should be arrayed as in Table 8.3, where $n = n_{12} + n_{21}$ and $m = m_{12} + m_{21}$. If treatments A and B are equally effective, the two proportions $p_1 = n_{12}/n$ and $p_2 = m_{21}/m$ should be close; if A and B are different, p_1 and p_2 should be different. The hypothesis of equal effectiveness of the two treatments may be tested by comparing p_1 with p_2 in the standard manner (see Problem 8.2).

Table 8.3. *Layout of data from Table 8.2 to test hypothesis of equal treatment effectiveness*

Order of Treatment	Outcome		Total
	First Treatment Better	Second Treatment Better	
AB	n_{12}	n_{21}	n
BA	m_{21}	m_{12}	m
Total	$n_{12} + m_{21}$	$n_{21} + m_{21}$	$n + m$

A possibility to be guarded against in crossover studies is that a treatment's effectiveness is long-lasting and hence may affect the response to the treatment given after it. When this so-called *carry-over effect* operates, and when it is unequal for the two treatments, Grizzle (1965) has shown that for comparing their effectiveness, only the data from the first period may be used. Specifically, the responses by the subjects given one of the treatments first must be compared with the responses by the subjects given the other treatment first. The responses to the treatments given second shed light on the carry-over effects, but might just as well not have been determined if the simple effectiveness of the treatments is all that is of interest.

Differential carry-over effects may be eliminated by interposing a long dry-out period between the termination of the treatment given first and the beginning of the treatment given second. The longer the dry-out period, however, the greater the chances that patients drop out of the trial.

Crossover designs are safe when the treatments are short-acting. When the possibility exists that they are long-acting, the crossover design is to be avoided.

8.3. FACTORS AFFECTING POWER IN A RANDOMIZED CONTROLLED TRIAL

8.3.1. The Intent-to-Treat Principle

Randomized controlled trials often encounter a variety of serious problems that can compromise their validity and/or the statistical power of the hypothesis test to be conducted at the end of the trial. These problems should be anticipated in the planning stages of the trial. Patients may need to be removed from study therapy by their physicians before the end of the trial, either temporarily or permanently. Subjects may not be fully adherent in taking study medications. They may try to break the blind, share their medications with others, or take unprescribed supplements. The assigned treatment may not be delivered in a timely manner, or as intended, as when an acute treatment (e.g., for stroke) has a narrow window of application. Crossovers occur when a patient assigned to one treatment arm in fact receives all or part of the intervention from another arm. For example, a patient assigned to a surgical intervention dies before the surgery can be performed; or, vice versa, a patient assigned to a medical intervention is given surgery before the end of follow-up due to worsening symptoms. The list goes on.

In all these cases, there is an understandable temptation to "adjust" for such problems, for example, by analyzing the data according to the actual treatments received by the subjects instead of according to the groups into which they were randomized, or by excluding nonadherers from the analysis altogether. Such practices have been shown to be seriously biased, so much so that the main advantages of the randomized design (balance and avoidance of confounding bias), indeed, the entire validity of the trial, can be lost completely. See, for example, Peduzzi et al. (1991) in the context of crossovers in randomized clinical trials for treatment of ischemic heart disease comparing medical with surgical treatment. The only analytic technique known to preserve a valid Type I error rate in the presence of these deficiencies, which thereby preserves the advantages of the randomized design, follows the so-called *intent-to-treat* principle, also called the intention-to-treat principle (Peto et al., 1976). All other attempts to redress what happened after randomization are potentially biased, some more seriously than others (Peduzzi et al., 1991).

The intent-to-treat principle has two components: (i) all patients, once randomized, are analyzed; (ii) patients are analyzed as members of the group to which they were initially randomized, irrespective of any nonadherence, treatment crossovers, behavior, or anything else. Component (i) rules out so-called *completers-only* and *compliers-only* analyses. Component (ii) rules out so-called *as-treated* analyses. The intent-to-treat principle calls for *as-randomized* analysis.

Another way to interpret the as-randomized analysis is that it compares a *policy* of treatment with one therapy versus another, rather than actual treatment with one therapy versus another. Whether this is merely a semantic distinction or an important substantive distinction depends on context. From a public health or outcome effectiveness perspective, it may be exactly the *policy* of treatment that is important, in the real world where therapies are not given or received under ideal laboratory conditions. How many people will *actually* be cured if we follow the policy of prescribing *A* versus *B*? From an etiologic or purely clinical perspective, the intent-to-treat analysis may be of less interest. If the treatment regimen were followed perfectly, how well could we do? Whatever one's perspective, it may suffice to point out that most, if not all, modern, large-scale, randomized clinical trials follow the intent-to-treat principle for their primary analysis.

So the statistical arguments (for preserving the validity of a randomized trial's test of the null hypothesis) strongly favor analysis under the intent-to-treat principle. That said, it should also be clear that there is an attendant inflation of Type II error and dilution of statistical power associated with the intent-to-treat analysis when crossovers and nonadherence exist. Therefore, the best procedure when conducting trials is to make every effort to minimize the rate of crossovers and nonadherence. When they are few in number, analysis by intent to treat has only a minimal effect on power, and is well worth that cost in exchange for validity of the primary test of the null hypothesis. This was the context originally envisaged by Peto and colleagues, to accommodate a relatively small number of patients who could not tolerate the side effects of active chemotherapy. On the other hand, when crossover or nonadherence is massive, failure to reject the null hypothesis on the basis of an intent-to-treat analysis should not be misinterpreted as evidence of no effect, because the power of the test can be severely impaired. But as-treated analyses may be fraught with bias, so the best that might be said of such a disastrous situation is that the randomized trial failed to meet its objectives of clarifying the science and altering clinical equipoise. See Weinstein and Levin (1989) for an example and discussion of the problems of large-scale crossover in the context of a coronary artery surgery trial.

To illustrate the effect of crossover on statistical power, consider the following simple example. A two-arm randomized trial is being planned to compare an experimental drug with a standard drug. The expected success rate with the standard treatment is $P_1 = 0.60$, and the investigators deem it important to declare as statistically significant an improvement in the success rate with the experimental treatment to $P_2 = 0.80$ (the *design alternative*). They choose the level of significance at 0.05, two-tailed, and require 80% power at the design alternative. Consulting Table A.4, equal sample sizes of $n = 91$ per group are required.

Suppose now that the experimental drug has unpleasant side effects, such that 25% of participants on that therapy cross over to standard treatment, and assume none on the standard drug cross over to the experimental treatment. What is the effective power of the test of the null hypothesis of no treatment difference under the intent-to-treat principle, assuming the design alternative is true? (Or, more precisely, what is the effective power of the test of the null hypothesis of no difference between the *policy*, or intention, to treat with one drug versus the other?) If those who do not cross over experience the hypothesized success rate P_2 of the experimental treatment, while those who do cross over experience the expected success rate P_1 of the standard treatment, then the group initially randomized to the experimental drug can be expected to have a success rate of $0.75 \times 0.80 + 0.25 \times 0.60 = 0.75 = P_2'$. From Table A4 we find the power of the test has fallen to approximately 50% . In order to recoup 80% power, $n = 165$ subjects per group would have to be enrolled, an increase in sample size of over 80%.

An actual trial can have crossovers in both directions, further reducing power. We note from expression (4.19) that because $P_1 - P_2$ appears as a *squared* term in the denominator of the sample size formula, the impact of the dilution of effect by crossover is much greater than might be intuited, and is generally inadequately counteracted by increasing the original sample size by the fraction of crossovers anticipated. Note also that the assumption made in the illustration (that those crossing over to standard treatment would have success rate P_1 while those not crossing over would remain with success rate P_2) is speculative and would require substantiation in practice. The subgroups of crossovers and noncrossovers are not randomized, and can exhibit selection biases of unknown magnitude and direction.

For example, in the Coronary Artery Surgery Study discussed in Weinstein and Levin (1989), patients were randomized to medical therapy or coronary artery bypass graft (CABG) surgery. If a patient's symptoms of coronary artery disease worsened, the treating physician was at liberty to recommend surgery. Of the patients initially randomized to medical therapy, about 25% had received CABG surgery (i.e., were crossovers) after five years of follow-up; crossover was as high as 38% among patients with triple vessel disease. Of those randomized to the surgery group 11% did not receive the surgery. One might think that the patients assigned to medical therapy who crossed over to surgery would have a higher mortality rate than those originally assigned to surgery, due to their selection as patients with worsening symptoms. In fact, the medical-to-surgical crossover subgroup had a substantially lower mortality rate than those initially assigned to surgery. This might have been due to a *survivor effect*, that is, candidates for late operation years after entering the study who are still well enough to undergo operation may have lower mortality than others. Whatever the clinical explanation, such *post hoc* rationalizations for the direction and magnitude of bias are difficult to predict or defend. The intent-to-treat analysis produced a valid test of the null hypothesis (in terms of Type I error) unaffected by any subgroup biases. In terms of statistical power, however, the effect of the crossovers was startling.

By one calculation, the intent-to-treat analysis had a power of only 33% to detect a true mortality difference equal to that observed in the trial. Five-year mortality was estimated at 8.0% for the medically assigned group versus 5.5% for the surgically assigned group. The difference of 2.5 percentage points is of considerable public health significance, amounting to a saving of about 25,000 lives per one million patients at risk with this common disease (Weinstein and Levin, 1989). To make matters worse, the published finding of no significant difference was misconstrued in the popular media as evidence supporting a policy of deferred surgery. For further discussion of this particular clinical trial, see Weinstein and Levin (1985), Fisher et al. (1989), Weinstein and Levin (1990), and Kannel (1990).

The lesson to be learned from this and cases like it is that the intent-to-treat principle should be reported as the primary analysis, because of its general validity, but the results should always be accompanied by careful interpretation, especially in the presence of nonnegligible crossover or other nonadherence. Well in advance of the trial, investigators need to plan to enroll sufficiently many participants to maintain good statistical power in the face of likely crossovers, which will be substantially more than the expected number of nonadherers. Interim analyses are useful during the trial to assess the magnitude of the problem and to make appropriate sample size corrections. On this point, see also Bigger et al. (1998).

8.3.2. Noninferiority and Equivalence Trials

A *noninferiority trial* is designed to show that a new treatment is not substantially worse than a standard treatment. A definition is required for "not substantially worse," which we will call the *limit of indifference*. For example, the success rate for standard treatment might be 75%, but because of unpleasant side effects, an alternative medication without those side effects would have better adherence, and therefore might be acceptable for general use even if its efficacy were slightly less than 75%. If a success rate of 70% or more is deemed "not substantially worse" than the standard, but below 70% unacceptable, the limit of indifference would be 5 percentage points. The limit of indifference could also be expressed in terms of a rate ratio or an odds ratio.

An *equivalence trial* is designed to show that a new treatment is neither substantially worse nor substantially better than another treatment. Again, a definition is required, and in this case, a *zone of indifference* is identified such that two treatments with success rate differences (or ratios) falling within it are regarded as effectively equivalent. The zone of indifference has a lower and an upper limit of indifference. In the above example, the zone of indifference might be taken as plus or minus 5 percentage points, to reflect a clinical judgment that if the new treatment had a true success rate less than 70%, it would be considered inferior to the standard treatment, and if more than 80%, it would be considered superior, assuming the standard had a true success rate of 75%. Otherwise the new treatment would be considered clinically equivalent to the standard.

For a noninferiority trial, the sample size required to achieve a given power under the alternative hypothesis when $P_1 = P_0$ is *not necessarily larger* than the sample size for the corresponding one-tailed test of the null hypothesis of no difference which gives the same power when the difference between the success rates is at the limit of indifference. This is contrary to a popular myth that noninferiority trials, like equivalence trials, require larger sample sizes than conventional tests. An example is given below. The biggest factor causing a large sample size is the choice of an indifference zone that is too narrow. For an equivalence trial, the sample size required to achieve a given power under the alternative hypothesis when $P_1 = P_0$ tends to be somewhat larger at typical error rates than the sample size for the corresponding two-tailed test of the null hypothesis of no difference which gives the same power when the difference between the success rates is at the limit of indifference. The increase in sample size, however, is not as great as is sometimes assumed, and depends on the Type I and II error rates. Therefore, these designs deserve full and careful consideration. In particular, in situations where a placebo-controlled trial would be deemed unethical because an active-control therapy is available, the hypotheses tested by a noninferiority or equivalence trial would become the relevant ones to consider.

A novel feature of the noninferiority or equivalence trial is the transposition of what might be expected to be the null and alternative hypothses. For a two-arm, randomized noninferiority trial, the null hypothesis is that the new treatment is inferior to the standard, and one seeks to reject that hypothesis in favor of the alternative that the new treatment is not inferior. If $\Delta > 0$ denotes the limit of indifference, P_0 the success rate for the standard treatment, and P_1 the success rate for the new treatment, then we can write $H_0: P_1 \leq P_0 - \Delta$ and $H_1: P_1 > P_0 - \Delta$.

Suppose a noninferiority trial is planned with a maximum Type I error rate of $\alpha = 0.05$ (for incorrectly declaring the new treatment noninferior to the standard when in fact it is inferior, i.e., $P_1 \leq P_0 - \Delta$), and power $1 - \beta = 0.80$ (for correctly declaring the new treatment noninferior to the standard when in fact $P_1 = P_0$). For large sample sizes n_1 and n_0, and corresponding sample proportions p_1 and p_0, the critical region is $z \geq z_\alpha$, where

$$z = \frac{p_1 - p_0 + \Delta - \frac{1}{2}\left(\frac{1}{n_0} + \frac{1}{n_1}\right)}{\sqrt{\dfrac{\hat{P}_0 \hat{Q}_0}{n_0} + \dfrac{(\hat{P}_0 - \Delta)(\hat{Q}_0 + \Delta)}{n_1}}}, \qquad (8.17)$$

where $\hat{P}_0$ is the maximum likelihood estimate of the standard treatment success rate subject to the constraint that the difference between success rates is at the limit of indifference. $\hat{P}_0$ satisfies the likelihood equation

$$\frac{p_0 - \hat{P}_0}{\hat{P}_0(1 - \hat{P}_0)/n_0} + \frac{p_1 - (\hat{P}_0 - \Delta)}{(\hat{P}_0 - \Delta)(1 - \hat{P}_0 + \Delta)/n_1} = 0. \qquad (8.18)$$

Expression (8.18) is a cubic equation in $\hat{P}_0$, and expresses the relation that when the theoretical proportions are at the maximum likelihood estimates $P_0 = \hat{P}_0$ and $P_1 = \hat{P}_0 - \Delta$, a weighted average of the differences between observed and theoretical proportions (with weights proportional to the squared standard errors of the differences) equals zero. The z-score in (8.17) has a standard normal distribution, approximately, under the null hypothesis when the difference in success rates is at the limit of indifference.

The power of the test for arbitrary P_0 and P_1 in large samples is given approximately by

$$\text{power} = \Phi\left(\frac{\Delta + (P_1 - P_0) - \frac{1}{2}\left(\frac{1}{n_0} + \frac{1}{n_1}\right)}{\sqrt{\dfrac{P_0 Q_0}{n_0} + \dfrac{P_1 Q_1}{n_1}}} \right.$$

$$\left. -z_\alpha \sqrt{\frac{\dfrac{P_0^* Q_0^*}{n_0} + \dfrac{(P_0^* - \Delta)(Q_0^* + \Delta)}{n_1}}{\dfrac{P_0 Q_0}{n_0} + \dfrac{P_1 Q_1}{n_1}}} \right), \qquad (8.19)$$

where $\Phi(x)$ is the area under the standard normal density function to the left of x, and where P_0^* is the solution of (8.18) when p_0 is replaced by P_0 and

p_1 is replaced by P_1. For equal sample sizes $n_1 = n_0 = n$, say, at the alternative hypothesis of perfect equivalence, $P_1 = P_0 = P$, say, (8.19) reduces to

power (at $P_1 = P_0 = P$)

$$= \Phi\left(\frac{\Delta\sqrt{n} - 1/\sqrt{n} - z_\alpha\sqrt{P^*Q^* + (P^* - \Delta)(Q^* + \Delta)}}{\sqrt{2PQ}} \right). \quad (8.20)$$

Consider the example at the beginning of this section, with $\Delta = 0.05$. Taking equal sample sizes of $n_0 = n_1 = n$ per group, the solution of (8.18) when 0.75 replaces both p_0 and p_1 is $P^* = 0.7733$, with $P^* - \Delta = 0.7233$. Substituting this in (8.20), one finds that the test will have power 80% at $P_0 = P_1 = P = 0.75$ when $n = 968$ per group.

How does this compare to a conventional test of the null hypothesis H_0: $P_1 \geq P_0$ versus the alternative hypothesis H_1: $P_1 < P_0$ for a one-sided "inferiority" trial? Entering Table A4 with $\alpha = 0.10$ (for a one-sided test at the 0.05 level of significance), we find the required sample size for 80% power when $P_1 = 0.70$ and $P_0 = 0.75$ to be *greater* than 968 per group ($n = 1025$ subjects per group are required). This can be explained by comparing expression (8.19) with the corresponding expression for the power of the conventional test:

$$\Phi\left(\frac{(P_0 - P_1) - \frac{1}{2}\left(\frac{1}{n_0} + \frac{1}{n_1}\right)}{\sqrt{\frac{P_0 Q_0}{n_0} + \frac{P_1 Q_1}{n_1}}} - z_\alpha \sqrt{\frac{\overline{PQ}\left(\frac{1}{n_0} + \frac{1}{n_1}\right)}{\frac{P_0 Q_0}{n_0} + \frac{P_1 Q_1}{n_1}}} \right), \quad (8.21)$$

where $\overline{P} = 1 - \overline{Q} = (n_0 P_0 + n_1 P_1)/(n_0 + n_1)$. The only difference between (8.19), with $P_1 = P_0 = P$, and (8.21), with $P_0 - P_1 = \Delta$, is the quantity $P^*Q^*/n_0 + (P^* - \Delta)(Q^* + \Delta)/n_1$ in the first expression versus $\overline{PQ}(1/n_0 + 1/n_1)$ in the second. For this illustration with equal sample sizes, the numerator of the first quantity is $0.7733 \times 0.2267 + 0.7233 \times 0.2767 = 0.3754$, which is less than the numerator of the second quantity, $2\overline{PQ} = 2 \times 0.725 \times 0.275 = 0.3988$. Consequently the power in (8.19) or (8.20) is greater than the power in (8.21).

The situation is a little different for an equivalence trial. The null hypothesis is that the new treatment is not equivalent to the standard, and one seeks to reject that hypothesis in favor of the alternative hypothesis of equivalence. Note in this case that the null hypothesis is a composite region for the difference of the success rates, consisting of two disjoint intervals. For a symmetric zone of indifference of the form $|P_1 - P_0| < \Delta$, we have H_0: $P_1 \leq P_0 - \Delta$ or $P_1 \geq P_0 + \Delta$, and H_1: $|P_1 - P_0| < \Delta$. Now one rejects H_0 when *both* of the one-sided components of H_0 would be rejected, such that, when $z' \geq z_\alpha$ and $z'' \leq -z_\alpha$, where z' is given by (8.17) and z'' is given by

$$z'' = \frac{p_1 - p_0 - \Delta + \frac{1}{2}\left(\frac{1}{n_0} + \frac{1}{n_1}\right)}{\sqrt{\frac{\left(\hat{P}_1 - \Delta\right)\left(\hat{Q}_1 + \Delta\right)}{n_0} + \frac{\hat{P}_1\hat{Q}_1}{n_1}}}.$$ (8.22)

In (8.22), $\hat{P}_1$ is the maximum likelihood estimate of the new treatment success rate subject to the constraint that the difference between success rates is at the upper limit of indifference with $P_1 - P_0 = \Delta$, and satisfies the likelihood equation

$$\frac{p_0 - \left(\hat{P}_1 - \Delta\right)}{\left(\hat{P}_1 - \Delta\right)\left(1 - \hat{P}_1 + \Delta\right)/n_0} + \frac{p_1 - \hat{P}_1}{\hat{P}_1\left(1 - \hat{P}_1\right)/n_1} = 0.$$ (8.23)

Let us assume that the sample size is large enough so that the critical value which $p_1 - p_0$ must be no less than in the first-component test, that is, the right-hand side of

$$p_1 - p_0 \geq -\Delta + \tfrac{1}{2}\left(n_0^{-1} + n_1^{-1}\right) + z_\alpha \mathrm{se}'(p_1 - p_0),$$

is negative [with $\mathrm{se}'(p_1 - p_0)$ given by the denominator of (8.17)], while the critical value which $p_1 - p_0$ must be no greater than in the second-component test, that is, the right-hand side of

$$p_1 - p_0 \leq \Delta - \tfrac{1}{2}\left(n_0^{-1} + n_1^{-1}\right) - z_\alpha \mathrm{se}''(p_1 - p_0),$$

is positive [with $\mathrm{se}''(p_1 - p_0)$ given by the denominator of (8.22)]. Under this assumption, to conduct the test of H_0 one only needs to check one of the inequalities, $z' \geq z_\alpha$ (when $p_1 - p_0$ is negative) or $z'' \leq -z_\alpha$ (when $p_1 - p_0$ is positive); the other inequality will follow automatically, and one need not calculate $\hat{P}_1$ from (8.23) in the first case or $\hat{P}_0$ from (8.18) in the second case.

Note that the critical values for z' and z'' are $\pm z_\alpha$, not $\pm z_{\alpha/2}$. This is because rejection only occurs when both component tests reject, so that under the null hypothesis, $P(\text{reject } H_0) = P(z' \geq z_\alpha \text{ and } z'' \leq -z_\alpha)$ which is no greater than the smaller of the two probabilities $P(z' \geq z_\alpha)$ and $P(z'' \leq z_\alpha)$, each of which is no greater than α. Thus the test is slightly conservative.

The power of the test of the null hypothesis of nonequivalence is

$$P\Big[-\Delta + \tfrac{1}{2}\left(n_0^{-1} + n_1^{-1}\right) + z_\alpha \mathrm{se}'(p_1 - p_0) \leq p_1 - p_0$$

$$\leq \Delta - \tfrac{1}{2}\left(n_0^{-1} + n_1^{-1}\right) - z_\alpha \mathrm{se}''(p_1 - p_0)\Big]$$

and is given approximately in large samples for arbitrary P_0 and P_1 by

$$\text{power} = \Phi\left(\frac{\Delta - (P_1 - P_0) - \frac{1}{2}\left(\frac{1}{n_0} + \frac{1}{n_1}\right)}{\sqrt{\frac{P_0 Q_0}{n_0} + \frac{P_1 Q_1}{n_1}}}\right.$$

$$-z_\alpha\sqrt{\frac{\frac{(P_1^* - \Delta)(Q_1^* + \Delta)}{n_0} + \frac{P_1^* Q_1^*}{n_1}}{\frac{P_0 Q_0}{n_0} + \frac{P_1 Q_1}{n_1}}}\left.\right)$$

$$-\Phi\left(\frac{-\Delta - (P_1 - P_0) + \frac{1}{2}\left(\frac{1}{n_0} + \frac{1}{n_1}\right)}{\sqrt{\frac{P_0 Q_0}{n_0} + \frac{P_1 Q_1}{n_1}}}\right.$$

$$+z_\alpha\sqrt{\frac{\frac{P_0^* Q_0^*}{n_0} + \frac{(P_0^* - \Delta)(Q_0^* + \Delta)}{n_1}}{\frac{P_0 Q_0}{n_0} + \frac{P_1 Q_1}{n_1}}}\left.\right). \quad (8.24)$$

In the case of equal sample sizes, $n_1 = n_0 = n$, say, at the alternative hypothesis of perfect equivalence, $P_1 = P_0 = P$, say, (8.24) reduces to

power (at $P_1 = P_0 = P$)

$$= 2\Phi\left(\frac{\Delta\sqrt{n} - 1/\sqrt{n} - z_\alpha\sqrt{P^* Q^* + (P^* - \Delta)(Q^* + \Delta)}}{\sqrt{2PQ}}\right) - 1, \quad (8.25)$$

where P^* satisfies (8.18) or (8.23) with p_0 and p_1 replaced by P, and n_1 and n_0 replaced by n (or canceled from the equation altogether).

Returning to the example, suppose an equivalence trial is planned with the symmetrical zone of indifference $|P_1 - P_0| < \Delta$ with $\Delta = 0.05$. Taking equal sample sizes of $n_0 = n_1 = n$ per group, the solution of (8.18) with $P_0 = P_1 = P = 0.75$ replacing p_0 and p_1 is $P^* = 0.7733$ as before, and substituting this in (8.25), one finds that the test will have power 80% at $P_0 = P_1 = P = 0.75$ when $n = 1,326$ per group.

How does this compare to a conventional test of the null hypothesis $H_0: P_1 = P_0$ versus the alternative hypothesis $H_0: P_1 \neq P_0$ for a two-sided "efficacy" trial? Entering Table A4 with $\alpha = 0.05$ (for a *two-sided* test at the

0.05 level of significance), we find the required sample size for 80% power when, say, $P_1 = 0.70$ and $P_0 = 0.75$ now to be less than 1,326 per group ($n = 1,291$ subjects per group are required), but the relative difference in sample sizes is not large. Problem 8.3 explores these relations further.

8.3.3. Selection Trials

A final factor that affects the power of a trial is the study goal itself. There are occasions, represented by the class of *selection problems*, when control of the Type I error rate at the conventional levels of 0.10, 0.05, or 0.01 is totally beside the point; rather, the goal of the study shifts away from hypothesis testing and towards making a necessary selection. Suppose, for example, one of two treatments, A or B, must be given to patients with a certain condition (at least until a better therapeutic choice is found), and the goal of the study is to select the better of the two treatments. If one therapy is truly superior to the other, then we seek a selection procedure that assures the correct selection with high probability if the level of superiority exceeds the prespecified limit of indifference. If the two treatments are of equal efficacy, however, then we might be indifferent as to which treatment we select (assuming other factors like cost and side effects are equal). If the two treatments had identical success rates in the sample, for example, we might even select one of them at random. In this example, when A and B are truly equivalent, no real error would be made by selecting A or B as the apparent best treatment, and so control of such a Type I error would miss the mark of relevance. The selection problem can be framed in terms of hypothesis testing, but now with complete indifference under the null hypothesis we have $\alpha = 0.50$ (not 0.05). This allows a selection trial to be conducted with smaller sample sizes than the corresponding efficacy test that controls the Type I error rate in a conventional manner.

In the example we have been considering, suppose the purpose of the trial is not to test efficacy or to test equivalence, but rather to select either the new or the standard treatment for future care of patients with the given condition. Patients will be randomized to the two treatment arms in equal numbers, and at the end of the trial, the treatment in the group with the higher sample success rate will be declared the winner and selected for subsequent use. (In the rare event that the two success rates are exactly equal, flip a coin to select the winner. In practice, one would regard both as equivalent.) Taking the zone of indifference again to be $|P_1 - P_0| < \Delta$ with $\Delta = 0.05$, we require the procedure to have an 80% chance of correctly selecting the truly superior treatment if $|P_1 - P_0| = \Delta$, for example, if $P_1 = 0.80$ and $P_0 = 0.75$. If the sample size is n per group, the probability of correct selection is then $P(p_1 > p_0) + \frac{1}{2}P(p_1 = p_0)$ assuming the new treatment is truly better than the standard, and $P(p_1 < p_0) + \frac{1}{2}P(p_1 = p_0)$ assuming the standard treatment is truly better than the new one. In large samples the probability of the $\frac{1}{2}P(p_1 = p_0)$ term is negligible, and so the power is given approximately by

$$\Phi\left(\frac{\Delta\sqrt{n} - 1/\sqrt{n}}{\sqrt{P_1 Q_1 + P_0 Q_0}}\right). \tag{8.26}$$

For this to exceed 80% when $P_1 = 0.80$ and $P_0 = 0.75$ requires $n \geq 136$ per group. Even if the investigators could not prespecify the approximate true success rates, the trial could still be designed conservatively using the values $P_1 = 0.525$ and $P_0 = 0.475$ that maximize the denominator of (8.26), in which case a sample size of 180 per group would suffice.

From the example, it can be seen that the selection trial is an appealing design in limited-sample-size situations, especially when there is justification for the selection goal as superseding the goal of controlling the Type I error rate in a hypothesis test paradigm. The selection trial design also lends itself easily to modifications such as sequential monitoring rather than fixed sample size, and adaptive allocation (see Section 8.4 below). The interested reader may consult the textbook by Gibbons, Olkin, and Sobel (1999) for fixed-sample-size designs for selecting the best of two or more treatments or for selecting a subset of treatments with high probability of containing the best; and Lai et al. (1980) for some theory of sequential selection procedures.

8.4. ALTERNATIVES TO SIMPLE RANDOMIZATION

The need always to randomize the assignment of treatments to patients in clinical trials continues to be debated. Gehan and Freireich (1974) and Weinstein (1974), for example, offer criticisms of and propose some alternatives to the strictly randomized clinical trial, whereas Byar et al. (1976) and Peto et al. (1976) come to its defense. Levine (1999) summarizes the debate over whether or not the current reliance on randomized trials is excessive. There appear to be some instances in which competitors to randomization should be seriously considered, but these are few. One instance arises when only a small number of patients is available for study, so that recent historical controls may have to be relied upon. An Institute of Medicine report on small clinical trials considers this case (IOM Committee, 2001). Another instance is when the disease in question has a uniformly lethal outcome when untreated, and for which there is no effective therapy (Levine, 1999). We return to this issue at the end of the section.

Debate and research continues, too, with respect to the need to stratify or to match patients on prognostic factors (e.g., age, sex, and initial severity), and just how to assure comparable distributions across the strata in the two treatment groups. On one side of the debate are Peto et al. (1976), who recommend not bothering to stratify the eligible sample of patients before randomizing them to one or the other treatment group, especially when the number of patients is large. The consensus among those responsible for the design of clinical trials, however, seems to be that some degree of control, preferably stratification, is desirable to guard against unlikely but devastating imbalances between the two groups (see, e.g., Simon, 1979). Separate and independent randomizations of the patients falling into the several strata will usually suffice, but some recently proposed modifications in simple stratified randomization should be borne in mind.

These modifications are intended especially for studies in which patients enter the trial serially over time, so that it is impossible to determine at the start of the trial exactly how many patients will end up in each stratum. Suppose, for example, that a patient enters the trial at a point at which, within his stratum, more patients have been assigned treatment A than to treatment B. Instead of assigning this new patient to one treatment group or the other independently of the current imbalance in his stratum, one may adopt an allocation method that seeks to bring the numbers in the two groups closer to each other.

One method for balancing is Efron's (1971) *biased-coin* scheme, which, in the current example, would assign this patient treatment B (the underrepresented one) with a fixed, prespecified probability that is greater than $\frac{1}{2}$ but less than 1. An essentially nonrandomized method is Taves' (1974) *minimization* scheme, which would assign this patient treatment B with certainty. Randomization plays no role in minimization except for the first group of patients to enter the trial, unless the two treatment groups are balanced at the time a new patient enters the trial. Other schemes have been proposed by Pocock and Simon (1975) and simplified by Freedman and White (1976).

As Pocock (1979) has pointed out, however, the ability to execute a design is at least as important as the design's theoretical optimality. Complexity of execution plus the likely sufficiency in most instances of simple stratified randomization appear to rule out the large-scale adoption of these proposed schemes for establishing balance between the two treatment groups.

Other alternatives to the simple comparative study, termed *adaptive trials*, have been proposed because of the uniqueness of comparative clinical trials as studies aimed as much at the testing of scientific hypotheses as at the alleviation of symptoms of the patients being studied. Whereas the classic design and its modifications summarized in the preceding call for assigning the different treatments to approximately equal numbers of patients, adaptive designs call for assigning to an increasing proportion of patients the treatment that, on the basis of the accumulated data, appears to be superior.

Adaptive designs are still in the process of development and have been adopted in only a small number of trials in spite of their intuitive appeal. The interested reader is referred to Anscombe (1963), Colton (1963), Cornfield, Halperin, and Greenhouse (1969), Zelen (1969), Canner (1970), Robbins (1974), Simon (1977), and Lai et al. (1980) for some suggested means of balancing the statistical requirement of equal sample sizes with the ethical requirement of applying the superior treatment to as many patients as possible as quickly as possible. For a discussion of an application of an adaptive allocation rule in a life-threatening situation, and the ethical problems the investigators faced, see Ware (1989) and Truog (1992).

Zelen (1979) introduced a daring idea into the design of clinical trials in seeking to overcome the reluctance of many patients and the physicians responsible for their care to consent to participate in a randomized experiment. This reluctance is especially prevalent when the patients suffer from life-threatening conditions such as cancer or heart disease. Zelen's idea was to randomize eligible patients into one of the two groups characterized as follows.

All patients in the first group will receive the currently accepted standard treatment. Because this is the treatment they would receive in any event, their informed consent to participate in an experiment (it was argued) is not required. All patients in the second group will be asked whether they consent to be treated with the experimental treatment. If they consent, they will be so treated. If they refuse, they will be treated with the standard treatment. At the end of the trial, the results for *all* patients in the second group, regardless of treatment, will be compared with the results for all those in the first, that is, according to the intent-to-treat principle.

Operating to reduce the power associated with Zelen's proposed design is the fact that the response rate estimated for the second group is an average of the rate for those patients receiving the experimental treatment and the rate for those patients receiving the standard treatment. If the experimental treatment is superior to the standard, this average will be closer to the response rate in the first group than the response rate would be in a group of patients treated exclusively with the experimental treatment.

Operating in favor of the proposed design is the presumption that much larger numbers of patients will be studied. The traditional design requires that an eligible patient give informed consent to participate in the trial before that patient is randomized. The proposed design would permit all eligible patients to be randomized; a patient's refusal to give consent would not result in that patient's being dropped from the study. The enrolled patients would represent a wider cross section of the population, and thus make the trial more "pragmatic" (Schwartz and Lellouch, 1967). The increased power due to the larger numbers of patients might overcome the decreased power due to the attenuated difference between the two groups.

The last twenty years have not seen widespread use of Zelen's (1979) proposal. In response to criticisms on ethical grounds, namely, that therapy would be assigned by chance without the participant's knowledge or consent, Zelen (1981) proposed a modified design in which randomization before consent would still take place, but would be followed by securing of informed consent from participants in each treatment group. This design has been used in several major randomized trials (Ellenberg, 1984), but is not without its own difficulties, to wit, the potential for major bias to be introduced in the unblinded negotiation of informed consent by clinicians and subjects, and whether or not participation at all in the trial is presented as an option.

Ellenberg (1984) finds the evidence lacking to support the presumed gains in efficiency in these so-called *prerandomization* designs. Insofar as enrollment is not substantially increased with these modified designs, power considerations alone would dictate against their use. In addition, current standards for the ethical conduct of research with human subjects generally require informed consent whenever patients participate in an experiment in which their therapy is chosen by chance, that is., informed consent is required explicitly for the randomized assignment of therapy (Levine, 1999).

We mentioned at the beginning of this section the existence of circumstances under which a randomized controlled trial might not be feasible or ethical to conduct from the start. One design for a clinical trial that avoids the considerable problems of historical controls was discussed by Finkelstein, Levin, and Robbins (1996a, 1996b), and we consider it briefly here, even though it is a nonrandomized design. Called an *assured allocation design*, or *risk-based allocation design* by these authors, it was proposed for use in situations where it is overwhelmingly clear that the randomized design would fail, either because subject enrollment would be close to zero, or when ethical concerns dictate against randomization in life-threatening illnesses.

The first situation arises, for example, when a therapy is readily available outside the study protocol, or when a treatment has been in use for a long time and is perceived to be efficacious, even though it has never been subjected to a randomized trial. Bone marrow transplantation (BMT) in the treatment of advanced breast disease is an illustration. A nationwide, multi-center, randomized trial was designed to test the efficacy of bone marrow extraction prior to aggressive chemotherapy followed by BMT in women with at least ten underarm nodes of tumor involvement. The comparison group was "standard of care" omitting the bone marrow procedures. BMT was widely available outside the clinical trial, which drastically slowed down patient enrollment: the target sample size of 982 women took over seven years to achieve (between 1991 and 1998), while more than 15,000 procedures were administered during this time period. If only one-half of the women receiving off-protocol BMTs could have been enrolled in the trial, the target sample size would have been reached before two years. The difficulty was that when subjects were informed they faced a 50% chance of being randomized to the comparison group, they withheld consent in order to obtain BMT elsewhere, often just across town (e.g., in New York City). It is a tribute to the investigators' and funding agency's perseverance to have followed this trial to its conclusion. Yet one has to wonder if the same answer achieved after seven years (no survival benefit) might not have been reached much sooner with a risk-based allocation design, saving many women from undergoing a very painful, expensive, and—ultimately—questionable surgical procedure.

Other examples exist of desperately ill patients or their caregivers seeking experimental treatments as their perceived last hope who would refuse to be randomized, e.g., in the early days of AIDS trials and with extracorporeal membrane oxygenation (ECMO) for premature infants. Other therapies, such as pulmonary artery catheterization (Swan–Ganz), estrogen treatment for Alzheimer's disease, or radical surgery for prostate cancer, have all been next to impossible to test in randomized trials because subjects convinced of therapeutic benefits do not want the placebo or standard therapy. These therapies have often been cited in the news media for the difficulty or near-impossibility of recruiting subjects into randomized trials—see Kolata (1995), Altman (1996), Kolata (1997), Brody (1997), and Kolata and Eichenwald (1999).

In the risk-based allocation design, all participants who exceed a prespecified threshold of risk measured at baseline are assigned to the experimental therapy. Nothing about the experimental therapy is assumed known beyond the usual preliminary safety and efficacy checks. Those who do not exceed the prespecified threshold of risk are assigned, as *concurrent controls*, to the standard therapy, about which much prior experience is assumed known. Specifically, one requires a *model* for the standard treatment (but only the standard treatment) that relates the average or expected outcome to specific values of the baseline measure of risk used for the allocation. For example, the model might specify that the standard treatment affects the expected outcome multiplicatively on a patient-by-patient basis. Only the functional form of the model is required, not specific values of the model parameters, because the parameters of the model are estimated from the concurrent control data, and then extrapolated to the high-risk patients. This is a real advantage over historical controlled studies. One need not rely on historical estimates of expected outcome means or proportions, which are notoriously untrustworthy for transport to other times or patient populations. All one needs to assume for the risk-based design is that the mathematical form of the model relating outcome to risk is correctly specified throughout the entire range of the risk measure. This is a strong assumption, to be sure, but with sufficient experience and prior data on the standard treatment, the form of the model can be validated. In addition, the validity of the predictive model can be checked against the concurrent control data in the risk-based trial, at least below threshold.

Because of the biased allocation of subjects to treatment arms, a simple comparison of outcomes between the two groups is *not* appropriate, as it is for a randomized trial. Rather, the appropriate analysis utilizes empirical Bayes methods of estimation to provide a valid estimate of the treatment effect among the high-risk patients. As indicated above, the heart of the analysis is an estimation of the expected outcome the high-risk patients would have had on average under the standard therapy. Empirical Bayes methods are ideally suited for these purposes because of their characteristic ability to use information from one group of subjects to make valid inferences about another group, even when the two groups are not directly comparable, as in the present case, by design.

Further discussion of the analytic technique is beyond the scope of this chapter, but for details, the interested reader should see: Finkelstein, Levin, and Robbins (1996a, 1996b) for examples and a demonstration of feasibility of the method in the context of controlled clinical trials, and the IOM (2001) report cited above for further discussion; Robbins (1956, 1977) for a series of landmark papers on the theory of general empirical Bayes estimation, also contained in the collection of papers by Robbins edited by Lai and Siegmund (1985); and Robbins and Zhang (1988, 1989, 1991) and Robbins (1993) for development of statistical methods adapted to the needs of a risk-based allocation design. The risk-based allocation design has often been used to evaluate social or behavioral interventions, in which fields it goes under the somewhat misleading name of "regression discontinuity" (see Campbell and Stanley, 1963, and Cook and Campbell, 1979). Cappelleri and Trochim (1994) and Trochim and Cappelleri (1992) discuss the method in the context of randomized clinical trials. Whether risk-based allocation will be used in clinical research when a randomized trial would not be feasible remains to be seen.

PROBLEMS

8.1. Suppose that the two treatments contrasted in Table 8.1 are compared in a second hospital, with the following results:

	Number of Patients	Proportion Improved
Treatment 1	100	0.35
Treatment 2	100	0.75
Overall	200	0.55

(a) Is the difference between the improvement rates significant in the second hospital?

(b) What is the simple difference [see (8.2)] between the two improvement rates in the second hospital? What is its estimated standard error [see (8.3)]? Is the difference found in the second hospital significantly different from that found in the first? [*Hint.* Denote the difference and its estimated standard error found in (8.4) and (8.5) by d_1 and $\widehat{se}(d_1)$, and denote the corresponding statistics just calculated by d_2 and $\widehat{se}(d_2)$. Refer the value of

$$z = \frac{|d_2 - d_1|}{\sqrt{\left\{\widehat{se}(d_1)\right\}^2 + \left\{\widehat{se}(d_2)\right\}^2}}$$

to Table A.1 of the normal distribution.]

(c) What is the relative difference [see (8.10)] between the two improvement rates in the second hospital? Is it significantly different from the relative difference found in the first hospital? [*Hint*. Define $L_1 = \ln\{1 - p_{e(1)}\}$ and $L_2 = \ln\{1 - p_{e(2)}\}$. Refer the value of

$$z = \frac{|L_2 - L_1|}{\sqrt{\left\{\widehat{se}(L_1)\right\}^2 + \left\{\widehat{se}(L_2)\right\}^2}}$$

to Table A.1.]

8.2. Suppose two treatments were compared in a two-period crossover design, with results as follows:

	Order AB			Order BA	
Response to A	Response to B		Response to A	Response to B	
	Good	Poor		Good	Poor
Good	20	15	Good	30	10
Poor	5	10	Poor	5	5

(a) Consider first the sample of patients given the treatments in the order AB. What is the value of n (i.e., how many of these patients gave responses that were informative about a difference between A and B)? What is the value of p_1 (i.e., what proportion of these n patients had a good response to the treatment given first)?

(b) Consider next the sample of patients given the treatments in the order BA. What is the value of m? What is the value of p_2?

(c) Test whether treatments A and B are equally effective by comparing p_1 with p_2.

8.3. When does a noninferiority or an equivalence trial require a larger sample size than a conventional one-sided or two-sided efficacy trial design? In this problem we abstract from the difficulties of nonconstant standard errors and consider the following idealized situation. We observe normally distributed random variables with known, constant standard deviation σ, in two groups of equal sample size n. We obtain the sample mean difference, $\bar{X}_1 - \bar{X}_0$, which has a normal distribution with mean $\mu_1 - \mu_0$ and standard error $\sigma(2/n)^{1/2}$. Larger values of the mean are considered better than smaller values.

(a) The null hypothesis in a noninferiority trial is H_0: $\mu_1 - \mu_0 \leq -\Delta$, and the alternative is H_1: $\mu_1 - \mu_0 > -\Delta$. Show that the sample size necessary to achieve power $1 - \beta$ when the alternative of perfect equivalence $\mu_1 = \mu_0$ holds is $n = 2\sigma^2(z_\alpha + z_\beta)^2/\Delta^2$.

(b) The null hypothesis in a one-sided efficacy trial is H_0: $\mu_1 - \mu_0 \leq 0$, and the alternative hypothesis is H_1: $\mu_1 - \mu_0 > 0$. Show that the sample size necessary to achieve power $1 - \beta$ when the alternative $\mu_1 - \mu_0 = \Delta$ holds is the same, $n = 2\sigma^2(z_\alpha + z_\beta)^2/\Delta^2$. Conclude that the two trial designs are equivalent under these assumptions.

(c) The null hypothesis in an equivalence trial is H_0: $\mu_1 - \mu_0 \leq -\Delta$ or $\mu_1 - \mu_0 \geq \Delta$, and the alternative hypothesis is H_1: $|\mu_1 - \mu_0| < \Delta$. Show that the sample size necessary to achieve power $1 - \beta$ when the alternative of perfect equivalence $\mu_1 = \mu_0$ holds is $n = 2\sigma^2(z_\alpha + z_{\beta/2})^2/\Delta^2$. [*Hint*. A rejection of H_0 occurs when both of the following inequalities are true:

$$-\Delta + z_\alpha \sigma\sqrt{2/n} \leq \bar{X}_1 - \bar{X}_0 \leq \Delta - z_\alpha \sigma\sqrt{2/n} .$$

so the power under the alternative $\mu_1 = \mu_0$ is

$$\Phi\left(\frac{\Delta\sqrt{n}}{\sigma\sqrt{2}} - z_\alpha\right) - \Phi\left(\frac{-\Delta\sqrt{n}}{\sigma\sqrt{2}} + z_\alpha\right) = 2\Phi\left(\frac{\Delta\sqrt{n}}{\sigma\sqrt{2}} - z_\alpha\right) - 1.$$

For this to equal $1 - \beta$, the argument of Φ on the right-hand side must equal $z_{\beta/2}$.]

(d) The null hypothesis in a two-sided efficacy trial is H_0: $\mu_1 - \mu_0 = 0$, and the alternative hypothesis is H_1: $\mu_1 - \mu_0 \neq 0$. Show that the sample size necessary to achieve power $1 - \beta$ when the alternative $\mu_1 - \mu_0 = \Delta$ holds is $n = 2\sigma^2(z_{\alpha/2} + z_\beta)^2/\Delta^2$.

(e) Comparing (c) and (d), conclude that the equivalence trial in this idealized situation requires a greater sample size than the two-sided efficacy trial if and only if $z_\alpha + z_{\beta/2} \geq z_{\alpha/2} + z_\beta$. Evaluate these expressions for $\alpha = 0.05$ and $\beta = 0.20$. Which trial requires the greater sample size? What happens if $\alpha = \beta$?

REFERENCES

Altman, L. K. (1996). Safety of catheter into the heart is questioned, startling doctors. *The New York Times*, September 18, A1.

Anscombe, F. J. (1963). Sequential medical trials. *J. Am. Statist. Assoc.*, **58**, 365–384.

Anturane Reinfarction Trial Research Group (1978). Sulfinpyrazone in the prevention of cardiac death after myocardial infarction: The anturane reinfarction trial. *New Engl. J. Med.*, **298**, 290–295.

Armitage, P. (1975). *Sequential medical trials*, 2nd ed. New York: Wiley.

Bigger, J. T., Parides, M. K., Rolnitzky, L. M., Meier, P., Levin, B., and Egan, D. A. (1998). Changes in sample size and length of follow-up to maintain power in the coronary artery bypass graft (CABG) patch trial. *Controlled Clinical Trials*, **19**, 1–14.

Brody, J. (1997). Alzheimer studies thwarted. *The New York Times*, March 5, C10.

Byar, D. P., Simon, R. H., Friedewald, W. T., Schlesselman, J. J., DeMets, D. L., Ellenberg, J. H., Gail, M. H., and Ware, J. H. (1976). Randomized clinical trials: Perspectives on some recent ideas. *New Engl. J. Med.*, **295**, 74–80.

Campbell, D. T. and Stanley, J. C. (1963). *Experimental and quasi-experimental designs for research*. Chicago: Rand McNally.

Canner, P. L. (1970). Selecting one of two treatments when the responses are dichotomous. *J. Am. Statist. Assoc.*, **65**, 293–306.

Cappelleri, J. C. and Trochim, W. M. K. (1994). An illustrative statistical analysis of cutoff-based randomized clinical trials. *J. Clin. Epidemiol.*, **47**, 261–270.

Colton, T. (1963). A model for selecting one of two medical treatments. *J. Am. Statist. Assoc.*, **58**, 388–401.

Cook, T. D. and Campbell, D. T. (1979). *Quasi-experimentation: Design and analysis issues for field settings*. Boston: Houghton Mifflin.

Cornfield, J., Halperin, M., and Greenhouse, S. W. (1969). An adaptive procedure for sequential clinical trials. *J. Am. Statist. Assoc.*, **64**, 759–770.

Dunnett, C. W., and Gent, M. (1977). Significance testing to establish equivalence between treatments with special reference to data in the form of 2×2 tables. *Biometrics*, **33**, 593–602.

Efron, B. (1971). Forcing a sequential experiment to be balanced. *Biometrika*, **58**, 403–417.

Ellenberg, S. S. (1984). Randomization designs in comparative clinical trials. *New Engl. J. Med.*, **310**, 1404–1408.

Ellenberg, S. S., Fleming, T. R., and DeMets, D. L. (2002). *Data monitoring committees in clinical trials: A practical perspective*. New York: John Wiley and Sons.

Everitt, B. S. and Pickles, A. (2000). *Statistical aspects of the design and analysis of clinical trials*. London: Imperial College Press.

Finkelstein, M. O., Levin, B., and Robbins, H. (1996a). Clinical and prophylactic trials with assured new treatment for those at greater risk. Part I—introduction. *Am. J. Public Health*, **86**, 691–695.

Finkelstein, M. O., Levin, B., and Robbins, H. (1996b). Clinical and prophylactic trials with assured new treatment for those at greater risk. Part II—examples. *Am. J. Public Health*, **86**, 696–705.

Fisher, L. D., Kaiser, G. C., Davis, K. B., and Mock, M. B. (1989). Crossovers in coronary artery bypass grafting trials: Desirable, undesirable, or both? (Editorial). *Ann. Thorac. Surg.*, **48**, 465–466.

Fox, T. F. (1959). The ethics of clinical trials. Pp. 222–229 in D. R. Laurence (Ed.), *Quantitative methods in human pharmacology and therapeutics*. New York: Pergamon Press.

Freedman, L. S. and White, S. J. (1976). On the use of Pocock and Simon's method for balancing treatment numbers over prognostic factors in the controlled clinical trial. *Biometrics*, **32**, 691–694.

Friedman, J. A., Chalmers, T. C., Smith, H., and Kuebler, R. R. (1978). The importance of Beta, the type II error and sample size in the design and interpretation of the randomized control trial: Survey of 71 "negative" trials. *New Engl. J. Med.*, **299**, 690–694.

Friedman, L. M. and DeMets, D. L. (1981). The data monitoring committee: How it operates and why. *IRB: Rev. Human Subjects Res.*, **3**, 6–8.

Friedman, L. M., Furberg, C., and DeMets, D. L. (1998). *Fundamentals of clinical trials*, 3rd ed. New York: Springer-Verlag.

Gart, J. J. (1969). An exact test for comparing matched proportions in crossover designs. *Biometrika*, **56**, 75–80.

Gehan, E. A. and Freireich, E. J. (1974). Non-randomized controls in cancer clinical trials. *New Engl. J. Med.*, **290**, 198–203.

Gibbons, J. D., Olkin, I., and Sobel, M. (1999). *Selecting and ordering populations: A new statistical methodology*. Classics in Applied Mathematics, #26. Philadelphia: SIAM.

Grizzle, J. E. (1965). The two-period change-over design and its use in clinical trials. *Biometrics*, **21**, 467–480.

Hill, A. B. (1962). *Statistical methods in clinical and preventive medicine*. New York: Oxford University Press.

Institute of Medicine Committee on Strategies for Small-Number-Participant Clinical Research Trials (2001). *Small clinical trials—issues and challenges*, C. H. Evans and S. T. Ildstad (Eds.). Washington: National Academy Press.

Jennison, C. and Turnbull, B. (1999). *Group sequential methods with applications to clinical trials*. Boca Raton, Fla.: Chapman & Hall/CRC Press.

Kannel, W. B. (1990). Coronary Artery Surgery Study revisited—limitation of the intent-to-treat principle. *Circulation*, **82**, 1859–1862.

Kolata, G. (1995). Women resist trials to test marrow transplants. *The New York Times*, February 15, C8.

Kolata, G. (1997). Lack of volunteers thwarts research on prostate cancer. *The New York Times*, February 12, A18.

Kolata, G. and Eichenwald, K. (1999). Business thrives on unproven care, leaving science behind. *The New York Times*, October 3, A1.

Lai, T.-L., Levin, B., Robbins, H., and Siegmund, D. O. (1980). Sequential medical trials. *Proc. Nat. Acad. Sci. U.S.A.*, **77**, 3135–3138.

Lai, T.-L. and Siegmund, D. O. (1985). *Herbert Robbins Selected Papers*. New York: Springer-Verlag.

Levin, B. (2003). No, *not* another IRB. Review of Ellenberg, Fleming, and DeMets, 2002. *IRB: Ethics and Human Research*, **25**, 17–18.

Levine, R. J. (1999). Randomized clinical trials: Ethical considerations. *Advances in Bioethics*, Vol. 5. Pp. 114–115 in R. B. Edwards and E. E. Bittar (Eds.) Stamford: JAI Press.

Mainland, D. (1960). The clinical trial—some difficulties and suggestions. *J. Chronic. Dis.*, **11**, 484–496.

Meier, P. (1975). Statistics and medical experimentation. *Biometrics*, **31**, 511–529.

Meier, P. (1979). Terminating a trial—The ethical problem. *Clin. Pharmacol. Ther.*, **25**, 633–640.

Meier, P., Free, S. M., and Jackson, G. L. (1958). Reconsideration of methodology in studies of pain relief. *Biometrics*, **14**, 330–342.

Peduzzi, P., Detre, K., Wittes, J., and Holford, T. (1991). Intent-to-treat analysis and the problem of crossovers—an example from the Veterans Administration coronary bypass surgery study. *J. Thorac. Cardiovasc. Surg.*, **101**, 481–487.

Peto, R., Pike, M. C., Armitage, P., Breslow, N. E., Cox, D. R., Howard, S. V., Mantel, N., McPherson, K., Peto, J., and Smith, P. G. (1976). Design and analysis of randomized clinical trials requiring prolonged observation of each patient. I. Introduction and design. *Brit. J. Cancer*, **34**, 585–612.

Piantadosi, S. (1997). *Clinical trials: A methodologic perspective*. New York: Wiley.

Pocock, S. J. (1979). Allocation of patients to treatment in clinical trials. *Biometrics*, **35**, 183–197.

Pocock, S. J. (1984). *Clinical trials: A practical approach*. New York: Wiley.

Pocock, S.J. and Simon, R. (1975). Sequential treatment assignment with balancing for prognostic factors in the controlled clinical trial. *Biometrics*, **31**, 103–115.

Report of the Committee for the Assessment of Biometric Aspects of Controlled Trials of Hypoglycemic Agents. (1975). *J. Am. Med. Assoc.*, **231**, 583–608.

Robbins, H. (1956). An empirical Bayes approach to statistics. Pp. 157–163 in *Proc. Third Berkeley Symposium Math. Statist. Probab.*, Vol 1. Univ. of Calif. Press.

Robbins, H. (1974). A sequential test for two binomial populations. *Proc. Natl. Acad. Sci.*, **71**, 4435–4436.

Robbins, H. (1977). Prediction and estimation for the compound Poisson distribution. *Proc. Natl. Acad. Sci. U.S.A.*, **74**, 2670–2671.

Robbins, H. and Zhang, C.-H. (1988). Estimating a treatment effect under biased sampling. *Proc. Natl. Acad. Sci. U.S.A.*, **85**, 3670–-672.

Robbins, H. and Zhang, C.-H. (1989). Estimating the superiority of a drug to a placebo when all and only those patients at risk are treated with the drug. *Proc. Natl. Acad. Sci. U.S.A.*, **86**, 3003–3005.

Robbins, H. and Zhang, C.-H. (1991). Estimating a multiplicative treatment effect under biased allocation. *Biometrika*, **78**, 349–354.

Robbins H. (1993). Comparing two treatments under biased allocation. *Gazette Sci. Math. Quebec*, **15**, 35–41.

Roth, H. P. and Gordon, R. S. (Eds.) (1979). Proceedings of the National Conference on Clinical Trials Methodology. *Clin. Pharmacol. Ther.*, **25**, 629–766.

Royall, R. M. (1991). Ethics and statistics in randomized clinical trials [with discussion]. *Statist. Sci.*, **6**, 52–88.

Schwartz, D. and Lellouch, J. (1967). Explanatory and pragmatic attitudes in therapeutic trials. *J. Chronic Dis.*, **20**, 637–648.

Sheps, M. C. (1958). Shall we count the living or the dead? *New Engl. J. Med.*, **259**, 1210–1214.

Sheps, M. C. (1959). An examination of some methods of comparing several rates or proportions. *Biometrics*, **15**, 87–97.

Siegmund, D. (1985). *Sequential analysis.* New York: Springer-Verlag.

Simon, R. H. (1977). Adaptive treatment assignment methods and clinical trials. *Biometrics*, **33**, 743–749.

Simon, R. (1979). Restricted randomization designs in clinical trials. *Biometrics*, **35**, 503–512.

Smith, R. (1998). Fifty years of randomised controlled trials. (Editor's choice.) *Brit. Med. J.*, **317**, 1166.

Taves, D. R. (1974). Minimization: A new method of assigning patients to treatment and control groups. *Clin. Pharmacol. Ther.*, **15**, 443–453.

Trochim, W. M. K. and Cappelleri, J. C. (1992). Cutoff assignment strategies for enhancing randomized clinical trials. *Controlled Clin. Trials*, **13**, 190–212.

Truog, R. D. (1992). Randomized controlled trials: Lessons from ECMO. *Clin. Res.*, **40**, 519–527.

Walter, S. D. (1975). The distribution of Levin's measure of attributable risk. *Biometrika*, **62**, 371–374.

Ware, J. H. (1989). Investigating therapies of potentially great benefit: ECMO [with discussion]. *Statist. Sci.*, **4**, 298–340.

Weinstein, G. S. and Levin, B. (1985). The Coronary Artery Surgery Study (CASS)—A critical appraisal. *J. Thorac. Cardiovasc. Surg.*, **90**, 541–548.

Weinstein, G. S. and Levin, B. (1989). The effect of crossover on the statistical power of randomized studies. *Ann. Thorac. Surg.*, **48**, 490–495.

Weinstein, G. S. and Levin, B. (1990). Crossovers in coronary artery bypass grafting trials (letter). *Ann. Thorac. Surg.*, **49**, 847–854.

Weinstein, M. C. (1974). Allocation of subjects in medical experiments. *New Engl. J. Med.*, **291**. 1278–1285.

Whitehead, J. (1997). *The design and analysis of sequential clinical trials*, 2nd rev. ed. New York: Wiley.

Zelen, M. (1969). Play the winner rule and the controlled clinical trial. *J. Am. Statist. Assoc.*, **64**, 131–146.

Zelen, M. (1979). A new design for randomized clinical trials. *New Engl. J. Med.*, **300**, 1242–1245.

Zelen, M. (1981). Alternatives to classic randomized trials. *Surg. Clin. N. Amer.*, **61**, 1425–1430.

CHAPTER 9

The Comparison of Proportions from Several Independent Samples

With only a few exceptions, we have restricted our attention to the comparison of two proportions. In this chapter we consider the comparison of a larger number of proportions. In Sections 9.1 through 9.3 we are concerned with comparing m independent sample binomial proportions. In Section 9.1 we study the analysis of an $m \times 2$ contingency table, where $m > 2$ and where there is no necessary ordering to the m groups. Sections 9.2 and 9.3 are devoted to the case where an intrinsic ordering to the m groups exists. We consider in Section 9.2 the hypothesis that the proportions vary monotonically (i.e., steadily increase or steadily decrease) with m quantitatively ordered groups, and in Section 9.3 that they vary monotonically with m qualitatively ordered groups. In Sections 9.4 and 9.5 we compare proportions from two independent multinomial samples with $m > 2$ mutually exclusive, qualitatively ordered categories. Section 9.4 discusses ridit analysis for the probability that an ordered categorical response from a study sample is shifted up or down in comparison with an identified reference population. Section 9.5 presents some more advanced logit models for qualitatively ordered response outcomes. Section 9.6 considers the analysis of m independent sample proportions when there is randomness among the true proportions. Because of the complexity of the exact analysis of an $m \times 2$ table, we postpone discussion of this topic until Chapter 11, Section 4.

The procedures of this chapter are suitable for each of the three methods of sampling presented previously (see Section 3.1). In randomized trials (method III sampling), the m samples represent groups treated by m different treatments, with subjects assigned to groups at random. In comparative studies (method II sampling), either the investigator selects prespecified

Statistical Methods for Rates and Proportions, Third Edition
By Joseph L. Fleiss, Bruce Levin, and Myunghee Cho Paik
ISBN 0-471-52629-0   Copyright © 2003 John Wiley & Sons, Inc.

Table 9.1. *Proportions from m independent samples*

Sample	Total in Sample	Number with Characteristic	Number without Characteristic	Proportion with Characteristic
1	$n_{1.}$	n_{11}	n_{12}	p_1
2	$n_{2.}$	n_{21}	n_{22}	p_2
$\vdots$	$\vdots$	$\vdots$	$\vdots$	$\vdots$
m	$n_{m.}$	n_{m1}	n_{m2}	p_m
Overall	$n_{..}$	$n_{.1}$	$n_{.2}$	$\bar{p}$

numbers of subjects from each of the m groups and observes a binary outcome for each subject, or the investigator selects prespecified numbers of subjects with and without a given characteristic and observes a multinomial outcome for each subject. In cross-sectional surveys (method I sampling), these numbers become known only after the study is completed. As was the case for the comparison of $m = 2$ samples (see Sections 7.1 and 7.2), method II sampling with equal sample sizes is superior in power and precision to method I sampling when $m > 2$. The methods of Section 9.6 are appropriate when each subject provides several binary responses.

9.1. THE COMPARISON OF m PROPORTIONS

Suppose that m independent samples of subjects are studied with each subject characterized by the presence or absence of some characteristic. The resulting data might be presented as in Table 9.1, where

$$p_i = \frac{n_{i1}}{n_{i.}} \tag{9.1}$$

and

$$\bar{p} = \frac{n_{.1}}{n_{..}} = \frac{\Sigma n_{i.} p_i}{\Sigma n_{i.}}. \tag{9.2}$$

For testing the significance of the differences among the m proportions, the value of

$$\chi^2 = \sum_{i=1}^{m} \sum_{j=1}^{2} \frac{\left(n_{ij} - n_{i.} n_{.j}/n_{..}\right)^2}{n_{i.} n_{.j}/n_{..}} \tag{9.3}$$

may be referred to tables of chi squared (see Table A.2) with $m - 1$ degrees of freedom (df). An equivalent and more suggestive formula for the test

Table 9.2. *Smoking status among lung cancer patients in four studies*

Study	Number of Patients	Number of Smokers	Proportion of Smokers
1	$86\ (=n_1.)$	83	$0.965\ (=p_1)$
2	$93\ (=n_2.)$	90	$0.968\ (=p_2)$
3	$136\ (=n_3.)$	129	$0.949\ (=p_3)$
4	$82\ (=n_4.)$	70	$0.854\ (=p_4)$
Overall	$397\ (=n_{..})$	372	$0.937\ (=\bar{p})$

statistic is

$$\chi^2 = \frac{1}{\bar{p}\bar{q}} \sum_{i=1}^{m} n_i.(p_i - \bar{p})^2, \tag{9.4}$$

where $\bar{q} = 1 - \bar{p}$.

Consider, as an example, the data in Table 9.2 from four studies cited by Dorn (1954). In each study, the number of smokers among lung cancer patients was recorded. For these data, the value of χ^2 (9.4) is

$$\chi^2 = \frac{1}{0.937 \times 0.063} \{ 86 \times (0.965 - 0.937)^2 + 93 \times (0.968 - 0.937)^2$$

$$+ 136 \times (0.949 - 0.937)^2 + 82 \times (0.854 - 0.937)^2 \}$$

$$= 12.56, \tag{9.5}$$

which, with 3 df, is significant at the 0.01 level.

Having found the proportions to differ significantly, one would next proceed to identify the samples or groups of samples that contributed to the significant difference. Methods for isolating sources of significant differences in the context of a general contingency table are given by Irwin (1949), Lancaster (1950), Kimball (1954), Kastenbaum (1960), Castellan (1965), and Knoke (1976). Here we illustrate the simplest method for the $m \times 2$ table.

Suppose that it is planned in advance of the data to compare the m samples when they are partitioned into two groups, the first containing m_1 samples and the second m_2, where $m_1 + m_2 = m$. Define

$$n_{(1)} = \sum_{i=1}^{m_1} n_i. \tag{9.6}$$

to be the total number of subjects in the first group of samples, and

$$n_{(2)} = \sum_{i=m_1+1}^{m} n_i. \tag{9.7}$$

to be the total number of subjects in the second group.

Let the proportion in the first group be denoted $\bar{p}_1$, where

$$\bar{p}_1 = \frac{\sum_{i=1}^{m_1} n_i.\,p_i}{n_{(1)}}, \tag{9.8}$$

and that in the second group be denoted $\bar{p}_2$, where

$$\bar{p}_2 = \frac{\sum_{i=m_1+1}^{m} n_i.\,p_i}{n_{(2)}}. \tag{9.9}$$

Then

$$\chi_{\text{diff}}^2 = \frac{1}{\bar{p}\bar{q}} \times \frac{n_{(1)} n_{(2)}}{n_{..}} (\bar{p}_1 - \bar{p}_2)^2, \tag{9.10}$$

with 1 df, may be used to test for the significance of the difference between $\bar{p}_1$ and $\bar{p}_2$. Note that χ_{diff}^2 is identical to the chi squared, without the continuity correction, that one would calculate on the fourfold table obtained by combining all the data from the first m_1 samples into one single set and all the data from the remaining m_2 samples into a second.

The statistic

$$\chi_{\text{group 1}}^2 = \frac{1}{\bar{p}\bar{q}} \sum_{i=1}^{m_1} n_i.(p_i - \bar{p}_1)^2, \tag{9.11}$$

with $m_1 - 1$ df, may be used to test the significance of the differences among the m_1 proportions in the first group, and the statistic

$$\chi_{\text{group 2}}^2 = \frac{1}{\bar{p}\bar{q}} \sum_{i=m_1+1}^{m} n_i.(p_i - \bar{p}_2)^2, \tag{9.12}$$

with $m_2 - 1$ df, may be used to test the significance of the differences among the m_2 proportions in the second group. It may be checked that the three statistics given by (9.10)–(9.12) sum to the overall value of χ^2 in (9.4).

If $\bar{p}_1$ and $\bar{p}_2$ differ appreciably, then the product $\bar{p}_1\bar{q}_1 = \bar{p}_1(1 - \bar{p}_1)$ should replace $\bar{p}\bar{q}$ in (9.11), and $\bar{p}_2\bar{q}_2 = \bar{p}_2(1 - \bar{p}_2)$ should replace $\bar{p}\bar{q}$ in (9.12). These adjustments have little effect on the magnitudes of χ^2, but the sum of the adjusted chi squareds plus the chi squared in (9.10) will no longer generally recapture the overall value of chi squared in (9.4).

A more serious modification is called for, however, if the partitioning of the samples into groups is suggested by the data instead of being planned beforehand. Of the four samples in Table 9.2, for example, the first three appear, on the basis of the similarity of their proportions, to form one homogeneous group, whereas the fourth sample seems to stand by itself as a second group. To control for the erroneous inferences possible by making comparisons suggested by the data, each of the χ^2 values in (9.10) to (9.12) should be referred to the critical value of chi squared with $m-1$ degrees of freedom and *not* to the critical values of chi squared with 1, $m_1 - 1$, and $m_2 - 1$ degrees of freedom (Miller, 1981, Section 6.2).

For the data of Table 9.2, for example, the first set of $m_1 = 3$ studies consists of

$$n_{(1)} = 86 + 93 + 136 = 315$$

lung cancer patients, of whom the proportion smoking is

$$\bar{p}_1 = \frac{83 + 90 + 129}{315} = 0.959.$$

The second set of $m_2 = 1$ study alone consists of $n_{(2)} = 82$ patients, of whom the proportion smoking is $\bar{p}_2 = 0.854$.

The significance of the difference between $\bar{p}_1$ and $\bar{p}_2$ is assessed by the magnitude of χ^2_{diff} [see (9.10)]:

$$\chi^2_{\text{diff}} = \frac{1}{0.937 \times 0.063} \times \frac{315 \times 82}{397} (0.959 - 0.854)^2$$

$$= 12.15. \tag{9.13}$$

The significance of the differences among p_1, p_2 and p_3—all from group 1—is assessed by the magnitude of $\chi^2_{\text{group 1}}$ [see (9.11)]:

$$\chi^2_{\text{group 1}} = \frac{1}{0.937 \times 0.063} \Big[86 \times (0.965 - 0.959)^2$$

$$+ 93 \times (0.968 - 0.959)^2 + 136 \times (0.949 - 0.959)^2 \Big]$$

$$= 0.41. \tag{9.14}$$

Because group 2 consists of but a single study sample, the statistic $\chi^2_{\text{group 2}}$ [see (9.12)] is inapplicable here.

Note first of all that

$$\chi^2_{\text{diff}} + \chi^2_{\text{group 1}} = 12.15 + 0.41 = 12.56,$$

which is equal to the value of the overall chi squared statistic given in (9.5). Note next that, with $\bar{p}_1 \bar{q}_1 = 0.959 \times 0.041$ replacing 0.937×0.063 in (9.14), the value of $\chi^2_{\text{group 1}}$ increases only slightly, to 0.62. Recall, finally, that the partitioning was suggested by the data and not planned *a priori*. The values of both χ^2_{diff} and $\chi^2_{\text{group 1}}$ must therefore be referred to the critical value of chi squared with $m-1 = 4-1 = 3$ df. Since the critical value for a significance level of 0.05 is 7.81, the conclusion would be that the proportion of

Table 9.3. *Prevalence of reported insomnia among women by age*

Age Interval	Number in Interval $(= n_{i.})$	Proportion Reporting Insomnia $(= p_i)$	Midpoint Age $(= x_i)$
18–24	534	0.280	21.5
25–34	746	0.335	30.0
35–44	784	0.337	40.0
45–54	705	0.428	50.0
55–64	443	0.538	60.0
65–74	299	0.590	70.0
Overall	3511 $(= n_{..})$	0.393 $(= \bar{p})$	42.15 $(= \bar{x})$

smokers among the patients in study 4 differed from the proportions in studies 1 to 3 (because $\chi^2_{\text{diff}} = 12.15 > 7.81$), but that there were no differences among the proportions in studies 1 to 3 (because $\chi^2_{\text{group 1}} = 0.41 < 7.81$).

9.2. GRADIENT IN PROPORTIONS: SAMPLES QUANTITATIVELY ORDERED

The analysis of the preceding section is of quite general validity, but lacks sensitivity when the m samples possess an intrinsic ordering. We assume in this section that the ordering is quantitative; specifically, that a measurement x_i is naturally associated with the ith sample. Data from the National Center for Health Statistics (1970, Tables 1 and 6) are used for illustration (Table 9.3).

Different methods of analysis are called for depending on how the proportions are hypothesized to vary with x (Yates, 1948). Here we consider only the simplest kind of variation, a linear one. In Chapter 11 we discuss the more common, and in many respects preferable, linear logistic model to describe the variation in proportions.

Let P_i denote the proportion in the population from which the ith sample was drawn. We hypothesize that

$$P_i = \alpha + \beta x_i, \tag{9.15}$$

where β, the slope of the line, indicates the amount of change in the proportion per unit change in x, and α, the intercept, indicates the proportion expected when $x = 0$.

The two parameters of (9.15) may be estimated as follows. Define

$$\bar{x} = \sum_{i=1}^{m} \frac{n_{i.} x_i}{n_{..}}, \tag{9.16}$$

the mean value of x in the given series of data. The slope is estimated as

$$b = \frac{\sum\limits_{i=1}^{m} n_{i.}(p_i - \bar{p})(x_i - \bar{x})}{\sum\limits_{i=1}^{m} n_{i.}(x_i - \bar{x})^2}, \tag{9.17}$$

and the intercept as

$$a = \bar{p} - b\bar{x}. \tag{9.18}$$

The calculation of b is simplified somewhat by noting that its numerator is

$$\text{numerator}(b) = \sum\limits_{i=1}^{m} n_{i.}p_i x_i - n_{..}\bar{p}\bar{x} \tag{9.19}$$

and that its denominator is

$$\text{denominator}(b) = \sum\limits_{i=1}^{m} n_{i.}x_i^2 - n_{..}\bar{x}^2. \tag{9.20}$$

A simple expression for the fitted line is

$$\hat{p}_i = \bar{p} + b(x_i - \bar{x}). \tag{9.21}$$

For the data of Table 9.3, $\bar{p} = 0.393$, $\bar{x} = 42.15$, and

$$b = 0.0064. \tag{9.22}$$

The fitted straight line becomes

$$\hat{p}_i = 0.393 + 0.0064(x_i - 42.15), \tag{9.23}$$

implying an increase of 0.64% in the proportion of adult women reporting insomnia per yearly increase in age, or 6.4% per decade.

It is useful to calculate the estimated proportion corresponding to each x_i in order to compare it with the actual proportion, p_i. If p_i and $\hat{p}_i$ are close in magnitude for all or most categories, then one can conclude that (9.15) provides a good fit to the data, that is, P_i tends to vary linearly with x_i. If p_i and $\hat{p}_i$ tend to differ, then the conclusion is that the association between P_i and x_i is more complicated than a linear one. Having the differences $p_i - \hat{p}_i$ available serves also to identity those categories for which the departures from linearity are greatest.

Table 9.4 contrasts the actual proportions of Table 9.3 with those yielded by (9.23). The fit appears to be a good one.

Table 9.4. *Observed and linearly predicted age-specific rates of insomnia*

x_i	$n_{i.}$	p_i	$\hat{p}_i$
21.5	534	0.280	0.261
30.0	746	0.335	0.315
40.0	784	0.337	0.379
50.0	705	0.428	0.443
60.0	443	0.538	0.507
70.0	299	0.590	0.571

A chi squared statistic due to Cochran (1954) and Armitage (1955) is available for testing whether the association between P_i and x_i is a linear one. This chi squared statistic is

$$\chi^2_{\text{linearity}} = \sum_{i=1}^{m} n_{i.}(p_i - \hat{p}_i)^2 / \overline{p}\,\overline{q}. \tag{9.24}$$

Under the hypothesis of linearity, when the $n_{i.}$'s are large, $\chi^2_{\text{linearity}}$ has an approximate chi squared distribution with $m - 2$ df, and the hypothesis of linearity would be rejected if $\chi^2_{\text{linearity}}$ were found to be large. The power of this test was studied by Chapman and Nam (1968).

The calculation of $\chi^2_{\text{linearity}}$ is simplified if one first calculates the statistic

$$\chi^2_{\text{slope}} = b^2 \sum_{i=1}^{m} n_{i.}(x_i - \bar{x})^2 / \overline{p}\,\overline{q}, \tag{9.25}$$

because it may be shown that

$$\chi^2_{\text{linearity}} = \chi^2 - \chi^2_{\text{slope}}, \tag{9.26}$$

where χ^2 is given by (9.4). The statistic χ^2_{slope} has 1 df and may be used to test the significance of the slope, b. If χ^2_{slope} is large, the inference is that the slope is significantly different from zero, indicating that there is a tendency for increasing values of x_i to be associated with increasing values of P_i if b is positive or with decreasing values of P_i if b is negative.

For the data of Table 9.3, the value of the overall chi squared statistic in (9.4) for testing the hypothesis that the proportion reporting insomnia is constant for all age groups is

$$\chi^2 = 140.72. \tag{9.27}$$

The magnitude of this chi squared, which has 5 df, indicates highly significant differences among the age-specific proportions, but fails to describe the steady increase with age of the proportion reporting insomnia.

The chi squared statistic for linearity [see (9.24)] is, for the data from Table 9.4,

$$\chi^2_{\text{linearity}} = \frac{534 \times (0.280 - 0.261)^2 + \cdots + 299 \times (0.590 - 0.571)^2}{0.393 \times 0.607}$$

$$= 10.76, \tag{9.28}$$

which, with 4 df, is significant at the 0.05 level. The association with age of the proportion of women reporting insomnia is thus not precisely a linear one, but the departures from linearity (i.e., the differences between the observed and linearly predicted proportions) are sufficiently small to make the hypothesis of linearity plausible and the predictions useful.

The chi squared statistic of (9.25) assumes the value

$$\chi^2_{\text{slope}} = \frac{0.0064^2 \times 757,964.7975}{0.393 \times 0.607} = 130.15, \tag{9.29}$$

which, with 1 df, indicates that the slope of the fitted line, $b = 0.0064$, is significantly different from zero. The difference between the overall chi squared of 140.72 and the chi squared for testing the significance of the slope, 130.15, should, by (9.26), be equal to the chi squared for linearity, 10.76. Except for errors due to rounding, this is seen to be the case.

The inferences to be drawn from this more detailed chi squared analysis are that there is a significant tendency for the proportion of women reporting insomnia to increase steadily with age and that this tendency is, approximately, a linear one. Had the chi squared for linearity been significant at, say, the 0.01 or 0.005 level instead of merely at the 0.05 level, the latter inference would not have been warranted.

Slightly different versions of the estimators and of the test statistics given above have been derived by Mantel (1963), Chapman and Nam (1968), and Wood (1978), who also consider the comparison and combination of fitted regression lines across several independent samples. The procedure presented here is valid when, as in the example, the p_i's are not close to 0 or to 1. For p_i's close to 0 or to 1, or extrapolations of x far from $\bar{x}$, the linear model may fail to give reasonable values for the fitted probabilities (below 0 or above 1). The methods of Chapter 11 should be used instead.

9.3. GRADIENT IN PROPORTIONS: SAMPLES QUALITATIVELY ORDERED

We assumed in Section 9.2 that the m samples could be ordered on a quantitative scale. We assume in this section that the ordering is merely qualitative. Suppose, for example, that one has data as in Table 9.5. The

Table 9.5. *Hypothetical one-month release rates as a function of initial severity*

Initial Severity	Total	Number Released within One Month	Proportion Released within One Month
Mild	$30\,(=n_{1.})$	25	$0.83\,(=p_1)$
Moderate	$25\,(=n_{2.})$	22	$0.88\,(=p_2)$
Serious	$20\,(=n_{3.})$	12	$0.60\,(=p_3)$
Extreme	$25\,(=n_{4.})$	6	$0.24\,(=p_4)$
Overall	$100\,(=n_{..})$	65	$0.65\,(=\bar{p})$

value of χ^2 in (9.4) for these data is

$$\chi^2 = 28.74 \tag{9.30}$$

with 3 df, clearly significant beyond the 0.001 level (see Table A.2).

The inference that the four release rates differ significantly is a valid one, but is clearly insufficient in that it fails to describe the almost steady decline in release rates as initial severity worsens. Because it would have been reasonable to hypothesize beforehand a gradient of release rate with severity, an alternative method of analysis is called for. The method of the preceding section is not appropriate, because no numerical values can naturally be assigned to the four levels of severity.

Chassan (1960, 1962) proposed a simple test of the hypothesis that m proportions were arrayed in a prespecified order, but his test was shown by Bartholomew (1963) to lack adequate power. Specifically, Chassan's test may be applied only when the sample proportions are arrayed *without exception* in the same order as hypothesized. It would therefore be inapplicable whenever there were slight departures (as, e.g., for p_1 and p_2 in Table 9.5) from the hypothesized order. A more powerful procedure due to Bartholomew (1959a, 1959b) will be described.

Suppose that the hypothesis predicts the ordering $p_1 > p_2 > \cdots > p_m$, but that departures from this ordering are observed. For the proportions in Table 9.5, for example, the ordering $p_1 > p_2 > p_3 > p_4$ was predicted, but instead we obtained $p_1 < p_2$ and then, as predicted, $p_2 > p_3 > p_4$.

When departures are found, weighted averages of those adjacent proportions that are out of order are taken until, when the averages replace the original proportions, the hypothesized ordering is observed. The revised proportions are denoted p'. For the proportions in Table 9.5, the weighted average of p_1 and p_2 must be taken. It is

$$\bar{p}_{1,2} = \frac{30 \times 0.83 + 25 \times 0.88}{30 + 25} = 0.85. \tag{9.31}$$

When p_1 and p_2 are replaced by $\bar{p}_{1,2}$, Table 9.6 results.

Table 9.6. *Proportions from Table 9.5 revised to be in hypothesized order*

Initial Severity	Total	Revised Proportion
Mild	$30 \, (= n_{1.})$	$0.85 \, (= p'_1)$
Moderate	$25 \, (= n_{2.})$	$0.85 \, (= p'_2)$
Serious	$20 \, (= n_{3.})$	$0.60 \, (= p_3 = p'_3)$
Extreme	$25 \, (= n_{4.})$	$0.24 \, (= p_4 = p'_4)$
Overall	$100 \, (= n_{..})$	$0.65 \, (= \bar{p})$

The revised proportions are no longer out of order. If they were, the process would have to be continued. When the process has been completed, the statistic

$$\bar{\chi}^2 = \frac{1}{\bar{p}\bar{q}} \sum_{i=1}^{m} n_{i.}(p'_i - \bar{p})^2 \tag{9.32}$$

is calculated. For the revised proportions of Table 9.6,

$$\bar{\chi}^2 = \frac{1}{0.65 \times 0.35} \left[30 \times (0.85 - 0.65)^2 + 25 \times (0.85 - 0.65)^2 \right.$$

$$\left. + 20 \times (0.60 - 0.65)^2 + 25 \times (0.24 - 0.65)^2 \right] = 28.27. \tag{9.33}$$

The value of $\bar{\chi}^2$ may no longer be referred to tables of chi squared, however. Instead, Tables A.7 to A.9 are to be used. When $m = 3$ proportions are compared, calculate

$$c = \sqrt{\frac{n_{1.} n_{3.}}{(n_{1.} + n_{2.})(n_{2.} + n_{3.})}}, \tag{9.34}$$

and enter Table A.7 under the desired significance level, interpolating if necessary. When $m = 4$, calculate

$$c_1 = \sqrt{\frac{n_{1.} n_{3.}}{(n_{1.} + n_{2.})(n_{2.} + n_{3.})}} \tag{9.35}$$

and

$$c_2 = \sqrt{\frac{n_{2.} n_{4.}}{(n_{2.} + n_{3.})(n_{3.} + n_{4.})}}, \tag{9.36}$$

and enter Table A.8 under the desired significance level, interpolating in both c_1 and c_2 if necessary. If all sample sizes are equal, and if $m \leq 12$, Table A.9 may be used.

For the data of Table 9.6, for which $m = 4$,

$$c_1 = \sqrt{\frac{30 \times 20}{(30 + 25)(25 + 20)}} = 0.49$$

and

$$c_2 = \sqrt{\frac{25 \times 25}{(25 + 20)(20 + 25)}} = 0.56.$$

Visual interpolation in Table A.8 (c_1 is approximately equal to 0.5, and c_2 is nearly midway between 0.5 and 0.6) shows that $\bar{\chi}^2$ would have to exceed 9.0 in order for significance to be declared at the 0.005 level. The obtained value of $\bar{\chi}^2 = 28.27$ from (9.33) is far beyond this critical value.

What is noteworthy, however, is the comparison of the value just found from Table A.8 with the corresponding value from Table A.2 for the standard chi squared test with $m - 1 = 3$ degrees of freedom. If no ordering is hypothesized, χ^2 would have to exceed 12.8 (instead of 9.0) for significance to be declared at the 0.005 level. Thus, *if the hypothesized ordering actually obtains in the population*, Bartholomew's test is more powerful than the standard chi squared test. If the hypothesized ordering is not true, however, the averaging process necessary before the calculation of $\bar{\chi}^2$ in (9.32) could well reduce its magnitude to insignificance. Further analyses and generalizations of Bartholomew's test have been made by Barlow et al. (1972).

9.4. RIDIT ANALYSIS

Suppose that one has data available from two or more samples, with the subjects from each sample distributed across a number of ordered categories. Let k denote the number of categories. For example, let us consider automobile accidents, with the phenomenon studied being the degree of injury sustained by the driver. The degree of injury might be graded from none through severe to fatal. Such a grading is clearly subjective and probably not too reliable. It nevertheless seems preferable to the adoption of the simple dichotomy, little or no injury versus severe or fatal injury, because it both possesses some degree of reliability and succeeds in describing the phenomenon more completely than the cruder yes-no system.

There exists the problem, however, of summarizing the data and making comparisons among different samples in an intelligible way. When two samples are being compared, the data may be arrayed as in Table 9.7. The proportions $(p_{11}, \ldots, p_{k1})$ represent the frequency distribution in sample 1, and the proportions $(p_{12}, \ldots, p_{k2})$ represent the frequency distribution in

Table 9.7. *Relative frequency distributions from two samples*

Outcome Category	Sample 1 (sample size $= n_1$)	Sample 2 (sample size $= n_2$)	Combined Sample (sample size $= n_.$)
1	p_{11}	p_{12}	$\bar{p}_1$
2	p_{21}	p_{22}	$\bar{p}_2$
$\vdots$	$\vdots$	$\vdots$	$\vdots$
k	p_{k1}	p_{k2}	$\bar{p}_k$
Total	1	1	1

sample 2. The frequency distribution in the combined sample is $(\bar{p}_1, \ldots, \bar{p}_k)$, where

$$\bar{p}_i = \frac{n_1 p_{i1} + n_2 p_{i2}}{n_.} \tag{9.37}$$

$(i = 1, \ldots, k)$ and $n_. = n_1 + n_2$, the total sample size. The value of chi squared with $k - 1$ degrees of freedom may be found using the formula

$$\chi^2 = \frac{n_1 n_2}{n_.} \sum_{i=1}^{k} \frac{(p_{i1} - p_{i2})^2}{\bar{p}_i} \tag{9.38}$$

(see Problem 9.4), but crucial information on the natural ordering of the k categories would be lost.

A frequently employed device is to number the categories from 0 for the least serious to some highest number for the most serious, and then calculate means and standard deviations and apply t tests or analyses of variance. This device of concocting a seemingly numerical measurement system has many drawbacks. For one thing, one is giving the impression of greater accuracy than really exists. For another, the results one gets depend on the particular system of numbers employed. The choice of a system is by no means a simple one.

Consider again the study of automobile accidents, and suppose that we have seven categories of injury, the first two being None and Mild, and the last two, Critical and Fatal. The straightforward system of numbering assigns the seven integers from 0 to 6 successively to the seven categories. This system is hard to justify, for it implies that the difference between no injury and a mild one is equivalent to the difference between a critical injury and a fatal one. The latter difference is obviously more important, but this greater importance can be picked up only by assigning a value in excess of 6 to the final category. Just what this value should be can, however, only be decided arbitrarily. If an underlying logistic model (see Chapter 11) may be assumed, a procedure due to Snell (1964) is appropriate. We return to the problem of assigning scores to categories in Section 9.5.

Table 9.8. *An Illustration of the calculation of ridits for degrees of injury*

Severity	(1)	(2)	(3)	(4)	(5) = ridit
None	17	8.5	0	8.5	0.047
Minor	54	27.0	17	44.0	0.246
Moderate	60	30.0	71	101.0	0.564
Severe	19	9.5	131	140.5	0.785
Serious	9	4.5	150	154.5	0.863
Critical	6	3.0	159	162.0	0.905
Fatal	14	7.0	165	172.0	0.961

For now, let us abandon the attempt to quantify the categories and instead agree to work only with the natural ordering that exists. A technique that takes advantage of this natural ordering is *ridit analysis*. Virtually the only assumption made in ridit analysis is that the discrete categories represent intervals of an underlying but unobservable continuous distribution. No assumption is made about normality or any other form for the distribution.

Ridit analysis is due to Bross (1958) and has been applied to the study of automobile accidents (Bross, 1960), of cancer (Wynder, Bross, and Hirayama, 1960), and of schizophrenia (Spitzer et al., 1965). A mathematical study of ridit analysis was made by Kantor, Winkelstein, and Ibrahim (1968). A critique of ridit analysis has been offered by Mantel (1979).

Ridit analysis begins with the selection of a population to serve as a standard or reference group. The term ridit is derived from the initials of "relative to an identified distribution." For the reference group, we estimate the proportion of all individuals with a value on the underlying continuum falling at or below the midpoint of each interval, that is, each interval's *ridit*. This initial arithmetic is illustrated in Table 9.8, using data from Bross (1958, p. 20).

1. In general, column 1 contains the distribution over the various categories for the reference group. In Table 9.8, the distribution is over seven categories of injury for the 179 members of a selected sample.
2. The entries in column (2) are simply half the corresponding entries in column (1).
3. The entries in column (3) are the accumulated entries in column (1), but displaced one category downwards.
4. The entries in column (4) are the sums of the corresponding entries in columns (2) and (3).
5. The entries in column (5), finally, are those in column (4) divided by the total sample size, in this case 179.

The final values are the ridits associated with the various categories. The ridit for a category, then, is nothing but the proportion of all subjects from the reference group falling in the lower-ranking categories plus half the proportion falling in the given category. If, in the model of an underlying continuum, we assume that the distribution is uniform in each interval, then a category's ridit is the proportion of all subjects from the reference group with an underlying value at or below the midpoint of the corresponding interval.

Given the distribution of any other group over the same categories, the mean ridit for that group may be calculated. The resulting mean value is interpretable as a probability. The mean ridit for a group is the probability that a randomly selected individual from it has a value indicating greater severity or seriousness than a randomly selected individual from the standard group.

In our example, if this probability is 0.50, we infer that the comparison group tends to sustain neither more nor less serious injuries than the reference group. For the reference group itself, by the way, the mean ridit is necessarily 0.50. This is consistent with the fact that, if two subjects are randomly selected from the same population, then the second subject will have a more extreme value half the time and will have a less extreme value also half the time.

If the mean ridit for a comparison group is greater than 0.50, then more than half of the time a randomly selected subject from it will have a more extreme value than a randomly selected subject from the reference group. In our example, we would infer that the comparison group tends to sustain more serious injuries than the reference group. If, finally, a comparison group's mean ridit is less than 0.50, we would infer that its subjects tend to have less extreme values than the subjects of the reference group.

As an example, consider the hypothetical data of Table 9.9, giving the distribution of seriousness of injury to the driver when he was involved in an accident and had been slightly intoxicated.

The mean ridit for a group is simply the sum of the products of observed frequencies times corresponding ridits, divided by the total frequency. For

Table 9.9. *Seriousness of injury sustained by slightly intoxicated drivers of automobiles involved in accidents*

Severity	Number	Ridit	Product
None	5	0.047	0.235
Minor	10	0.246	2.460
Moderate	16	0.564	9.024
Severe	5	0.785	3.925
Serious	3	0.863	2.589
Critical	6	0.905	5.430
Fatal	5	0.961	4.805
Total	50		28.468

slightly intoxicated drivers the mean is

$$\bar{r} = \frac{28.468}{50} = 0.57. \tag{9.39}$$

Thus the odds are 4 to 3 ($= 0.57/0.43$) that a slightly intoxicated driver will sustain a more serious injury than a driver from the reference group if both are involved in accidents.

Selvin (1977) has shown how ridit analysis is closely connected with so-called rank order analysis used in nonparametric statistics and thus how standard errors of mean ridits can be found. Let N_i denote the number of individuals from the reference group in category i, $N = \Sigma N_i$ the total number of individuals in the reference group, n_i the number of individuals from the comparison group in category i, and $n = \Sigma n_i$ the total number of individuals in the comparison group. If the reference group is not too much larger than the comparison group, the standard error of the mean for the comparison group is given by

$$se(\bar{r}) = \frac{1}{2\sqrt{3n}} \sqrt{1 + \frac{n+1}{N} + \frac{1}{N(N+n-1)} - \frac{\Sigma(N_i + n_i)^3}{N(N+n)(N+n-1)}} \, . \tag{9.40}$$

The two frequency distributions for the current problem are presented in Table 9.10. The standard error of the mean ridit for slightly intoxicated drivers involved in accidents is, by (9.40),

$$se(\bar{r}) = \frac{1}{2\sqrt{150}} \sqrt{1 + \frac{51}{179} + \frac{1}{179 \times 228} - \frac{735,907}{179 \times 229 \times 228}} = 0.045. \tag{9.41}$$

Table 9.10. *Frequency distributions from reference and comparison groups*

Severity	Reference Group (N_i)	Comparison Group (n_i)	Total $(N_i + n_i)$
None	17	5	22
Minor	54	10	64
Moderate	60	16	76
Severe	19	5	24
Serious	9	3	12
Critical	6	6	12
Fatal	14	5	19
Total	179 ($= N$)	50 ($= n$)	229 ($= N + n$)

The significance of the difference between an obtained mean ridit and the standard value of 0.5 may be tested by referring the value of

$$z = \frac{\bar{r} - 0.5}{\text{se}(\bar{r})} \qquad (9.42)$$

to Table A.1 of the normal distribution. For our example,

$$z = \frac{0.57 - 0.50}{0.045} = 1.56. \qquad (9.43)$$

Because z failed to reach significance, we would have to conclude that the seriousness of injuries to slightly intoxicated drivers might equal that of the injuries to members of the reference group.

When N, the size of the reference group, is very large relative to that of any possible comparison group, the standard error of the mean ridit simplifies to

$$\text{se}(\bar{r}) \approx \frac{1}{2\sqrt{3n}}. \qquad (9.44)$$

For the current data, this simple approximation yields an estimated standard error of 0.041, slightly smaller than the correct value 0.045 from (9.41).

As another example of the use of ridit analysis, suppose we have data on a sample of 50 extremely intoxicated drivers who were involved in accidents, and suppose that their mean ridit is 0.73. An important comparison is between slightly and extremely intoxicated drivers. Instead of identifying a new reference group, a simple approximation is to subtract one of the two mean ridits from the other and add 0.50. Thus we obtain $(0.73-0.57) + 0.50 = 0.66$ as the chances that a driver who is extremely intoxicated will sustain a more severe injury than one who is slightly so, when they are involved in accidents. Problem 9.6 shows the rationale for this simple approximation.

If one mean ridit is based on N_1 subjects and the other on N_2, the standard error is approximately

$$\text{se}(\bar{r}_2 - \bar{r}_1) = \frac{\sqrt{N_1 + N_2}}{2\sqrt{3N_1 N_2}}. \qquad (9.45)$$

This formula provides a good approximation to the standard error of the mean ridit for a single comparison group when N and n are of comparable magnitudes [see expression (9.40)], provided N and n replace N_1 and N_2. It *overapproximates* the standard error, but usually by only a very slight amount [see Problem 9.5, parts (c) and (d)].

With $N_1 = N_2 = 50$, the approximate standard error is

$$se(\bar{r}_2 - \bar{r}_1) = \frac{\sqrt{100}}{2\sqrt{3 \times 50 \times 50}} = 0.06. \tag{9.46}$$

The significance of the difference between $\bar{r}_1$ and $\bar{r}_2$ may be tested by referring the value of

$$z = \frac{\bar{r}_2 - \bar{r}_1}{se(\bar{r}_2 - \bar{r}_1)} \tag{9.47}$$

to Table A.1. For our example,

$$z = \frac{0.73 - 0.57}{0.06} = 2.67, \tag{9.48}$$

which indicates a difference significant at the 0.01 level. We can therefore infer that extremely intoxicated drivers involved in accidents tend to sustain more serious injuries than slightly intoxicated drivers involved in accidents.

The reader is warned of the possibility of an anomalous result using the approximate approach just described for contrasting two comparison groups, that is, the estimated probability may be less than zero or greater than unity. Consider the hypothetical data in Table 9.11, where one frequency distribution is the mirror image of the other. It is easily checked using the ridits of Table 9.8 that the two mean ridits are $\bar{r}_A = 0.25$ and $\bar{r}_B = 0.89$. The above approach yields an impossible value of $(0.89 - 0.25) + 0.50 = 1.14$ for the probability that a randomly selected member of group B will sustain a more severe injury than a randomly selected member of group A. Problem 9.6 reveals the difficulty with the approximation.

When, as in this hypothetical case, frequency distributions in the two contrasted comparison groups are widely different, it is appropriate to ignore

Table 9.11. *Hypothetical data on seriousness of injury in two comparison groups*

Severity	Group A	Group B
None	46	1
Minor	34	2
Moderate	9	3
Severe	5	5
Serious	3	9
Critical	2	34
Fatal	1	46
Total	100	100

the original reference group entirely and to calculate the desired probability as a mean ridit, with either of the two groups serving as the ad hoc reference group. Problem 9.5 is devoted to the appropriate analysis of the data from Table 9.11. We may also proceed as in the next section.

9.5.* LOGIT MODELS FOR QUALITATIVELY ORDERED OUTCOMES

The methods of Chapter 11 for polytomous logistic regression are applicable here. Our purpose in this section is to illustrate the kind of results available with these methods.

Consider the two columns of relative frequency distributions in Table 9.7. Here we take the view that each column is an independent sample from a multinomial distribution with sample sizes n_1 and n_2, respectively, and true cell probabilities given by the vectors $(P_{11}, \ldots, P_{k1})$ and $(P_{12}, \ldots, P_{k2})$, with $P_{1j} + \cdots + P_{kj} = 1$ for $j = 1$ and 2. The multinomial distributions can be reparameterized by an equivalent system of parameters which reflect the qualitative ordering of the categories. One such system uses *adjacent logit parameters*, defined by

$$L_i^{(j)} = \ln \frac{P_{i+1,j}}{P_{ij}} \qquad \text{for } i = 1, \ldots, k-1 \text{ and } j = 1, 2. \qquad (9.49)$$

The adjacent logit parameter $L_i^{(j)}$ specifies the odds on an accident in group j falling in category $i + 1$ versus i as $\exp(L_i^{(j)})$ for $i = 1, \ldots, k-1$. This is also the conditional odds given that an accident in group j falls in either category i or $i + 1$.

For many applications, a very useful model specifies that the differences between corresponding adjacent logits in groups 1 and 2 are constant:

$$L_i^{(2)} - L_i^{(1)} = \Delta \qquad \text{for } i = 1, \ldots, k-1. \qquad (9.50)$$

Assumption (9.50) defines the *proportional adjacent odds model*, so named because the adjacent odds $\exp(L_i^{(2)})$ in group 2 are proportional to the adjacent odds $\exp(L_i^{(1)})$ in group 1, with constant of proportionality $\exp(\Delta)$, which is the *common adjacent odds ratio*:

$$\frac{P_{i+1,2}}{P_{i2}} = \exp(\Delta) \cdot \frac{P_{i+1,1}}{P_{i1}} \qquad \text{for } i = 1, \ldots, k-1. \qquad (9.51)$$

Model (9.50) gives Δ the interpretation of a shift parameter, indicating how much moderate drinking shifts the log odds toward more serious injuries at each categorical level of severity. Whether or not a single parameter Δ suffices for each comparison in (9.50) or (9.51) is an empirical question. When it does, the analysis is greatly simplified. Otherwise the complete set of odds ratios $\exp(\Delta_i) = \exp(L_i^{(2)} - L_i^{(1)})$ for $i = 1, \ldots, k-1$ should be reported.

Using methods of Chapter 11, we can test the goodness of fit of the proportional adjacent odds model. If we do not reject the assumption of a constant difference in (9.50), or of a common adjacent odds ratio $(P_{i+1,2}/P_{i2})/(P_{i+1,1}/P_{i1}) = \exp(\Delta)$, we can assess the null hypothesis of homogeneous multinomial cell probabilities by testing H_0: $\Delta = 0$, and give a confidence interval for the common adjacent odds ratio $\exp(\Delta)$.

For the data in Table 9.10, the chi squared goodness-of-fit statistic for the proportional adjacent odds model is $\chi^2 = 3.67$ on 5 df, indicating a good fit. There are 5 df because there are 6 adjacent logit parameters for each comparison group under the alternative hypothesis of no relationship, for 12 parameters, minus 7 parameters under the null hypothesis, comprising the 6 adjacent logit parameters for one of the groups plus the parameter of interest, Δ. The difference in the number of parameters, $12 - 7 = 5$, is the number of degrees of freedom. Table 9.12 shows the observed and fitted frequencies and proportions. Although the observed adjacent odds ratios show substantial variation, the fitted frequencies are, on the whole, quite close to the sample frequencies, yet have a constant adjacent odds ratio. (The largest relative deviation between observed and fitted frequencies occurs in the critical severity category.) The chi squared statistic indicates that such small-sample fluctuations are not uncommon.

The maximum likelihood estimate of Δ is $\hat{\Delta} = 0.1568$, corresponding to a constant adjacent odds ratio of $\exp(\hat{\Delta}) = 1.17$. The estimated standard error of $\hat{\Delta}$ is $\widehat{\text{se}}(\hat{\Delta}) = 0.0924$, and the Wald z-score, $z = \hat{\Delta}/\widehat{\text{se}}(\hat{\Delta}) = 1.70$, with two-tailed p-value equal to 0.09, slightly less than, but in general agreement with, that of the ridit z-score (9.43) at the 0.05 level of significance. An approximate 95% confidence interval for Δ is given by $\hat{\Delta} \pm 1.96 \, \widehat{\text{se}}(\hat{\Delta})$, yielding $(-0.024, 0.338)$, and exponentiating the interval endpoints yields $(0.98, 1.40)$ as an approximate 95% confidence interval for the common adjacent odds ratio.

Another version of the proportional odds model, discussed by McCullagh (1980), replaces the adjacent logits in (9.49) with *cumulative logit parameters*, defined by

$$H_i^{(j)} = \ln \frac{G_{i+1,l}}{F_{ij}} \qquad \text{for } i = 1, \ldots, k-1 \text{ and } j = 1, 2, \qquad (9.52)$$

where $F_{ij} = P_{1j} + \cdots + P_{ij}$ is the cumulative probability of a person in group j having an injury in category i or any category less severe, and $G_{i+1,j} = P_{i+1,j} + \cdots + P_{kj}$ is the cumulative probability of having an injury strictly more severe than category i. The model corresponding to (9.50) is now

$$H_i^{(2)} - H_i^{(1)} = \Delta' \qquad \text{for } i = 1, \ldots, k-1 \qquad (9.53)$$

and is called the *proportional cumulative odds* model. The numerical results

Table 9.12. *Observed and fitted frequencies and proportions for the data of Table 9.10*

| Severity | Observed Frequencies | | | Observed Adjacent Odds Ratio | Fitted Frequencies | | Fitted Proportions | |
	Reference	Comparison	Total		Reference	Comparison	Reference	Comparison
None	17	5	22		18.4	3.6	0.103	0.071
				0.63				
Minor	54	10	64		52.2	11.8	0.292	0.236
				1.44				
Moderate	60	16	76		60.1	15.9	0.336	0.318
				0.99				
Severe	19	5	24		18.3	5.7	0.102	0.114
				1.27				
Serious	9	3	12		8.8	3.2	0.049	0.064
				3.00				
Critical	6	6	12		8.4	3.6	0.047	0.071
				0.36				
Fatal	14	5	19		12.7	6.2	0.071	0.126
Total	179	50	229		179.0	50.0	1.000	1.000

The common adjacent odds ratios among the fitted expected frequencies and proportions is 1.17.

of fitting (9.53) to the data of Table 9.10 are very similar to those for the proportional adjacent odds model, and are not presented.

There are other ways to model multinomial responses, which are discussed in Section 11.4. The reader may find Figure 11.9 with a conceptual diagram of each model helpful.

There is a relation between the proportional adjacent odds model and the problem of assignment of scores $1, 2, 3, \ldots$ to categories that was raised in Section 9.4. To motivate the discussion, suppose we ask whether or not sample 2 could be considered to have arisen as a random sample without replacement from the finite population consisting of the two samples pooled together. To operationalize this further, consider assigning any set of specific scores a_i for $i = 1, 2, \ldots, k$ to the categories, and then ask whether or not the difference in mean scores would be statistically significant between the two groups. We could address this question with a randomization test; it remains to decide on a set of scores.

Our choice of scores could be guided by the locally most powerful score test for a given model thought to apply under the alternative hypothesis. The *conditional score test* for the null hypothesis $H_0: \Delta = 0$ under the proportional adjacent odds model (9.50) or (9.51) takes the form (with continuity correction)

$$
z_c = \frac{\left| \sum_{i=1}^{k} a_i (p_{i2} - p_{i1}) \right| - \frac{1}{2} \left(\frac{1}{n_1} + \frac{1}{n_2} \right)}{s_a \sqrt{\left(\frac{1}{n_1} + \frac{1}{n_2} \right)}} \sqrt{\frac{n_. - 1}{n_.}}, \tag{9.54}
$$

where the scores a_i multiplying the differences in relative frequencies take the simple form of integer scoring,

$$
a_i = i \qquad (i = 1, \ldots, k) \tag{9.55}
$$

(see Problem 9.7). In (9.54) the denominator contains the finite-population standard deviation of the scores, s_a, given in squared form by

$$
s_a^2 = \frac{\sum_{j=1}^{n_.} (a_j - \bar{a})^2}{n_.} = \sum_{i=1}^{k} \bar{p}_i (a_i - \bar{a}_w)^2, \tag{9.56}
$$

where $\bar{a}$ is the average score per injury over all $n_.$ observations (a_j denoting the score for the jth injury out of $n_.$), equivalently expressed as a weighted average score per category, with weights given by the marginal proportions $\bar{p}_i$:

$$
\bar{a}_w = \sum_{j=1}^{n_.} a_j / n_. = \sum_{i=1}^{k} \bar{p}_i a_i. \tag{9.57}
$$

The test statistic z_c is referred to the standard normal distribution under H_0. The factor $\{(n_{.}-1)n_{.}\}^{1/2}$ in (9.54) reflects the exact conditional variance of the difference in mean scores given fixed margins and may be omitted for large sample sizes n_1 and n_2. The same statistic z_c in (9.54) is used as a normal approximation to the exact randomization or urn model test that is used to assess the randomness hypothesis using scores (9.55).

We conclude from these considerations that assignment of the simple scores $a_i = i$ to the severity categories can be justified as an optimal scoring for the locally most powerful score test with respect to an assumed proportional adjacent odds model. Use of these scores need not imply that we are attempting to equate the severity difference of level 0 versus 1 with level $k-1$ versus k; it is, rather, that we behave in the same way simply for purposes of optimizing the power of the hypothesis test in a certain direction (that of proportional adjacent odds).

For the proportional cumulative odds model (9.53), the locally optimal scores are

$$a_i = n_{1.} + \cdots + n_{(i-1).} + \frac{n_{i.}+1}{2} \qquad (i=1,\ldots,k). \qquad (9.58)$$

These scores are the same as the tied ranks used in the Wilcoxon rank sum test with all outcomes in the same severity category tied. Note that they depend on the marginal frequencies $N_i + n_i = n_{i1} + n_{i2} = n_{i.}$ in the notation of Section 9.4 and Problems 9.4 and 9.7, and so vary from sample to sample.

For ridit analysis, (9.54) gives the ridit z-score (9.42) with use of the ridit scores. The ridit scores depend only on the reference group proportions, and therefore not on all the data. If the ridits were computed on the basis of the *combined* group of data, i.e., from $n_{1.},\ldots,n_{k.}$, the ridit scores would be equivalent to those in (9.58).

The score statistic in (9.54)–(9.56) was introduced by Cochran (1954) and Armitage (1955). It was discussed by Mantel (1963) and also goes under the name of an extended Mantel-Haenszel statistic ("extended" referring to the use of a given scoring system). The urn model is a commonly used device for testing null hypotheses. See Gail, Tan, and Piantadosi (1988) for an application in clinical trials; Hatch et al. (1990) give an application in epidemiology; and Levin and Robbins (1983) and Finkelstein and Levin (2001) give some applications in the law.

9.6.* THE EFFECT OF RANDOMNESS IN TRUE PROPORTIONS

In Section 9.1 we presented the chi-squared test of homogeneity of m binomial proportions. When the χ^2 statistic (9.4) is large, we infer that two or more of the true proportions differ among the populations, subgroups, or units sampled. How we further interpret the data depends on whether we view the true proportions as constants or as random variables. When viewed as constants, we interpret the differences as indicating systematic or *fixed effects*, the causes of which one tries to discover and explain. In other situations, especially those in which the sampling units are numerous and have many sources of variability, it makes sense to regard the true proportions themselves as random variables, and to view differences between them as *random effects*. As the search for systematic explanations for such differences continues, additional statistical tasks arise: (i) to characterize and/or quantify the unexplained random variation, (ii) to estimate the population average proportion with appropriate standard errors reflecting that variation, and (iii) to provide estimates for individual true proportions or odds which might improve upon the individual sample proportions by taking advantage of the "strength in numbers" in the ensemble of sampling units.

For example, during her reproductive years, a woman may have a number of pregnancies that result in a livebirth and some that result in other outcomes such as stillbirth, miscarriage (spontaneous abortion), or induced abortion. The proportion of livebirths among pregnancies could be called the woman's livebirth rate. This is a sample version of what demographers call a pregnancy outcome probability (Mode, 1985) on a per woman basis, or the woman's *true* livebirth rate. In a sample of m women with a given number of pregnancies, say n with $n \geq 2$, the livebirth rates for individual women can be observed empirically to have a variance larger than that implied by the binomial distribution with index n and parameter π, where π is the average livebirth pregnancy outcome probability in the group of women under consideration. A natural interpretation of this empirical fact is that, for whatever reasons, true livebirth rates vary from woman to woman as a random variable in the population. In that case, the average true livebirth rate should be estimated with a standard error greater than $\{\pi(1 - \pi)/(mn)\}^{1/2}$, which reflects only binomial variation. It is also of interest to estimate the true livebirth rate for a woman who has had x miscarriages among her first n pregnancies, for counseling on the chances of delivering a livebirth on her next pregnancy.

In the context of a clinical trial, subjects evaluated posttreatment with n binary assessments of health status in a given period would provide m independent sample proportions in each treatment group. To properly test the significance of the treatment effect, a random effects model would be required to allow for the natural variation in true health status from subject to subject. This and the previous example illustrate the *large sparse* case in which the number of proportions, m, is large but each proportion is based on a small number of binary observations, n.

In general, whenever observations have a hierarchical structure with nontrivial statistical variation operating at two or more levels, such as independent binary trials within subjects and subjects within populations, true proportions at the lower level (level 1) become random variables at the higher level (level 2). As a result, a test of the hypothesis of homogeneity for m binomial proportions ought to reject that hypothesis because the true proportions do truly differ. This is the view adopted in Section 10.8 on random effects meta-analysis. In that application, subjects constitute the sampling unit within studies (level 1), and studies constitute the sampling unit within groups of studies or within the hypothetical universe of all studies (level 2). The fixed effects estimated within a single study become random effects across the group of studies. For example, the significant variation in the proportion of smokers among the studies of lung cancer patients presented in Table 9.2 (or between the groups of studies identified as nonhomogeneous) might reflect random, unexplained variation across study populations. In that case, estimates of the average proportion of smokers in the universe of studies of lung cancer patients should reflect this additional source of variation.

Drawing statistical inferences when parameters are regarded as random variables is known as *Bayesian inference*, and also goes under the name of random effects modeling. The foregoing examples illustrate the *empirical Bayes* problem of estimation, in which there are many units each providing sample data governed by individual true parameters, and in which the data themselves are used to derive information about the distribution of the true parameters and other quantities of interest. *Parametric* empirical Bayes methods work with specific parametric families of distributions for the random parameters, and use the data to estimate the *hyper-parameters* of the assumed family. This in turn allows estimation of other quantities of interest. The choice of parametric families should be guided by experience with previous data sets of similar nature. *General* empirical Bayes methods provide nonparametric estimates of the quantities of interest directly, without first estimating the actual prior distribution of true parameters. Although they require a larger number of sampling units than parametric Bayes methods for a given level of precision, general empirical Bayes methods, when available, are attractive because they provide valid (consistent) estimates of quantities of interest for any prior distribution of true parameters in the population, even in ignorance of that distribution.

Subjective Bayesian inference refers to the use of subjective probability distributions to quantify a person's beliefs about a parameter regarded as a random variable. The subjective prior distribution governing the random parameter is to be identified through introspection or structured interview to elicit an individual's odds on the possible values he or she believes the true parameter may assume. For a subjective Bayesian analysis to be coherent, the prior distribution should reflect the subjective views of the decision-maker, not the convenience of the analyst. Therefore the common practice of adopting a simple prior distribution for mathematical convenience is not recommended except as illustrative.

Bayesian methods are enjoying renewed interest thanks to the continuing development of modern computers and algorithms for executing the complex computations required for applied problems. A full treatment of Bayesian methods is beyond the scope of this book. The interested reader may consult the textbooks by Berry (1996), Box and Tiao (1992), Carlin and Louis (2000), Gelman et al. (1995), Kadane (1996), and Press (1989). The subject of empirical Bayes inference and the closely related problem of compound decision theory was pioneered by Herbert Robbins; see, for example, Robbins (1956) and the collection of Robbins' papers selected by Lai and Siegmund (1985). Interesting applications of general empirical Bayes methods are contained in Robbins (1977, 1993), Robbins and Zhang (1988, 1989, and 1991), and Finkelstein, Levin, and Robbins (1996a, 1996b). The parametric empirical Bayes approach was popularized by Efron and Morris in a series of influential papers (1971, 1972a, 1972b, 1973a, 1973b, 1975). Below we present a few results to give the reader a taste of the problems encountered and the analyses that are possible.

9.6.1. Estimation of the Marginal Mean Proportion

Suppose we observe m binomial sample proportions $p_1, \ldots, p_m$, based on sample sizes $n_1, \ldots, n_m$, respectively. To simplify the notation, we write n_i instead of $n_{i.}$ and $n_. = n_1 + \cdots + n_m$ instead of $n_{..}$ in this section. We assume for simplicity that the true proportions P_i vary at random, independently of the sample sizes n_i. If a correlation did exist between P_i and n_i, as evidenced by a correlation between the observed p_i and n_i, the analysis below would require stratification on the binomial index. For example, the independence assumption might not hold for a pregnancy outcome analysis for women with complete reproductive histories: women with a higher likelihood of a live-birth versus other pregnancy outcomes may complete their desired family size with fewer pregnancies than those with a higher risk of termination. Estimates of π for women of specified gravidities (numbers of pregnancies) would be obtained separately.

We can write $E(p_i|n_i, P_i) = P_i$ and $\text{Var}(p_i|n_i, P_i) = P_i(1 - P_i)/n_i$ for the sample proportions from units at the first level, and $E(P_i|n_i) = \pi$ and $\text{Var}(P_i|n_i) = \pi(1 - \pi)D^2$ at the second level. We choose this form for the variance of P_i because $\pi(1 - \pi)$ is the maximum possible variance for a random variable on the unit interval with mean π; thus D^2 is a constant between 0 and 1. We first consider estimating π, the population average true proportion, and D^2. It follows from the assumptions that

$$E(p_i|n_i) = E\{E(p_i|n_i, P_i)|n_i\} = E(P_i|n_i) = \pi \tag{9.59}$$

and

$$\text{Var}(p_i|n_i) = E\{\text{Var}(p_i|n_i, P_i)|n_i\} + \text{Var}\{E(p_i|n_i, P_i)|n_i\}$$

$$= E\{P_i(1 - P_i)/n_i|n_i\} + \text{Var}(P_i|n_i)$$

$$= \frac{\pi(1 - \pi)\{1 + (n_i - 1)D^2\}}{n_i} \tag{9.60}$$

(see Problem 9.8).

The pooled average proportion is $\bar{p} = \sum_{i=1}^{m} n_i p_i / \sum_{i=1}^{m} n_i = \sum_{i=1}^{m} n_i p_i / n_.$, as in (9.2); it is a weighted average of the sample proportions, with weights $n_i / n_.$. This $\bar{p}$ is an unbiased estimate of π, because given the collection of sample sizes, which will be denoted by $\underline{n}$, we have from (9.59) that $E(\bar{p}|\underline{n}) = \sum_{i=1}^{m} n_i E(p_i|n_i)/n_. = \pi$. The variance of $\bar{p}$ is

$$\text{Var}(\bar{p}|\underline{n}) = \frac{\pi(1-\pi)\{1 + (\bar{n}_w - 1)D^2\}}{n_.}, \qquad (9.61)$$

where $\bar{n}_w$ is the weighted average sample size,

$$\bar{n}_w = \sum_{i=1}^{m} \left(\frac{n_i}{n_.}\right) n_i = \sum_{i=1}^{m} n_i^2 \bigg/ \sum_{i=1}^{m} n_i \qquad (9.62)$$

(see Problem 9.9). Expression (9.61) shows that compared to the fixed-effects variance, $\pi(1-\pi)/n_.$, in the presence of random variation in true proportions, the variance of $\bar{p}$ is magnified by the *variance inflation factor*, VIF $= 1 + (\bar{n}_w - 1)D^2$. Note that D^2 can be interpreted as an intraclass correlation coefficient (see Chapter 15). The larger the average sample size $\bar{n}_w$, or the larger the intraclass correlation coefficient D^2, the greater is the variance inflation factor. The variance inflation factor is also called an *overdispersion* parameter.

To estimate π with minimum variance when the n_i's are not all equal, we must generally use a different weighted average, one that uses weights proportional to the reciprocal of (9.60). Assuming π and D^2 were known, the optimal estimator would be

$$\hat{\pi} = \sum_{i=1}^{m} w_i p_i \bigg/ \sum_{i=1}^{m} w_i \qquad (9.63)$$

with

$$w_i = \frac{n_i}{\pi(1-\pi)\{1 + (n_i - 1)D^2\}}. \qquad (9.64)$$

(See Chapter 10, Section 1 for some general theory related to weighted average estimators with minimum variance.) The variance of $\hat{\pi}$ would be

$$\text{Var}(\hat{\pi}|\underline{n}) = \frac{\sum_{i=1}^{m} w_i^2 \text{Var}(p_i|\underline{n})}{\left(\sum_{i=1}^{m} w_i\right)^2} = \frac{1}{\sum_{i=1}^{m} w_i}$$

$$= \frac{1}{\sum_{i=1}^{m} \dfrac{n_i}{\pi(1-\pi)\{1 + (n_i - 1)D^2\}}}. \qquad (9.65)$$

Problem 9.10 demonstrates that (9.65) is no greater than (9.61) and is strictly less than (9.61) unless all n_i's are equal, in which case (9.63) is the same as $\bar{p}$.

In order to use the formulas (9.61)–(9.65) for standard errors and confidence intervals, we need to estimate the unknown variance components $\pi(1 - \pi)$ and D^2. Estimates of these quantities may be used in (9.64) to produce approximately optimal weights (call them $\hat{w}_i$), and then the weights $\tilde{w}_i$ may be used in (9.63) to produce an estimate of π with approximately minimum variance:

$$\tilde{\pi} = \sum_{i=1}^{m} \tilde{w}_i p_i \bigg/ \sum_{i=1}^{m} \tilde{w}_i. \tag{9.66}$$

The standard error of $\tilde{\pi}$ is estimated by

$$\widetilde{se}(\tilde{\pi}|\underline{n}) = \frac{1}{\sqrt{\sum_{i=1}^{m} \tilde{w}_i}}. \tag{9.67}$$

To estimate $\pi(1 - \pi)$ and D^2 we proceed as follows. Let

$$Q_1 = \frac{\chi^2 \overline{pq}}{m - 1} = \frac{\sum_{i=1}^{m} n_i (p_i - \bar{p})^2}{m - 1}, \tag{9.68}$$

where χ^2 is the chi squared statistic (9.4). Problem 9.11 asks the reader to show that

$$E(Q_1|\underline{n}) = \pi(1 - \pi)(1 + c_1 D^2), \tag{9.69}$$

where

$$c_1 = \frac{(n_. - m) - (\bar{n}_w - 1)}{m - 1} = \frac{m(\bar{n}_a - 1) - (\bar{n}_w - 1)}{m - 1}, \tag{9.70}$$

In (9.70), $\bar{n}_a = n_./m$ is the arithmetic-average sample size, which is always less than or equal to the weighted-average sample size $\bar{n}_w$.

Now let

$$Q_2 = \bar{p}(1 - \bar{p})\frac{n_.}{n_. - 1}. \tag{9.71}$$

Problem 9.12 is to show that

$$E(Q_2|\underline{n}) = \pi(1 - \pi)(1 - c_2 D^2), \tag{9.72}$$

where

$$c_2 = \frac{\bar{n}_w - 1}{n_. - 1} = \frac{\bar{n}_w - 1}{m\bar{n}_a - 1}. \tag{9.73}$$

Note that because m appears in the denominator of (9.73), c_2 becomes small as m becomes large, i.e., Q_2 is approximately unbiased for $\pi(1 - \pi)$ for a large number of proportions. By solving the pair of equations (9.69) and (9.72) for $\pi(1 - \pi)$ and D^2, it follows that an unbiased estimate of $\pi(1 - \pi)$ is given by

$$\frac{c_1 Q_2 + c_2 Q_1}{c_1 + c_2} \tag{9.74}$$

and an unbiased estimate of $\mathrm{Var}(P) = \pi(1 - \pi)D^2$ is given by

$$\widetilde{\mathrm{Var}}(P) = \frac{Q_1 - Q_2}{c_1 + c_2}. \tag{9.75}$$

Thus a ratio-unbiased estimate of D^2 is given by

$$\widetilde{D^2} = \frac{Q_1 - Q_2}{c_1 Q_2 + c_2 Q_1}, \tag{9.76}$$

and substituting (9.74) and (9.76) in (9.61) yields an estimate of $\mathrm{Var}(\bar{p} \mid \underline{n})$:

$$\widetilde{\mathrm{Var}}(\bar{p}) = \left[\frac{c_1 Q_2 + c_2 Q_1}{c_1 + c_2} \left\{ 1 + (\bar{n}_w - 1)\widetilde{D^2} \right\} \right] \Big/ n_{.} \tag{9.77}$$

This estimate is unbiased, because it can be written equivalently as

$$
\begin{aligned}
\mathrm{Var}(\bar{p}) &= \frac{\{c_2 + (\bar{n}_w - 1)\}Q_1 - \{(\bar{n}_w - 1) - c_1\}Q_2}{n_{.}(c_1 + c_2)} \\
&= \frac{(\bar{n}_w - 1)\dfrac{n_{.}}{n_{.} - 1}Q_1 - (\bar{n}_w - \bar{n}_a)\dfrac{m}{m - 1}Q_2}{n_{.}\left\{(\bar{n}_w - 1)\dfrac{n_{.}}{n_{.} - 1} - (\bar{n}_w - \bar{n}_a)\dfrac{m}{m - 1}\right\}},
\end{aligned}
\tag{9.78}
$$

and taking expectations yields (9.61). In the above expression, and in (9.71) and (9.73), $n_{.}$ may be used instead of $n_{.} - 1$ with negligible bias when $n_{.}$ is large.

If we ignore terms of order $1/n_{.}$, we can write $\widetilde{D^2}$ alternatively as

$$
\begin{aligned}
\widetilde{D^2} &= \frac{Q_1 - Q_2}{c_1 Q_2 + c_2 Q_1} \\
&= \frac{\left(\dfrac{x^2}{m - 1}\right)\left(\dfrac{n_{.} - 1}{n_{.}}\right) - 1}{c_1 + c_2\left(\dfrac{x^2}{m - 1}\right)\left(\dfrac{n_{.} - 1}{n_{.}}\right)} \approx \frac{\left(\dfrac{x^2}{m - 1}\right) - 1}{c_1 + c_2\left(\dfrac{x^2}{m - 1}\right)}.
\end{aligned}
$$

From this we arrive at the following large-sample estimate of the variance inflation factor, $\text{VIF} = 1 + (\bar{n}_w - 1)D^2$ (continuing to ignore terms of order $1/n.$):

$$\widetilde{\text{VIF}} = \frac{\dfrac{\chi^2}{m-1} - b}{1 - b}, \qquad \text{where } b = \frac{\bar{n}_w - \bar{n}_a}{\bar{n}_w - 1}\frac{m}{m-1} \qquad (9.79)$$

is a correction for imbalance in the sample sizes n_i. If the sample sizes are all equal to n, say, then $c_1 = \bar{n}_w - 1 = \bar{n}_a - 1 = n - 1$, the unbiased estimate of the variance of $\bar{p}$ in (9.77) reduces to $Q_1/n. = Q_1/(mn)$, and the estimate for the VIF in (9.79) reduces simply to $\chi^2/(m - 1)$.

Although (9.69) and (9.72) show that the expected value of Q_1 is at least as large as the expected value of Q_2, the sample difference of Q_1 and Q_2 in the unbiased estimator (9.76) for D^2 may be negative. Indeed, if there were no heterogeneity in the true proportions ($D^2 = 0$), we would expect $\widetilde{D}^2$ to be negative roughly half of the time. Because D^2 must be nonnegative a truncated version of $\widetilde{D}^2$ is often used in place of (9.76):

$$\widetilde{D}^{2+} = \max\left(\widetilde{D}^2, 0\right).$$

When $\widetilde{D}^2 < 0$, the fixed effects hypothesis $D^2 = 0$ is usually adopted; $\bar{p}$ estimates the now constant true proportion P, and, from (9.61) and (9.72), $Q_2/n. = \bar{p}(1 - \bar{p})/(n - 1)$ estimates $\text{Var}(\bar{p}|\underline{n})$. While (9.77) with $\widetilde{D}^2 = 0$ is an unbiased estimate of $\text{Var}(\bar{p}|\underline{n})$ under the fixed-effects hypothesis $D^2 = 0$, generally $\bar{p}(1 - \bar{p})/(n - 1)$ is a more precise estimate of $\text{Var}(\bar{p}|\underline{n})$ than is (9.77) with $\widetilde{D}^2$ set equal to zero. For the weighted average estimator (9.66), when $\widetilde{D}^2 < 0$ and $\widetilde{D}^{2+} = 0$ is used instead, the weights (9.64) are proportional to n_i, (9.66) reduces to $\bar{p}$, and the variance formula (9.65) reduces to $\pi(1 - \pi)/n.$, which again may be estimated by $Q_2/n. = \bar{p}(1 - \bar{p})/(n. - 1)$.

Several models for overdispersed binomial or multinomial data have been considered in the literature; see, e.g., Banerjee and Paul (1999) and Morel and Nagaraj (1993). Morton (1991) represents an overdispersed multinomial as a set of independent overdispersed Poisson random variables conditioned on a fixed sum. Analyses of such data have been discussed in the two-sample problem by Neerchal and Morel (1998) and Cook and Lawless (1991), and in log linear models by Waller and Zelterman (1997). Goodness-of-fit test statistics of a multinomial model against overdispersion alternatives have been proposed by Kim and Margolin (1992), Paul, Liang, and Self (1989), Wilson (1989), and Whittemore et al. (1987), and, in the case of large sparse data sets, by Zelterman (1987). Overdispersion models appear in diverse application areas, particularly in toxicology (Ibrahim and Ryan, 1996; O'Hara-Hines and Lawless, 1993).

Table 9.13. *Pregnancy outcomes for women with one, two, or three pregnancies*

Gravidity	Frequency of Livebirths				No. of Women (m_g)	No. of Pregnancies (n_g)	No. of Livebirths (X_g)	Livebirth Proportion $(\bar{p}_g = X_g / n_g)$
$(g = n_i)$	0	1	2	3				
1	433	737	—	—	1170	1170	737	0.630
2	168	436	368	—	972	1944	1172	0.603
3	52	215	229	131	627	1881	1066	0.567
Total	653	1388	597	131	2769	4995	2975	0.596

9.6.2. An Example

To illustrate these ideas, consider the data in Table 9.13 from a case-control study of spontaneous abortion (Kline et al., 1995). Cases were women presenting to one of three New York City hospitals with a miscarriage (spontaneous abortion). Controls were women who were recruited from a prenatal care setting before 22 weeks gestation and delivered at 28 weeks or later. The table presents livebirth outcomes from 2,769 women in the control group with one, two, or three pregnancies prior to the index pregnancy that led to their enrollment in the study.

The first row gives the frequencies of women whose only prior pregnancy resulted in 0 or 1 livebirth. The second row gives the frequencies of women having 0, 1, or 2 livebirths for women with two pregnancies, and the third row similarly gives frequencies of women having 0, 1, 2, or 3 livebirths among those with three pregnancies. In the first row, the estimated average livebirth proportion is $\bar{p}_1 = 0.63$; in the second row, the pooled estimate is $\bar{p}_2 = 0.60$, and in the third row, the pooled estimate is $\bar{p}_3 = 0.57$. Do the average livebirth outcome probabilities differ significantly by gravidity?

The first row comprises only binary outcomes, so the standard error of the livebirth proportion for gravidity 1 is $\{\bar{p}_1(1 - \bar{p}_1)/(n_{1.} - 1)\}^{1/2} = 0.0141$. For gravidity 2, we have $Q_1 = 0.2548$, $Q_2 = 0.2395$, $c_1 = 1$, and $c_2 = 1/1169 = 0.000515$, so that from (9.75), the estimated variance of P is 0.0153, implying that the true livebirth proportions have a standard deviation of 0.1237. The variance inflation factor is estimated as $\widehat{\text{VIF}} = \chi^2/(m - 1) \approx Q_1/Q_2 = 1.064$, and from (9.78), the standard error of $\bar{p}_2$ is estimated as $(Q_1/n_{2.})^{1/2} \approx \{\widehat{\text{VIF}} \cdot Q_2/n_{2.}\}^{1/2} = 0.0114$. For gravidity 3, we have $Q_1 = 0.2650$, $Q_2 = 0.2456$, $c_1 = 2$, and $c_2 = 2/1880 = 0.00106$, so that from (9.75), the estimated variance of P is $(0.2650 - 0.2456)/2.00106 = 0.00969$, implying that the true livebirth proportions have a standard deviation of 0.0985. The variance inflation factor is estimated as $\widehat{\text{VIF}} \approx Q_1/Q_2 = 1.079$, and from this the standard error of $\bar{p}_3$ is estimated as 0.0119.

The difference between livebirth proportions for gravidity 1 and 2 is $\bar{p}_1 - \bar{p}_2 = 0.027$ with standard error $(0.0141^2 + 0.0114^2)^{1/2} = 0.0181$, so the difference has z-score $z = 0.027/0.0181 = 1.49$ and is not statistically significant. If we estimate a single pooled livebirth proportion, $\bar{p}_{1+2}$, for gravidities 1 and 2, we find $\bar{p}_{1+2} = (737 + 1172)/(1170 + 1944) = 0.613$. Now $Q_1 = 0.2432$, $Q_2 = 0.2373$, $c_1 = 0.4558$ from (9.70), and $c_2 = 0.0002916$ from (9.73), so that from (9.75), the estimated variance of P is $(0.2432 - 0.2373)/(0.4558 + 0.0002916) = 0.01294$, implying that the true livebirth proportions would have a standard deviation of 0.1137. The variance inflation factor is estimated from (9.79) with $b = 0.2732$ as $\widehat{\text{VIF}} = 1.034$. From this, or directly from (9.77), the standard error of $\bar{p}_{1+2}$ is estimated as 0.008877.

For comparison, the weighted average (9.66) for gravidity 1 and 2 is $\tilde{\pi} = 0.613$, with optimal weights from (9.64) estimated by substituting the estimates of $\pi(1 - \pi)$ and D^2 from (9.74) and (9.76), respectively. $\tilde{\pi}$ is essentially the same as $\bar{p}_{1+2}$, and the standard error of $\tilde{\pi}$ is 0.008874, trivially less than that of the pooled estimate $\bar{p}_{1+2}$. The variance reduction is negligible in this case because the n_i's only take values 1 or 2, and $\text{Var}(P)$ is small.

The methods of Section 10.1 may be used to test the homogeneity hypothesis $\pi_1 = \pi_2 = \pi_3$ with a 2 df test. Here we simply point out that $\bar{p}_3$ is significantly less than $\bar{p}_{1+2}$ with critical ratio $z = (\bar{p}_{1+2} - \bar{p}_3)/\widehat{\text{se}}(\bar{p}_{1+2} - \bar{p}_3)$ $= (0.613 - 0.567)/(0.008877^2 + 0.0119^2)^{1/2} = 3.10$. If we do not pool the livebirth proportions for gravidity 1 and 2, we find $\bar{p}_3$ to be significantly smaller than both $\bar{p}_1$ and $\bar{p}_2$, with z-scores 3.41 $(p < 0.001)$ and 2.18 $(p < 0.05)$, respectively.

9.6.3. General Empirical Bayes Estimation of Posterior Odds, and a Test of Homogeneity of Proportions in the Large Sparse Case

Next we consider estimation of the odds $P/(1 - P)$ for subjects with given observed outcomes. Suppose that, given n_i and P_i, X_i has a binomial distribution with index n_i and parameter P_i, and write $p_i = x_i/n_i$ for observed $X_i = x_i$. The following fundamental relation, due to Herbert Robbins, is called the *general empirical Bayes identity* for binomial distributions. See Robbins (1956), Cressie (1982), and Robbins and Zhang (1991). It states that for $j = 0, \ldots, n_i - 1$,

$$E\left(\frac{P_i}{1 - P_i}\bigg| n_i, X_i = j\right) = \frac{P(X_i = j + 1|n_i)\bigg/\binom{n_i}{j + 1}}{P(X_i = j|n_i)\bigg/\binom{n_i}{j}}$$

$$= \frac{P(X_i = j + 1|n_i)}{P(X_i = j|n_i)}\left(\frac{j + 1}{n_i - j}\right). \tag{9.80}$$

Problem 9.13 gives a proof of (9.80). In words, the identity says that for the group of subjects with j successes out of n_i trials, the average of the true odds is given by the expression on the right-hand side of (9.80). The beauty of the identity is that it expresses the posterior expected odds, an otherwise unobservable quantity, in terms of the marginal probabilities of the frequencies X_i, which can be estimated directly from the data when m is large.

For the data in the second row of Table 9.13, the values of (9.80) for $j = 0$ and 1 are $(436/2)/168 = 1.298$ and $368/(436/2) = 1.688$. We infer that the average odds on a livebirth among those with one previous livebirth out of two pregnancies are about 30% greater than the average odds on a livebirth among those with no livebirths in two pregnancies. Estimates of the average livebirth probabilities are considered below.

The fundamental identity (9.80) suggests that if there is random variation in the true P, the quantities on the right-hand side should increase as j increases from 0, because in the expected odds on the left-hand side, the conditioning on the event $[X = j]$ selects for those individuals with increasingly larger values of P. This assertion can be proved by Jensen's inequality. If there is no heterogeneity in P, the quantities on the right-hand side remain constant, which can be verified by substituting the terms from the binomial probability function. These considerations can be used to construct a test for heterogeneity in P in the large sparse case. Such a test is useful because the usual chi squared statistic (9.4) for m proportions does not have good power in the large sparse case (because there are too many degrees of freedom); in fact, (9.4) does not even have a χ^2 distribution in this case (because the sample sizes n_i need to be large with m remaining fixed, just the opposite of the large sparse case).

Other methods for testing homogeneity in the large-sparse case have been proposed (see, e.g., Paul et al., 1989). A simple test is provided by the chi squared goodness-of-fit statistic for the hypothesis that the multinomial cell probabilities underlying the frequencies in Table 9.13 agree with the binomial probability function. The goodness-of-fit test will generally have degrees of freedom more than 1, however, so a 1 df statistic that capitalizes on the increasing sequence of posterior expected odds in (9.80) for $j = 0, \ldots, n_i - 1$ due to random variation in P should do better.

To motivate the test, consider again the second row of data in Table 9.13. The identity states that $2P(X_i = 2)/P(X_i = 1) \geq P(X_i = 1)/\{2P(X_i = 0)\}$ with equality if and only if there is no variation in the true proportions, in which case $P(X_i = j) = \binom{2}{j} \pi^j (1 - \pi)^{2-j}$ and $\pi/(1 - \pi) = 2P(X_i = 2)/P(X_i = 1) = P(X_i = 1)/\{2P(X_i = 0)\}$. When m_2 is large, we may test whether the sample quantity

$$\hat{\delta} = \ln \frac{2f_{22}}{f_{21}} - \ln \frac{f_{21}}{2f_{20}} = \ln f_{20} - 2\ln f_{21} + \ln f_{22} + \ln 4 \qquad (9.81)$$

has zero mean, where f_{20}, f_{21}, and f_{22} are the frequencies of women of gravidity 2 with 0, 1, and 2 livebirths, respectively, with $f_{20} + f_{21} + f_{22} = m_2$. By the delta method, $\tilde{\delta}$ has estimated standard error

$$\widehat{se}(\tilde{\delta}) = \sqrt{\frac{1}{f_{20}} + \frac{4}{f_{21}} + \frac{1}{f_{22}}}, \tag{9.82}$$

and the critical ratio $z = \tilde{\delta}/\widehat{se}(\tilde{\delta})$ can be referred to the standard normal distribution. For the data in Table 9.13, we find $\tilde{\delta} = \ln 1.688 - \ln 1.298 = 0.2631$ with $\widehat{se}(\tilde{\delta}) = \{(1/168) + (4/436) + (1/368)\}^{1/2} = 0.1336$ and critical ratio $z = 0.2631/0.1336 = 1.97$. A one-sided test is appropriate here due to the inequality in (9.80). We infer that the 30% increase in odds mentioned above for those with one livebirth relative to those with no livebirths is significant at the one-sided 0.025 level.

The empirical Bayes test for heterogeneity of proportions in the general large sparse case proceeds as follows. The form of the fundamental identity (9.80) leads us to parameterize the multinomial distribution governing the frequencies of outcomes f_{gj} for given g by adjacent logits (see Section 9.5). Under the null hypothesis of no variation in P, the adjacent logits plus offsets $\ln\{(j+1)/(g-j)\}$ are constant in j for $j = 0, \ldots, g-1$. For a wide variety of prior distributions for P under the alternative hypothesis, these quantities increase in a remarkably linear manner. It is thus reasonable to fit a linear model in j to the adjacent logits plus offsets and test the hypothesis of zero slope versus the one-sided alternative that the slope is positive. Assuming a common slope for all gravidity groups $g \geq 2$ yields a test with a single degree of freedom (see Parides, 1995). Levin (1992) uses the same method to derive a test of odds-ratio homogeneity with improved power in the large sparse case of many fourfold tables with small margins.

Fitting the logit model

$$\ln \frac{P(X_i = j+1 \mid n_i = g) \Big/ \binom{g}{j+1}}{P(X_i = j \mid n_i = g) \Big/ \binom{g}{j}} = \alpha_g + \beta j \qquad \text{for } g = 1, 2, 3$$

$$\text{and } j = 0, \ldots, g-1 \quad (9.83)$$

to the data in Table 9.13, we find $\hat{\beta} = 0.1866$ with $\widehat{se}(\hat{\beta}) = 0.0745$. The critical ratio $z = \hat{\beta}/\widehat{se}(\hat{\beta}) = 2.50$ has one-tailed p-value 0.006. Compare this with the chi squared goodness-of-fit statistic for multinomial cell probabilities given by the binomial probability function with index g and parameter $\bar{p}_g$. For $g = 2$, chi squared is 3.94 on 1 df, and for $g = 3$, chi squared is 7.72 on 2

Table 9.14. *Observed and fitted cell probabilities for the empirical Bayes logit model (9.83) and the binomial model*

	Gravidity $(g = n_i)$	Cell Probabilities (for Frequency of Livebirths)			
		0	1	2	3
Observed	1	0.370	0.630	—	—
Model (9.83)		0.370	0.630	—	—
Binomial model		0.370	0.630		
Observed	2	0.173	0.449	0.379	—
Model (9.83)		0.168	0.457	0.374	—
Binomial model		0.160	0.480	0.360	—
Observed	3	0.083	0.343	0.365	0.209
Model (9.83)		0.097	0.308	0.393	0.202
Binomial model		0.084	0.319	0.418	0.182

df. The sum of these is 11.66 on 3 df (p-value 0.009). That the p-value is not as small as that for the one-sided critical ratio test for the slope coefficient β in model (9.83) reflects the greater power of the latter test.

The intercept terms $\exp(\alpha_g) = E\{P/(1 - P)|X_i = 0, \ n_i = g\}$ are also of interest. The expected odds on livebirth decrease strongly with gravidity among those with no livebirths: $\hat{\alpha}_1 = 0.5319$ (expected odds 1.702), $\hat{\alpha}_2 = 0.3058$ (expected odds 1.358), and $\hat{\alpha}_3 = 0.0581$ (expected odds 1.060). Unlike the test for equality of the marginal proportions $\bar{p}_1$ and $\bar{p}_2$, there is a significant difference between $\hat{\alpha}_1$ and $\hat{\alpha}_2$: $\hat{\alpha}_1 - \hat{\alpha}_2 = 0.2261$, $\widehat{se}(\hat{\alpha}_1 - \hat{\alpha}_2) = 0.0877$, $z = 2.58$, p-value = 0.01, two-tailed. The difference between $\hat{\alpha}_1$ and $\hat{\alpha}_3$ is also significant: $\hat{\alpha}_1 - \hat{\alpha}_3 = 0.4738$, $\widehat{se}(\hat{\alpha}_1 - \hat{\alpha}_3) = 0.1124$, $z = 4.22$, p-value < 0.001, two-tailed.

Table 9.14 shows the observed and fitted cell probabilities for the logit model (9.83) and for the binomial model with separate average livebirth probabilities. The logit model fits the data significantly better than does the binomial model: the chi squared goodness-of-fit statistic is 11.66 on 3 df for the binomial model, compared to 5.49 on 2 df for model (9.83), and the difference of 6.17 on 1 df agrees well with the square of the critical ratio for the β coefficient ($z^2 = 2.50^2 = 6.25$). Both models fit the data for the primigravidae perfectly, because there is only one degree of freedom in the first row of Table 9.13, and there is one free parameter for row 1 in each model. The logit model fits the data in row 2 better than the null binomial model in each cell. The logit model fits the data in row 3 a little better than the null binomial model: $\chi^2 = 7.72$ for the binomial compared to 5.16 for model (9.83); but the residuals from the model suggest that there are too few women of gravidity 3 with no livebirths in the data compared to women with one livebirth. This may reflect a relation between obstetric history and patterns of seeking routine prenatal care.

9.6.4. Parametric Models

If the prior distribution of P belongs to the family of beta distributions, calculations are dramatically simplified. A beta distribution with parameters $a > 0$ and $b > 0$ has probability density function

$$f(P) = \frac{\Gamma(a+b)}{\Gamma(a)\Gamma(b)} P^{a-1}(1-P)^{b-1} \qquad (9.84)$$

for $0 < P < 1$. The normalizing constant involves the gamma function, defined as $\Gamma(a) = \int_0^\infty x^{a-1} e^{-x}\, dx$, taking values $\Gamma(a) = (a-1)!$ for positive integer values of a, and satisfying the recursive relation $\Gamma(a) = (a-1)\Gamma(a-1)$ for arbitrary values of $a > 0$. The mean and variance of the beta distribution are

$$E(P) = \pi = \frac{a}{a+b} \quad \text{and} \quad \text{Var}(P) = \frac{ab}{(a+b)^2(a+b+1)} = \frac{\pi(1-\pi)}{a+b+1}.$$

$$(9.85)$$

The beta family of density functions encompasses a wide variety of shapes. When $a = b = 1$, P has the uniform distribution on the unit interval. When $0 < a < 1$ and $0 < b < 1$, the density of P is U-shaped. When $a > 1$ and $0 < b < 1$, the density of P is J-shaped, or reverse J-shaped when $0 < a < 1$ and $b > 1$. When $a > 1$ and $b > 1$, the density of P is unimodal and roughly bell-shaped. As a and b become large with $a/(a+b) = \pi$, the distribution of P becomes concentrated around π as the variance approaches zero. As a and b approach zero, P approaches a binary random variable, taking values 1 or 0 with probability π or $1 - \pi$, respectively.

Suppose, given integer n, P has a beta distribution with parameters a and b, independent of n, and further suppose that given n and P, X has a binomial distribution with index n and parameter P. Then the marginal distribution of X has the *beta-binomial* distribution with index n and parameters a and b. Its probability function is

$$P(X = j \mid n) = \binom{n}{j} \frac{\Gamma(a+b)}{\Gamma(a)\Gamma(b)} \cdot \frac{\Gamma(a+j)\Gamma(b+n-j)}{\Gamma(a+b+n)}$$

$$= \binom{n}{j} \frac{(a+j-1)\cdots(a+1)a\cdot(b+n-j-1)\cdots(b+1)b}{(a+b+n-1)\cdots(a+b+1)(a+b)}.$$

$$(9.86)$$

For example, when $a = b = 1$, the marginal distribution of X is uniform on the integers $0, \dots, n$, such that, $P(X = j \mid n) = 1/(n+1)$. The marginal mean and variance of X are

$$E(X|n) = n\pi \quad \text{and} \quad \text{Var}(X|n) = n\pi(1-\pi)\frac{a+b+n}{a+b+1}, \quad (9.87)$$

As the prior parameters a and b become large with $a/(a+b)=\pi$, the beta-binomial distribution of X approaches the ordinary binomial distribution with index n and parameter π, with minimum variance $n\pi(1-\pi)$. As the prior parameters approach zero, the beta-binomial distribution of X approaches a polarized distribution, taking values n or 0 with probability π and $1-\pi$, respectively, with maximum variance $n^2\pi(1-\pi)$.

The sample proportion $p = X/n$ has mean $E(p|n) = \pi$ and variance

$$\text{Var}(p|n) = \frac{\pi(1-\pi)}{n}\{1+(n-1)D^2\}, \quad \text{where } D^2 = \frac{1}{a+b+1}. \quad (9.88)$$

Given m independent proportions p_i based on sample sizes n_i $(i=1,\ldots,m)$ with numerators following the beta-binomial distribution with index n_i and parameters a and b, the average proportion π may be estimated by the methods in the preceding subsection, but it is more efficient to estimate a, b, and π by maximum likelihood (see Appendix B).

For the livebirth data, the maximum likelihood estimates of π and $a+b$ are, for gravidity 1, $\hat{\pi}_1 = 0.630$ and $\hat{a}+\hat{b} = \infty$ (because the beta-binomial and binomial models are identical for $n=1$); for gravidity 2, $\hat{\pi}_2 = 0.603$ and $\hat{a}+\hat{b} = 14.82$; and for gravidity 3, $\hat{\pi}_3 = 0.567$ and $\hat{a}+\hat{b} = 24.48$. The overdispersion parameters are 0, $1+(1/15.82) = 1.063$, and $1+(2/24.48) = 1.082$, respectively. Although $D^2 = 1/(a+b+1)$ is estimated to be larger for gravidity 2 than gravidity 3, note that multiplication by $n-1$ in the variance inflation factor causes greater overdispersion for gravidity 3 than gravidity 2. The overdispersion parameters agree well with the VIF estimates found in Section 9.6.2 using (9.79).

The most useful property of the beta-binomial model is that the posterior distribution of P_i given X_i has an especially simple form: that of another beta distribution, with parameters $a+X_i$ and $b+n_i-X_i$. It follows that the conditional mean of P_i given X_i is

$$E(P_i|n_i, X_i) = \frac{a+X_i}{a+b+n_i} = \pi\left(\frac{a+b}{a+b+n_i}\right) + p_i\left(\frac{n_i}{a+b+n_i}\right). \quad (9.89)$$

Expression (9.89) shows that the posterior mean of P_i is a weighted average of the *a priori* average π and the sample proportion p_i, with relatively more weight on the sample proportion for larger n_i, and relatively more weight on the prior mean for smaller n_i. When used to estimate P_i or to predict a future value of X_i, expression (9.89) is called a *shrinkage estimator*, because the sample proportion p_i is "shrunk" toward the prior mean π. Although (9.89) is a biased estimate for P_i, it can be shown that the mean squared error of (9.89) as an estimate for P_i is smaller than that for p_i: the mean squared error for the former is $ab/\{(a+b)(a+b+1)(a+b+n_i)\}$, while that for p_i is $ab/\{(a+b)(a+b+1)n_i\}$. This holds true both for individual estimates and for the total mean squared error for the ensemble of women. Thus the shrinkage estimator has an optimality property when the beta-binomial model holds. Further results from empirical Bayes theory show that as m becomes large, (9.89) with a, b, and π estimated by maximum likelihood performs as well in terms of mean squared error as knowing the true values of a and b. Remarkably, the same is true of the general empirical Bayes estimates of posterior odds: as m becomes large, (9.80) does as well as actually knowing the true prior distribution of P (without having to estimate it).

In the livebirth data, from (9.89) and the maximum likelihood estimates of π and $a+b$ given above, for a woman with no livebirths, the estimate of her true livebirth probability for gravidity 1, $E(P|n=1, X=0)$, is 0.630; for gravidity 2, the estimate of $E(P|n=2, X=0)$ is 0.531, and for gravidity 3, the estimate of $E(P|n=3, X=0)$ is 0.505. How do these expectations compare with the posterior expected odds found in Section 9.6.3 using model (9.83)?

We note that by Jensen's inequality, for any prior distribution for P_i,

$$E\left(\frac{P}{1-P}\middle| n, X=j\right) \geq \frac{E(P|n, X=j)}{1-E(P|n, X=j)} \tag{9.90}$$

and

$$E\left(\frac{1-P}{P}\middle| n, X=j\right) \geq \frac{E(P|n, X=j)}{1-E(P|n, X=j)}. \tag{9.91}$$

For $j=0,\ldots,n-1$, define the numbers

$$r_j = \frac{E\left(\frac{P}{1-P}\middle| n, X=j\right)}{1+E\left(\frac{P}{1-P}\middle| n, X=j\right)} = \frac{P(X=j+1|n)\bigg/\binom{n}{j+1}}{P(X=j|n)\bigg/\binom{n}{j}} \Bigg/ \left(1 + \frac{P(X=j+1|n)\bigg/\binom{n}{j+1}}{P(X=j|n)\bigg/\binom{n}{j}}\right). \tag{9.92}$$

The r_j are proportions obtained by "back-transforming" the posterior expected odds; they can be estimated from the marginal data as shown on the right-hand side of (9.92). From the inequalities in (9.90) and (9.91), the general empirical Bayes identity (9.80) for $E\{P/(1-P)|n, X=j\}$, and the corresponding identity for the reciprocal odds, namely,

$$E\left(\frac{1-P}{P}\Bigg|n,\ X=j\right) = \frac{P(X=j-1|n)\Big/\binom{n}{j-1}}{P(X=j|n)\Big/\binom{n}{j}}, \tag{9.93}$$

it follows that for $j = 0,\ldots,n$,

$$r_{j-1} \le E(P|n,\ X=j) \le r_j. \tag{9.94}$$

In (9.94), we need a definition of r_{-1} and r_n, which are not covered by (9.92), so for the moment let us take the simple bounds $r_{-1} = 0$ and $r_n = 1$ (we improve on this choice below). (9.94) shows that the r_j bracket the desired posterior expected probabilities, but we need to specify suitable values between the r_j in order to estimate $E(P|n,\ X=j)$ without the bias produced by Jensen's inequality. Following work by Robbins, Cressie (1982) argued that a reasonable choice for an estimate $\hat{E}_j$ of $E(P|n,\ X=j)$ that falls between r_{j-1} and r_j would be obtained by choosing a "self-weighted" average of r_{j-1} and r_j, i.e., by defining $\hat{E}_j$ such that $\hat{E}_j = \hat{E}_j r_{j-1} + (1 - \hat{E}_j)r_j$. When the prior distribution for P is beta with parameters a and b, $\hat{E}_j$ agrees perfectly with (9.89). In practice, we estimate $E(P|n,\ X=j)$ by replacing r_{j-1} and r_j by estimates $\hat{r}_{j-1}$ and $\hat{r}_j$. For $j = 0,\ldots,n$, this produces the estimates

$$\hat{E}_j = \frac{\hat{r}_j}{1 + \hat{r}_j - \hat{r}_{j-1}}. \tag{9.95}$$

The estimates $\hat{r}_j$ may be obtained directly from the marginal data for each value of n, or from a model estimate. Here we illustrate the latter using model (9.83). From the maximum likelihood estimates of α_g and β, for gravidity $g = 2$ or 3 and $j = -1, 0, \ldots, g-1, g$, we obtain the estimates

$$\hat{r}_j = \frac{\exp\left(\hat{\alpha}_g + \hat{\beta}j\right)}{1 + \exp\left(\hat{\alpha}_g + \hat{\beta}j\right)}. \tag{9.96}$$

Note that for $\hat{r}_{-1}$ and $\hat{r}_g$ we use the extrapolated values from the model for $j = -1$ and $j = g$. These produce better estimates of $\hat{E}_0$ and $\hat{E}_g$ than the crude bounds $\hat{r}_{-1} = 0$ and $\hat{r}_g = 1$.

Table 9.15. *Conditional expected livebirth probabilities for women with given numbers of livebirths among two or three pregnancies, estimated from the empirical Bayes logit model (9.83) and the beta-binomial model (9.89)*

Gravidity g	Estimate	\multicolumn{5}{c}{Number of Livebirths among g Pregnancies}
		-1	0	1	2	3
2	$\hat{r}_j$	0.5298*	0.5759	0.6207	0.6635*	
	$\hat{E}_j$	—	0.5505	0.5941	0.6363	
	Beta-binomial	—	0.5312	0.5906	0.6501	
3	$\hat{r}_j$	0.4679*	0.5145	0.5609	0.6062	0.6497*
	$\hat{E}_j$	—	0.4916	0.5360	0.5799	0.6226
	Beta-binomial	—	0.5049	0.5413	0.5777	0.6141

*Extrapolated from model (9.83) for $j = -1$ and $j = g$.

Table 9.15 shows the estimates from (9.92), (9.95), and (9.96) for the livebirth data. There is good agreement between the estimates $\hat{E}_j$ and the beta-binomial estimates, which are (9.89) with maximum likelihood estimates substituted for π and $a + b$.

PROBLEMS

9.1. Prove the equality of expressions (9.3) and (9.4) for χ^2.

9.2. The estimate of the slope b is given by (9.17). Prove that its numerator is given by (9.19) and that its denominator is given by (9.20).

9.3. Three samples of New York mental hospital patients were studied as part of a collaborative project (Cooper et al., 1972). The numbers of hospital diagnoses of affective disorders were as follows:

Sample	Age Range	Number of Patients	Number Diagnosed Affective	Proportion
1	20–34	105	2	
2	20–59	192	13	
3	35–59	145	24	
Overall		442	39	

(a) Calculate the proportions diagnosed affective, and test whether they differ significantly.

(b) Test whether the proportion diagnosed affective in the first two samples combined differs significantly from the proportion in the third sample. Test whether the proportions in the first two samples differ.

(c) The patients in sample 1 tend to be younger than those in sample 2, who in turn tend to be younger than those in sample 3. Because the chances of an affective disorder increase with age, it might be hypothesized that p_1 should be less than p_2, and that p_2 in turn should be less than p_3. Are the proportions in this order? What is the value of χ^2 in (9.32)? What is the value of c in (9.34)? Refer to Table A.7 to test the hypothesized ordering.

9.4. Let the frequencies underlying the data in Table 9.7 be $(n_{11}, \ldots, n_{k1})$ and $(n_{12}, \ldots, n_{k2})$, so that $p_{i1} = n_{i1}/n_1$ and $p_{i2} = n_{i2}/n_2$, $i = 1, \ldots, k$. Define $n_{i.} = n_{i1} + n_{i2}$, so that $\bar{p}_i = n_{i.}/n_.$. The classic formula for chi squared is

$$\chi^2 = \sum_{i=1}^{k} \frac{\left(n_{i1} - \frac{n_{i.}n_1}{n_.}\right)^2}{\frac{n_{i.}n_1}{n_.}} + \sum_{i=1}^{k} \frac{\left(n_{i2} - \frac{n_{i.}n_2}{n_.}\right)^2}{\frac{n_{i.}n_2}{n_.}}.$$

Prove that this formula is equal to the one in (9.38).

9.5. Consider the data of Table 9.11.

(a) Taking group A as the reference group, find the mean ridit for group B.

(b) Taking group B as the reference group, find the mean ridit for group A. What is the relation between answers in (a) and (b)?

(c) Use formula (9.40) to find the standard error of the mean ridit contrasting groups A and B.

(d) Use formula (9.45) to estimate the same standard error. How do the values in (c) and (d) compare?

9.6. (a) Prove that for any three continuous random variables, X_0, X_1, and X_2,

$$P(X_2 > X_1) + P(X_1 > X_0) - P(X_2 > X_0)$$
$$= P(X_1 > X_0 > X_2) + P(X_0 > X_2 > X_1) + P(X_2 > X_1 > X_0).$$

Thus if ridit r_1 estimates $P(X_1 > X_0)$, where X_0 is an observation from the reference population, and ridit r_2 estimates $P(X_2 > X_0)$, then $r_2 - r_1 + \frac{1}{2}$ estimates $P(X_2 > X_1)$ with error term

$$\tfrac{1}{2} - \{P(X_1 > X_0 > X_2) + P(X_0 > X_2 > X_1) + P(X_2 > X_1 > X_0)\}.$$

(b) If X_0, X_1, and X_2 are identically distributed, show that the error term in part (a) equals 0, so that $r_2 - r_1 + \frac{1}{2}$ estimates $P(X_2 > X_1)$ without bias, even if the three variables are not independent.

(c) Suppose the distribution of X_1 is entirely supported below that of X_0, which in turn is entirely supported below that of X_2; that is, suppose $P(X_0 > X_1) = 1 = P(X_2 > X_0)$. Then $r_2 = 1$, $r_1 = 0$, and $P(X_2 > X_1) = 1$, but $r_2 - r_1 + \frac{1}{2} = \frac{3}{2}$, a nonsensical estimate of $P(X_2 > X_1)$. Show that the error term in part (a) is as large as possible, viz., $\frac{1}{2}$. [*Hint.* $P(X_1 > X_0 > X_2) = P(X_0 > X_2 > X_1) = P(X_2 > X_1 > X_0) = 0$.] Thus if the comparison groups are widely separated in this sense, or nearly this sense, the error term in part (a) will be large and lead to error in estimating $P(X_2 > X_1)$. Apply this reasoning to the data in Table 9.11 with reference distribution data in Table 9.8.

(d) Use the inequalities $P(X_1 > X_0 > X_2) \le P(X_1 > X_2)$, $P(X_0 > X_2 > X_1) \le P(X_0 > X_2)$, and $P(X_2 > X_1 > X_0) \le P(X_1 > X_0)$ to show that the error term in part (a) is at least

$$\frac{1}{2} - \{P(X_1 > X_2) + (1 - r_2) + r_1\}$$

$$= r_2 - r_1 - \frac{1}{2} - P(X_1 > X_2) \approx r_2 - r_1 - \frac{1}{2},$$

where the last approximate equality holds if the two comparison groups are widely separated in the sense that $P(X_1 > X_2) \approx 0$. For the two comparison groups in Table 9.11, with $r_1 = 0.25$ and $r_2 = 0.89$, show that the error in estimating $P(X_1 > X_2)$ by $r_2 - r_1 + \frac{1}{2} = 1.14$ is (approximately) at least $0.89 - 0.25 - 0.5 = 0.14$.

9.7.* **(a)** State the conditional log-likelihood function given all margins fixed for the two-sample multinomial problem under the proportional adjacent odds model. [*Hint.* Using the notation of Problem 9.4, the appropriate conditional distribution for the comparison group frequencies $n_{12}, \ldots, n_{k2}$ given all margins fixed is the noncentral multiple hypergeometric distribution (see Section 13.2) with probability function

$$P(n_{12}, \ldots, n_{k2} | n_1, n_1, \ldots, n_k, \lambda_2, \ldots, \lambda_k)$$

$$= \frac{\binom{n_1.}{n_{12}} \cdots \binom{n_k.}{n_{k2}} \exp(\lambda_2 n_{22} + \cdots + \lambda_k n_{k2})}{\sum\limits_{u_1, \ldots, u_k \in D} \binom{n_1.}{u_1} \cdots \binom{n_k.}{u_k} \exp(\lambda_2 u_2 + \cdots + \lambda_k u_k)},$$

where the sum in the denominator is taken over the set $D = D(n_1; n_1, \ldots, n_k.)$ of all vectors of nonnegative integers $0 \le u_i \le n_i$ such that $n_1 = u_1 + \cdots + u_k$. The parameters $\lambda_2, \ldots, \lambda_k$ are the log odds ratios relating row category i to the first row category, for the comparison group versus the reference group, i.e., $\lambda_i = \ln\{(P_{i2}/P_{12})/(P_{i1}/P_{11})\}$ for $i = 2, \ldots, k$. Express these log odds ratios in terms of Δ from the proportional adjacent odds model, and collect the terms in the exponent multiplying Δ.]

(b) Prove that the statistic $S = \Sigma a_i(n_{i2} - n_2 \bar{p}_i)$ with $a_i = i$ for $i = 1, \ldots, k$ results from differentiating the conditional log-likelihood function derived in part (a) with respect to Δ when the derivative is evaluated at the null hypothesis value $\Delta = 0$. This is a score statistic, and takes the typical form of an observed sum of scores from group 2 minus an expected sum of scores under the null hypothesis. Because the observed sum of scores is integer-valued, it is appropriate to subtract $\frac{1}{2}$ from the absolute value of S. The result is a scaled version of the numerator of the score test z_c in (9.54).

(c) The conditional variance of S under H_0: $\Delta = 0$ is simply the variance of a sum of n_2 scores randomly selected without replacement from a finite population containing $n.\bar{p}_i = n_i.$ scores with value a_i for $i = 1, \ldots, k$. Reexpress S in terms of $p_{i2} - p_{i1}$, and rescale the continuity corrected statistic $|S| - \frac{1}{2}$ to derive (9.54)–(9.57).

9.8. Use the definition $\mathrm{Var}(P_i | n_i) = E(P_i^2 | n_i) - \{E(P_i | n_i)\}^2$ to confirm expression (9.60).

9.9. Write $\mathrm{Var}(\bar{p} | n) = \Sigma_i n_i^2 \mathrm{Var}(p_i | n_i)/n^2$, and use (9.60) to confirm expression (9.61) for the variance of $\bar{p}$.

9.10. Demonstrate that $(9.65) \le (9.61)$ with equality if and only if $n_1 = \cdots = n_m$. [*Hint.* Let V be a random variable taking values $1/[\pi(1 - \pi)\{1 + (n_i - 1)D^2\}]$ with probability $n_i/n.$ for $i = 1, \ldots, m$, and let $f(x) = 1/x$. Use Jensen's inequality to argue that

$$n.\times(9.61) = \sum_{i=1}^{m} \frac{n_i}{n.} \pi(1 - \pi)\{1 + (n_i - 1)D^2\} = Ef(V)$$

$$\ge f(EV) = \cfrac{1}{\sum_{i=1}^{m} \left(\cfrac{n_i}{n.}\right) \cfrac{1}{\pi(1 - \pi)\{1 + (n_i - 1)D^2\}}}$$

$$= n.\times(9.65).]$$

9.11. Prove expression (9.69). [*Hint.* Write $\sum_{i=1}^{m} n_i(p_i - \bar{p})^2 = \sum_{i=1}^{m} n_i p_i^2 - n \bar{p}^2$, and take expectations, using the relations $E(p_i^2|\underline{n}) = \text{Var}(p_i|\underline{n}) + \{E(p_i|\underline{n})\}^2$ and (9.60), and similarly, $E(\bar{p}^2|\underline{n}) = \text{Var}(\bar{p}|\underline{n}) + \{E(\bar{p}|\underline{n})\}^2$ and (9.61); then simplify.]

9.12. Prove expression (9.72).

9.13. Prove expression (9.80). [*Hint.* Omitting subscripts, the posterior distribution of P given $X = j$ has density proportional to the binomial likelihood times the prior distribution for P; specifically, the posterior density is $P^j(1 - P)^{n-j}g(P)/\int P^j(1 - P)^{n-j}g(P)\,dP$, where $g(P)$ is the prior density for P. The left-hand side of (9.80) is

$$\frac{\int (P/Q)P^j(1 - P)^{n-j}g(P)\,dP}{\int P^j(1 - P)^{n-j}g(P)\,dP} = \frac{\int P^{j+1}(1 - P)^{n-j-1}g(P)\,dP}{\int P^j(1 - P)^{n-j}g(P)\,dP}.$$

Express the numerator and denominator in terms of the marginal probabilities $P(X = j|n) = \int P(X = j|n, P)g(p)\,dP.$]

REFERENCES

Armitage, P. (1955). Tests for linear trends in proportions and frequencies. *Biometrics*, **11**, 375–385.

Banerjee, T. and Paul, S. R. (1999). An extension of Morel-Nagaraj's finite mixture distribution for modelling multinomial clustered data. *Biometrika*, **86**, 723–727.

Barlow, R. E., Bartholomew, D. J., Bremner, J. M., and Brunk, H. D. (1972). *Statistical inference under order restrictions*. New York: Wiley.

Bartholomew, D. J. (1958a). A test of homogeneity for ordered alternatives. *Biometrika*, **46**, 36–48.

Bartholomew, D. J. (1959b). A test of homogeneity for ordered alternatives II. *Biometrika*, **46**, 328–335.

Bartholomew, D. J. (1963). On Chassan's test for order. *Biometrics*, **19**, 188–191.

Berry, D. A. (1996). *Statistics: A Bayesian perspective*. North Scituate, Mass.: Duxbury Press.

Box, G. E. P. and Tiao, G. C. (1992). *Bayesian inference in statistical analysis* (Classics Edition). New York: Wiley.

Bross, I. D. J. (1958), How to use ridit analysis. *Biometrics*, **14**, 18–38.

Bross, I. D. J. (1960). How to cut the highway toll in half in the next ten years. *Public Health Rep.*, **75**, 573–581.

Carlin, B. P. and Louis, T. A. (2000). *Bayes and empirical Bayes methods for data analysis*, 2nd ed. Boca Raton, Fla.: Chapman & Hall/CRC Press.

Castellan, N. J. (1965). On the partitioning of contingency tables. *Psychol. Bull.*, **64**, 330–338.

Chapman, D. G. and Nam, J. (1968). Asymptotic power of chi square tests for linear trends in proportions. *Biometrics*, **24**, 315–327.

Chassan, J. B. (1960). On a test for order. *Biometrics*, **16**, 119–121.

Chassan, J. B. (1962). An extension of a test for order. *Biometrics*, **18**, 245–247.

Cochran, W. G. (1954). Some methods of strengthening the common χ^2 tests. *Biometrics*, **10**, 417–451.

Cook, J. A. and Lawless, J. F. (1991). Two-sample tests with multinomial or grouped failure time data. *Biometrics*, **47**, 445–459.

Cooper, J. E., Kendell, R. E., Garland, B. J., Sharpe, L., Copeland, J. R. M., and Simon, R. (1972). *Psychiatric diagnosis in New York and London*. London: Oxford University Press.

Cressie, N. (1982). A useful empirical Bayes identity. *Ann. Statist.*, **10**, 625–629.

Dorn, H. F. (1954). The relationship of cancer of the lung and the use of tobacco. *Am. Statist.*, **8**, 7–13.

Efron, B. and Morris, C. (1971). Limiting the risk of Bayes and empirical Bayes estimators. Part I: The Bayes case. *J. Am. Statist. Assoc.*, **66**, 807–815.

Efron, B. and Morris, C. (1972a). Limiting the risk of Bayes and empirical Bayes estimators. Part II: The empirical Bayes case. *J. Am. Statist. Assoc.*, **67**, 130–139.

Efron, B. and Morris, C. (1972b). Empirical Bayes on vector observations: an extension of Stein's method. *Biometrika*, **59**, 335–347.

Efron, B. and Morris, C. (1973a). Stein's estimation rule and its competitor—an empirical Bayes approach. *J. Am. Statist. Assoc.*, **68**, 117–130.

Efron, B. and Morris, C. (1973b). Combining possibly related estimation problems (with discussion). *J. R. Statist. Soc., Ser. B*, **35**, 379–421.

Efron, B. and Morris, C. (1975). Data analysis using Stein's estimator and its generalizations. *J. Am. Statist. Assoc.*, **70**, 311–319.

Finkelstein, M. O., and Levin, B. (2001). *Statistics for lawyers*, 2nd ed. New York: Springer-Verlag.

Finkelstein, M. O., Levin, B., and Robbins, H. (1996a). Clinical and prophylactic trials with assured new treatment for those at greater risk. Part I—introduction. *Am. J. Public Health*, **86**, 691–695.

Finkelstein, M. O., Levin, B., and Robbins, H. (1996b). Clinical and prophylactic trials with assured new treatment for those at greater risk. Part II—Examples. *Am. J. Public Health*, **86**, 696–705.

Gail, M. H., Tan, W. Y., and Piantadosi, S. (1988). Tests for no treatment effect in randomized clinical trials. *Biometrika*, **75**, 57–64.

Gelman, A., Carlin, J. B., Stern, H. S., and Rubin, D. B. (1995). *Bayesian data analysis*. Boca Raton, Fla.: Chapman & Hall/CRC Press.

Hatch, M., Kline, J., Levin, B., Hutzler, M., and Warburton, D. (1990). Paternal age and trisomy among spontaneous abortions. *Human Genetics*, **85**, 335–361.

Ibrahim, J. G. and Ryan, L. M. (1996). Use of historical controls in time-adjusted trend tests for carcinogenicity. *Biometrics*, **52**, 1478–1485.

Irwin, J. O. (1949). A note on the subdivision of chi-square into components. *Biometrika*, **36**, 130–134.

Kadane, J. B. (1996). *Bayesian methods and ethics in a clinical trial design*. New York: Wiley.

Kantor, S., Winkelstein, W. and Ibrahim, M. A. (1968). A note on the interpretation of the ridit as a quantile rank. *Am. J. Epidemiol.*, **87**, 609–615.

Kastenbaum, M. A. (1960). A note on the additive partitioning of chi-square in contingency tables. *Biometrics*, **16**, 416–422.

Kim, B. S. and Margolin, B. H. (1992). Testing goodness of fit of a multinomial model against overdispersed alternatives. *Biometrics*, **48**, 711–719.

Kimball, A. W. (1954). Short-cut formulas for the exact partition of χ^2 in contingency tables. *Biometrics*, **10**, 452–458.

Kline, J., Levin, B., Kinney, A., Stein, Z., Susser, M., and Warburton, D. (1995). Cigarette smoking and spontaneous abortion of known karyotype: Precise data but uncertain inferences. *Am. J. Epidemiol*, **141**, 417–427.

Knoke, J. D. (1976). Multiple comparisons with dichotomous data. *J. Am. Statist. Assoc.*, **71**, 849–853.

Lai, T. L. and Siegmund, D., Eds. (1985). *Herbert Robbins selected papers*. New York: Springer-Verlag.

Lancaster, H. O. (1950). The exact partitioning of chi-square and its application in the problem of pooling small expectations. *Biometrika*, **37**, 267–270.

Levin, B. (1992). Tests of odds ratio homogeneity with improved power in sparse fourfold tables. *Commun. Statist.—Theory Meth.*, **21**, 1469–1500.

Levin, B. and Robbins, H. (1983). Urn models for regression analysis, with applications to employment discrimination studies. *Law and Contemporary Problems*, **83**, 247–267.

Liang, K.-Y. and Self, S. G. (1985). Tests for homogeneity of odds ratios when the data are sparse. *Biometrika*, **72**, 353–358.

Mantel, N. (1963). Chi-square tests with one degree of freedom: Extensions of the Mantel-Haenszel procedure. *J. Am. Statist. Assoc.*, **58**, 690–700.

Mantel, N. (1979). Ridit analysis and related ranking procedures—use at your own risk. *Am. J. Epidemiol.*, **109**, 25–29.

McCullagh, P. (1980). Regression models for ordinal data (with discussion). *J. R. Statist. Soc. B*, **42**, 109–142.

Miller, R. G. (1981). *Simultaneous statistical inference*, 2nd ed., New York: Springer-Verlag.

Mode, C. J. (1985). *Stochastic processes in demography and their computer implementation*. New York: Springer-Verlag.

Morel, J. G. and Nagaraj, N. K. (1993). A finite mixture distribution for modelling multinomial extra variation. *Biometrika*, **80**, 363–371.

Morton, R. (1991). Analysis of extra-multinomial data derived from extra-Poisson variables conditional on their total. *Biometrika*, **78**, 1–6.

National Center for Health Statistics (1970). Selected symptoms of psychological distress in the United States. *Data from National Health Survey*, Series 11, No. 37.

Neerchal, N. K., and Morel, J. G. (1998). Large cluster results for two parameter multinomial extra variation models. *J. Am. Statist. Assoc.*, **93**, 1078–1087.

O'Hara-Hines, R. J. and Lawless, J. F. (1993). Modelling overdispersion in toxicological mortality data grouped over time. *Biometrics*, **49**, 107–121.

Parides, M. K. (1995). Testing homogeneity of discrete exponential families in the large-sparse case. Unpublished doctoral dissertation, Department of Biostatistics, Columbia University.

Paul, S. R., Liang, K.-Y., and Self, S. G. (1989). On testing departure from the binomial and multinomial assumptions. *Biometrics*, **45**, 231–236.

Press, S. J. (1989). *Bayesian statistics*: *Principles, models, and applications*. New York: Wiley.

Robbins, H. (1956). An empirical Bayes approach to statistics. In J. Neyman (Ed.), *Proceedings of the third Berkeley symposium on mathematics and statistical probability*, 1954–1955. Berkeley: University of California Press.

Robbins, H. (1977). Prediction and estimation for the compound Poisson distribution. *Proc. Natl. Acad. Sci. U.S.A.*, **74**, 2670–2671.

Robbins, H. (1993). Comparing two treatments under biased allocation. *Gazette Sci. Math. Québec*, **15**, 35–41.

Robbins, H. and Zhang, C.-H. (1988). Estimating a treatment effect under biased sampling. *Proc. Natl. Acad. Sci. U.S.A.*, **85**, 3670–3672.

Robbins, H. and Zhang, C.-H. (1989). Estimating the superiority of a drug to a placebo when all and only those patients at risk are treated with the drug. *Proc. Natl. Acad. Sci. U.S.A.*, **86**, 3003–3005.

Robbins, H. and Zhang, C.-H. (1991). Estimating a multiplicative treatment effect under biased allocation. *Biometrika*, **78**, 349–354.

Selvin, S. (1977). A further note on the interpretation of ridit analysis. *Am. J. Epidemiol.*, **105**, 16–20.

Snell, E. J. (1964). A scaling procedure for ordered categorical data. *Biometrics*, **20**, 592–607.

Spitzer, R. L., Fleiss, J. L., Kernohan, W., Lee, J., and Baldwin, I. T. (1965). The Mental Status Schedule: Comparing Kentucky and New York schizophrenics. *Arch. Gen. Psychiatry*, **12**, 448–455.

Waller, L. A. and Zelterman, D. (1997). Loglinear modeling with the negative multinomial distribution. *Biometrics*, **53**, 971–982.

Whittemore, A. S., Friend, N., Brown, B. W., and Holly, E. A. (1987). A test to detect clusters of disease. *Biometrika*, **74**, 631–635. Correction, **75**, 396.

Wilson, J. R. (1989). Chi-square tests for overdispersion with multiparameter estimates. *Appl. Statist.*, **38**, 441–453.

Wood, C. L. (1978). Comparison of linear trends in binomial proportions. *Biometrics*, **34**, 496–504.

Wynder, E. L., Bross, I. D. J., and Hirayama, T. (1960). A study of the epidemiology of cancer of the breast. *Cancer*, **13**, 559–601.

Yates, F. (1948). The analysis of contingency tables with groupings based on quantitative characteristics. *Biometrika*, **35**, 176–181.

Zelterman, D. (1987). Goodness-of-fit tests for large sparse multinomial distributions. *J. Am. Statist. Assoc.*, **82**, 624–629.

CHAPTER 10

Combining Evidence from Fourfold Tables

There are a number of ways in which data relevant to the association between a risk factor A and a disease B might end up arrayed in several fourfold tables. If the possibility of an association between A and B is strong, interesting, or important enough, it is virtually guaranteed that a number of investigators will study the association. Similarly, if an association has been found to exist in one kind of population, it is to be expected that the possibility of association in other kinds of populations will be studied. As a final example, a single given study might call for stratifying the samples being compared on variables known to be associated with the outcome variable under investigation; each stratum would then provide its own four-fold table.

Suppose that the association between A and B has been studied in each of g groups, with each group generating its own fourfold table. The following questions can be asked:

1. Is there evidence that the degree of association, whatever its magnitude, is consistent from one group to another?

2. Assuming that the degree of association is found to be consistent, is the common degree of association statistically significant?

3. Assuming that the common degree of association is significant, what is the best estimate of the common value for the measure of association? What is its standard error? How does one construct a confidence interval for the underlying measure?

Statistical Methods for Rates and Proportions, Third Edition
By Joseph L. Fleiss, Bruce Levin, and Myunghee Cho Paik
ISBN 0-471-52629-0   Copyright © 2003 John Wiley & Sons, Inc.

Section 10.1 provides a simple statistical framework within which these questions can be answered. Section 10.2 describes how to use methods with the logarithm of the odds ratio. Section 10.3 gives the foundations of exact inference about a common odds ratio, and Section 10.4 describes approximate methods based on results of Cornfield and Gart. Section 10.5 describes the Mantel-Haenszel method. Section 10.6 compares these methods for different kinds of study designs, and Section 10.7 indicates how they can be used as alternatives to matching in the control of confounding factors. Section 10.8 describes some popular but generally invalid methods of comparing and combining data from several fourfold tables. Section 10.9 concludes with some matters related to the material presented earlier on confounding, meta-analysis, and tests for homogeneity of odds ratios in the large sparse case.

The methods reviewed in this chapter are special cases of those available for the analysis of complex cross-classification tables. The texts by Cox and Snell (1989), Bishop, Fienberg, and Holland (1975), Everitt (1992), Breslow and Day (1993, 1994), and Hosmer and Lemeshow (2000) are excellent references to the general methods of log linear and logistic regression analysis. Muñoz and Rosner (1984) discuss power and sample size for a collection of 2×2 tables.

10.1. THE CONSTRUCTION AND INTERPRETATION OF SOME CHI SQUARED TESTS

To answer the questions posed above, some knowledge of the theory of chi squared tests is necessary. For a single one of the g groups, say the ith, let y_i denote the value of the chosen measure of association. The measure might be the difference between two proportions, the logarithm of the odds ratio, and so on.

Whatever y_i is, let $se(y_i)$ denote its standard error, and define

$$w_i = \frac{1}{[se(y_i)]^2}, \tag{10.1}$$

so that w_i is the reciprocal of the squared standard error of y_i. The quantity w_i is the weight to be attached to y_i. If the standard error of y_i is large, implying that y_i is not too precise, then w_i is small. This is reasonable, since imprecise estimates should not be given great weight. If, on the other hand, the standard error of y_i is small, implying that y_i is rather precise, then w_i is large. This, too, is reasonable, since precise estimates should be given great weight.

Let us suppose that y_i is such that a value of zero indicates no association. When the hypothesis of no association in the ith group is true, suppose that the quantity

$$\frac{y_i}{\text{se}(y_i)} = y_i\sqrt{w_i} \qquad (10.2)$$

has, approximately, the standard normal distribution. Then the quantity

$$\chi_i^2 = w_i y_i^2 \qquad (10.3)$$

has, approximately, the chi squared distribution with 1 df. If the hypothesis of no association in the ith group is false, χ_i^2 may be expected to be large, so that the hypothesis is likely to be rejected if a chi squared test is applied.

We are not so much interested in the ith group, or in any other single group, however, as in all the groups together. The analysis of all groups conveniently begins with the calculation of

$$\chi_{\text{total}}^2 = \sum_{i=1}^{g} \chi_i^2 = \sum_{i=1}^{g} w_i y_i^2. \qquad (10.4)$$

If there is no association in any of the g groups, then χ_{total}^2 has a chi squared distribution with g df. This follows because the sum of g independent chi squareds, each with 1 df, has a chi squared distribution with g df, and because the g groups are assumed to be independent.

If we calculate χ_{total}^2 and find it to be significantly large, we may validly conclude that there is association somewhere within the g groups. We do not, however, know whether the association is consistent across all groups or whether it varies from one group to another. χ_{total}^2 is not, therefore, informative by itself. Rather, its calculation serves the purpose of simplifying other calculations, as will now be indicated.

χ_{total}^2 is subdivided, or partitioned, into two components,

$$\chi_{\text{total}}^2 = \chi_{\text{homog}}^2 + \chi_{\text{assoc}}^2. \qquad (10.5)$$

The quantity χ_{homog}^2 assesses the degree of homogeneity, or equality, among the g measures of association, and the quantity χ_{assoc}^2 assesses the significance of the average degree of association. The subdivision indicated by (10.5) is most easily effected by calculating χ_{assoc}^2 first and determining χ_{homog}^2 by simple subtraction.

The term χ_{assoc}^2 is calculated as follows. The overall measure of association across all groups is taken as the weighted average of the g individual measures, with the weights being those defined in (10.1):

$$\bar{y} = \frac{\sum_{i=1}^{g} w_i y_i}{\sum_{i=1}^{g} w_i}. \qquad (10.6)$$

Under the hypothesis that the overall association is zero, $\bar{y}$ has an average value of zero and a standard error of

$$\text{se}(\bar{y}) = \frac{1}{\sqrt{\sum_{i=1}^{g} w_i}}. \qquad (10.7)$$

Hence

$$\frac{\bar{y}}{\mathrm{se}(\bar{y})} = \frac{\sum_{i=1}^{g} w_i y_i}{\sqrt{\sum_{i=1}^{g} w_i}} \tag{10.8}$$

is distributed approximately as a standard normal variate under the hypothesis, and

$$\chi^2_{\mathrm{assoc}} = \left\{ \frac{\bar{y}}{\mathrm{se}(\bar{y})} \right\}^2 = \bar{y}^2 \sum_{i=1}^{g} w_i = \frac{\left(\sum_{i=1}^{g} w_i y_i \right)^2}{\sum_{i=1}^{g} w_i} \tag{10.9}$$

is distributed approximately as chi squared with 1 df.

The term χ^2_{homog} is then easily obtained by subtraction:

$$\chi^2_{\mathrm{homog}} = \chi^2_{\mathrm{total}} - \chi^2_{\mathrm{assoc}} = \sum_{i=1}^{g} w_i y_i^2 - \bar{y}^2 \sum_{i=1}^{g} w_i. \tag{10.10}$$

An equivalent expression for χ^2_{homog} is

$$\chi^2_{\mathrm{homog}} = \sum_{i=1}^{g} w_i (y_i - \bar{y})^2. \tag{10.11}$$

This expression for χ^2_{homog} is useful for two purposes. One is to provide a numerical check on the arithmetic. The other is to point out that χ^2_{homog} actually measures the degree of variability among the separate values of y_i. χ^2_{homog} is uncorrelated with χ^2_{assoc}, and is approximately distributed as chi squared with $g-1$ df under the hypothesis of consistent (homogeneous) association.

Means are therefore provided for answering the three questions posed at the beginning of this chapter.

1. Consistency of association can be tested by referring χ^2_{homog} to tables of chi squared with $g-1$ df. If χ^2_{homog} is significant, the next step in the analysis is to partition χ^2_{homog} into appropriate components in order to identify those groups in which the association is different from that in the remaining groups (see Problem 10.1).

2. If χ^2_{homog} is not significant, the significance of the overall degree of association can be tested by referring χ^2_{assoc} to tables of chi squared with 1 df.

3. The best estimate of the overall degree of association is $\bar{y}$ [see (10.6)]. Its standard error is given by (10.7). An approximate $100(1-\alpha)\%$

confidence interval for the underlying overall degree of association is

$$\bar{y} \pm z_{\alpha/2} \, se(\bar{y}),\qquad (10.12)$$

where $z_{\alpha/2}$ is the value cutting off the proportion $\alpha/2$ in the upper tail of the standard normal curve.

In general, one hopes to find that the value of χ^2_{homog} is small, so that homogeneous association may be inferred, and that the value of χ^2_{assoc} is large, so that real overall association may be inferred.

The issue of whether a test of the hypothesis of homogeneous association should ever be performed has been debated. Bishop, Fienberg, and Holland (1975, p. 147), for example, state that homogeneity of association must always be verified before inferences are made about a purportedly common degree of association. Mantel, Brown, and Byar (1977), on the other hand, suggest caution in interpreting the results of such tests; they point out that the presence or absence of homogeneous association is strongly dependent on which measure of association is used.

In practice, it would seem prudent before proceeding too far with the analysis both to inspect the data to confirm that the g measures are at least pointing to association in the same direction even if not of exactly the same magnitude, and to use χ^2_{homog} to confirm that the several measures of association are not widely divergent and that subsequent inferences about a supposedly common measure actually tend to apply to the individual groups.

What remains, then, is to apply these results to particular choices of the measure of association. The following notation will be used consistently in this chapter. In the ith group, n_{i1} is the number of observations in the first sample and p_{i1} is the proportion of the first sample having the studied characteristic. The quantity n_{i2} is the number of observations in the second sample, and p_{i2} is the proportion of the second sample having the studied characteristic. The total number of observations in the ith group is denoted by $n_{i.} = n_{i1} + n_{i2}$, and the overall proportion in the ith group having the characteristic is denoted by

$$\bar{p}_i = \frac{n_{i1} p_{i1} + n_{i2} p_{i2}}{n_{i.}}.\qquad (10.13)$$

The complementary proportion is $\bar{q}_i = 1 - \bar{p}_i$.

10.2. COMBINING THE LOGARITHMS OF ODDS RATIOS

The sample odds ratio itself,

$$o_i = \frac{p_{i1}(1 - p_{i2})}{p_{i2}(1 - p_{i1})},\qquad (10.14)$$

does not have the property that a value of zero indicates no association. The logarithm of the odds ratio does have this property. Thus consider taking as the measure of association

$$y_i = L_i = \ln o_i. \tag{10.15}$$

The squared standard error of L_i is approximately

$$\left[\widehat{se}(L_i)\right]^2 = \frac{1}{w_i} = \frac{1}{n_{i1} p_{i1}(1 - p_{i1})} + \frac{1}{n_{i2} p_{i2}(1 - p_{i2})}, \tag{10.16}$$

which is equal to the sum of the reciprocals of the frequencies within the cells. The weight w_i is then the reciprocal of this sum of reciprocals.

The chi squared analyses of Section 10.1 have been applied to the logarithm of the odds ratio by Gart (1962) and Sheehe (1966). They will now be illustrated with the data of Table 10.1, which presents the proportions of patients diagnosed as schizophrenic by resident hospital psychiatrists in New York and London (see Cooper et al., 1972).

Table 10.2 outlines the arithmetic required to perform the analysis of the log odds ratios. To reduce bias (Naylor, 1967; Gart, 1970, 1971), the constant 0.5 was added to each frequency, as in (6.20) and (6.33), in calculating $L_i' = \ln o_i'$ and $w_i' = 1/[\widehat{se}(L_i')]^2$. The values of the individual chi squareds $[= w_i'(L_i')^2]$ are all approximately equal to the values given by the standard 1-df chi squareds incorporating the continuity correction and are all highly significant.

Table 10.1. *Diagnoses of schizophrenia by resident hospital psychiatrists in three studies in New York and London*

| Study | New York | | London | |
	n_{i1}	p_{i1}	n_{i2}	p_{i2}
$i = 1$ (ages 20–34)	105	0.771	105	0.324
$i = 2$ (ages 20–59)	192	0.615	174	0.397
$i = 3$ (ages 35–59)	145	0.566	145	0.359

Table 10.2. *Analysis of logarithms of odds ratios applied to data of Table 10.1*

Study	o_i'	L_i'	w_i'	$w_i'L_i'$	$w_i'(L_i')^2$
1	6.894	1.931	10.410	20.102	38.816
2	2.415	0.881	21.868	19.266	16.973
3	2.314	0.839	17.357	14.563	12.218
Total			49.635	53.931	68.007

The value of the total chi squared is

$$\chi^2_{total} = \sum_{i=1}^{3} w_i'(L_i')^2 = 68.01, \tag{10.17}$$

and the value of the chi squared statistic for testing the homogeneity of the odds ratios is

$$\chi^2_{homog} = \sum_{i=1}^{3} w_i'(L_i')^2 - \frac{\left(\sum_{i=1}^{3} w_i' L_i'\right)^2}{\sum_{i=1}^{3} w_i'}$$

$$= 68.01 - \frac{(53.931)^2}{49.635}$$

$$= 9.41 \tag{10.18}$$

with 2 df, indicating the existence of significant differences at the 0.01 level among the three odds ratios. Problem 10.1 is devoted to a detailed analysis of the heterogeneity of the odds ratios in Table 10.2.

While not equal, the three odds ratios are at least all in the same direction. Further analysis of all the data, in terms of a hypothetical common underlying odds ratio, might be justified if the conclusions are understood to apply to hospital diagnoses made on psychiatric patients in New York and London in general, not to diagnoses made on patients of any specific age group. Problem 10.2 carries the following kind of analysis forward on the data from studies $i = 2$ and $i = 3$ only, where the patients tended to be older and the odds ratios were similar.

The estimate of the logarithm of the supposedly common odds ratio is

$$\bar{L}' = \frac{\sum_{i=1}^{3} w_i' L_i'}{\sum_{i=1}^{3} w_i'} = \frac{53.931}{49.635}$$

$$= 1.087, \tag{10.19}$$

with an estimated standard error of

$$\widehat{se}(\bar{L}') = \frac{1}{\sqrt{\sum_{i=1}^{3} w_i'}} = \frac{1}{\sqrt{49.635}}$$

$$= 0.142. \tag{10.20}$$

The value of chi squared for testing the significance of the mean log odds ratio is then

$$\chi^2_{assoc} = \left(\frac{\bar{L}'}{\widehat{se}(\bar{L}')}\right)^2 = \left(\frac{1.087}{0.142}\right)^2 = 58.60 \tag{10.21}$$

with 1 df, which is obviously highly significant. The inference may therefore be drawn that the odds that a mental patient hospitalized in New York will be diagnosed schizophrenic by a hospital psychiatrist are significantly greater than the corresponding odds for a mental patient hospitalized in London.

An approximate 95% confidence interval for λ, the logarithm of the supposed common odds ratio, is

$$\overline{L}' - 1.96\,\widehat{\text{se}}(\overline{L}') \leq \lambda \leq \overline{L}' + 1.96\,\widehat{\text{se}}(\overline{L}'),$$

$$1.087 - 1.96 \times 0.142 \leq \lambda \leq 1.087 + 1.96 \times 0.142,$$

or

$$0.809 \leq \lambda \leq 1.365. \tag{10.22}$$

It is usually desirable to report the final results in terms of the odds ratio itself rather than in terms of its logarithm. The mean odds ratio is estimated by

$$\overline{o}' = e^{\overline{L}'} = \text{antilog}(\overline{L}'), \tag{10.23}$$

and an approximate 95% confidence interval for ω, the supposed common odds ratio, is given by

$$\text{antilog}\left[\overline{L}' - 1.96\,\widehat{\text{se}}(\overline{L}')\right] \leq \omega \leq \text{antilog}\left[\overline{L}' + 1.96\,\widehat{\text{se}}(\overline{L}')\right]. \tag{10.24}$$

For the data at hand,

$$\overline{o}' = \text{antilog}(1.087) = 2.97, \tag{10.25}$$

and an approximate 95% confidence interval for ω is, from (10.22),

$$\text{antilog}(0.809) \leq \omega \leq \text{antilog}(1.365),$$

or

$$2.25 < \omega < 3.92. \tag{10.26}$$

10.3.* EXACT INFERENCE FOR A COMMON ODDS RATIO

An outline of the theory to be applied here was presented in Section 6.4. Readers who wish to use approximate methods only may proceed directly to Section 10.4.

Let the data from group i be reexpressed as in Table 10.3, where we have written $l_i = m_i + n_{i1} - n_{i.}$. If all four marginal frequencies are held fixed, and if ω is the underlying odds ratio, then each X_i has a noncentral hypergeometric distribution—see expression (6.35) in Section 6.2. The joint conditional probability of observing the collection of g independent 2×2 tables

Table 10.3. *Notation for data from group I*

	Outcome Variable		
Sample	Present	Absent	Total
1	X_i	$n_{i1} - X_i$	n_{i1}
2	$m_i - X_i$	$X_i - l_i$	n_{i2}
Total	m_i	$n_{i.} - m_i$	$n_{i.}$

given all margins as observed is the product of these g noncentral hypergeometric probabilities. Under the assumption of a common odds ratio ω, the product of terms of the form (6.35) depends on the individual reference cells X_i only through their sum, $S = \sum_{i=1}^{g} X_i$, that is, the sum is a sufficient statistic for drawing inferences about ω. Hypothesis tests about the common odds ratio, and confidence intervals for it, can be constructed in the same way as described in Sections 6.4 and 6.5. The only change required is that the noncentral hypergeometric distribution for a single X must be replaced by the distribution of S. Using the notation $H(j_i | n_{i.}, n_{i1}, m_i, \omega) = P(X_i = j_i | n_{i.}, n_{i1}, m_i, \omega)$ from (6.35) for the probability function for each component distribution, the probability function of the sum is defined as

$$P\left(\sum_{i=1}^{g} X_i = s | \underline{n}_., \underline{n}_1, \underline{m}, \omega \right) = \sum_{\{j_1, \ldots, j_g\} \in R_g(s)} \prod_{i=1}^{g} H(j_i | n_{i.}, n_{i1}, m_i, \omega),$$

(10.27)

where $\underline{n}_. = (n_{1.}, \ldots, n_{g.})$, $\underline{n}_1 = (n_{11}, \ldots, n_{g1})$, $\underline{m} = (m_1, \ldots, m_g)$, and where the sum is taken over the set $R_g(s)$ of all g-fold partitions of s into nonnegative integers $(j_1, \ldots, j_g)$ with $j_1 + \cdots + j_g = s$.

This distribution is called a *convolution* of noncentral hypergeometric distributions. The convolution of two vectors $\underline{a} = (a_0, \ldots, a_u)$ and $\underline{b} = (b_0, \ldots, b_v)$ is defined as the vector $\underline{a} * \underline{b} = (c_0, \ldots, c_{u+v})$ where, for $j = 0, \ldots, u + v$,

$$c_j = \sum_{i=0}^{j} a_i b_{j-i} = a_0 b_j + a_1 b_{j-1} + \cdots + a_{j-1} b_1 + a_j b_0. \quad (10.28)$$

In practice one calculates the probability function (10.27) iteratively by obtaining the convolution of the vectors $h^{(i)} = h^{(i)}(\omega) = \{h_0^{(i)}(\omega), \ldots, h_{r_i}^{(i)}(\omega)\}$, where for $i = 1, \ldots, g$, $r_i = \min(m_i, n_{i1})$, and for $j = 0, \ldots, r_i$, $h_j^{(i)}(\omega) = H(j | n_{i.}, n_{i1}, m_i, \omega)$. In this notation, (10.27) can be written as

$$P\left(\sum_{i=1}^{g} X_i = s | \underline{n}_., \underline{n}_1, \underline{m}, \omega \right) = h^{(1)}(\omega) * \cdots * h^{(g)}(\omega). \quad (10.29)$$

The convolution operations in (10.29) may be carried out by starting with $h^{(1)} * h^{(2)}$ and then recursively calculating $h^{(1)} * \cdots * h^{(k+1)} = \{h^{(1)} * \cdots * h^{(k)}\} * \{h^{(k+1)}\}$. The order of entering the vectors $h^{(i)} = h^{(i)}(\omega)$ into the calculation does not matter. For efficient calculation of $P(S = s | \underline{n}_{.}, \underline{n}_1, \underline{m}, \omega)$, the terms in the sum (10.28) need only be found for indices i and j for which a_i and b_{j-i} do not equal 0. Problem 10.3 specifies which indices these are.

The fast Fourier transform provides an alternative way to calculate the convolution. We find the simplicity of programming (10.28) attractive for personal computing, and relatively rapid for tables of small to moderate sample sizes where exact computation is of special interest.

Once the convolution distribution of $S = \sum_{i=1}^{g} X_i$ is in hand, conditional inference about ω is straightforward given the table margins and the observed reference values $X_1 = x_1, \ldots, X_g = x_g$. For example, as shown by Gart (1970), two-tailed $100(1 - \alpha)\%$ confidence limits for ω are the solutions to the two polynomial equations

$$P\left(\sum_{i=1}^{g} X_i \geq \sum_{i=1}^{g} x_i \middle| \underline{n}_{.}, \underline{n}_1, \underline{m}, \omega_L \right) = \frac{\alpha}{2}$$

and

$$P\left(\sum_{i=1}^{g} X_i \leq \sum_{i=1}^{g} x_i \middle| \underline{n}_{.}, \underline{n}_1, \underline{m}, \omega_U \right) = \frac{\alpha}{2}.$$

Just as for the binomial distribution, smaller p-values and narrower confidence regions are achievable using one of the other methods described in Section 2.7 that work assuredly. For example, the two-tailed p-value by the point probability method is

$$\text{pval}\left(\sum_{i=1}^{g} x_i, \omega \right) = \sum_{s} P(S = s | \underline{n}_{.}, \underline{n}_1, \underline{m}, \omega),$$

where the sum is taken over all s such that $P(S = s | \underline{n}_{.}, \underline{n}_1, \underline{m}, \omega) \leq P(S = \sum x_i | \underline{n}_{.}, \underline{n}_1, \underline{m}, \omega)$.

The conditional maximum likelihood estimate of ω, cmle(ω), is the solution of the likelihood equation

$$\sum_{i=1}^{g} X_i - \sum_{i=1}^{g} E(X_i | n_{i.}, n_{i1}, m_i, \omega) = 0, \qquad (10.30)$$

where the second term is the sum of the expectations of the respective noncentral hypergeometric distributions [see (6.43)]. Iterative solution of (10.30) is generally required to find cmle(ω). This is a prototype example of the kind of calculation found in the *odds ratio regression model* or, more generally, in *conditional logistic regression analysis* (see Section 14.2).

How does one test exactly the assumption of a common odds ratio underlying each of the g tables? Zelen (1971) specified an exact test of odds ratio homogeneity. Because $S = \sum_{i=1}^{g} X_i$ is sufficient for ω, conditioning the joint distribution of $X_1, \ldots, X_g$ on S as well as on all four margins of each fourfold table eliminates the nuisance parameter ω from the conditional distribution, and produces a simple (point) null hypothesis distribution for the data. This is in exact analogy to the way conditioning on the sum of two binomial distributions with equal probability parameters produces Fisher's exact (central hypergeometric) distribution. The joint conditional distribution of $X_1, \ldots, X_g$ given $\sum_{i=1}^{g} X_i = s$ is

$$P\left(X_1 = x_1, \ldots, X_g = x_g \middle| \sum_{i=1}^{g} X_i = s, \underline{n}_., \underline{n}_1, \underline{m}\right) = \frac{\prod_{i=1}^{g} H(x_i | n_{i.}, n_{i1}, m_i, \omega = 1)}{P(\sum_{i=1}^{g} X_i = s | \underline{n}_., \underline{n}_1, \underline{m}, \omega = 1)}$$

$$= \frac{\prod_{i=1}^{g} \binom{n_{1i}}{x_i}\binom{n_{2i}}{m_i - x_i} \middle/ \binom{n_{i.}}{m_i}}{P\left(\sum_{i=1}^{g} X_i = s \middle| \underline{n}_., \underline{n}_1, \underline{m}, \omega = 1\right)}. \tag{10.31}$$

On the right-hand side of (10.31), use of any odds ratio ω is permissible, since the conditional distribution does not depend on ω. The choice $\omega = 1$ is merely one of convenience. Then the two-tailed p-value by the point probability method for Zelen's test of homogeneity is the sum of terms (10.31) over all g-fold partitions $(j_1, \ldots, j_g)$ of s with $j_1 + \cdots + j_g = s$, and

$$P\left(X_1 = j_1, \ldots, X_g = j_g \middle| \sum_{i=1}^{g} X_i = s, \underline{n}_., \underline{n}_1, \underline{m}\right)$$

$$\leq P\left(X_1 = x_1, \ldots, X_g = x_g \middle| \sum_{i=1}^{g} X_i = s, \underline{n}_., \underline{n}_1, \underline{m}\right).$$

As a simple illustration, we consider an extension of Fisher's example of "The Lady Tasting Tea" (Fisher, 1971) to a comparison of three tea tasters. In the original story, delightfully retold by Sir Cyril Clarke (1991) with punchline supplied by Fisher's daughter and biographer, Joan Fisher Box (1978), at a now famous tea party at Rothamsted Research Station, Sir Ronald poured a cup of tea for a lady, Dr. Muriel Bristol, who declined it, saying she liked the milk poured in first, before the tea. "Surely it makes no difference," said Fisher, but the lady claimed she could taste the difference. Fisher devised an experiment on the spot to test the claim: he presented her with eight cups of tea, four with tea before milk, four with milk before tea, in a randomized order. The lady tasted all eight cups before making her declarations, and, with full knowledge of the design, she was asked to identify the four cups of each kind. Such an experimental design results in a fourfold table with all four margins fixed at four: the rows are the true orderings (tea before milk versus milk before tea) and the columns are the lady's declarations. The elegance of Fisher's experiment is that only getting all eight declarations correct would yield a significant result: $P(X = 4 \mid n_{.}, n_1 = 4,$ $m = 4, \omega = 1) = 1 / \binom{8}{4} = \frac{1}{70}$, whereas if any choice was incorrect, $P(X \geq 3) =$ $(1 + 16)/70 \approx 0.24$. According to Joan Fisher Box, in the actual experiment, Dr. Bristol got all eight declarations correct!

Let us entertain the noncentral hypergeometric distribution as a model for such data, where the odds ratio serves as a measure of ability: $\omega = 1$ is pure guesswork, $\omega = \infty$ would be perfect ability, and $\omega = 0$ would be perfect anti-ability (reminiscent of the claim of "anti-ESP" when the psychics get it wrong!). Now suppose there were three tea tasters, with the following results: (a) all eight declarations correct ($X_1 = 4$), (b) guesswork ($X_2 = 2$), and (c) all eight wrong ($X_3 = 0$). What is the exact p-value for the null hypothesis of equal odds ratios? The sum $S = X_1 + X_2 + X_3 = 6$ has probability 0.3023 from the threefold convolution $h(1) * h(1) * h(1)$ of $h(1)$ with itself, where $h(1) = (\frac{1}{70}, \frac{16}{70}, \frac{36}{70}, \frac{16}{70}, \frac{1}{70})$ with $h_j(1) = H(j \mid 8, 4, 4, \omega = 1)$ for $j = 0, \ldots, 4$. There are 19 partitions of 6 into three integers between 0 and 4: $(4, 2, 0)$, $(4, 1, 1)$, $(4, 0, 2)$, $(3, 3, 0)$, $(3, 2, 1)$, $(3, 1, 2)$, $(3, 0, 3)$, $(2, 4, 0)$, $(2, 3, 1)$, $(2, 2, 2)$, $(2, 1, 3)$, $(2, 0, 4)$, $(1, 4, 1)$, $(1, 3, 2)$, $(1, 2, 3)$, $(1, 1, 4)$, $(0, 4, 2)$, $(0, 3, 3)$, and $(0, 2, 4)$. Then (10.31) gives $P(X_1 = 4, X_2 = 2, X_1 = 0 \mid S = 6, (8, 8, 8), (4, 4, 4), (4, 4, 4), \omega = 1) =$ 0.0003471. Of all the partitions listed above, only the 6 permutations of $(4, 2, 0)$ have the same probability as $(4, 2, 0)$, and no other partition has smaller probability. Thus the two-tailed p-value by the point probability method is $6 \times 0.0003471 = 0.00208$. The data are significant in their rejection of the null hypothesis. Note that the presence of extreme sample odds ratios of 0 and ∞ was no impediment to calculation of the p-value. The reader might enjoy Problem 10.4, which asks for the significance of the results from only the first two tasters.

Much literature has been devoted to developing efficient computational algorithms for finding exact p-values and confidence intervals for a common odds ratio. The network algorithm plays a large role in this area. See, e.g., Mehta and Patel (1983); Mehta, Patel, and Gray (1985); Hirji, Mehta, and Patel (1987); Mehta, Patel, and Senchaudhuri (1988, 1992); Agresti, Mehta, and Patel (1990); and Vollset, Hirji, and Elashoff (1991). Various exact and asymptotic tests for homogeneity of several odds ratios were compared by Reis, Hirji, and Afifi (1999). Agresti (1992) gives a nice review of exact methods for contingency tables.

Exact methods become computationally infeasible after a certain point, even though the steady improvement in computing speed and memory keeps pushing that envelope out. Well before the breaking point, fortunately, saddlepoint approximations to exact quantities become highly accurate. Levin (1990) gives a double saddlepoint approximation to the exact conditional score statistic on the left-hand side of (10.30), and discusses its use in conditional logistic regression analysis. The approximation applies a correction term to the profile score function, which is the result of starting with the two-independent-binomial model in each fourfold table, and substituting into the corresponding score statistic maximum likelihood estimates for the nuisance parameters, one per table, under the assumed common odds ratio. Bartlett (1953, 1955) had provided a general bias correction for such profile score statistics, and Gart (1970) notes the high accuracy of the bias correction for fourfold tables. Levin and Kong (1990) explain why Bartlett's bias correction to the profile score function gives such accurate approximations to the exact conditional score function for fourfold tables, by pointing out that in canonical exponential families, Bartlett's correction is actually a double saddlepoint correction, which is known to have a higher order of accuracy. Strawderman and Wells (1998) give a saddlepoint approximation to the exact distribution of cmle(ω). Their method is based on a novel way of calculating the exact mean of the noncentral hypergeometric distribution introduced by Kou and Ying (1996).

10.4. APPROXIMATE INFERENCE FOR A COMMON ODDS RATIO

An outline of the theory to be applied here was presented in Section 6.6. As proven by Cornfield (1956), X_i in Table 10.3 is approximately normally distributed with approximate mean x_i and approximate standard error

$$se(X_i) = \frac{1}{\sqrt{W_i(x_i)}}. \tag{10.32}$$

In (10.32),

$$W_i(x_i) = \frac{1}{x_i} + \frac{1}{m_i - x_i} + \frac{1}{n_{i1} - x_i} + \frac{1}{x_i - l_i} \tag{10.33}$$

with $l_i = m_i + n_{i1} - n_{i.}$, and x_i is the unique root in the admissible interval

$$\text{larger of } (l_i, 0) \leq x_i \leq \text{smaller of } (m_i, n_{i1}) \tag{10.34}$$

of the quadratic equation

$$\frac{x_i(x_i - l_i)}{(m_i - x_i)(n_{i1} - x_i)} = \omega. \tag{10.35}$$

The approximate mean x_i of X_i is the same as N_{11} in the notation of Table 6.5. Explicitly, the quadratic equation is

$$x_i^2(\omega - 1) - x_i\{\omega(m_i + n_{i1}) - l_i\} + \omega m_i n_{i1} = 0. \tag{10.36}$$

Gart (1970) has taken these results and extended them to the case of several fourfold tables. An examination of the data for heterogeneous odds ratios begins by estimating the hypothesized common odds ratio, say $\hat{\omega}$. The appropriate estimate, which cannot be obtained by means of an explicit equation, is such that, when $\hat{x}_i$ is the admissible root of

$$\frac{\hat{x}_i(\hat{x}_i - l_i)}{(m_i - \hat{x}_i)(n_{i1} - \hat{x}_i)} = \hat{\omega} \qquad (i = 1, \ldots, g), \qquad (10.37)$$

[the solution of which is given in (6.52) for given $\hat{\omega}$], then

$$\sum_{i=1}^{g} X_i - \sum_{i=1}^{g} \hat{x}_i = 0. \qquad (10.38)$$

The estimate $\hat{\omega}$ may be found either by trial and error or by any one of the standard iteration methods available for the solution of complicated equations; either $\bar{o}'$ from (10.23) or the Mantel-Haenszel estimate (see Section 10.5) can serve as the initial approximation of $\hat{\omega}$. Note that (10.38) has the same form as (10.30). The only difference is whether the sum of expectations is approximate or exact.

For the data of Table 10.1, the desired estimate is

$$\hat{\omega} = 3.04, \qquad (10.39)$$

which is only slightly larger than the estimate based on the log odds ratio given in (10.25). Table 10.4 presents the associated values of $\hat{x}_i$ and $W_i(\hat{x}_i)$. Note that $\Sigma X_i = \Sigma \hat{x}_i = 281$.

The hypothesis that the underlying odds ratios are equal may be tested by referring the quantity

$$\chi^2_{\text{homog}} = \sum_{i=1}^{g} W_i(\hat{x}_i)(X_i - \hat{x}_i)^2 \qquad (10.40)$$

to the chi squared distribution with $g - 1$ degrees of freedom. For the data of Table 10.4,

$$\chi^2_{\text{homog}} = 9.70 \qquad (10.41)$$

Table 10.4. *Values associated with $\hat{\omega} = 3.04$ for data of Table 10.1*

Study	n_{i1}	n_{i2}	m_i	X_i	$\hat{x}_i$	$W_i(\hat{x}_i)$
1	105	105	115	81	71.601	0.0832
2	192	174	187	118	122.856	0.0473
3	145	145	134	82	86.543	0.0600
Total				281	281.000	

with 2 df, indicating statistically significant differences ($p < 0.01$) among the odds ratios for the three studies of Table 10.1. The chi squared value in (10.41) happens to be slightly larger than the corresponding value in (10.18) based on the log odds ratios.

A test for the significance of the overall odds ratio is performed as follows. If ω, the underlying supposed common odds ratio, is equal to unity, (10.36) becomes linear, and its unique solution is

$$x_i = \frac{n_{i1} m_i}{n_{i.}}.$$ (10.42)

The corresponding value of $W_i(x_i)$ is

$$W_i(x_i) = \frac{n_{i.}^3}{n_{i1} n_{i2} m_i (n_{i.} - m_i)}.$$ (10.43)

Under the hypothesis that $\omega = 1$, the quantity

$$\chi^2_{assoc} = \frac{\left(\left| \sum_{i=1}^{g} X_i - \sum_{i=1}^{g} x_i \right| - 0.5 \right)^2}{\sum_{i=1}^{g} \frac{1}{W_i(x_i)}}$$ (10.44)

has, approximately, a chi squared distribution with 1 df. As pointed out in Section 10.5, this statistic is closely related to the Mantel-Haenszel chi squared statistic.

The values of x_i and $W_i(x_i)$ associated with the hypothesis that $\omega = 1$ are presented in Table 10.5. The value of the statistic in (10.44) for testing whether the overall degree of association is significant is

$$\chi^2_{assoc} = \frac{(|281 - 222.598| - 0.5)^2}{53.836} = 62.28.$$ (10.45)

The inference may therefore be drawn that the supposed common value of the underlying odds ratio is different from unity. The value of chi squared in

Table 10.5. *Values associated with the hypothesis that $\omega = 1$ for data of Table 10.1*

Study	n_{i1}	n_{i2}	m_i	X_i	x_i	$W_i(x_i)$	$1/W_i(x_i)$
1	105	105	115	81	57.500	0.0769	13.006
2	192	174	187	118	98.098	0.0438	22.809
3	145	145	134	82	67.000	0.0555	18.021
Total				281	222.598		53.836

(10.45) happens to be somewhat larger than the value of the corresponding chi squared statistic in (10.21) based on the log odds ratio.

An approximate $100(1 - \alpha)\%$ confidence interval for the supposed common underlying odds ratio is determined as follows. The lower confidence limit, say ω_L, is such that, if x_{iL} is the admissible root of

$$\frac{x_{iL}(n_{i2} - m_i + x_{iL})}{(n_{i1} - x_{iL})(m_i - x_{iL})} = \omega_L \tag{10.46}$$

and if

$$W_i(x_{iL}) = \frac{1}{x_{iL}} + \frac{1}{m_i - x_{iL}} + \frac{1}{n_{i1} - x_{iL}} + \frac{1}{x_{iL} - l_i}, \tag{10.47}$$

then

$$\frac{\left[\left(\sum_{i=1}^{g} X_i - \sum_{i=1}^{g} x_{iL}\right) - 0.5\right]^2}{\sum_{i=1}^{g} \dfrac{1}{W_i(x_{iL})}} = z_{\alpha/2}^2. \tag{10.48}$$

The upper limit, say ω_U, is found similarly, except that the continuity correction in (10.48) is taken as $+0.5$ instead of -0.5.

As with the estimation of the common odds ratio described earlier in this section, the upper and lower limits must be found either by trial and error or by means of a formal iterative procedure. The limits based on the log odds ratio, given in (10.24), may be used as first approximations.

Table 10.6 presents values associated with the lower 95% confidence limit, $\omega_L = 2.28$. Note that

$$\frac{[(281 - 266.421) - 0.5]^2}{51.606} = 3.84, \tag{10.49}$$

the value required for a confidence coefficient of 95%.

Table 10.6. *Values associated with lower 95% confidence limit,*
$\omega_L = 2.28$, *for data of Table 10.1*

Study	n_{i1}	n_{i2}	m_i	X_i	x_{iL}	$W_i(x_{iL})$	$1/W_i(x_{iL})$
1	105	105	115	81	68.083	0.0803	12.453
2	192	174	187	118	116.672	0.0457	21.882
3	145	145	134	82	81.666	0.0579	17.271
Total				281	266.421		51.606

Table 10.7. *Values associated with upper 95% confidence limit,*
$\omega_U = 4.06$, *for data of Table 10.1*

Study	n_{i1}	n_{i2}	m_i	X_i	x_{iU}	$W_i(x_{iU})$	$1/W_i(x_{iU})$
1	105	105	115	81	74.985	0.0870	11.494
2	192	174	187	118	128.811	0.0494	20.243
3	145	145	134	82	91.237	0.0627	15.949
Total				281	295.033		47.686

Table 10.7 presents values associated with the upper 95% confidence
limit, $\omega_U = 4.06$. Note that

$$\frac{[(281 - 295.033) + 0.5]^2}{47.686} = 3.84, \qquad (10.50)$$

as required.

Using Cornfield's results, then, the approximate 95% confidence interval
for the supposed common odds ratio is

$$2.28 \le \omega \le 4.06. \qquad (10.51)$$

This interval is shifted slightly to the right of, and is slightly wider than, the
interval based on the log odds ratio given in (10.26).

10.5. THE MANTEL-HAENSZEL METHOD

A procedure due to Mantel and Haenszel (1959), and extended by Mantel
(1963), permits one to estimate the assumed common odds ratio and to test
whether the overall degree of association is significant. Curiously, it is not the
odds ratio itself but another measure of association that directly underlies
the test for overall association; Radhakrishna (1965) has shown that such an
approach is valid. The fact that the methods use simple, closed-form formulas has much to recommend it. We start with the Mantel-Haenszel summary
estimate of the common odds ratio, present a simple confidence interval for
the log odds ratio, briefly consider tests of homogeneity of the odds ratio, and
finally present the test of overall association.

The Mantel-Haenszel summary estimate of the odds ratio is, say,

$$\hat{\omega}_{MH} = \frac{\displaystyle\sum_{i=1}^{g} \frac{n_{i1}n_{i2}}{n_{i.}} p_{i1}(1 - p_{i2})}{\displaystyle\sum_{i=1}^{g} \frac{n_{i1}n_{i2}}{n_{i.}} p_{i2}(1 - p_{i1})} = \frac{\displaystyle\sum_{i=1}^{g} X_i(X_i - l_i)/n_{i.}}{\displaystyle\sum_{i=1}^{g} (m_i - X_i)(n_{i1} - X_i)/n_{i.}}; \qquad (10.52)$$

$\hat{\omega}_{MH}$ is a weighted average of the separate odds ratios from the g groups (see Problem 10.5). Note that $\hat{\omega}_{MH}$ is the solution of the estimating equation (see Section 15.5)

$$\sum_{i=1}^{g} \frac{n_{i1}n_{i2}}{n_{i.}} p_{i1}(1 - p_{i2}) - \omega \cdot \sum_{i=1}^{g} \frac{n_{i1}n_{i2}}{n_{i.}} p_{i2}(1 - p_{i1}) = 0. \qquad (10.53)$$

This is an unbiased estimating equation because the conditional expectation of the left-hand side of (10.53) given fixed margins is equal to zero by the result of Mantel and Hankey (1975) discussed in Section 6.4.

For the data of Table 10.1,

$$\hat{\omega}_{MH} = \frac{87.516}{29.143} = 3.00, \qquad (10.54)$$

which happens to be slightly greater than the estimate given in (10.25) based on the log odds ratio, and slightly smaller than the estimate given in (10.39) based on the approximate approach of Cornfield and Gart.

Mantel and Haenszel (1959) referred to Cornfield (1956) for calculation of interval estimates for the common odds ratio without presenting standard error formulas for $\hat{\omega}_{MH}$. The Mantel-Haenszel estimator is important because of its consistency in two different large-sample situations: (i) a fixed, possibly small, number of tables, each with large marginal frequencies; and (ii) a large number of tables, each with possibly small frequencies. The latter is the large sparse case, and frequently arises in matched-sample or finely stratified studies. Robins, Breslow, and Greenland (1986) and Phillips and Holland (1987) proposed an asymptotic variance formula that is a consistent estimator of the variance of $\ln \hat{\omega}_{MH}$ under both situations and other, intermediate ones. For $i = 1, \ldots, g$, let

$$R_i = X_i(X_i - l_i)/n_{i.} \quad \text{and} \quad R = \sum_{i=1}^{g} R_i, \qquad (10.55)$$

$$S_i = (m_i - X_i)(n_{i1} - X_i)/n_{i.} \quad \text{and} \quad S = \sum_{i=1}^{g} S_i, \qquad (10.56)$$

and

$$P_i = (X_i + X_i - l_i)/n_{i.} \quad \text{and} \quad Q_i = 1 - P_i = (m_i - X_i + n_{i1} - X_i)/n_{i.}. \qquad (10.57)$$

P_i is the proportion of data on the main diagonal of the ith table, and Q_i is the proportion of data off the diagonal. Then the Mantel-Haenszel estimate of the common odds ratio is $\hat{\omega}_{MH} = R/S$, and the variance of $\ln \hat{\omega}_{MH}$ is consistently estimated by

$$\widehat{\text{Var}}(\ln \hat{\omega}_{\text{MH}}) = \frac{1}{2} \left\{ \frac{\displaystyle\sum_{i=1}^{g} P_i R_i}{R^2} + \frac{\displaystyle\sum_{i=1}^{g} (P_i S_i + Q_i R_i)}{RS} + \frac{\displaystyle\sum_{i=1}^{g} Q_i S_i}{S^2} \right\}. \quad (10.58)$$

For a single 2×2 table, (10.58) reduces to the familiar formula for the estimated variance of the log odds ratio, namely, the sum of reciprocal cell frequencies, or (6.33) without the $\frac{1}{2}$ bias correction. At the same time, for matched pair data (the most extreme form of sparse data, corresponding to a set of g 2×2 tables each with margins of $n_{i1} = n_{i2} = 1$), formula (10.58) reduces to the familiar formula for the estimated variance $(1/b) + (1/c)$ for the log odds ratio estimate $\ln(b/c)$ (see Chapter 13). Thus (10.58) is a generally useful formula. A modified formula is given by Sato (1990). An alternative formula that works in asymptotic framework (i) is given by Hauck (1979) and in framework (ii) by Breslow (1981).

A confidence interval for the common log odds ratio may be constructed from (10.58) in the usual way:

$$\ln \hat{\omega}_{\text{MH}} \pm z_{\alpha/2} \widehat{\text{se}}(\ln \hat{\omega}_{\text{MH}}), \quad (10.59)$$

where the estimated standard error is the square root of (10.58), giving a $100(1 - \alpha)\%$ confidence interval for $\ln \omega$. Exponentiating (10.59) yields a $100(1 - \alpha)\%$ confidence interval for the common odds ratio itself.

Tests of homogeneity of the assumed common underlying odds ratio require different methods for the two large-sample situations identified above. For situation (i), Tarone (1985) proposed a statistic that corrects for the fact that (10.30) is not satisfied exactly by the Mantel-Haenszel estimator. Tarone's test statistic is

$$\sum_{i=1}^{g} \frac{\left\{ X_i - E(X_i | n_{i.}, m_i, n_{i1}, \hat{\omega}_{\text{MH}}) \right\}^2}{\text{Var}(X_i | n_{i.}, m_i, n_{i1}, \hat{\omega}_{\text{MH}})}$$

$$- \frac{\left[\displaystyle\sum_{i=1}^{g} \left\{ X_i - E(X_i | n_{i.}, m_i, n_{i1}, \hat{\omega}_{\text{MH}}) \right\} \right]^2}{\displaystyle\sum_{i=1}^{g} \text{Var}(X_i | n_{i.}, m_i, n_{i1}, \hat{\omega}_{\text{MH}})}, \quad (10.60)$$

where the first term is the score test statistic evaluated at the Mantel-Haenszel odds ratio, and the second term is the correction for bias. Under the hypothesis of a common underlying odds ratio, (10.60) has an approximate chi-squared distribution on $g - 1$ df. The assumption of large samples within each table is used for the approximate normality of each squared term on the left of expression (10.60).

Tests for odds ratio homogeneity in situation (ii), the large sparse case, are best handled by random effects methods, and will be taken up in Section 10.9.3.

The Mantel-Haenzel chi squared test for the significance of the overall degree of association is based on a weighted average of the g differences between proportions, say

$$\bar{d} = \frac{\displaystyle\sum_{i=1}^{g} \frac{n_{i1}n_{i2}}{n_{i.}}(p_{i1} - p_{i2})}{\displaystyle\sum_{i=1}^{g} \frac{n_{i1}n_{i2}}{n_{i.}}}. \tag{10.61}$$

The Mantel-Haenszel chi squared statistic is given by

$$\chi^2_{\mathrm{MH}} = \frac{\left(\left|\displaystyle\sum_{i=1}^{g} \frac{n_{i1}n_{i2}}{n_{i.}}(p_{i1} - p_{i2})\right| - 0.5\right)^2}{\displaystyle\sum_{i=1}^{g} \frac{n_{i1}n_{i2}}{n_{i.} - 1}\bar{p}_i\bar{q}_i}, \tag{10.62}$$

with 1 df. Note that the numerator of (10.62) without continuity correction is the left-hand side of (10.53) evaluated at $\omega = 1$.

For the data of Table 10.1, the value of χ^2_{MH} is

$$\chi^2_{\mathrm{MH}} = \frac{(|58.374| - 0.5)^2}{54.024} = 62.00, \tag{10.63}$$

which is slightly smaller than the value given in (10.45) for the chi squared statistic for association based on the Cornfield-Gart approach. In fact, if $n_{i.} - 1$ were replaced by $n_{i.}$ in the denominator of (10.62), the two chi squared statistics would be identical.

Closely related to the Mantel-Haenszel chi squared statistic is one due to Cochran (1954):

$$\chi^2_{\mathrm{C}} = \frac{\left(\displaystyle\sum_{i=1}^{g} \frac{n_{i1}n_{i2}}{n_{i.}}(p_{i1} - p_{i2})\right)^2}{\displaystyle\sum_{i=1}^{g} \frac{n_{i1}n_{i2}}{n_{i.}}\bar{p}_i\bar{q}_i}. \tag{10.64}$$

The statistics in (10.62) and (10.64) differ not only in the former's inclusion of the continuity correction but, more seriously, in the former's taking $n_{i.} - 1$ rather than $n_{i.}$ in the denominator. When the sample sizes in the g groups are all large, the difference is trivial. When, however, the sample sizes in the g groups are small, the difference becomes substantial.

Consider again the extreme case of matched pairs, in which, each group consists of two individuals, one from each sample. It is easy to check that McNemar's chi squared statistic, given in (13.3), is identical to the Mantel-Haenszel chi squared statistic given in (10.62). See Problem 10.6. Cochran's statistic in (10.64) with the continuity correction, on the other hand, would yield a value twice as large as McNemar's statistic.

The classic criterion for whether the sample sizes in a fourfold table are large enough to warrant referring the value of the standard chi squared statistic to tables of the chi squared distribution with 1 df is that each expected cell frequency must be at least equal to 5 (see Section 3.2). A similar criterion has been proposed for the Mantel-Haenszel chi squared statistic by Mantel and Fleiss (1980). It is that each of the four sums of expected cell frequencies,

$$\sum_{i=1}^{g} n_{i1}\bar{p}_i, \qquad \sum_{i=1}^{g} n_{i2}\bar{p}_i, \qquad \sum_{i=1}^{g} n_{i1}\bar{q}_i, \qquad \sum_{i=1}^{g} n_{i2}\bar{q}_i,$$

must differ by 5 or more from its maximum and from its minimum.

It is therefore not necessary that each table have large marginal frequencies in order for the statistic in (10.62) to be safely referred to the chi squared distribution with 1 df; in fact, as in the case of matched pairs, the total frequency in each table can be as small as 2. All that is required is that there be sufficiently many tables so that each sum of cell expectations is large.

10.6. A COMPARISON OF THE THREE PROCEDURES

Gart (1962, 1970), Odoroff (1970), and McKinlay (1975b, 1978) have compared the procedures described in the three preceding sections as well as procedures due to Birch (1964) and Goodman (1969). Two cases must be distinguished.

In one case, the number of groups or strata is small or moderate, and the sample sizes within each are large. This would be the case if the samples being compared were stratified into a limited number of strata, with additional subjects being assigned to existing strata, or if a limited number of replicate studies were being analyzed. For this case, procedures based on the logarithms of the odds ratios perform either better than or only slightly poorer than their competitors. Given their fair to good precision and accuracy, together with their relative simplicity, the methods of Section 10.2 are recommended for addressing, in a unified manner, all the major inference problems for the odds ratios in each of a small number of strata.

In the second case, each group or stratum is of small or moderate size, but the number of groups or strata is large. This would be the case if the samples being compared were stratified (usually after the data were collected) on several dimensions, or if matching were employed and the number of matched individuals possibly varied (e.g., some matched sets consisting of a pair of individuals, others of a single member from one sample and two members from the other, etc.), or, in general, if the recruitment of additional subjects meant the creation of additional groups or strata.

In this case, the Mantel-Haenszel estimate of the overall odds ratio [see (10.52)], the Mantel-Haenszel 1 df chi squared statistic for testing its significance [see (10.62)], and the confidence interval (10.59) for the overall odds ratio are the methods of choice. Testing for the equality of the several odds ratios may be conducted by Tarone's test (10.60) for a fixed number of tables, or by random effects methods for the large sparse case. In contrast to the case of few groups each of large size, the procedures in Section 10.2 based on the log odds ratio perform terribly in the case of many groups each of small size. Exact methods are useful for checking on the accuracy of approximate ones, and for small-sample-size inferences.

10.7. ALTERNATIVES TO MATCHING

McKinlay (1975a) conducted a historical review of methods that have been used to control for biasing factors in nonrandomized studies such as comparative prospective and comparative retrospective studies, and also reviewed statistical studies of these methods. Her bibliography consists of 165 items, and Fienberg adds others in his Comment on her paper. There are three relatively simple methods available for the control of biasing factors: matching (for which the analytic procedures described in Chapter 13 are appropriate), stratification (for which the procedures described in this chapter are appropriate), and covariance or regression control (for which the analytical procedures described in Chapters 11 and 12 are appropriate).

Suppose, for example, that a retrospective study is contemplated of the association between cigarette smoking and lung cancer, with control for the possible confounding effects of age and sex. One method of control is to pair each lung cancer case with one or more controls of the same sex and of a similar age and to apply the methods of Section 13.1 or 13.3.

Another method of control is to draw a cross-sectional sample of cases and a cross-sectional sample of controls, to stratify the two samples by sex and by age intervals, and then, separately for each resulting stratum, to set up a fourfold table contrasting the rates of smoking for the cases and controls. If there are, say, five age intervals, the total number of fourfold tables is $g = 10$: five for the males plus five for the females. The resulting set of tables may be viewed as coming from g distinct groups, and the methods of Sections 10.2 to 10.5 may be applied.

If only a small number (two or three) of biasing factors out of several are actually controlled, the possible effects of those factors not controlled (and perhaps not even measured) may be assessed by criteria suggested by Bross

(1966) and Schlesselman (1978). If simultaneous control over several biasing factors (more than three) is desired, the composite "multivariate confounder score" of Miettinen (1976) may be used as the basis for stratification; Miettinen suggests five as a reasonable number of strata. A multivariate procedure such as discriminant function analysis must be applied first, however, in order to determine how the composite score is to be calculated.

The multivariate confounder score has been largely supplanted by the *propensity score* of Rosenbaum and Rubin (1983, 1984, 1985a, 1985b). The propensity score has become an indispensible tool in drawing causal inferences in observational studies. Holland (1986) gives a nice overview of causal inference.

Matching has the advantage of assuring that the two samples are comparable on the factors used for matching, but has as a major disadvantage the practical difficulty of finding a matched control for each case if the number of cases is large. Other disadvantages are cited in Section 13.5.

Stratifying the samples after they have been drawn has the advantage of not requiring a specification beforehand of the composition of the two samples, as well as the advantage of permitting an examination of the consistency of association across the various strata. A disadvantage is that, if the sample sizes are not large, the number of individuals in a stratum from one sample may be small compared to the number of individuals in it from the other sample. The power and precision of the comparisons may therefore suffer.

Research on the effectiveness of matching versus the effectiveness of stratification in controlling for confounding factors has been performed by Cochran (1968) and Rubin (1973) for quantitative measurements and by McKinlay (1975c) for dichotomous measurements. Based on their results, we may view matching as the method of choice only for moderate sample sizes and cross-sectional sampling followed by stratification as the method of choice for large sample sizes.

10.8. METHODS TO BE AVOIDED

A Test Described by Fleiss

In the first edition of this book, a test for homogeneity originally proposed by Yates (1955) was described. It calls for summing the values of the standard single-degree-of-freedom chi squareds for the individual groups (without the continuity correction) and for subtracting from this sum the value of Cochran's (1954) single-degree-of-freedom summary chi squared given in (10.64). The procedure is based on the following application of the theory of Section 10.1.

Let the measure of association in the ith group be the so-called *standardized difference*,

$$y_i = d_i = \frac{p_{i1} - p_{i2}}{\bar{p}_i \bar{q}_i}.$$ (10.65)

Its squared standard error is

$$\left[\widehat{se}(d_i)\right]^2 = \frac{1}{\bar{p}_i\bar{q}_i}\left(\frac{n_{i.}}{n_{i1}n_{i2}}\right), \tag{10.66}$$

so that

$$w_i = \frac{\bar{p}_i\bar{q}_in_{i1}n_{i2}}{n_{i.}} \tag{10.67}$$

and

$$\chi_i^2 = w_i d_i^2 = \frac{(p_{i1}-p_{i2})^2}{\bar{p}_i\bar{q}_i(1/n_{i1}+1/n_{i2})}, \tag{10.68}$$

which is precisely the usual chi squared value, aside from the continuity correction.

The mean standardized difference is

$$\bar{d} = \frac{\displaystyle\sum_{i=1}^{g}\frac{(p_{i1}-p_{i2})n_{i1}n_{i2}}{n_{i.}}}{\displaystyle\sum_{i=1}^{g}\frac{\bar{p}_i\bar{q}_in_{i1}n_{i2}}{n_{i.}}} \tag{10.69}$$

with a squared standard error of

$$\left[\widehat{se}(\bar{d})\right]^2 = \frac{1}{\displaystyle\sum_{i=1}^{g}\frac{\bar{p}_i\bar{q}_in_{i1}n_{i2}}{n_{i.}}}, \tag{10.70}$$

so the chi squared statistic for testing overall association is

$$\chi_{\text{assoc}}^2 = \frac{\bar{d}^2}{\left[\widehat{se}(\bar{d})\right]^2} = \frac{\left(\displaystyle\sum_{i=1}^{g}\frac{(p_{i1}-p_{i2})n_{i1}n_{i2}}{n_{i.}}\right)^2}{\displaystyle\sum_{i=1}^{g}\frac{\bar{p}_i\bar{q}_in_{i1}n_{i2}}{n_{i.}}}, \tag{10.71}$$

which is identical to Cochran's χ_C^2 in (10.64).

The error in the first edition was in suggesting that

$$\chi_{\text{homog}}^2 = \sum_{i=1}^{g}w_id_i^2 - \chi_C^2, \tag{10.72}$$

Table 10.8. *Data to illustrate previously suggested test for homogeneity*

Group	Sample 1		Sample 2		Overall	
	n_{i1}	p_{i1}	n_{i2}	p_{i2}	$n_{i.}$	$\bar{p}_i$
$i = 1$	230	0.87	50	0.20	280	0.75
$i = 2$	40	0.25	810	0.0123	850	0.0235

Table 10.9. *Summarization of data in Table 10.8*

Group	d_i	w_i	$w_i d_i$	$w_i d_i^2$
$i = 1$	3.57	7.70	27.489	98.136
$i = 2$	10.36	0.87	9.013	93.375
Total		8.57	36.502	191.511

with $g - 1$ df, always formed the basis of a valid test of homogeneity. Mantel, Brown, and Byar (1977) have shown that the standardized difference in (10.65), and therefore the test statistic in (10.72), is sensitive to the ratio of sample sizes as well as to the underlying degree of association, so that the test based on (10.72) may sometimes be invalid.

Consider the data in Table 10.8, taken from Mantel, Brown, and Byar (1977). It is easily checked that the odds ratio in both groups is equal to 26.7. Nevertheless, as shown in Table 10.9, the two standardized differences are markedly different, and the test based on (10.72) suggests, incorrectly, that association differs between the two groups:

$$\chi^2_{\text{homog}} = 191.511 - \frac{36.502^2}{8.57} = 36.04 \qquad (10.73)$$

with $g - 1 = 1$ df, which is highly significant.

Mantel, Brown, and Byar (1977) illustrate other possible anomalies associated with the statistic given in (10.72) (e.g., the odds ratios may vary markedly across the g groups, but χ^2_{homog} might nevertheless equal zero). The problem with χ^2_{homog} is the dependence of the standardized differences, which this statistic compares, on the sample sizes n_{i1} and n_{i2}. The sample sizes affect the values of $\bar{p}_i$ and $\bar{q}_i$; therefore, as seen in (10.65), they affect the value of d_i. Because of the above difficulties, the test for homogeneity based on (10.72) should be avoided.

The Summation-of-Chi Procedure

One of the more frequently employed methods for combining data from different fourfold tables is of the form outlined in Section 10.1, although not obviously so. The method, usually referred to as the summation-of-chi procedure, has long been known to have serious defects but keeps reappearing nevertheless (see, e.g., Finney, 1965). The method in effect takes as the measure of association

$$y_i = z_i = \frac{p_{i1} - p_{i2}}{\sqrt{\bar{p}_i \bar{q}_i (1/n_{i1} + 1/n_{i2})}}. \tag{10.74}$$

Because z_i has been standardized to have a standard error of unity, therefore

$$w_i = \frac{1}{[\text{se}(z_i)]^2} = 1. \tag{10.75}$$

The word "chi" in the name of the procedure derives from z_i's being the square root of a chi squared variate (without the correction for continuity), and hence being a chi variate.

When y_i is defined by (10.74),

$$\bar{y} = \frac{\sum_{i=1}^g z_i}{g} = \bar{z} \tag{10.76}$$

and

$$\sum_{i=1}^g w_i = g, \tag{10.77}$$

by (10.75). Therefore, by (10.9),

$$\chi^2_{\text{assoc}} = \frac{\left(\sum_{i=1}^g z_i\right)^2}{g} = g\bar{z}^2. \tag{10.78}$$

There is a serious flaw inherent in this chi squared statistic (see, e.g., Pasternack and Mantel, 1966). Consider the numerical example of Table 10.10. For group 1,

$$\chi_1^2 = z_1^2 = 8.00; \tag{10.79}$$

for group 2,

$$\chi_2^2 = z_2^2 = 80.00. \tag{10.80}$$

Table 10.10. *Data to illustrate summation-of-chi procedure*

Group	Sample 1		Sample 2		Overall		
	n_{i1}	p_{i1}	n_{i2}	p_{i2}	$n_{i.}$	$\bar{p}_i$	z_i
$i = 1$	100	0.60	100	0.40	200	0.50	2.83
$i = 2$	1000	0.60	1000	0.40	2000	0.50	8.94

The average value of z is

$$\bar{z} = \tfrac{1}{2}(2.83 + 8.94) = 5.88, \tag{10.81}$$

so that, by (10.78),

$$\chi^2_{\text{assoc}} = 2 \times (5.88)^2 = 69.15 \tag{10.82}$$

with 1 df. What is disquieting about this value for the overall test of association is that it is less than the value for one of the individual chi squareds for association, $\chi^2_2 = 80$. The addition of the evidence from group 1, in which the association was really the same as in group 2, would be expected to increase the statistical significance of the association. The summation-of-chi procedure failed to do so.

Any procedure for which an accumulation of evidence for association may lead to a reduction in chi squared is to be avoided. So be it with the summation-of-chi procedure.

Summation Observed versus Summation Expected
A relative lack of sensitivity to added evidence for association in a given direction characterizes the following method, too. Although it can be cast into the terms of the theory of Section 10.1, that would not be an aid to understanding.

The method calls first for generating a total fourfold table by summing the frequencies across the g individual tables. Let the observed frequencies for $g = 2$ groups be as in Table 10.11 Chi squared is calculated without the continuity correction. The association between A and B, measured by an odds ratio of 26.7, is the same in both groups.

The table of total frequencies is as shown in Table 10.12.

The next step is to determine, for each group, the set of frequencies expected under the hypothesis of no association. The expected frequency for a cell is calculated as the product of the total frequencies in a cell's row and column divided by the overall frequency in the table. Thus the expected

Table 10.11. *Data to illustrate procedure based on summation observed versus summation expected*

	Group 1			Group 2		
	B	$\bar{B}$	Total	B	$\bar{B}$	Total
A	200	30	230	40	120	160
$\bar{A}$	10	40	50	10	800	810
Total	210	70	280	50	920	970
		$\chi^2_1 = 98.20$			$\chi^2_2 = 154.35$	

Table 10.12. *Sum of frequencies for groups 1 and 2*

	B	$\overline{B}$	Total
A	240	150	390
$\overline{A}$	20	840	860
Total	260	990	1250

Table 10.13. *Expected frequencies for groups 1 and 2*

	Group 1			Group 2		
	B	$\overline{B}$	Total	B	$\overline{B}$	Total
A	172.5	57.5	230	8.25	151.75	160
$\overline{A}$	37.5	12.5	50	41.75	768.25	810
Total	210	70	280	50	920	970

frequency in the (A, B) cell for group 2 is $160 \times 50/970 = 8.25$. All expected frequencies are shown in Table 10.13.

Next, generate an overall table of expected frequencies by summing, as in Table 10.14, across the individual tables just determined.

Finally, calculate the summary chi squared for association by taking, for each cell, the difference between the total observed and total expected frequencies, squaring, dividing by the total expected frequency, and summing across all four cells. Thus from Tables 10.12 and 10.14,

$$\chi^2_{assoc} = \frac{(240 - 180.75)^2}{180.75} + \frac{(150 - 209.25)^2}{209.25}$$

$$+ \frac{(20 - 79.25)^2}{79.25} + \frac{(840 - 780.75)^2}{780.75}$$

$$= 84.99. \tag{10.83}$$

This value for chi squared is less than either of the two original chi squared values shown in Table 10.11. The procedure based on comparing the

Table 10.14. *Sum of expected frequencies for groups 1 and 2*

	B	$\overline{B}$	Total
A	180.75	209.25	390
$\overline{A}$	79.25	780.75	860
Total	260	990	1250

Table 10.15. *Association between A and B in two groups*

	Group 1			Group 2		
	B	$\overline{B}$	Total	B	$\overline{B}$	Total
A	10	40	50	60	40	100
$\overline{A}$	20	80	100	30	20	50
Total	30	120	150	90	60	150
		$\chi_1^2 = 0$			$\chi_2^2 = 0$	

sums of observed frequencies with the sums of expected frequencies therefore suffers from the same deficiency as the summation-of-chi procedure and
is to be avoided for the same reason.

Chi Squared on the Table of Totals (Pooling the Data)

A defect opposite in nature to that of the two preceding methods characterizes the following procedure for testing overall association. The method
cannot be described in terms of the theory of Section 10.1. It calls merely for
generating the table of total observed frequencies as described in the preceding section and then calculating a straightforward chi squared on it.

The method works quite well on the data of the two previous sections, and
in general for groups in which corresponding proportions are nearly equal.
Such a state of affairs is exceptional, however. Consider the data of Table
10.15. No association between A and B exists in either group, although the
basic rates are different in the two groups.

The table of total frequencies is as shown in Table 10.16. Its associated chi
squared is 5.01, indicating an association significant at the 0.05 level. The
pooling of data from tables with unequal proportions and with unequal ratios
of sample sizes, n_{i1}/n_{i2}, has created the impression of association where
none actually existed. See Section 10.9.1 for further discussion of such
confounding.

The procedures described in this section should be avoided for the reasons
indicated (see also Gart, 1962, and Sheehe, 1966). This necessarily means
that the calculations become more complicated, as was seen in Sections 10.2
to 10.5, but that is the price one must pay for a valid analysis.

Table 10.16. *Sum of frequencies for groups 1 and 2*

	B	$\overline{B}$	Total
A	70	80	150
$\overline{A}$	50	100	150
Total	120	180	300

10.9.   RELATED MATTERS

We close the chapter with some comments and results on matters related to the combination of evidence from fourfold tables. Section 10.9.1 continues the discussion of confounding illustrated at the end of the preceding section. Section 10.9.2 extends the methods of Section 10.1 to random effects meta-analysis. Section 10.9.3 covers tests for homogeneity of odds ratios in the large-sparse case.

10.9.1.   Potential Confounding and Operational Nonconfounding

The problem highlighted at the end of Section 10.8 is one of confounding. Generally, when the group or stratification variable C is associated with variable A (within fixed levels of variable B), and is also associated with B (within fixed levels of A), one should presume that the pooled odds ratio will be a biased estimate of the true odds ratio assumed constant across tables. Here we further distinguish between *potential confounding* and *operational nonconfounding*. In order to abstract the discussion from issues of sampling, let us assume in this subsection that the sample sizes per group are so large that the sample proportions p_{i1} and p_{i2} are essentially equal to the true proportions P_{i1} and P_{i2}, respectively. Then given a set of g 2×2 tables with a common odds ratio, $(p_{i1}q_{i2})/(p_{i2}q_{i1}) = \omega_{\text{common}}$, the *necessary and sufficient condition* for the pooled odds ratio,

$$\omega_{\text{pooled}} = \frac{\left(\displaystyle\sum_{i=1}^{g} n_{i1} p_{i1} \right)\left(\displaystyle\sum_{i=1}^{g} n_{i2} q_{i2} \right)}{\left(\displaystyle\sum_{i=1}^{g} n_{i2} p_{i2} \right)\left(\displaystyle\sum_{i=1}^{g} n_{i1} q_{i1} \right)}, \tag{10.84}$$

to equal ω_{common} is that

$$\sum_{i=1}^{g} w_{i1} \frac{p_{i2}}{q_{i2}} = \sum_{i=1}^{g} w_{i2} \frac{p_{i2}}{q_{i2}}, \tag{10.85}$$

where the two sets of weights are defined as $w_{i1} = n_{i1}q_{i1}/(\Sigma_i n_{i1} q_{i1})$ and $w_{i2} = n_{i2}q_{i2}/(\Sigma_i n_{i2} q_{i2})$. When the necessary and sufficient condition (10.85) holds, we say the collection of tables is *collapsible*, meaning that the pooled odds ratio from the collapsed set of tables equals the common odds ratio. It is easy to identify two special cases of (10.85):

(i) p_{i2}/q_{i2} is constant for $i = 1, \ldots, g$. In this case the stratum variable C is unassociated with the outcome variable B within level 2 of variable A, and, because of the assumption of a common odds ratio, C is also

Table 10.17. *Potential confounding with operational nonconfounding*

	Group 1			Group 2			Group 3			Pooled		
	B	$\bar{B}$	Total	B	$\bar{B}$	Total	B	$\bar{B}$	Total	B	$\bar{B}$	Total
A	79	79	158	36	18	54	270	90	360	385	187	572
$\bar{A}$	36	36	72	144	72	216	135	45	180	315	153	468
Total	115	115	230	180	90	270	405	135	540	700	340	1040

unassociated with B within level 1 of variable A. Briefly, C is conditionally unassociated with B given A; in symbols we write $B \perp C | A$.

(ii) The two sets of weights are identical: $w_{i1} = w_{i2}$ for $i = 1, \ldots, g$. In this case the odds on an observation at level 1 versus 2 of A among outcomes at level 2 of B are $(n_{i1}q_{i1})/(n_{i2}q_{i2}) = (\Sigma_i n_{i1}q_{i1})/(\Sigma_i n_{i2}q_{i2})$ and thus constant, and similarly for the odds at level 1 of B, i.e., C is conditionally unassociated with A given B, $A \perp C | B$.

Conditions (i) and (ii) are *sufficient* conditions for the pooled odds ratio to be unbiased for the common odds ratio. When either sufficient condition holds, the group or stratification variable is nonconfounding.

When neither condition holds, variable C is said to be *potentially confounding*. The qualifier is required because (i) and (ii) are sufficient but not necessary for collapsibility. Thus it is possible for neither (i) nor (ii) to hold while (10.85) nevertheless holds, in which case we say that the group variable is *operationally nonconfounding*. For example, consider the hypothetical data in Table 10.17. The reader may confirm that the odds ratio equals 1 in each table, as well as in the pooled table, so that C is operationally nonconfounding, even though neither sufficient condition (i) nor (ii) holds.

Our view of the situation illustrated in Table 10.17 is that the group variable should still be considered a confounding factor, notwithstanding its status as an operational non-confounder in the data. The reason is that with exactly the same proportions p_{i1} and p_{i2} and odds ratios, but merely different sample sizes n_{i1} and n_{i2}, collapsibility is usually lost. Consider the data of Table 10.18, which has precisely the same proportions and odds ratio relations as Table 10.17 for the three separate groups, but triples one sample size, n_{11}, in the first table. Now the pooled table odds ratio shows serious bias for the common odds ratio in one direction (pooled odds ratio = 0.76). Table 10.19 triples n_{12} in the first table and produces serious bias in the opposite direction (pooled odds ratio = 1.20). Thus if a researcher reported a finding of nonconfounding by the group variable in his or her analysis of the data in Table 10.17, other researchers who failed to control for the same potential confounder with a different design could be misled. In general, whenever a

Table 10.18. *Loss of operational nonconfounding in one direction*

	Group 1			Group 2			Group 3			Pooled		
	B	$\bar{B}$	Total	B	$\bar{B}$	Total	B	$\bar{B}$	Total	B	$\bar{B}$	Total
A	237	237	474	36	18	54	270	90	360	543	345	888
$\bar{A}$	36	36	72	144	72	216	135	45	180	315	153	468
Total	273	273	546	180	90	270	405	135	540	858	498	1356

Table 10.19. *Loss of operational nonconfounding in the other direction*

	Group 1			Group 2			Group 3			Pooled		
	B	$\bar{B}$	Total	B	$\bar{B}$	Total	B	$\bar{B}$	Total	B	$\bar{B}$	Total
A	79	79	158	36	18	54	270	90	360	385	187	572
$\bar{A}$	108	108	216	144	72	216	135	45	180	387	225	612
Total	187	187	374	180	90	270	405	135	540	772	412	1184

characterization of a relation between variables is sensitive to changes in a design feature under the control of the investigator, like sample size, the characterization should be avoided as unreliable. So it is with the notion of operational nonconfounding when the stratum variable is a potential confounder.

10.9.2. Fixed and Random Effects Meta-analysis

Section 10.1 presented general methods for combining evidence across several independent studies, and those methods have come to be called fixed-effects meta-analysis when they are applied to literature review and synthesis on a particular research question. An excellent review of the problems and methods in this area is given by Hedges and Olkin (1985), Fleiss (1993), and Olkin (1995a, 1995b, 1996). When the studies are viewed not as the entire population of studies but rather as a sample from a larger population of studies, then random effects meta-analysis is a better analytic framework to use. Here, paraphrasing liberally from Fleiss (1993), we present methods appropriate for random effects meta-analysis for combining the evidence about odds ratios from several independent studies. These extend the methods of Section 9.6 for a set of proportions with random heterogeneity to methods for a set of odds ratios with random heterogeneity.

Under the assumption that the g studies are a random sample from a larger population of studies, there is a mean population log odds ratio, say Λ, about which the true study-specific log odds ratios vary. Thus, even if each study's results were based on sample sizes so large that the standard errors of the sample log odds ratios were zero, there would still be study-to-study variation in the log odds ratios. Let D^2 denote the variance of the studies' true log odds ratios, and let χ^2_{homog} denote the statistic (10.11) or (10.18) for measuring study-to-study variation in effect size. Note that there is no concern in the random effects analysis about the statistical significance or not of χ^2_{homog}. On the contrary, it is taken as axiomatic that interstudy heterogeneity exists, and that it should automatically be taken into account in the analysis. Instead, χ^2_{homog} is used to estimate the true interstudy variance D^2, as follows.

Let $\bar{w} = \sum_{i=1}^{g} w_i / g$ be the average of the g weights $w_1, \ldots, w_g$, and let s_w^2 be the sample variance of the weights,

$$s_w^2 = \frac{\sum_{i=1}^{g}(w_i - \bar{w})^2}{g-1} = \frac{\sum_{i=1}^{g} w_i^2 - g\bar{w}^2}{g-1}. \tag{10.86}$$

The weights w_i are defined in (10.16), or, if the cell frequencies from the individual studies' fourfold tables are available, the bias-corrected version w_i' from Section 10.2 or (6.33) may be used; alternatively, if log odds ratios are adjusted for confounding factors in the individual studies and these are to be used in the meta-analysis, the general definition of w_i as the squared reciprocal of the estimated standard error for the adjusted log odds ratio will be used. We will not here further distinguish between these alternatives, and will simply write L_i for the estimated log odds ratio to be meta-analyzed, and w_i for its squared reciprocal standard error. We shall also ignore the fact that, technically, the weights themselves are random variables, both because they are estimated from data, and because they generally depend on the parameters from each study, which are variables in the random effects approach. We assume the sample sizes are large enough in each study to justify the assumption of an approximately normal distribution for L_i, and we shall treat the estimated standard errors, and hence the weights, as if they were known constants. This approach is justified on the grounds that the additional uncertainty introduced in the meta-analysis due to random weights is generally small, and ignoring it simplifies the analysis substantially. Results of Lin et al. (1997) support this approach, though they point out that the standard error of an estimate of D^2 is sensitive to random variation in the weights.

Now let

$$U = (g-1)\left(\bar{w} - \frac{s_w^2}{g\bar{w}}\right). \tag{10.87}$$

An estimate of D^2, the component of variance due to interstudy variation in effect size, is given by the following formula of Dersimonian and Laird (1986):

$$
\tilde{D}^2 =
\begin{cases}
\dfrac{\chi^2_{\text{homog}} - (g-1)}{U} & \text{if } \chi^2_{\text{homog}} > g - 1, \\
0 & \text{if } \chi^2_{\text{homog}} \le g - 1.
\end{cases}
\tag{10.88}
$$

Due to the interstudy variability in true log odds ratios, the marginal variance of each estimated log odds ratio is no longer simply w_i^{-1}, but $\text{Var}(L_i) = D^2 + w_i^{-1}$. Thus, for estimating Λ, we use the approximately optimal weights

$$
w_i^* = \frac{1}{\tilde{D}^2 + w_i^{-1}};
\tag{10.89}
$$

the random effects point estimate of Λ is then

$$
\tilde{L}^* = \frac{\sum_{i=1}^{g} w_i^* L_i}{\sum_{i=1}^{g} w_i^*},
\tag{10.90}
$$

with standard error

$$
\widetilde{\text{se}}(\tilde{L}^*) = \frac{1}{\sqrt{\sum_{i=1}^{g} w_i^*}}.
\tag{10.91}
$$

Thus an approximate $100(1 - \alpha)\%$ confidence interval for Λ is

$$
\tilde{L}^* - \frac{z_{\alpha/2}}{\sqrt{\sum_i w_i^*}} < \Lambda < \tilde{L}^* + \frac{z_{\alpha/2}}{\sqrt{\sum_i w_i^*}},
\tag{10.92}
$$

and a test for significance of the population average log odds ratio is provided by

$$
\chi^2_{\text{assoc}} = \tilde{L}^{*2} \sum_{i=1}^{g} w_i^*.
\tag{10.93}
$$

A consequence of the random effects analysis compared with the fixed-effects analysis is that the confidence interval for the population average log odds ratio Λ in the former is wider than that for the assumed constant log odds ratio in the latter. Specifically, $\sum_i w_i^* \le \sum_i w_i$, with equality only when $\tilde{D}^2$ in (10.88) equals zero, so that the standard error in (10.91) is at least as large as (10.7) in the fixed-effects analysis. A random effects analysis therefore suggests more uncertainty in estimating the population average parame-

Table 10.20. *Random effects analysis of logarithms of odds ratios applied to data of Table 10.1*

Study	o_i'	L_i'	w_i'	w_i^*	$w_i^* L_i'$
1	6.894	1.931	10.410	3.035	5.861
2	2.415	0.881	21.868	3.583	3.156
3	2.314	0.839	17.357	3.436	2.883
Total				10.054	11.900

ter than does a fixed-effects analysis, reflecting the additional variability in the true study-specific parameters.

Consider once again the data in Table 10.1. From (10.18), $\chi_{\text{homog}}^2 = 9.41$, and from Table 10.2, the average weight is $\bar{w} = 49.635/3 = 16.545$. The variance of the weights is $s_w^2 = 33.316$. Thus the quantity U in (10.87) is $U = 2\{16.545 - 33.316/(3 \times 16.545)\} = 31.748$, whence the estimated dispersion is $\tilde{D}^2 = (9.41 - 2)/31.748 = 0.2334$.

The fixed and random effects weights are displayed in Table 10.20 for comparison. Note how the weights w_i^* place more even weight on the three studies than do the weights w_i. (This is typical of the random effects analysis; in fact, as D^2 grows large, the optimal weights approach $1/g$, wherein all studies would be weighted equally.) The estimate of the population average log odds ratio is $\tilde{L}^* = 11.900/10.054 = 1.184$, slightly larger than the value of $\tilde{L}' = 1.087$ in (10.19), as a result of the greater weight placed on the first study than on the other two. The standard error of $\tilde{L}^*$ is estimated as $\widetilde{\text{se}}(\tilde{L}^*) = 1/\sqrt{10.054} = 0.315$, over twice as large as 0.142 in (10.20) from the fixed-effects analysis, reflecting the substantial variation in the odds ratios across the three studies. The test of overall association from (10.93) is $\chi_{\text{assoc}}^2 = 1.184^2 \times 10.054 = 14.09$, still highly significant, but substantially smaller than 58.60 from (10.21). An approximate 95% confidence interval for the population average log odds ratio from (10.92) is $1.184 \pm 1.96 \times 0.315 = (0.567, 1.801)$. Taking antilogs yields an approximate 95% confidence interval for $\exp(\Lambda)$: $1.76 < \exp \Lambda < 6.06$, which is substantially wider than the fixed-effects confidence interval for the assumed common odds ratio, $2.25 < \omega < 3.92$, from (10.26).

There has been controversy concerning how interstudy differences in the magnitudes of estimated effect sizes should be taken account of in a meta-analysis. Fleiss (1993) argues that the random effects model anticipates better than the fixed-effects model the possibility that some studies not included in the analysis are under way, are about to be published, were published in obscure places, or were never even reported, and that the results of the unincluded studies may show the same kind of variation as those of the included studies. DeMets (1987) and Bailey (1987) discuss the strengths and weaknesses of the two approaches. Bailey suggests that when the research question involves extrapolation to the future—*will* the treatment have an effect, on average—then the random effects model is the appropriate one. When the research question concerns whether treatment *has* produced an effect, on average, *in the set of studies being analyzed*, then the fixed-effects model is the appropriate one. Meier (1987) argues that study-to-study variation is a key feature of the data and should contribute to the analysis, and thus supports the random effects approach. Peto (1987), on the other hand, supports the view that only the studies currently being analyzed should be of interest.

On the whole, the present authors find the random effects model generally most appropriate. Crucial to remember, however, is that whichever statistical model is chosen, understanding the sources and causes of inter-study variation in effect sizes is as important (if not more so) to understanding the phenomena under study as is the mechanical calculation of a summary effect size and confidence interval for it, be it a constant or a population average. Summarization should follow understanding, not the other way around.

10.9.3.* Tests of Odds Ratio Homogeneity in the Large-Sparse Case

The large sparse case presents special challenges for detecting heterogeneity in odds ratios, because, like any test of a higher-order interaction, it has smaller power than the test of overall association. In addition, the usual approximation of the exact distribution of a test statistic for odds ratio homogeneity by the chi squared distribution, which is valid in the classic framework of a fixed number of tables each with large margins, breaks down when there are many degrees of freedom and each component is not accurately approximated by chi squared. To help address these issues, it makes good sense to seek methods that take advantage of the random effects model.

Ejigou and McHugh (1984) considered the case of 1-to-R matched sample studies, and Zelterman and Le (1991) considered chi-squared goodness-of-fit tests. Liang and Self (1985) considered several tests of odds ratio homogeneity in the large sparse case. One of their statistics, which had favorable operating characteristics in a Monte Carlo study, was the so-called mixture model score test. This test statistic is theoretically locally most powerful against nearby alternatives of a random mixture of odds ratios. Using the notation of Table 10.3, the numerator of the mixture model score statistic is

$$T = \sum_{i=1}^{g} \left[\{X_i - E(X_i|n_{i.}, n_{i1}, m_i, \hat{\omega}_c)\}^2 - \mathrm{Var}(X_i|n_{i.}, n_{i1}, m_i, \hat{\omega}_c) \right], \quad (10.94)$$

where the mean and variance of the reference cell X_i are the moments (6.43) and (6.44) of the noncentral hypergeometric distribution, evaluated at the conditional maximum likelihood estimate of the common odds ratio under the null hypothesis of homogeneity [see expression (10.30)]. Under the null hypothesis of a common odds ratio, the expected value of T is approximately zero [and would be exactly zero if ω were known and used in (10.94)]. Under the alternative hypothesis of random variation in true odds ratios, the leading terms of squared observed-minus-expected differences in (10.94) tend to exceed their null expectation of $\text{Var}(X_i)$, so T becomes large. As the number g of tables increases, T has an approximately normal distribution with zero mean under the null hypothesis, by the central limit theorem.

In order to operationalize the test procedure, one needs the standard error of T, which involves third and fourth moments of the noncentral hypergeometric distribution. Jones et al. (1989) give explicit formulas for the variance of T. Letting

$$\hat{\mu}_i^{(1)} = E\left(X_i | n_{i.}, n_{i1}, m_i, \hat{\omega}_c\right), \qquad \hat{\mu}_i^{(2)} = \text{Var}\left(X_i | n_{i.}, n_{i1}, m_i, \hat{\omega}_c\right),$$

$$\hat{\mu}_i^{(3)} = E\left\{\left(X_i - \mu_i^{(1)}\right)^3 | n_{i.}, n_{i1}, m_i, \hat{\omega}_c\right\}, \tag{10.95}$$

$$\hat{\mu}_i^{(4)} = E\left\{\left(X_i - \mu_i^{(1)}\right)^4 | n_{i.}, n_{i1}, m_i, \hat{\omega}_c\right\},$$

denote the first four moments evaluated at the conditional maximum likelihood estimate $\hat{\omega}_c$ the standard error of T is given by

$$\widehat{se}(T) = \left(\sum_{i=1}^{g}\left[\hat{\mu}_i^{(4)} - \left\{\left(\hat{\mu}_i^{(2)}\right)^2 + \frac{\left(\hat{\mu}_i^{(3)}\right)^2}{\left(\hat{\mu}_i^{(2)}\right)}\right\}\right]\right)^{1/2}. \tag{10.96}$$

The mixture model score test consists of referring $z = T/\widehat{se}(T)$ to the one-tailed critical value z_α from the standard normal distribution, and rejecting the null hypothesis of odds ratio homogeneity if $z \geq z_\alpha$.

To illustrate, consider the hypothetical data in Table 10.21, which simulates the results of a matched case-control study with a dichotomous antecedant exposure and with $2:2$ matching, that is, two cases matched with two

Table 10.21. *Data of 200 matched samples from a simulated matched sample case-control study with 2:2 matching*

Canonical Representation				Product Multinomial Representation			
Number of Exposed Cases	Number of Exposed Controls				Number of Exposed Cases		
	0	1	2	m	0	1	2
0	11	29	16	1	29	36	—
1	36	35	30	2	16	35	13
2	13	16	14	3	—	30	16

controls, with each of the four matched on given levels of strongly confounding factors. For the illustration, two hundred pairs of binomial variables with sample sizes $n_{i1} = n_{i2} = 2$ were generated, representing the number of exposed cases, X_i, or the number of exposed controls, $Y_i = m_i - X_i$. The binomial parameters were selected as follows. P_{i1} was held fixed at $P_1 = 0.5$, and ln ω_i was given a standard normal distribution. P_{i2} was then calculated as $P_{i2} = P_{i1}/(P_{i1} + \omega_i Q_{i1}) = 1/(1 + \omega_i)$. The results are displayed in two formats in Table 10.21. The first is the canonical presentation of data from matched samples (see Chapter 13), and cross-classifies the number of cases exposed (0, 1, or 2) by the number of controls exposed (0, 1, or 2). The second recasts the data into independent rows with fixed $m_i = 1$, 2, or 3. The uninformative matched sets with $X_i = Y_i = m_i = 0$ or $X_i = Y_i = 2$ and $m_i = 4$ have been omitted from the second format. These do not affect either the statistic (10.94) or its standard error (10.95) and may be deleted from the analysis.

For the mixture model score test, the first step is to obtain the conditional maximum likelihood estimate of the common odds ratio. Solution of (10.30) yields $\hat{\omega}_c = 0.8759$, with standard error for ln $\hat{\omega}_c$ equal to 0.1429 and 95% confidence interval for $\hat{\omega}_c$ equal to $(0.66, 1.16)$, all under the assumption of a constant odds ratio. [For comparison, the Mantel-Haenszel estimate of the common odds ratio is 0.8802, and the 95% confidence interval by (10.58) and (10.59) is $(0.67, 1.16)$.] Next one obtains the first four moments for the informative cases with $m_i = 1$, 2, or 3. We have the following results:

for $m_i = 1$: $\hat{\mu}_i^{(1)} = 0.4669$, $\hat{\mu}_i^{(2)} = 0.2489$, $\hat{\mu}_i^{(3)} = 0.01647$, and $\hat{\mu}_i^{(4)} = 0.06304$;

for $m_i = 2$: $\hat{\mu}_i^{(1)} = 0.9558$, $\hat{\mu}_i^{(2)} = 0.3333$, $\hat{\mu}_i^{(3)} = 0.00008578$, and $\hat{\mu}_i^{(4)} = 0.3314$;

for $m_i = 3$: $\hat{\mu}_i^{(1)} = 1.4669$, $\hat{\mu}_i^{(2)} = 0.2489$, $\hat{\mu}_i^{(3)} = 0.01647$, and $\hat{\mu}_i^{(4)} = 0.06304$.

(The distribution for $m_i = 3$ is the same as that for $m_i = 1$ shifted up by 1.) Then

$$T = 29\{(0 - 0.4669)^2 + - 0.2489\} + 36\{(1 - 0.4669)^2 - 0.2489\}$$
$$+ 16\{(0 - 0.9558)^2 - 0.3333\} + 35\{(1 - 0.9558)^2 - 0.3333\}$$
$$+ 13\{(2 - 0.9558)^2 - 0.3333\} + 30\{(1 - 1.4669)^2 - 0.2489\}$$
$$+ 16\{(2 - 1.4669)^2 - 0.2489\} = 7.54.$$

After a somewhat lengthy calculation the standard error of T is found to be 3.7616, for a z-score of $7.54/3.76 = 2.00$. The one-tailed p-value is thus 0.023, and the test has confirmed the substantial heterogeneity in odds ratios.

In the simulated data, the true odds ratios had a mean of 1.524 and a standard deviation of 1.817, with a highly skewed log-normal distribution.

Note that 1.524 is outside the 95% confidence interval $(0.66, 1.16)$ for the presumed common odds ratio. This highlights another point about varying odds ratios: when odds ratios are random, a confidence interval for an assumed constant odds ratio, constructed by exponentiating the endpoints of a confidence interval for its logarithm, will generally not be a confidence interval for the average of the random odds ratios, especially when there is skewness in their distribution. The constructed interval centers about the geometric mean odds ratio rather than the arithmetic mean, and these differ unless the odds ratios are constant.

Jones et al. (1989) conducted a Monte Carlo investigation comparing several tests for odds ratio homogeneity including the mixture model score test. Interestingly, these authors found substantially lower power for the mixture model score test than did Liang and Self (1985) in their Monte Carlo study. Levin (1992) explained the discrepancy between the two studies on the basis of how each set of authors generated their simulated data. Liang and Self (1985) generated random probabilities P_{i1} and odds ratios ω_i independently, implicitly defining $P_{i2} = P_{i1}/(P_{i1} + \omega_i Q_{i1})$. Then, given the pair of probabilities (P_{i1}, P_{i2}), they generated the reference cell X_i as a binomial random variable with sample size n_{i1} and parameter P_{i1}, and generated the count Y_i in the $(2, 1)$ cell independently as a binomial with sample size n_{2i} and parameter P_{i2}. They considered $1:R$ matched designs with $(n_{i1}, n_{i2}) = (1, R)$, and completely balanced designs with $n_{i1} = n_{i2} = n$, and also considered cases in which P_{i1} was fixed, not random, as in the illustration above.

By contrast, Jones et al. (1989) generated random variables P_{2i} and ω_i independently, implicitly defining $P_{i1} = P_{i2}/(P_{i2} + \omega_i^{-1} Q_{i2})$. They considered completely balanced designs and balanced designs with $n_{i1} = n_{i2}$ varying from table to table, and also considered cases in which P_{i2} was fixed, not random. Levin (1992) pointed out that there is a complete loss of power for the $1:R$ matched design when P_{i2} is fixed, even when ω_i is random, because one cannot distinguish a binary random variable X_i with $n_{i1} = 1$ and a random P_{i1}, on the one hand, from a binary random variable with a fixed P_1 equal to the expected value of the random P_{i1}. Thus the null and alternative hypotheses are indistinguishable. He also showed that there is a partial loss of power when $n_{i1} > 1$ and P_{i2} is fixed, based on consideration of an empirical Bayes model. We present this model next.

Let us start with the two-binomial model for each 2×2 table. Given (n_{i1}, n_{i2}) and (P_{i1}, P_{i2}), X_i and Y_i have conditionally independent binomial distributions with parameters P_{i1} and P_{i2} and sample sizes n_{i1} and n_{i2}, respectively; further conditioning on the sum $X_i + Y_i = m_i$ gives X_i the noncentral hypergeometric distribution $H(j|n_i, n_{i1}, m_i, \omega_i)$ as in (6.35), depending only on the odds ratio $\omega_i = (P_{i1}/Q_{i1})/(P_{i2}/Q_{i2})$. It is easy to check that

$$\frac{P(X_i = j + 1 | n_i, n_{i1}, m_i, \omega_i)}{P(X_i = j | n_i, n_{i1}, m_i, \omega_i)} = \frac{C(j + 1 | n_i, n_{i1}, m_i)}{C(j | n_i, n_{i1}, m_i)} \cdot \omega_i, \quad (10.97)$$

where we have written

$$C(j|n_{i.}, n_{i1}, m_i) = \binom{n_{i1}}{j}\binom{n_{i2}}{m_i - j} \qquad \text{for } j = 0, \ldots, \min(m_i, n_{i1}) - 1.$$

Now suppose G is any unknown joint distribution function for the pair of probabilities (P_{i1}, P_{i2}) over the unit square $(0, 1) \times (0, 1)$, which induces a distribution for the odds ratio ω_i. We assume that each pair of probability parameters (P_{i1}, P_{i2}) is independent of the corresponding pair of sample sizes (n_{i1}, n_{i2}), and that for $i = 1, \ldots, g$, the pairs (P_{i1}, P_{i2}) are an independently and identically distributed sample from G. Then from (10.97) it follows that for $j = 0, \ldots, \min(m_i, n_{i1}) - 1$ we have

$$E(\omega_i | X_i = j, n_{i.}, n_{i1}, m_i) = \frac{P(X_i = j + 1 | n_{i.}, n_{i1}, m_i)/C(j+1|n_{i.}, n_{i1}, m_i)}{P(X_i = j | n_{i.}, n_{i1}, m_i)/C(j|n_{i.}, n_{i1}, m_i)}$$

(10.98)

(see Problem 10.8). Expression (10.98) is the fundamental general empirical Bayes identity for the noncentral hypergeometric distribution, analogous to that presented in Section 9.6.3 for proportions. In words, the identity states that among all fourfold tables with the given margins and reference cell equal to j, the average value of the true odds ratio underlying those tables can be expressed as the ratio of the marginal conditional probabilities on the right-hand side, which can be estimated directly from the data. Given the complexity of the marginal conditional probabilities (marginal with respect to the unobserved odds ratio ω_i, conditional given the observed m_i),

$$P(X_i = j | n_{i.}, n_{i1}, m_i) = \frac{\int_0^\infty P(X_i = j, Y_i = m_i - j | n_{i1}, n_{i2}, P_{i1}, P_{i2})\, dG(P_{i1}, P_{i2})}{\int_0^\infty P(X_i + Y_i = m_i | n_{i1}, n_{i2}, P_{i1}, P_{i2})\, dG(P_{i1}, P_{i2})}$$

$$= \frac{\displaystyle\iint_{(P_{i1}, P_{i2}) \in (0,1)\times(0,1)} \binom{n_{i1}}{j} P_{i1}^j (1 - P_{i1})^{n_{i1}-j} \times \binom{n_{i2}}{m_i - j} P_{i2}^{m_i - j}(1 - P_{i2})^{j - l_i}\, dG(P_{i1}, P_{i2})}{\displaystyle\iint_{(P_{i1}, P_{i2}) \in (0,1)\times(0,1)} \sum_{u=\max(l_i, 0)}^{\min(m_i, n_{i1})} \binom{n_{i1}}{u} P_{i1}^u (1 - P_{i1})^{n_{i1}-u} \times \binom{n_{i2}}{m_i - j} P_{i2}^{m_i - u}(1 - P_{i2})^{u - l_i}\, dG(P_{i1}, P_{i2})},$$

(10.99)

it is remarkable that (10.98) offers such a simple and direct way to estimate the average odds ratio given $X_i = j$.

An application of Jensen's inequality shows that for any mixing distribution G, the quantities in (10.98) are nondecreasing in j for fixed margins, and are *strictly increasing* in j unless G is such that ω_i degenerates to a constant. This suggests the following approach. For ease of presentation, suppose we assume that $n_{i1} = n_1$ and $n_{i2} = n_2$ are fixed by design, as they would be in a matched sample design; the general case is a straightforward elaboration of this case. For each informative value of m from 1 to $n_. - 1 = n_1 + n_2 - 1$, classify the reference cell outcomes X_i into categories $0, \ldots, \min(m, n_1)$, thinking of them as multinomial responses. We then have one row of independent multinomial observations for each value of m. For this product multinomial data set, we specify a polytomous logistic regression model using adjacent logit parameterization (see Section 9.5). Let

$$\varphi_j(m|n_1, n_2) = \ln \frac{P(X_i = j + 1|n_., n_1, m)/C(j + 1|n_., n_1, m)}{P(X_i = j|n_., n_1, m)/C(j|n_., n_1, m)} \quad (10.100)$$

denote the adjacent logits $\ln\{P(X_i = j + 1|n_., n_i, m)/P(X_i = j|n_., n_i, m)\}$ plus the offsets $\ln\{C(j|n_., n_1, m)/C(j + 1|n_., n_1, m)\}$. The first model we consider is

$$\varphi_j(m|n_1, n_2) = \beta(m|n_1, n_2) + \delta j. \quad (10.101)$$

Under the null hypothesis H_0: $\omega = \text{constant}$, the slope coefficient $\delta = 0$ [in which case $\beta = \ln \omega$ by (10.97)], whereas under the random effects alternative, $\delta > 0$. Thus we can use the techniques of Chapter 11 to fit model (10.101) to the multinomial data, and then use a Wald z-score, $z = \hat{\delta}/\widehat{\text{se}}(\hat{\delta})$, as a test of H_0: $\delta = 0$, to carry out the test of odds ratio homogeneity.

Note that there is no real concern if the true dependence of $\varphi_j(m|n_1, n_2)$ on j is not exactly linear. Although many examples do confirm that the dependence is remarkably linear, what is important for the test to have good power is the monotonicity of φ_j.

An interesting feature of this problem is that often there is more evidence of odds ratio heterogeneity in the data than is represented by the coefficient δ. From the empirical Bayes identity (10.98), it would be plausible for the logit parameters $\varphi_j(m|n_1, n_2)$ to *decrease* monotonically in m for fixed j. Although this is not universally true, Levin (1992) identifies a certain wide class of joint distributions G for (P_{i1}, P_{i2}) [or equivalently, (P_{i1}, ω_i) or (P_{i2}, ω_i)], for which the logit parameters $\varphi_j(m|n_1, n_2)$ do decrease monotonically. The necessary and sufficient condition for $\varphi_j(m|n_1, n_2)$ to be decreasing in m for fixed j is that the odds P_{i2}/Q_{i2} and the odds ratio $\omega_i = (P_{i1}/Q_{i1})/(P_{i2}/Q_{i2})$ have a negative conditional covariance given $X_i = j$. If the covariance is zero, as when the odds ratio is constant, then $\varphi_j(m|n_1, n_2)$ is constant in m for fixed j. Sufficient conditions for $\varphi_j(m|n_1, n_2)$ to strictly decrease are any of the following: (a) P_{i1} and P_{i2} are initially independent with P_{i2} nondegenerate; (b) as a special case of (a), P_{i1} is constant with P_{i2} not constant; (c) P_{i2}/Q_{i2} is initially independent of ω_i; (d) P_{i1}/Q_{i1} is independent of ω_i, the support of P_{i1}/Q_{i1} is all of $(0, \infty)$, and the density of $\ln(P_{i1}/Q_{i1})$ is log-concave. Condition (d) includes, for example, the cases where P_{i1} has a beta distribution or $\ln(P_{i1}/Q_{i1})$ has a log-normal distribution. These sufficient conditions cover all the simulation scenarios considered by Liang and Self (1985) and Jones et al. (1989). Condition (a) ought not to occur in a properly designed matched sample study, due to the correlation between P_{i1} and P_{i2} induced by matching on strong confounding factors. It is nevertheless of interest to note that even with P_{i1} constant and ω_i nondegenerate, $\varphi_j(m|n_1, n_2)$ will decrease in m for fixed j.

Thus we consider a second model, even simpler than (10.101):

$$\varphi_j(m|n_1, n_2) = \beta(n_1, n_2) + \gamma m + \delta j. \qquad (10.102)$$

Under the null hypothesis, both δ and γ equal zero, whereas under the alternative hypothesis of random odds ratios satisfying the necessary and/or sufficient condition stated above, $\delta > 0$ and $\gamma < 0$. Levin (1992) provides a test statistic for the null hypothesis H_0: $\delta = \gamma = 0$ against alternatives in the parameter quadrant $\delta > 0$, $\gamma < 0$ based on the maximum likelihood estimates of δ and γ from the polytomous logistic regression model (10.102) and on a specialized likelihood ratio test given by Chernoff (1954) for parameter quadrant alternatives. A simpler procedure is to test the hypothesis H_0: $\delta - \gamma = 0$ versus the one-sided alternative H_1: $\delta - \gamma > 0$. This is accomplished with the z-score, $z = (\hat{\delta} - \hat{\gamma})/\widehat{\text{se}}(\hat{\delta} - \hat{\gamma})$. Another simple test, albeit with less power, is the Wald chi squared statistic, $(\hat{\delta}, \hat{\gamma})'\{\text{Cov}(\hat{\delta}, \hat{\gamma})\}^{-1}(\hat{\delta}, \hat{\gamma})$ with 2 df, which is a test of H_0: $\delta = \gamma = 0$ against omnibus alternatives.

The conditional covariance in the necessary and sufficient condition will be zero not only when there is a constant odds ratio, but also when P_{i2} is constant, in which case $\varphi_j(m|n_1, n_2)$ is constant in m for fixed j, and $\gamma = 0$ in model (10.102). Thus if P_{i2} is constant, there is only one-dimensional instead of two-dimensional evidence for odds ratio heterogeneity, and tests of odds ratio homogeneity based on both δ and γ will have lower power than tests based only on δ in this case. A preliminary test of homogeneity in P_{i2} as in Section 9.6.3 could be used to screen for this situation. Similarly, if $n_{i1} = n_1 = 1$ for all i, then there is only evidence from γ, and the Wald test for γ should be used.

For the illustrative data in Table 10.20, the sample estimates of the $\varphi_j(m|n_1, n_2)$ are as follows: for $\varphi_0(1|2, 2)$, we have $\ln\{(36/2)/(29/2)\} = 0.216$. For $\varphi_0(2|2, 2)$ we have $\ln\{(35/4)/(16/1)\} = -0.604$, and for $\varphi_1(2|2, 2)$ we have $\ln\{(13/1)/(35/4)\} = 0.396$. For $\varphi_1(3|2, 2)$ we have $\ln\{(16/2)/(30/2)\} = -0.629$. These display the trends suggested by heterogeneity: $\varphi_0(2|2, 2) < \varphi_1(2|2, 2)$, whereas $\varphi_0(1|2, 2) > \varphi_0(2|2, 2)$ and $\varphi_1(2|2, 2) > \varphi_1(3|2, 2)$. Fitting model (10.102) yields the following maximum likelihood estimates (± 1 standard error): $\hat{\beta} = 1.164 \pm 0.473$, $\hat{\gamma} = -0.905 \pm 0.317$, and $\hat{\delta} = 0.987 \pm 0.504$; each coefficient is nominally significant. The 2 df chi squared test of joint significance of $\hat{\delta}$ and $\hat{\gamma}$ is 8.346 with p-value 0.015, and the difference $\hat{\delta} - \hat{\gamma} = 1.892$ has z-score 2.43 with one-tailed p-value 0.008. The statistic based on Chernoff's generalized likelihood ratio test also has p-value 0.008. In this example the empirical Bayes test had a smaller p-value than did the mixture model score test.

PROBLEMS

10.1. It was found in Section 10.2 that the odds ratios in the three studies summarized in Table 10.1 were significantly different.

(a) The odds ratios o'_2 and o'_3 appear to be similar (see Table 10.2). Test whether they differ significantly, basing the test on the value of

$$\chi^2_{2 \text{ vs } 3} = \frac{w'_2 w'_3}{w'_2 + w'_3}(L'_2 - L'_3)^2.$$

(b) The odds ratios o'_2 and o'_3 differ by less than either does from o'_1. Test whether the mean of o'_2 and o'_3 differs significantly from o'_1. [*Hint.* The mean of L'_2 and L'_3 is $\bar{L}_{2,3} = (w'_2 L'_2 + w'_3 L'_3)/(w'_2 + w'_3)$. Refer the value of

$$\chi^2_{2 \text{ vs } (2,3)} = \frac{w'_1(w'_2 + w'_3)}{w'_1 + w'_2 + w'_3}(L'_1 - \bar{L}_{2,3})^2$$

to critical values of chi squared with 2 df rather than 1, because the comparison was suggested by the data.]

(c) How does the sum of the chi squared statistics determined in (a) and (b) compare with the value of χ^2_{homog} found in (10.18)?

10.2. Apply the methods of Section 10.2 to the data of groups 2 and 3 only in Tables 10.1 and 10.2. Specifically,

(a) What is the mean log odds ratio? What is its standard error? Is the mean log odds ratio significantly different from zero?

(b) Find an approximate 95% confidence interval for the underlying log odds ratio.

(c) What is the mean odds ratio? What is the approximate 95% confidence interval for the underlying odds ratio corresponding to the interval found in (b)?

10.3. Assume one is at stage k of the calculation of $h^{(1)} * \cdots * h^{(g)}$, and let $a = h^{(1)}(\omega) * \cdots * h^{(k)}(\omega)$ and $b = h^{(k+1)}(\omega)$. In (10.28), show that only terms with j satisfying

$$\sum_{h=1}^{k+1} \max(l_h, 0) \leq j \leq \sum_{h=1}^{k+1} \min(m_h, n_{h1})$$

are nonzero, and that, in the limits of the sum, only terms with i satisfying

$$\max\left\{ j - \min(m_{k+1}, n_{k+1,1}), \sum_{h=1}^{k} \max(l_h, 0) \right\}$$

$$\leq i \leq \min\left\{ j - \max(l_{k+1}, 0), \sum_{h=1}^{k} \min(m_h, n_{h1}) \right\}$$

need be included.

10.4. Refer to the discussion of the ladies tasting tea in Section 10.3*. Suppose two ladies are tested, and one gets all eight declarations right ($X_1 = 4$) while the other exhibits no better than chance accuracy ($X_2 = 2$). Calculate the two-tailed p-value.

10.5. While it perhaps is not obvious, $\bar{o}_{MH}$ (see 10.52) is actually a weighted average of the g individual odds ratios,

$$o_i = \frac{p_{i1}(1 - p_{i2})}{p_{i2}(1 - p_{i1})}, \quad i = 1, \ldots, g.$$

Show that this is so by finding a set of weights, $w_1, \ldots, w_g$, so that, with $\bar{o}_{MH}$ given by (10.52),

$$\bar{o}_{MH} = \frac{\sum_{i=1}^{g} o_i w_i}{\sum_{i=1}^{g} w_i}$$

10.6. Prove that, when $n_{i1} = n_{i2} = 1$, as in the study of matched pairs, the Mantel-Haenszel chi squared statistic given in (10.62) is identical to McNemar's chi squared statistic given in (13.3).

10.7. Kline et al. (1995) report the results of a case-control study of the association between cigarette smoking and miscarriage (spontaneous abortion). Cases were women who presented at one of three New York City hospitals with a spontaneous abortion prior to 28 weeks of gestation. Controls were women who were recruited from a prenatal care setting before 22 weeks of gestation and who delivered at 28 weeks or later. The study was conducted over a 12-year period, and changes in participating hospitals and sociodemographics suggested the need to stratify on time period in three phases as a potential confounder. The three fourfold tables shown below cross-classify women by case and control status and smoking in two categories: regular smokers (14 or more cigarettes per day at last menstrual period) and women who never smoked. (Ex-smokers and those who smoked fewer than 14 cigarettes per day are excluded from consideration here. Cases represent those with chromosomally normal fetuses. Fetuses with chromosomal aberrations are excluded.)

Phase of study:	1 1974–1979		2 1979–1982		3 1982–1986	
Smoking status:	14 +	Never	14 +	Never	14 +	Never
Cases:	70	333	40	211	23	273
Controls:	127	938	105	1011	60	794

(a) Test at level $\alpha = 0.05$ (two-sided) the hypothesis of no association between smoking and miscarriage given phase of study, against the alternative of a constant odds ratio relating smoking and miscarriage across the three phases of the study. Estimate the assumed common log odds ratio along with its standard error.

(b) Is the test in part (a) powerful? Test the hypothesis of a constant odds ratio relating smoking and miscarriage across the three phases of the study at level $\alpha = 0.05$ (two-sided).

(c) Calculate the odds ratio from the data pooled across all three phases. Was phase a potential confounder? Was phase an operational confounder?

[*Hint*. To help with calculations, use the following worksheet.]

Phase	Log Odds Ratio* L'	Weight w	Product wL'	wL'^2
1	0.4421	38.33	16.95	7.492
2	0.6076	25.07	15.23	9.254
3	0.1208	15.63	1.89	0.228
Total		79.03	34.06	16.974

*$\frac{1}{2}$ bias correction added.

10.8. Prove expression (10.98). [*Hint*. Use (10.97) and the definition of posterior density as proportional to the likelihood function times the prior to express the marginal probability $P(X_i = j + 1 | n_{i\cdot}, n_{i1}, m_i)$ in terms of the posterior expected value of ω_i given the margins and $X_i = j$.]

REFERENCES

Agresti, A. (1992). A survey of exact inference for contingency tables. *Statist. Sci.*, **7**, 131–153 (with discussion, 154–177).

Agresti, A., Mehta, C. R., and Patel, N. R. (1990). Exact inference for contingency tables with ordered categories. *J. Am. Statist. Assoc.*, **85**, 453–458.

Bailey, K. R. (1987). Inter-study differences: How should they influence the interpretation and analysis of results? *Statist. in Med.*, **6**, 351–358.

Bartlett, M. S. (1953). Approximate confidence intervals, II. More than one unknown parameter. *Biometrika*, **40**, 306–317.

Bartlett, M. S. (1955). Approximate confidence intervals, III. A bias correction. *Biometrika*, **42**, 201–204.

Birch, M. W. (1964). The detection of partial association. I: The 2×2 case. *J. R. Statist. Soc., Ser. B*, **26**, 313–324.

Bishop, Y. M. M., Fienberg, S. E., and Holland, P. W. (1975). *Discrete multivariate analysis: Theory and practice*. Cambridge, Mass.: MIT Press.

Box, J. F. (1978). *R. A. Fisher, the life of a scientist*. New York: Wiley.

Breslow, N. E. (1981). Odds ratio estimators when the data are sparse. *Biometrika*, **68**, 73–84.

Breslow, N. E. and Day, N. E. (1993). *Statistical methods in cancer research. Volume 1: The analysis of case-control studies*. IARC Scientific Publication No. 32, paperback reprint edition. London: Oxford University Press.

Breslow, N. E. and Day, N. E. (1994). *Statistical methods in cancer research. Volume 2: The design and analysis of cohort studies*. IARC Scientific Publication No. 82, paperback reprint edition. London: Oxford University Press.

Bross, I. D. J. (1966). Spurious effects from an extraneous variable. *J. Chronic Dis.*, **19**, 637–647.

Chernoff, H. (1954). On the distribution of the likelihood ratio. *Ann. Math. Statist.*, **25**, 573–578.

Clarke, C. (1991). Invited commentary on R. A. Fisher. *Am. J. Epidemiol.*, **134**, 1371–1374.

Cochran, W. G. (1954). Some methods of strengthening the common χ^2 tests. *Biometrics*, **10**, 417–451.

Cochran, W. G. (1968). The effectiveness of adjustment by subclassification in removing bias in observational studies. *Biometrics*, **24**, 295–313.

Cooper, J. E., Kendell, R. E., Gurland, B. J., Sharpe, L., Copeland, J. R. M., and Simon, R. (1972). *Psychiatric diagnosis in New York and London*. Oxford University Press.

Cornfield, J. (1956). A statistical problem arising from retrospective studies. Pp. 135–148 in J. Neyman (Ed.), *Proceedings of the third Berkeley symposium on mathematical statistics and probability*, Vol. 4. Berkeley: University of California Press.

Cox, D. R. (1970). *The analysis of binary data*. London: Methuen.

Cox, D. R. and Snell, E. J. (1989). *Analysis of binary data*, 2nd ed. Boca Raton, Fla.: Chapman & Hall/CRC Press.

DeMets, D. L. (1987). Methods for combining randomized clinical trials: Strengths and limitations. *Statist. in Med.*, **6**, 341–348.

Dersimonian, R. and Laird, N. (1986). Meta-analysis in clinical trials. *Controlled Clinical Trials*, **7**, 177–186.

Ejigou, A. and McHugh, R. (1984). Testing the homogeneity of the relative risk under multiple matching. *Biometrika*, **71**, 408–411.

Everitt, B. S. (1992). *The analysis of contingency tables*, 2nd ed. Boca Raton, Fla.: CRC Press.

Fienberg, S. E. (1977). *The analysis of cross-classified categorical data*. Cambridge, Mass.: MIT Press.

Finney, D. J. (1965). The design and logic of a monitor of drug use. *J. Chronic Dis.*, **18**, 77–98.

Fisher, R. A. (1971). *The design of experiments*, 9th ed. New York: Hafner.

Fleiss, J. L. (1993). The statistical basis of meta-analysis. *Statist. Methods Med. Res.*, **2**, 121–145.

Gart, J. J. (1962). On the combination of relative risks. *Biometrics*, **18**, 601–610.

Gart, J. J. (1970). Point and interval estimation of the common odds ratio in the combination of 2×2 tables with fixed marginals. *Biometrika*, **57**, 471–475.

Gart, J. J. (1971). The comparison of proportions: A review of significance tests, confidence intervals and adjustments for stratification. *Rev. Int. Statist. Inst.*, **39**, 16–37.

Goodman, L. A. (1969). On partitioning χ^2 and detecting partial association in three-way contingency tables. *J. R. Statist. Soc., Ser. B*, **31**, 486–498.

Hauck, W. W. (1979). The large sample variance of the Mantel-Haenszel estimator of a common odds ratio. *Biometrics*, **35**, 817–819.

Hedges, L. V. and Olkin, I. (1985). *Statistical methods for meta-analysis*. New York: Academic Press.

Hirji, K. F., Mehta, C. R., and Patel, N. R. (1987). Computing distributions for exact logistic regression. *J. Am. Statist. Assoc.*, **82**, 1110–1117.

Hirji, K. F., Tang, M.-L., Vollset, S. E., and Elashoff, R. M. (1994). Efficient power computation for exact and mid-p tests for the common odds ratio in several 2×2 tables. *Statist. in Med.*, **13**, 1539–1549.

Holland, P. W. (1986). Statistics and causal inference. *J. Am. Statist. Assoc.*, **81**, 945–960 (with discussion, 961–970).

Hosmer, D. W. and Lemeshow, S. (2000). *Applied logistic regression*, 2nd ed. New York: Wiley.

Jones, M. P., O'Gorman, T. W., Lemke, J. H., and Woolson, R. F. (1989). A Monte Carlo investigation of homogeneity tests of the odds ratio under various sample size configurations. *Biometrics*, **45**, 171–181.

Kline, J., Levin, B., Kinney, A., Stein, Z., Susser, M., and Warburton, D. (1995). Cigarette smoking and spontaneous abortion of known karyotype: Precise data but uncertain inferences. *Am. J. Epidemiol*, **141**, 417–427.

Kou, S. and Ying, Z. (1996). Asymptotics for a 2×2 table with fixed margins. *Statist. Sinica*, **6**, 809–830.

Levin, B. (1990). The saddlepoint correction in conditional logistic likelihood analysis. *Biometrika*, **77**, 275–285.

Levin, B. (1992). Tests of odds ratio homogeneity with improved power in sparse fourfold tables. *Commun. Statist.—Theory Meth.*, **21**, 1469–1500.

Levin, B. and Kong, F. (1990). Bartlett's bias correction to the profile score function is a saddlepoint correction. *Biometrika*, **77**, 219–221.

Liang, K.-Y. and Self, S. G. (1985). Tests for homogeneity of odds ratio when the data are sparse. *Biometrika*, **72**, 353–358.

Lin, X., Raz, J., and Harlow, S. D. (1997). Linear mixed models with heterogeneous within-cluster variances. *Biometrics*, **53**, 910–923.

Mantel, N. (1963). Chi-square tests with one degree of freedom: Extensions of the Mantel-Haenszel procedure. *J. Am. Statist. Assoc.*, **58**, 690–700.

Mantel, N. (1966). Evaluation of survival data and two new rank order statistics arising in its consideration. *Cancer Chemother. Rep.*, **50**, 163–170.

Mantel, N. (1977). Tests and limits for the common odds ratio of several 2×2 contingency tables: Methods in analogy with the Mantel-Haenszel procedure. *J. Statist. Plann. Inf.*, **1**, 179–189.

Mantel, N., Brown, C., and Byar, D. P. (1977). Tests for homogeneity of effect in an epidemiologic investigation. *Am. J. Epidemiol.*, **106**, 125–129.

Mantel, N. and Fleiss, J. L. (1980). Minimum expected cell size requirements for the Mantel-Haenszel one-degree-of-freedom chi square test and a related rapid procedure. *Am. J. Epidemiol.*, **112**, 129–134.

Mantel, N. and Haenszel, W. (1959). Statistical aspects of the analysis of data from retrospective studies of disease. *J. Natl. Cancer Inst.*, **22**, 719–748.

Mantel, N. and Hankey, B. F. (1975). The odds ratios of a 2×2 contingency table. *Am. Statistician*, **29**, 143–145.

McKinlay, S. M. (1975a). The design and analysis of the observational study—a review (with a comment by S. E. Fienberg). *J. Am. Statist. Assoc.*, **70**, 503–523.

McKinlay, S. M. (1975b). The effect of bias on estimators of relative risk for pair-matched and stratified samples. *J. Am. Statist. Assoc.*, **70**, 859–864.

McKinlay, S. M. (1975c). A note on the chi-square test for pair-matched samples. *Biometrics*, **31**, 731–735.

McKinlay, S. M. (1978). The effect of non-zero second order interaction on combined estimators of the odds-ratio. *Biometrika*, **65**, 191–202.

Mehta, C. R. and Patel, N. R. (1983). A network algorithm for performing Fisher's exact test in r $\times$ c contingency tables. *J. Am. Statist. Assoc.*, **78**, 427–434.

Mehta, C. R., Patel, N. R., and Gray, R. (1985). Computing an exact confidence interval for the common odds ratio in several 2×2 contingency tables. *J. Am. Statist. Assoc.*, **80**, 969–973 (with correction, **81**, 1132).

Mehta, C. R., Patel, N. R., and Senchaudhuri, P. (1988). Importance sampling for estimating exact probabilities in permutational inference. *J. Am. Statist. Assoc.*, **83**, 999–1005.

Mehta, C. R., Patel, N. R., and Senchaudhuri, P. (1992). Exact stratified linear rank tests for ordered categorical and binary data. *J. Comp. Graph. Statist.*, **1**, 21–40.

Meier, P. (1987). Commentary. *Statist. in Med.*, **6**, 329–331.

Miettinen, O. S. (1976). Stratification by a multivariate confounder score. *Am. J. Epidemiol.*, **104**, 609–620.

Muñoz, A. and Rosner, B. (1984). Power and sample size for a collection of 2×2 tables. *Biometrics*, **40**, 995–1004 (with correction, **42**, 229).

Naylor, A. F. (1967). Small sample considerations in combining 2×2 tables. *Biometrics*, **23**, 349–356.

Odoroff, C. L. (1970). A comparison of minimum logit chi-square estimation and maximum likelihood estimation in $2 \times 2 \times 2$ and $3 \times 2 \times 2$ contingency tables: Tests for interaction. *J. Am. Statist. Assoc.*, **65**, 1617–1631.

Olkin, I. (1995a). Meta-analysis: Reconciling the results of independent studies. *Statist. in Med.*, **14**, 457–472.

Olkin, I. (1995b). Statistical and theoretical considerations in meta-analysis. *J. Clin. Epidemiol.*, **48**, 133–146.

Olkin, I. (1996). Meta-analysis: Current issues in research synthesis. *Statist. in Med.*, **15**, 1253–1257.

Pasternack, B. S. and Mantel, N. (1966). A deficiency in the summation of chi procedure. *Biometrics*, **22**, 407–409.

Peto, R. (1987). Discussion of Peto R.: Why do we need systematic overviews of randomized trials? *Statist. in Med.*, **6**, 242.

Phillips, A. and Holland, P. W. (1987). Estimators of the variance of the Mantel-Haenszel log-odds-ratio estimate. *Biometrics*, **43**, 425–431.

Radhakrishna, S. (1965). Combination of results from several 2×2 contingency tables. *Biometrics*, **21**, 86–98.

Reis, I. M., Hirji, K. F., and Afifi, A. A. (1999). Exact and asymptotic tests for homogeneity in several 2×2 tables. *Statist. in Med.*, **18**, 893–906.

Robins, J., Breslow, N., and Greenland, S. (1986). Estimators of the Mantel-Haenszel variance consistent in both sparse data and large-strata limiting models. *Biometrics*, **42**, 311–323.

Rosenbaum, P. R. and Rubin, D. B. (1983). The central role of the propensity score in observational studies for causal effects. *Biometrika*, **70**, 41–55.

Rosenbaum, P. R. and Rubin, D. B. (1984). Reducing bias in observational studies using subclassification on the propensity score. *J. Am. Statist. Assoc.*, **79**, 516–524.

Rosenbaum, P. R. and Rubin, D. B. (1985a). Constructing a control group using multivariate matched sampling methods that incorporate the propensity score. *Am. Statistician*, **39**, 33–38.

Rosenbaum, P. R. and Rubin, D. B. (1985b). The bias due to incomplete matching. *Biometrics*, **41**, 103–116.

Rubin, D. B. (1973). The use of matched sampling and regression adjustment to remove bias in observational studies. *Biometrics*, **29**, 185–203.

Sato, T. (1990). Confidence limits for the common odds ratio based on the asymptotic distribution of the Mantel-Haenszel estimator. *Biometrics*, **46**, 71–80.

Schlesselman, J. J. (1978). Assessing effects of confounding variables. *Am. J. Epidemiol.*, **108**, 3–8.

Sheehe, P. R. (1966). Combination of log relative risk in retrospective studies of disease. *Am. J. Public Health*, **56**, 1745–1750.

Strawderman, R. L. and Wells, M. T. (1998). Approximately exact inference for the common odds ratio in several 2×2 tables (with discussion). *J. Am. Statist. Assoc.*, **93**, 1294–1320.

Tarone, R. E. (1985). On heterogeneity tests based on efficient scores. *Biometrika*, **72**, 91–95.

Vollset, S. E., Hirji, K. F., and Elashoff, R. M. (1991). Fast computation of exact confidence limits for the common odds ratio in a series of 2×2 tables. *J. Am. Statist. Assoc.*, **86**, 404–409.

Yates, F. (1955). The use of transformations and maximum likelihood in the analysis of quantal experiments involving two treatments. *Biometrika*, **42**, 382–403.

Zelen, M. (1971). The analysis of several 2×2 contingency tables. *Biometrika*, **58**, 129–137.

Zelterman, D. and Le, C. T. (1991). Tests of homogeneity for the relative risk in multiply-matched case-control studies. *Biometrics*, **47**, 751–755.

CHAPTER 11

Logistic Regression

11.1. INTRODUCTION

We use logistic regression to express relationships between a set of explanatory factors and one or more categorical outcomes. In much the same way as
the mean is the key quantity to be modeled in ordinary multiple regression,
so the *log odds parameter* plays a prominent role when outcome variables are
categorical. Good reasons exist for preferring to analyze discrete data in
terms of log odds parameters rather than probabilities or expectations. The
simplest reason is that the log odds parameter may take on any value
between plus and minus infinity, whereas a probability parameter is constrained to lie between zero and one. A binary outcome variable Y, taking
values zero or one, has a single probability parameter $P = P(Y = 1)$ governing
its distribution, and P is the mean value of Y. The log odds parameter is

$$\lambda = \ln \frac{P}{1 - P}. \tag{11.1}$$

We may pass back and forth between P and λ via that relation and

$$P = \frac{e^{\lambda}}{1 + e^{\lambda}} = \frac{1}{1 + e^{-\lambda}}. \tag{11.2}$$

For specifying the distribution of the binary variable Y, the two parameters P
and λ are equivalent, in the sense that equations (11.1) and (11.2) put them
into one-to-one correspondence. Because there is no constraint on λ, a
working model may assign any value to λ, which will automatically transform
via (11.2) into a proper probability between 0 and 1.

Statistical Methods for Rates and Proportions, Third Edition
By Joseph L. Fleiss, Bruce Levin, and Myunghee Cho Paik
ISBN 0-471-52629-0   Copyright © 2003 John Wiley & Sons, Inc.

The transformation from P to λ expressed in (11.1) is called the *logit transformation* of P, written $\text{logit}(P) = \ln\{P/(1-P)\}$. The transformation from λ back to P expressed in (11.2) is variously called the *inverse logit*, *logistic*, or *expit transform* of λ. Table A.10 contains the logit transformation and its inverse for selected values of P and λ. We examine more fundamental reasons for using the log odds parameter in the next section.

Due to its wide applicability, logistic regression has become the standard tool for analyzing categorical data. Here are three illustrations of how to use logistic regression.

1. A researcher wishes to study how the probability of contracting a sexually transmitted disease varies with the number of occasions of unprotected sexual intercourse within a one-year period. The researcher asks a sample of subjects, all of whom are initially free of disease, to keep personal diaries for one year. Thereupon the researcher observes X = number of unprotected occasions and, upon subject examination, observes disease status Y (1 = infected, 0 = not infected). While it would be straightforward to demonstrate an association between X and risk of infection by showing that the average of X among those infected differed from the average among those not infected, this comparison would not directly furnish an estimate of elevated risk per additional occasion. So the researcher fits a linear logistic regression model of the form $\text{logit}\{P(X)\} = \alpha + \beta X$, where $P(X) = P[Y = 1 | X]$ is the conditional probability of infection given X occasions. The coefficient β, found to be large and positive, indicates strong association. The magnitude of β allows the researcher to quantify the increased risk of infection per occasion and to extrapolate sensible estimates of risk for values of X larger than those observed in the sample.

2. Another researcher wishes to study how the risk of miscarriage among pregnant women above age 35 varies with the age of the woman at the time of conception. Instead of taking a random sample of all pregnant women above age 35, the researcher intentionally oversamples younger and older women in this age group, undersampling women in the middle range. For each subject selected, let X denote maternal age at conception, and let Y denote an outcome (1 = miscarriage, 0 = no miscarriage). Unlike the previous example, it is not clear that the researcher could quantify the association between maternal age and risk of miscarriage simply by comparing the mean age of women who miscarried with the mean age of women who did not, because any age differential found would merely reflect the researcher's choice of subjects. Instead, the researcher fits a logistic regression model of the form $\text{logit}\{P(X)\} = \alpha + \beta X$, where $P(X)$ is the age-specific risk of miscarriage for women of age X. The results are correct because the analysis conditions on the specific ages of the women sampled; just as in ordinary linear regression, the values of the X variable may be selected to accomplish the study's aims rather than to reflect the distribution in the population. The researcher's choice of X at the extreme age ranges allows a more precise

estimate of β than would a simple random sample of the same size. The model also allows the researcher to estimate the risk of miscarriage at intermediate ages not necessarily observed in the sample.

3. A retrospective study is conducted to examine multiple risk factors for breast cancer. Let Y denote the binary case-control indicator (1 = case, 0 = control), and let $\underline{X} = (X_1, X_2, \ldots)$ denote a vector of biologic risk factors such as familial history, age at menarche, nulliparity or age at first birth, and history of lactation for parous women, age at menopause, body mass index, etc. A multiple logistic regression model of the form $\text{logit}\{P(\underline{X})\} = \alpha + \beta_1 X_1 + \cdots$ is fitted to the data as if the data had been collected prospectively. After some preliminary model revisions, the coefficients $\beta_1, \ldots, \beta_k$ corresponding to selected variables $X_1, \ldots, X_k$ are estimated, furnishing useful information about the relative importance of the selected risk factors. Environmental factors such as exposure to organochlorine compounds or polyaromatic hydrocarbons are then entered into the model. The statistical significance of the environmental terms is assessed, and gene-environment interactions are explored.

11.2. THE LOG ODDS TRANSFORMATION REVISITED

Why is the log odds transformation so important to categorical data analysis? In this section we go a little deeper into the charms of logistic regression and make a few historical and terminological observations. The reader interested in applications may go directly to Section 11.3.

Historical Roots—Bioassay and Log-linear Models

The logistic regression model developed from two beginnings: first, as a mathematical formulation of bioassay models more convenient than probit analysis, and second, as a natural analog of analysis of variance methods suitable for contingency table analysis.

The bioassay model is similar to the second illustration of the previous section. In the laboratory a researcher administers a possibly toxic substance at various dose levels X to a sample of experimental animals and observes the proportion $P(X)$ of animals at each dose that exhibit a quantal response Y such as death or morbidity. The goal is to describe the ogival dose-response curve and from it to estimate certain quantities, such as the median lethal dose [that value of X with $P(X) = \frac{1}{2}$]. A hypothetical mechanism for generating the Y outcomes is to assume a latent threshold quantity τ such that the event $[Y = 1]$ occurs if and only if the dose exceeds the threshold, $[X \geq \tau]$. It is further assumed that τ is a random variable with some mean μ and standard deviation σ in the population of experimental animals, with a cumulative distribution function of the form $F\{(x - \mu)/\sigma\}$ for some standard cumulative distribution function $F(x)$. It follows that $P(X) = P(Y = 1|X) = P(\tau \leq X) = F\{(X - \mu)/\sigma.\}$ Inverting this relation gives $F^{-1}\{P(X)\} = \alpha + \beta X$, where $\alpha = -\mu/\sigma$ and $\beta = 1/\sigma$; i.e., the inverse F transform of $P(X)$ is linear in X.

The class of *probit* models arises by taking $F(x) = \Phi(x)$, where $\Phi(x)$ is the standard normal cumulative distribution function. It is traditional to add an arbitrary constant to the transformed probability to avoid negative values; for example, the probit transform of $P(X)$ is defined as probit $\{P(X)\} = \Phi^{-1}\{P(X)\} + 5$, where $\Phi^{-1}(p)$ gives the pth quantile of the standard normal distribution. Before computers were widely available, the logistic distribution function, $F(x) = e^x/(1 + e^x) = 1/(1 + e^{-x})$, was used as an alternative specification to $\Phi(x)$ (Finney, 1964). This distribution function is remarkably close to a suitably scaled version of $\Phi(x)$ for values of $F(x)$ between 0.1 and 0.9, although the logistic distribution has thicker tails than the normal (see Figures 11.1 and 11.2). The closed form expressions for $F(x)$ and its inverse, $F^{-1}(p) = \ln\{p/(1 - p)\} = \text{logit}(p)$, produce a class of logistic bioassay models, $F^{-1}\{P(X)\} = \text{logit}\{P(X)\} = \alpha + \beta X$, which are easily calculated by hand. Beyond computational convenience, however, there is little motivation for the assumption of a logistic distribution for the latent threshold τ. Even if the threshold model corresponds to a real biologic mechanism, there is no reason to expect its distribution to be logistic. However, the term "logistic regression" does derive from this origin.

In an entirely different vein, work by Leo Goodman and Frederick Mosteller and others in the late 1960s to adapt analysis-of-variance ideas to multiway contingency tables led to the development of *log-linear* models. See, for example, Goodman (1970) and Mosteller (1968). In a log-linear model, the logarithms of the table's cell probabilities are expressed as simple linear functions of certain main effect terms and higher-order interaction terms. In the case where one of the cross-classification variables is dichotomous, the difference between the log probabilities of the two possible outcomes, that is, the log odds parameter, is also a simple linear function of the main effects and other terms, so the log-linear model implies a certain linear logistic regression model. We discuss log-linear models further in Section 11.4, but a brief digression on terminology may be helpful here.

Terminology

Bishop (1969) asserts that log-linear analysis is more general than logistic regression analysis in the sense that the logit model can be represented as one kind of log-linear model, but not every log-linear model can be written as a logit model. See also Fienberg (1980). This characterization presupposes, however, a definition of logistic regression limited only to binary logistic regression. In fact, log-linear models and logistic regression models are both special cases of a more inclusive family of models called the *multinomial response model* (Bock, 1970, 1975; Levin and Shrout, 1981). Typically, we have

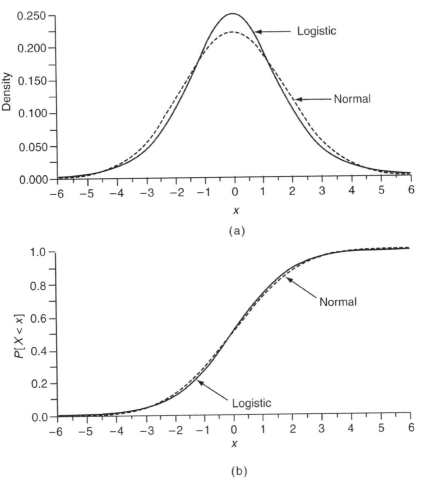

Figure 11.1. (a) Logistic and normal probability density functions; (b) logistic and normal cumulative distribution functions. Both distributions have mean 0 and variance $\pi^2/3$.

a set of discrete outcome variables whose joint distribution can be described in the language of log-linear analysis. In addition, we have a set of explanatory variables, some of which may be discrete, some continuous. The multinomial response model relates each of the log-linear parameters for the multivariate outcomes to each of the explanatory factors. Specifically, we speak of a model for a single dichotomous outcome variable as a *binary* logistic regression model, and a model for more complex outcomes as a *polytomous* logistic regression model. The polytomous model arises in the univariate case when a single outcome variable has three or more outcome categories, or in the multivariate case when several categorical outcome variables are jointly cross-classified. A log-linear model for a multiway contingency table is simply a multinomial response model with no explana-

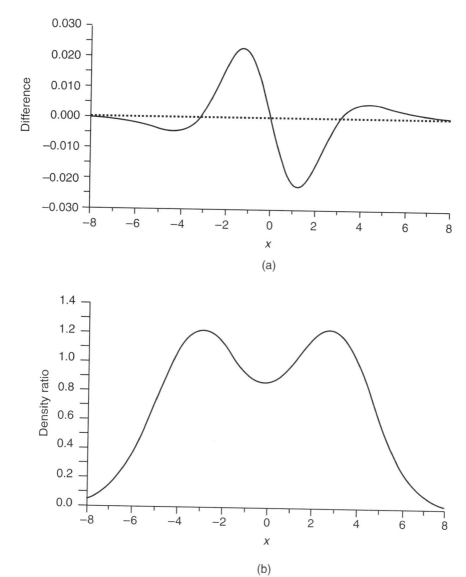

Figure 11.2. (a) Difference between $N(0, \pi^2/3)$ and unit logistic cumulative distribution functions. (b) Ratio of $N(0, \pi^2/3)$ to unit logistic density.

tory factors. In this way the multinomial response model contains both the classical log-linear model and the classical binary logistic regression model as special cases.

Log-linear models are most useful when all the categorical variables in a multiway table are regarded as outcome variables, and none as explanatory factors. This perspective is appropriate in the context of cross-sectional studies or survey data, where several cross-classification variables are considered interdependent outcomes and interest centers on describing their joint distribution. For univariate logistic regression models (either binary or polytomous), one variable is distinguished as the outcome variable, while all others are viewed as explanatory, and interest centers on describing the conditional distribution of the outcome given the explanatory factors. This perspective is most useful in etiologic investigations, where relations among the explanatory factors are of less interest than relations between an outcome variable and the explanatory factors. Section 11.4 has examples which combine features of both log-linear analysis and logistic regression analysis.

Henceforth we use the term *log-linear model* to refer to the parametric structure of the joint distribution of the dependent variables under consideration, and the term *logistic regression* to refer to the general multinomial response model which relates the log-linear structure to the explanatory factors. As in the case of classical linear regression, if the explanatory factor is a single variable, we call the model a *simple* logistic regression. If there are several explanatory factors, we call the model a *multiple* logistic regression. The context will make clear whether the dependent variable in a given logistic regression model is binary or polytomous, and, if the latter, the log-linear parameterization of the outcome variables will be specified.

Discriminant Problem

Returning to the question posed at the beginning of this section, we come to a fundamental reason that log-odds parameters and logistic models hold a central place in the analysis of categorical data.

Suppose a population has two subgroups identified by $Y = 1$ or $Y = 0$, with proportions $P(Y = 1) = \pi$ and $P(Y = 0) = 1 - \pi$. We assume that determination of Y for an individual is nontrivial, as occurs, for example, with a difficult diagnosis or an occult condition. We further assume that we have an easily observable variable X whose probability density function, for individuals with given group membership $Y = j$, is denoted by $f_j(x)$ for $j = 1$ or 0. We wish to classify Y for a randomly selected person on the basis of his or her value of X—this is the *discriminant* problem. By Bayes' theorem

$$\frac{P(Y = 1 | X = x)}{P(Y = 0 | X = x)} = \frac{f_1(x)}{f_0(x)} \cdot \frac{\pi}{1 - \pi}, \tag{11.3}$$

so that the log odds on outcome $Y = 1$ versus $Y = 0$ is of the form

$$\ln \frac{P(Y = 1 | X = x)}{P(Y = 0 | X = x)} = \ln \frac{\pi}{1 - \pi} + l(x), \tag{11.4}$$

where $l(x)$ is the log-likelihood ratio function, $l(x) = \ln\{f_1(x)/f_0(x)\}$. For example, if $f_j(x)$ is a normal density function with mean μ_j and variance σ_j^2, then $l(x)$ is of the form $l(x) = \alpha' + \beta x + \gamma x^2$ for some coefficients α', β, and γ which depend on the means μ_j and variances σ_j^2 [see Problem 11.1(a)]. This leads directly to the binary multiple logistic regression model logit$\{P(x)\} = \alpha + \beta x + \gamma x^2$, where we have written $P(x) = P(Y = 1 | X = x)$ and $\alpha = \alpha' + \ln\{\pi/(1 - \pi)\}$. In the special case $\sigma_1^2 = \sigma_0^2$, the coefficient of the quadratic term is zero, reducing the model to the simple linear logistic equation logit$\{P(x)\} = \alpha + \beta x$. See Figure 11.3.

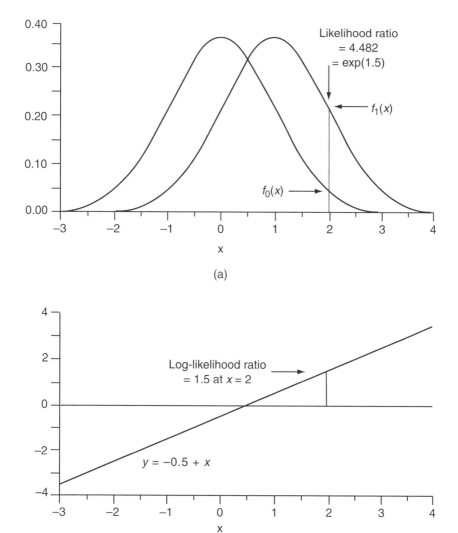

Figure 11.3. (a) $N(0, 1)$ and $N(1, 1)$ densities. (b) Log-likelihood ratio function for $N(0, 1)$ and $N(1, 1)$ densities.

Several points are worth noting. First, equation (11.4) exhibits a fundamental connection between log-odds parameters and the log-likelihood ratio
function, which is of central importance in statistical inference. Second, the
assumption of normal distributions for X in the example above can be
checked by simple examination of the data from the two groups, unlike the
situation in the bioassay model, where the threshold distribution is not
directly observable. If the normal assumption is inaccurate, then the appropriate sampling densities of X may be used and, with the corresponding
log-likelihood ratio function, (11.4) provides the correct logistic regression
model. Third, many common parametric families of densities for X besides
the normal have a linear log-likelihood ratio $l(x)$. For example, if X is a
Poisson random variable with mean μ_j in group $Y = j$, then $l(x)$ is linear in x
[see Problem 11.1(b)]. If X has a Gamma distribution with shape parameter
a_j and scale parameter b_j in group $Y = j$, then $l(x)$ is of the form $l(x) = \alpha' +
\beta x + \gamma \ln x$, which implies a multiple linear logistic regression model with
"carrier" variables X and $\ln X$. [The chi squared distribution is a member of
the Gamma family—see Problem 11.1(c). This example is further discussed
in Section 11.4.] Thus the logistic regression model has a certain robustness
against misspecification of the sampling densities for X, which explains why
linear logistic models so often provide excellent descriptions of data. Inas-
much as (thanks to the central limit theorem) the normal distribution is
ubiquitous in continuous data analysis, the linear logistic model is similarly
fundamental via (11.4).

11.3. A CLOSER LOOK AT SOME LOGISTIC REGRESSION MODELS

11.3.1. Simple Binary Logistic Regression

Let outcome Y take values 0 and 1, let X be a single explanatory factor, and
let $P(X) = P(Y = 1 | X)$ denote the conditional probability that $Y = 1$ given
X. Suppose X and Y are related via the model

$$\text{logit}\{P(X)\} = \alpha + \beta X. \tag{11.5}$$

The intercept term α represents the log odds on outcome $Y = 1$ versus $Y = 0$
when X takes the value 0. It is good practice to arrange the coding of X so
that $X = 0$ is meaningful as a reference value. In that case we call α the
reference or baseline log odds. A unit increase in X increases $\text{logit}\{P(X)\}$ by
the amount $\text{logit}\{P(X + 1)\} - \text{logit}\{P(X)\} = \alpha + \beta(X + 1) - (\alpha + \beta X) = \beta$,
so that β is the log odds ratio (per unit increase in X).

The simplest example of model (11.5) occurs in the two-group prospective
comparative study discussed in Chapter 7. We have a study group of exposed
subjects, coded $X = 1$, and a reference group of unexposed subjects, coded

$X = 0$. Model (11.5) specifies that the log odds on the outcome, or *response*, $Y = 1$ versus $Y = 0$ for any member of the reference group is α, and (11.2) gives the response probability $P(Y = 1 | X = 1) = e^{\alpha}/(1 + e^{\alpha}) = 1/(1 + e^{-\alpha})$. The response probability in the exposed group is $P(Y = 1 | X = 1) = e^{\alpha + \beta}/(1 + e^{\alpha + \beta}) = 1/\{1 + e^{-(\alpha + \beta)}\}$. The odds ratio comparing the response probabilities for group $X = 1$ versus 0 is e^{β}.

We illustrate model (11.5) with a subset of the data from the study of Kline et al. (1995) of risk factors for spontaneous abortion that was reported in Kline et al. (1983). As mentioned in Section 9.6 and Problem 10.6, cases were women presenting to one of three New York City hospitals with a spontaneous abortion; controls were women recruited from a prenatal care setting before 22 weeks of gestation who delivered at 28 weeks or later. The women were interviewed, and, with their consent, specimens of fetal cells were grown in culture and karyotyped. Karyotyping is a microscopic examination and classification procedure which determines characteristics of the fetal chromosomes. Fetal karyotypes may be numerically and morphologically normal (i.e., 23 pairs of chromosomes without rearrangements), or may manifest one of several kinds of chromosomal aberrations. Trisomy is a particular kind of chromosomal aberration in which one of the 23 chromosome pairs gains an extra member through an error of germ cell meiosis. Thus, trisomy actually refers to a collection of 23 possible aberrations. Down's syndrome, for example, is trisomy 21: the 21st chromosome pair has a third member. A well-known but little-understood phenomenon concerns the association between trisomic conception and increasing maternal age. Let us focus on the binary outcome of any trisomic aberration $(Y = 1)$ versus no chromosomal aberration $(Y = 0)$ among spontaneous abortions. For now we ignore other kinds of aberration, such as monosomies or triploidies. Trisomies plus chromosomally normal outcomes constitute about 75% of all spontaneous abortions, and the remaining aberrations are unrelated to age.

Table 11.1 shows the proportion of trisomy among chromosomally normal or trisomic karyotyped spontaneous abortions by maternal age. The data are presented in five-year intervals of maternal age for ease of presentation. The

Table 11.1. *Trisomy and maternal age among spontaneous abortions*

Age (years)	Coded Age X	Number of Trisomic Karyotypes	Number of Normal Karyotypes	Total Trisomy Plus Normal	Proportion with Trisomy	Fitted $P(X)$ from Model (11.5)
15–19	−2.5	9	70	79	0.114	0.107
20–24	−1.5	26	157	183	0.142	0.145
25–29	−0.5	42	163	205	0.205	0.194
30–34	0.5	37	130	167	0.222	0.254
35–39	1.5	33	59	92	0.359	0.325
40–44	2.5	12	18	30	0.400	0.405

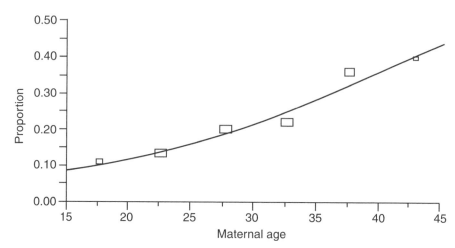

Figure 11.4. Observed and fitted proportions with trisomy. Area of symbol is proportional to sample size.

column headed "Coded Age (X)" gives the midpoint of each age interval minus 30 years, divided by 5; for example, the first entry is $(17.5 - 30)/5 = -2.5$. Thus the reference age is 30 years, and a unit increase in X represents five years. Although we analyze grouped data here, there is no necessity in practice to impose such an arbitrary grouping when individual values of X and Y are available. This is a virtue of the method of maximum likelihood estimation used to fit model (11.5) to these data (see Appendix B). An iterative computation is required to obtain maximum likelihood estimates in most problems; all major statistical software packages today provide the necessary numerical procedures.

The fitted model is $\text{logit}\{P(X)\} = -1.2536 + 0.3470X$. The intercept term -1.2536 corresponds to the proportion $1/\{1 + e^{-(-1.2536)}\} = 0.22$ trisomic at the reference age. The slope coefficient 0.3470 indicates that the odds on trisomy increase by a factor of $e^{0.3470} = 1.41$ per five years of age, or $e^{0.3470/5} = 1.072$ per year. The final two columns of Table 11.1 demonstrate a remarkably good fit, so the model gives reasonable estimates for probabilities at given ages of interest. For example, what does the model predict for the proportion of trisomies in women at age 45 (among miscarriages which are either trisomic or chromosomally normal)? The coded age is $(45 - 30)/5 = 3$, so the estimated log odds is $-1.2536 + 0.3470 \times 3 = -0.2126$, and the estimated proportion is $1/\{1 + e^{-(-0.2126)}\} = 0.447$. See Figure 11.4.

How precise are the estimates? Formulas for standard errors of the estimates are available from the theory of maximum likelihood. Given a sample of n pairs $(X_1, Y_1), \ldots, (X_n, Y_n)$, let $\hat{\alpha}$ and $\hat{\beta}$ be the maximum likelihood estimates (mle's) of α and β, respectively. Let $\hat{P}(X)$ be the estimated model probability at a given value of X, that is, $\hat{P}(X) = \exp(\hat{\alpha} + \hat{\beta}X)/\{1 + \exp(\hat{\alpha} + \hat{\beta}X)\}$, and let $\hat{P}_i = \hat{P}_i(X_i)$ for $i = 1, \ldots, n$. For each observation, define the weight $w_i = \hat{P}_i(1 - \hat{P}_i)$. Let $\bar{X}_w$ denote the weighted average of the X_i's, $\bar{X}_w = \sum_{i=1}^{n} w_i X_i / \sum_{i=1}^{n} w_i$, and let SS_w denote the weighted sum of squared deviations about the mean, $SS_w = \sum_{i=1}^{n} w_i (X_i - \bar{X}_w)^2$. Then

$$\widehat{se}(\hat{\alpha}) = \sqrt{\frac{1}{\sum_{i=1}^{n} w_i} + \frac{\bar{X}_w^2}{SS_w}}, \tag{11.6}$$

$$\widehat{se}(\hat{\beta}) = \frac{1}{\sqrt{SS_w}}, \tag{11.7}$$

and the covariance between the estimates $\hat{\alpha}$ and $\hat{\beta}$ is

$$\widehat{Cov}(\hat{\alpha}, \hat{\beta}) = -\frac{\bar{X}_w}{SS_w}. \tag{11.8}$$

The last expression is used to obtain standard errors and confidence intervals for probabilities predicted from the model. At a given value of X, say $X = x_0$, the log odds is estimated as $\text{logit}\{\hat{P}(x_0)\} = \hat{\alpha} + \hat{\beta}x_0$, with estimated standard error

$$\widehat{se}\left[\text{logit}\{\hat{P}(x_0)\}\right] = \sqrt{\{\widehat{se}(\hat{\alpha})\}^2 + 2x_0\widehat{Cov}(\hat{\alpha}, \hat{\beta}) + x_0^2\{\widehat{se}(\hat{\beta})\}^2}. \tag{11.9}$$

The delta method then gives the standard error for $\hat{P}(x_0)$ (see Problem 11.2):

$$\widehat{se}\{\hat{P}(x_0)\} = \hat{P}(x_0)\{1 - \hat{P}(x_0)\}\widehat{se}\left[\text{logit}\{\hat{P}(x_0)\}\right]. \tag{11.10}$$

Approximate $100(1 - \alpha)\%$ confidence limits for $\text{logit}\{P(x_0)\}$ are

$$\text{logit}\{\hat{P}(x_0)\} \pm z_\alpha \widehat{se}\left[\text{logit}\{\hat{P}(x_0)\}\right]. \tag{11.11}$$

Taking the inverse logit transform (11.2) of these limits provides a confidence interval for $P(x_0)$. Using (11.11) to obtain confidence intervals for $P(x_0)$ is more accurate than taking the crude interval $\hat{P}(x_0) \pm z_\alpha \widehat{se}\{\hat{P}(x_0)\}$, especially when $\hat{P}(x_0)$ is far from one-half.

For the trisomy example, $\widehat{se}(\hat{\alpha}) = 0.0909$, $\widehat{se}(\hat{\beta}) = 0.0699$, and $\widehat{Cov}(\hat{\alpha}, \hat{\beta}) = 0.0001936$. The small value for the covariance results from coding X so that the reference value $X = 0$ is near the central value of the explanatory variable. Thus, an approximate 95% confidence interval for β is $\hat{\beta} \pm 1.96 \times \widehat{se}(\hat{\beta}) = 0.347 \pm 1.96 \times 0.0699 = (0.21, 0.48)$. The slope coefficient is highly significant: $z = \hat{\beta}/\widehat{se}(\hat{\beta}) = 4.96$. At maternal age 45, $x_0 = 3$, and the predicted log odds has standard error $\{0.0909^2 + 2 \times 3 \times 0.0001936 + 9 \times 0.06992^2\}^{1/2} = 0.231$ from (11.9). From (11.10), the standard error for the predicted probability $\hat{P}(x_0) = 0.447$ is $0.447(1 - 0.447) \times 0.231 = 0.057$. An approximate 95% confidence interval for logit$\{\hat{P}(x_0)\}\}$ is $-0.2126 \pm 1.96 \times 0.231 = (-0.665, 0.240)$, and (11.2) yields the corresponding interval $(0.340, 0.560)$ for $\hat{P}(x_0)$. In this example, the crude confidence interval $0.447 \pm 1.96 \times 0.057$ is in good agreement, because $\hat{P}(x_0)$ is close to one-half.

In the special case of the two-group comparative binomial study, the mle's and standard errors have a closed form. Let n_k denote the sample size in group $k = 0$ or 1, and let p_k be the sample proportion of outcome $Y = 1$ in group k. The mle of the reference log odds α is the sample log odds, $\hat{\alpha} = \ln\{p_0/(1 - p_0)\}$, and the mle of β is the sample log odds ratio, $\beta = \ln[\{p_1/(1 - p_1)\}/\{p_0/(1 - p_0)\}]$. Algebra then shows that

$$\sum_{i=1}^{n} w_i = n_1 p_1(1 - p_1) + n_0 p_0(1 - p_0), \tag{11.12}$$

$$\bar{X}_w = \frac{n_1 p_1(1 - p_1)}{n_1 p_1(1 - p_1) + n_0 p_0(1 - p_0)}, \tag{11.13}$$

and

$$SS_w = n_1 p_1(1 - p_1) - \frac{\{n_1 p_1(1 - p_1)\}^2}{n_1 p_1(1 - p_1) + n_0 p_0(1 - p_0)}$$

$$= \frac{n_1 p_1(1 - p_1) n_0 p_0(1 - p_0)}{n_1 p_1(1 - p_1) + n_0 p_0(1 - p_0)}. \tag{11.14}$$

The reader may check that the standard error for $\hat{\beta}$ given by (11.7) specializes to formula (6.33) without the $\frac{1}{2}$ correction term. See Problem 11.3.

11.3.2. Multiple Binary Logistic Regression: Additive and Interactive Models

Given explanatory factors $\underline{X} = (X_1, \ldots, X_r)$ and binary outcome Y, the multiple binary logistic regression model is

$$\text{logit}\{P(\underline{X})\} = \beta_0 + \beta_1 X_1 + \cdots + \beta_r X_r, \tag{11.15}$$

where $P(\underline{X}) = P(Y = 1 | \underline{X})$. When the explanatory factors are all functionally independent variables, the model is said to be *additive*, in which case the regression coefficients have straightforward interpretations analogous to those in the simple binary case. In particular, β_0 is the reference log odds on event $[Y = 1]$ versus $[Y = 0]$ when all $X_j = 0$, and β_j is the log odds ratio per unit increase in X_j, holding all other variables constant. For additive models, these interpretations hold irrespective of the levels at which the other explanatory variables are held constant.

An example of an additive multiple logistic regression model was discussed in Section 6.3. In the present notation, we take X_1 to be the mean pollution level in a subject's community, X_2 to be a smoking indicator (1 = smoker, 0 = nonsmoker), and Y to be mortality from lung cancer (1 = yes, 0 = no). Then equations (6.25) and (6.26) may be written logit$\{P(\underline{X})\} = \beta_0 + \beta_1 X_1 + \beta_2 X_2$. Coefficient β_0 gives the reference log odds on mortality for a non-smoker who lives in a pollution-free community. Coefficient β_1 is the log odds ratio on mortality per unit increase in pollution, which applies for smokers and nonsmokers alike. Coefficient β_2 is the log odds ratio on mortality for smokers versus nonsmokers, which applies at any pollution level. We refer to β_1 as the log odds ratio for pollution *adjusted* for smoking, and β_2 as the log odds ratio for smoking adjusted for pollution.

Another example of an additive model derives from a generalization of the discussion of Section 11.2. Suppose (X_1, X_2) has a bivariate normal distribution with means (μ_{11}, μ_{12}) in group $Y = 1$ and (μ_{01}, μ_{02}) in group $Y = 0$, and assume (X_1, X_2) has the same variance-covariance structure in the two groups. Then among all individuals with explanatory factor (X_1, X_2), the proportion $P(\underline{X})$ in group $Y = 1$ is given by logit$\{P(\underline{X})\} = \beta_0 + \beta_1 X_1 + \beta_2 X_2$ (see Problem 11.4).

The presence of several expanatory factors introduces two new features of the model. One is the effect of interaction between Y and two or more explanatory factors. The other is the need to test for joint significance of two or more coefficients β_j.

An interaction between Y and X_1 and X_2 means that the magnitude of the effect of X_1 on Y depends on the level of X_2, and vice versa, the magnitude of the effect of X_2 on Y depends on the level of X_1. Suppose, for example, X_1 is a continuous variable, X_2 is a binary indicator variable, and $X_3 = X_1 X_2$ is the product of X_1 and X_2. We call X_3 an *interaction variable*, and (11.15) is then called an *interactive* model. The interpretation of β_1 changes because it is no longer possible to hold X_3 constant as X_1 changes. Now, β_1 has the interpretation of a log odds ratio *only when X_2 is at its reference value $X_2 = 0$*. When $X_2 = 1$, however, subtraction of (11.15) with X_1 at a given value, say x_1, from (11.15) with $X_1 = x_1 + 1$, produces a change in logit $\{P(\underline{X})\}$ equal to $\{\beta_0 + \beta_1(x_1 + 1) + \beta_2 + \beta_3(x_1 + 1)\} - \{\beta_0 + \beta_1 x_1 + \beta_2 + \beta_3 x_1\} = \beta_1 + \beta_3$. Thus, nonzero values of X_2 modify the effect of X_1 from β_1 to $\beta_1 + \beta_3$, and we speak of X_2 as an *effect modifier*. Similarly, X_1 acts as an effect modifier for the relation between Y and X_2: coefficient β_2 describes the log odds ratio associating Y with X_2 only when $X_1 = 0$. When X_1 takes some nonzero value x_1, the difference between logit$\{P(\underline{X})\}$ for $X_2 = 1$ and for $X_2 = 0$ is the modified log odds ratio $\beta_2 + \beta_3 x_1$.

The interaction coefficient thus has the interpretation of a difference in log odds ratios, and exp(β_3) corresponds to a ratio of odds ratios. In particular, β_3 is the difference between the log odds ratio (on $Y = 1$ versus $Y = 0$ per unit increase in X_1) at level $X_2 = 1$ versus that at level $X_2 = 0$. β_3 is also the difference between the log odds ratio (on $Y = 1$ versus $Y = 0$ comparing $X_2 = 1$ with $X_2 = 0$) when X_1 takes value $x_1 + 1$ versus that when $X_1 = x_1$. Then $\exp(\beta_3)$ is the multiplicative factor by which the odds ratio associating Y with X_1 increases per unit increment in X_2, and it is also the factor by which the odds ratio associating Y with X_2 increases per unit increment in X_1.

The interaction term $\beta_3 X_1 X_2$ in the above example is called a *first-order* interaction. Higher-order interactions are constructed by including extended product terms as explanatory factors. For example, a second-order interaction between Y and variables X_1, X_2, and X_3 would be modeled by including $\beta_0 + \beta_1 X_1 + \beta_2 X_2 + \beta_3 X_3 + \beta_{12} X_1 X_2 + \beta_{13} X_1 X_3 + \beta_{23} X_2 X_3 + \beta_{123} X_1 X_2 X_3$ in model (11.15). The coefficients β_1, β_2, and β_3 are log odds ratios when the other variables not included in the subscript are at reference value; coefficients β_{12}, β_{13}, and β_{23} represent first-order interactions when the third variable not in the subscript is at reference value; and β_{123} represents the second-order interaction. Thus $\exp(\beta_{123})$ is a ratio of ratios of odds ratios. And so on.

A word of caution is in order here. It is always good practice to assess the impact of potential effect modifiers on important coefficients in the model. However, interactions such as β_{12} are generally not estimated as precisely as main effect terms like β_1 or β_2 in an additive model, and higher-order interactions are even more difficult to estimate precisely. Similarly, tests of significance of first- and higher-order interactions generally have less statistical power than tests of main effects. When screening for interactions, therefore, one can often get a clearer picture by setting confidence interval widths at lower confidence levels and conducting tests at less stringent Type I error rates, such as $\alpha = 0.10$ or higher.

As an example of an interactive model, consider the data in Table 11.2, which elaborate on the trisomy example of Section 11.3.1. Maternal smoking before and around the time of conception was determined by detailed interview shortly after occurrence of the miscarriage, but before either the subject or her interviewer were aware of the fetal karyotype. For illustrative purposes, we classify smoking status in three categories: (a) "current smokers"—primarily women who smoked at the time of their last menstrual period (LMP), plus a small number of "probable" smokers, women whose exact smoking status in relation to their LMP was uncertain, but who probably smoked around the time of conception based on other interview information; (b) "ex-smokers"—women who quit smoking prior to their LMP; and (c) "nonsmokers"—women who reported never having smoked. We take nonsmokers as the reference category. Maternal age is coded linearly in the variable $X_1 = (\text{age} - 30)/5$ as before. Two additional indicator variables for smoking status are needed: $X_2 = 1$ if current smoker, otherwise 0; and $X_3 = 1$ if ex-smoker, otherwise 0. Thus all women are coded uniquely as $(X_2, X_3) = (1, 0)$ for current smokers, $(0, 1)$ for ex-smokers, or $(0, 0)$ for

Table 11.2. *Trisomy and smoking and maternal age among spontaneous abortions*

| Age (years) | Outcome | Smoking Status | | | Total |
		Current Smoker	Ex-smoker	Non-smoker	
15–19	Trisomy	5	0	4	9
	Normal	43	4	23	70
20–24	Trisomy	6	0	20	26
	Normal	81	9	67	157
25–29	Trisomy	10	6	26	42
	Normal	64	17	82	163
30–34	Trisomy	13	8	16	37
	Normal	40	21	69	130
35–39	Trisomy	10	5	18	33
	Normal	13	7	39	59
40–44	Trisomy	5	0	7	12
	Normal	7	2	9	18

nonsmokers. In general, one constructs $c - 1$ indicator variables to encode a c-category explanatory factor, excluding the reference category indicator. We fit the model

$$\text{logit}\{P(\underline{X})\} = \beta_0 + \beta_1 X_1 + \beta_2 X_2 + \beta_3 X_3 + \beta_{12} X_1 X_2 + \beta_{13} X_1 X_3 \quad (11.16)$$

to these data, with the results shown in Table 11.3. Note the interaction coefficient for age by current smoking, β_{12}: it is numerically large and

Table 11.3. *Model-fitting results for the trisomy and smoking data*

Model	Coefficient	Maximum Likelihood Estimate	Standard Error	Critical Ratio z	$-2 \times$ (Maximized Log Likelihood)	Goodness of Fit (df)
(11.16)	β_0	−1.1300	0.1210	−9.3422	743.121	14.127
unconstrained	β_1	0.1727	0.0942	1.8345		(12)
(interactive	β_2	−0.3016	0.2031	−1.4852		
model H_1)	β_3	−0.1069	0.3071	−0.3481		
	β_{12}	0.3670	0.1531	2.3971		
	β_{13}	0.3089	0.2800	1.1034		
(11.16) with	β_0	−1.1280	0.1222	−9.2276	749.351	20.357
$\beta_{12} = \beta_{13} = 0$	β_1	0.3304	0.0710	4.6533		(14)
(additive	β_2	−0.3393	0.2016	−1.6827		
model H_0)	β_3	−0.0668	0.2933	−0.2279		

Joint test of significance of interaction terms: $G^2(H_0 : H_1) = 6.230$ on 2 df.

statistically significant (nearly 2.4 standard errors above zero). The age-by-ex-smoking interaction coefficient β_{13} is also substantial although, with its larger standard error, not statistically significant. One interpretation of these results is that the effect of current smoking on the trisomy versus normal outcome is modified by age: at the reference age or younger, current smokers have smaller risk of trisomy than those who never smoked (because $\beta_2 < 0$), but at older ages current smoking is associated with elevated risk of trisomy. For example, at age 45, the model estimates the odds ratio for current smoking to be $\exp(\beta_2 + \beta_{12} X_1) = \exp(-0.3016 + 0.3670 \times 3) = 2.22$. Similar remarks pertain to ex-smokers. An equivalent interpretation is that smoking appears to modify the trisomy–maternal-age relation: women who never smoked have a modest age slope coefficient ($\beta_1 = 0.1727$) compared to current smokers (with age slope $\beta_1 + \beta_{12} = 0.54$) or to ex-smokers (with age slope $\beta_1 + \beta_{13} = 0.48$).

The lower panel in Table 11.3 shows the effect of omitting the interaction terms and fitting a purely additive model. Both smoking effects are negative, suggesting an inverse association of smoking with trisomy, irrespective of age. This conclusion is incomplete and misleading, as visual inspection of Table 11.2 confirms.

11.3.3. Generalized Likelihood Ratio Tests

How do we assess whether or not some subset of coefficients are jointly significant? In the trisomy data, for example, would the two interaction coefficients survive a joint test of significance? Likelihood theory with maximum likelihood estimation again provides an answer. We observe n vectors, $(\underline{X}_1, Y_1), \ldots, (\underline{X}_n, Y_n)$, where for subject i, $\underline{X}_i = (X_{i1}, \ldots, X_{ir})$ is the vector of r explanatory factors ($i = 1, \ldots, n$). Suppose we call (11.15) model hypothesis H_1. First, estimate the coefficients for H_1 by maximum likelihood; let $\hat{\beta}_j^{(1)}$ denote the mle of β_j under H_1 for $j = 0, \ldots, r$. Next record the log likelihood for H_1, which in this case is

$$L(H_1) = \sum_i \left\{ Y_i \ln \hat{P}^{(1)}(\underline{X}_i) + (1 - Y_i) \ln \hat{Q}^{(1)}(\underline{X}_i) \right\}$$

$$= \sum_i Y_i \ln \frac{\hat{P}^{(1)}(\underline{X}_i)}{\hat{Q}^{(1)}(\underline{X}_i)} + \sum_i \ln \hat{Q}^{(1)}(\underline{X}_i), \qquad (11.17)$$

where

$$\hat{P}^{(1)}(\underline{X}_i) = 1 - \hat{Q}^{(1)}(\underline{X}_i) = 1 / \left[1 + \exp\left\{ -\left(\hat{\beta}_0^{(1)} + \hat{\beta}_1^{(1)} X_{i1} + \cdots + \hat{\beta}_r^{(1)} X_{ir} \right) \right\} \right]$$

is the fitted model probability under H_1 for the ith observation. $L(H_1)$ is simply the sum of fitted model log probabilities corresponding to the observed outcome for each subject: $\hat{P}^{(1)}(X_i)$ for those with $Y_i = 1$, or $\hat{Q}^{(1)}(\underline{X}_i)$ for those with $Y_i = 0$.

Now suppose we hypothesize that certain coefficients equal zero; for example, that model H_0 specifies $\beta_{s+1} = \cdots = \beta_r = 0$ for some index $s < r$.

We call H_0 a reduced model nested within H_1, because it contains the $s + 1$ parameters $\beta_0, \ldots, \beta_s$ from H_1, but constrains the remaining parameters to be zero. Next, fit the reduced model H_0 by maximum likelihood to obtain mle's $\hat{\beta}_0^{(0)}, \ldots, \hat{\beta}_s^{(0)}$ and the corresponding log likelihood $L(H_0)$ from (11.17) using the fitted probabilities from model H_0, $\hat{P}_0^{(0)}(\underline{X}_i) = 1/[1 + \exp\{-(\hat{\beta}_0^{(0)} + \hat{\beta}_1^{(0)} X_{i1} + \cdots + \hat{\beta}_s^{(0)} X_{is})\}]$, instead of $\hat{P}^{(1)}(\underline{X}_i)$. Finally, obtain the *generalized log-likelihood ratio statistic* $G^2(H_0 : H_1)$, which is defined as twice the difference in log-likelihoods:

$$G^2(H_0 : H_1) = 2\{L(H_1) - L(H_0)\}$$

$$= 2\sum_i \left(Y_i \ln \frac{\hat{P}^{(1)}(\underline{X}_i)}{\hat{P}_0^{(0)}(\underline{X}_i)} + (1 - Y_i) \ln \frac{\hat{Q}^{(1)}(\underline{X}_i)}{\hat{Q}^{(0)}(\underline{X}_i)} \right). \quad (11.18)$$

Summarizing, we construct the log-likelihood ratio statistic for a pair of nested models by subtracting twice the maximized log likelihood for the reduced model from that of the full model.

When the sample size n is large, $G^2(H_0 : H_1)$ has an approximate chi squared distribution with $r - s$ df under H_0. We therefore reject H_0 when $G^2(H_0 : H_1)$ exceeds the critical value $\chi^2_{r-s;\alpha}$, cutting off probability α in the upper tail of the chi squared distribution with $r - s$ df.

Let H_s represent the *saturated* model, which allows the probability $P(\underline{X})$ to be arbitrary for each i. Then $G^2(H_j : H_s)$ is called the *deviance* of the model H_j ($j = 1$ or 0), in which case $G^2(H_0 : H_1)$ is the difference between the deviances for models H_0 and H_1. Unlike $G^2(H_0 : H_1)$, $G^2(H_j : H_s)$ is not distributed as chi squared, even in large samples, because the number of parameters associated with H_s increases as the sample size increases.

Log likelihoods are often numerically large and a bit cumbersome. We can dodge that problem because the statistic $G^2(H_0 : H_1)$ is a difference of two log-likelihood terms, and therefore equivalent results may be obtained if each of the terms $L(H_1)$ and $L(H_0)$ is shifted by the same amount. It is most convenient, for example, to replace $L(H_1)$ and $L(H_0)$ by the deviance expressions $G^2(H_1 : H_s) = 2\{L(H_s) - L(H_1)\}$ and $G^2(H_0 : H_s) = 2\{L(H_s) - L(H_0)\}$, respectively, and then to write $G^2(H_0 : H_1)$ as the difference of the deviances for model H_0 and H_1, $G^2(H_0 : H_1) = G^2(H_0 : H_s) - G^2(H_1 : H_s)$. The term $L(H_s)$, defined later in this section, is usually of the same order of magnitude as $L(H_1)$ and $L(H_0)$, so the deviances $G^2(H_0 : H_s)$ and $G^2(H_1 : H_s)$ are less awkward to tabulate. Of greater importance is the following: although $G^2(H_0 : H_s)$ and $G^2(H_1 : H_s)$ do not generally play the role of goodness-of-fit statistics, under appropriate circumstances they do, as we shall soon see.

In the trisomy example, the penultimate column of Table 11.3 gives minus two times the log-likelihood, $-2L(H_1)$, for model (11.16) in the upper panel, and $-2L(H_0)$ in the lower panel for the null hypothesis that the interaction coefficients equal zero, H_0: $\beta_{12} = \beta_{13} = 0$. Thus $G^2(H_0 : H_1) = 749.351 - 743.121 = 6.23$ or, equivalently, $G^2(H_0 : H_1) = G^2(H_0 : H_s) - G^2(H_1 : H_s) = 20.357 - 14.127 = 6.23$, using the goodness-of-fit statistics in the final column. Under H_0, $G^2(H_0 : H_1)$ has an approximate chi squared distribution on 2 df. Since the $\alpha = 0.05$ critical value for this distribution is 5.99 and is exceeded by $G^2(H_0 : H_1)$, we reject H_0 and conclude that the interaction terms are jointly significant.

The reader may have noticed that for hypotheses about an individual parameter, say H_0: $\beta_j = 0$, we now have two test statistics: the log-likelihood ratio statistic, $G^2(H_0 : H_1)$, and the critical ratio, $z = \hat{\beta}_j^{(1)} / \widehat{\text{se}}\{\hat{\beta}_j^{(1)}\}$, also called the Wald test critical ratio, or its square, z^2, called the Wald test statistic. $G^2(H_0 : H_1)$ is asymptotically equivalent to z^2, as is a third variety of test statistic, the score test statistic X^2, which is the square of the partial derivative of the log-likelihood function with respect to β_j, evaluated at the maximum likelihood estimate of $\beta_1, \ldots, \beta_r$ subject to the constraint $\beta_j = 0$. Asymptotic equivalence means that while the various test statistics are not arithmetically identical, they have the same approximating distribution in large samples under the null hypothesis, so that with high probability they all result in the same inference.

As a simple illustration, consider a single binomial variable $Y \sim \text{Bin}(n, P)$. Y may be viewed as the sufficient statistic $\Sigma_i Y_i$ based on a sample $Y_1, \ldots, Y_n$ from the trivial logit model logit$\{P\} = \beta_0$; call this model H_1. The maximum likelihood estimate of β_0 under H_1 is the sample log odds $\hat{\beta}_0^{(1)} = \ln(p/q)$ with estimated standard error $\widehat{\text{se}}\{\hat{\beta}_0^{(1)}\} = (npq)^{-1/2}$, where $p = 1 - q = Y/n$ is the sample proportion, which is the mle of P, $\hat{P}^{(1)} = p$. To test the null hypothesis H_0: $P = \frac{1}{2}$, equivalent to H_0: $\beta_0 = 0$, we have the following three test statistics: (i) the log-likelihood ratio statistic, $G^2(H_0 : H_1) = 2\{Y \ln 2p + (n - Y) \ln 2q\}$; (ii) the Wald test statistic, $z^2 = [\hat{\beta}_0^{(1)} / \widehat{\text{se}}\{\hat{\beta}_0^{(1)}\}]^2 = \{\ln(p/q)\}^2 npq$; and (iii) the score test statistic, $X^2 = (Y - n/2)^2 / (n/4) = 4n(p - \frac{1}{2})^2$. Problem 11.5 demonstrates the asymptotic equivalence of these three statistics by showing they are all approximately chi squared on one degree of freedom under H_0 in large samples.

For the remainder of this chapter, the log-likelihood ratio statistic will be our main tool for drawing inferences about model hypotheses. For convenience in informal discussions of the significance of individual regression coefficients, we also quote the Wald test critical ratios $z = \hat{\beta}_j^{(1)} / \widehat{\text{se}}\{\hat{\beta}_j^{(1)}\}$ and their associated p-values.

As another illustration of multiple logistic regression, interactive models, and the use of log-likelihood ratio tests, let us reconsider the test of homogeneity of odds ratios in a set of g independent 2×2 tables discussed in Chapter 10. The test statistic χ^2_{homog}, given in Section 10.1 at (10.10) and (10.11) or in Section 10.2 at (10.18), is based on Wald test procedures; the test statistic χ^2_{homog} given in Section 10.4 at (10.40) is based on score test procedures. For the log-likelihood ratio test procedure, we view the problem in the context of a multiple logistic regression model for binary outcome Y and explanatory variables $X_1, \ldots, X_g$, where X_1 is the binary risk factor of interest in each 2×2 table, and $X_2, \ldots, X_g$ are indicator variables for tables 2 through g, taking the first table as reference. The full model, with no constraints on the g odds ratios, is H_1:

$$\text{logit}\{P(\underline{X})\} = \beta_0 + \beta_1 X_1 + \beta_2 X_2 + \cdots + \beta_g X_g + \beta_{12} X_1 X_2 + \cdots + \beta_{1g} X_1 X_g. \tag{11.19}$$

The log odds ratio associating outcome Y with exposure X_1 is β_1 in the reference table, and $\beta_1 + \beta_{1j}$ in table $j = 2, \ldots, g$, due to the presence of the interaction variables $X_1 X_j$. Thus, the hypothesis of constant odds ratio is represented in this model as $H_0: \beta_{12} = \cdots = \beta_{1g} = 0$. To test H_0 versus H_1, we first require the mle's of the parameters under each model. Under H_1, the mle of β_1 is the sample log odds ratio in the reference table, while the mle of β_{1j} is the difference between the sample log odds ratio in table j and that in the reference table. It follows that the fitted model probabilities are simply the sample proportions in each row of each table. Then (11.17) gives the log likelihood $L(H_1)$, which simplifies slightly in this case as follows. Let y_{ij} be the frequency of the outcome $Y = 1$ in row $i = 1$ or 0 of table $j = 1, \ldots, g$, and let n_{ij} be the sample size in row i of table j. Then

$$L(H_1) = \sum_{i=0}^{1} \sum_{j=1}^{g} y_{ij} \ln \frac{y_{ij}}{n_{ij}} + (n_{ij} - y_{ij}) \ln \frac{n_{ij} - y_{ij}}{n_{ij}}. \tag{11.20}$$

To cover the case in which a row has a zero cell frequency, we define $0 \ln 0$ to be 0 in (11.20). Under H_0, the model is $\text{logit}\{P(\underline{X})\} = \beta_0 + \beta_1 X_1 + \beta_2 X_2 + \cdots + \beta_g X_g$, for which one must calculate the maximum likelihood estimates iteratively. Call these $\hat{\beta}_0^{(0)}, \ldots, \hat{\beta}_g^{(0)}$. The common log odds ratio estimated under H_0 is $\hat{\beta}_1^{(0)}$. Using the fitted probabilities $\hat{P}(\underline{X})$ from H_0 in (11.17) yields $L(H_0)$, and then $G^2(H_0 : H_1) = 2\{L(H_1) - L(H_0)\}$ is the log-likelihood ratio statistic. Model H_1 has a total of $1 + g + (g - 1) = 2g$ parameters, while model H_0 has $g + 1$ parameters. Therefore $G^2(H_0 : H_1)$ has an approximate chi squared distribution under H_0 with $2g - (g + 1) = g - 1$ df.

For the data in Table 10.1, $Y = 1$ denotes diagnosis of schizophrenia. X_1 is hospital location ($1 = $ New York, $0 = $ London); $X_2 = 1$ for study 2, else 0; $X_3 = 1$ for study 3, else 0. Under H_1, the log-likelihood is $L(H_1) = -561.303$. The mle's under H_0 are $\hat{\beta}_0^{(0)} = -0.3502$, $\hat{\beta}_1^{(0)} = 1.1128$, $\hat{\beta}_2^{(0)} = -0.1878$, and $\hat{\beta}_3^{(0)} = -0.3702$. The estimated common odds ratio is $\exp(\hat{\beta}_1^{(0)}) = \exp(1.1128) = 3.04$, in excellent agreement with (10.39). Under H_0, the log likelihood is $L(H_0) = -566.310$. Thus $G^2(H_0 : H_1) = 2\{(-561.303) - (-566.310)\} = 1132.620 - 1122.606 = 10.01$ on 2 df ($p < 0.01$). This result should be compared with the value of the Wald test statistic of 9.41 given in (10.18) and the score test statistic of 9.70 given in (10.41).

11.3.4. Log-Likelihood Ratio Goodness-of-Fit Tests and the Analysis of Information

Another important use of the log-likelihood ratio statistic is to test the global goodness of fit of a model. Suppose we wish to test whether model (11.15) fits the data $(\underline{X}_1, Y_1), \ldots, (\underline{X}_n, Y_n)$ adequately, or whether there are important but unspecified departures in the data from the model. We assume for the moment that only a fixed number of explanatory factor combinations occur even as n becomes large. This would occur, for example, with grouped data, such as in the trisomy example, or with purely categorical explanatory factors. In essence, model (11.15), which we shall continue to call H_1, now becomes a null hypothesis which we desire to test against another model, H_s say, that allows the probability $P(\underline{X})$ to be arbitrary for each combination of factors. Such a model is called *fully saturated*, because it possesses as many parameters as there are distinct combinations of factors and corresponding probabilities. As mentioned in the previous section, $G^2(H_0 : H_s)$ is not generally distributed as chi squared. In the present case of grouped data, however, we can appeal to the central limit theorem when group sizes are large, in which case $G^2(H_0 : H_s)$ does have a chi squared distribution. To distinguish the general saturated model H_s with individual-level data from the saturated model with grouped data, we denote the latter by H_2, and then the chi squared approximation for $G^2(H_0 : H_2)$ can be made. For example, in the preceding discussion of g fourfold tables, model (11.19), which was fully saturated, would play the role of H_2 in the present discussion. The hypothesis of constant odds ratio, previously called H_0, is now the model H_1 of interest; this leaves room to consider a reduced model, H_0, such as the hypothesis of no association in any table, $H_0 : \beta_1 = \beta_{12} = \cdots = \beta_{1k} = 0$.

In order to test H_1 versus H_2, we construct the test statistic $G^2(H_1 : H_2) = 2\{L(H_2) - L(H_1)\}$, which is called the *log-likelihood ratio goodness-of-fit statistic* to emphasize its use in checking the fit of a model (and which explains the choice of the symbol G^2). Specifically, suppose there are c distinct possible combinations of explanatory factors. Let n_i denote the number of observations at the ith combination, and let y_i denote the frequency of the event $[Y = 1]$ at that combination; thus $n_i - y_i$ is the frequency of the event $[Y = 0]$. Under the saturated model, the sample proportions y_i/n_i are maximum likelihood estimates of the unrestricted probabilities, so that the maximized log likelihood $L(H_2)$ is

$$L(H_1) = \sum_{i=1}^{c} y_i \ln \frac{y_i}{n_i} + (n_i - y_i) \ln \frac{n_i - y_i}{n_i}, \qquad (11.21)$$

where, as above, $0 \ln 0$ is defined as 0 wherever it appears. Then the log-likelihood ratio goodness-of-fit statistic is given explicitly by

$$G^2(H_1 : H_2) = 2 \sum_{i=1}^{c} y_i \ln \frac{y_i}{n_i \hat{P}_i^{(1)}} + (n_i - y_i) \ln \frac{n_i - y_i}{n_i \hat{Q}_i^{(1)}}, \qquad (11.22)$$

where $\hat{P}_i^{(1)} = 1 - \hat{Q}_i^{(1)}$ is the fitted model probability under H_1 at the ith combination of explanatory factors. Under H_1, as the n_i become large, $G^2(H_1 : H_2)$ has an approximate chi squared distribution with $c - (r + 1)$ degrees of freedom [because the saturated model has c parameters, one for the probability $P(X) = P(Y = 1|X)$ at each combination of X].

In similar fashion, $G^2(H_0 : H_2) = 2\{L(H_2) - L(H_0)\}$ is the log-likelihood ratio goodness-of-fit statistic for testing the reduced model H_0: $\beta_{s+1} = \cdots = \beta_r = 0$ against the saturated model H_2. Under H_0, $G^2(H_0 : H_2)$ has an approximate chi squared distribution with $c - (s + 1)$ degrees of freedom. We have seen the difference between the two goodness-of-fit statistics as the log-likelihood ratio statistic for testing H_0 versus H_1 in (11.18), with $\{c - (s + 1)\} - \{c - (r + 1)\} = r - s$ df:

$$G^2(H_0 : H_1) = G^2(H_0 : H_2) - G^2(H_1 : H_2) = 2\{L(H_1) - L(H_0)\}. \quad (11.23)$$

In the trisomy example, the saturated logit model for the data in Table 11.2 has $c = 18$ parameters, corresponding to the $18 = 6 \times 3$ combinations of maternal age interval and smoking status. The log likelihood for H_2 is $L(H_2) = 5 \ln(5/48) + 43 \ln(43/48) + \cdots = -364.497$, with $-2L(H_2) = 728.994$. From the penultimate column of Table 11.3, $-2L(H_1) = 743.121$. Thus $G^2(H_1 : H_2) = 743.121 - 728.994 = 14.127$ with $18 - 6 = 12$ df, as indicated in the final column of Table 11.3. We do not reject model H_1 at (11.16) at the $\alpha = 0.05$ level, because, from Table A.2, the critical value for χ^2 on 12 df is $21.03 > G^2(H_1 : H_2)$. The model is formally judged adequate. We recognize, though, that the power to reject H_1 against H_2 may not be high, so it is good practice also to consider the agreement between observed and fitted probabilities. Figure 11.5 illustrates this, and confirms a reasonably

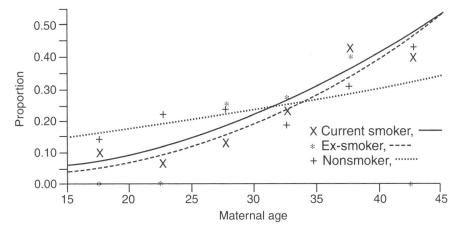

Figure 11.5. Observed and fitted proportions with trisomy by smoking status.

close fit. We discuss the formal comparison of observed and fitted probabilities in Section 11.5.

Note that the goodness-of-fit statistic $G^2(H_0 : H_2) = 20.357$ in the lower panel of Table 11.3 also does not exceed the $\alpha = 0.05$ level critical value for chi squared on 14 df, so that, judging from the global goodness-of-fit statistic alone, we might conclude that H_0 is adequate, even though we have already rejected H_0 in favor of H_1. This illustrates an important point: a test of H_0 against a parametric (unsaturated) alternative like H_1, which fits the data well, using a statistic having few degrees of freedom, will typically be *more powerful* than a test of H_0 against a nonparametric (fully saturated) hypothesis like H_2, using a goodness-of-fit statistic with many degrees of freedom. The analysis of g fourfold tables also illustrates the point. To test the null hypothesis H_0 of no association in any table, we would rather test against H_1: constant odds ratio with a 1 df test than against H_2 with a g df test, assuming, of course, that H_1 fits the data well. (If there are substantial variations in the odds ratios in both directions around unity, then the test of H_0 against H_2 may well be more powerful.) For example, the Mantel-Haenszel 1 df procedure, a conditional score test which is locally most powerful for testing H_0 versus H_1, is not necessarily powerful at all if H_1 is false. In Problem 11.6 the reader will conduct the log-likelihood ratio goodness-of-fit test of H_0 versus H_2 and the log-likelihood ratio test of H_0 versus H_1 for the data in Table 10.1. In this exercise, the odds ratios are all substantially greater than unity, in which case the power of $G^2(H_0 : H_1)$ is maintained even though H_1 does not fit the data well.

Rearranging terms in equation (11.23) yields a relation analogous to the analysis-of-variance decomposition for continuous outcome variables,

$$G^2(H_0 : H_2) = G^2(H_0 : H_1) + G^2(H_1 : H_2), \qquad (11.24)$$

but (11.24) does not parcel out components of explained and unexplained variance. Instead, we interpret the log-likelihood ratio as a measure of the *weight of evidence* contained in the data in favor of one hypothesis and against another. This interpretation is valid because $\exp\{\frac{1}{2}G^2(H_0 : H_2)\}$ describes how many times more likely the data are under an optimized form of H_2 than under an optimized form of H_0. Measures of the weight of evidence, like other measures of information content, are usually expressed logarithmically. Thus if $\frac{1}{2}G^2(H_0 : H_2)$ represents the total weight of evidence against H_0, then (11.24) apportions this total to the weight of evidence against H_0 explained by model H_1, $\frac{1}{2}G^2(H_0 : H_1)$, plus the weight of evidence against H_0 or any other version of model H_1 explained by model lack of fit, $\frac{1}{2}G^2(H_1 : H_2)$. An *analysis-of-information* table may be constructed as in Table 11.4. The fractions $G^2(H_0 : H_1)/G^2(H_0 : H_2)$ and $G^2(H_1 : H_2)/G^2(H_0 : H_2)$ are roughly analogous to R^2 and $1 - R^2$ from the analysis of variance, but instead of proportions of variance in Y explained and unexplained by model

Table 11.4. *Analysis-of-information table*

Source of Evidence against H_0	G^2	No. of df	p-Value
Explained by H_1	$G^2(H_0 : H_1)$	$r - s$	$P[\chi^2_{r-s} > G^2(H_0 : H_1)]$
Unexplained by H_1	$G^2(H_1 : H_2)$	$c - (r + 1)$	$P[\chi^2_{c-(r+1)} > G^2(H_1 : H_2)]$
Total	$G^2(H_0 : H_2)$	$c - (s + 1)$	$P[\chi^2_{c-(s+1)} > G^2(H_0 : H_2)]$

H_1, respectively, the log-likelihood ratio fractions describe the proportions of evidentiary weight against H_0 explained and unexplained by model H_1.

Goodness-of-fit tests break down when explanatory factors are continuous, i.e., $H_2 = H_s$, for then the number of distinct combinations of $\underline{X}$ may grow essentially as fast as the sample size n, instead of remaining fixed. When there are n distinct combinations, each with $n_i = 1$ observation of Y_i, the expression for $L(H_s)$ reduces to 0, $G^2(H_1 : H_s)$ reduces to $-2L(H_1)$, and $G^2(H_0 : H_s)$ reduces to $-2L(H_0)$. That does not alter the relation (11.23), and $G^2(H_0 : H_1)$ is still a valid and useful test statistic for H_0 versus H_1. However, the individual components $G^2(H_0 : H_s)$ and $G^2(H_1 : H_s)$ no longer have approximate chi squared distributions, so other methods must be employed to assess the models' goodness of fit.

Such methods fall into two broad categories: grouping methods and model embedding methods. In a grouping method, the data are grouped in some specific way and a corresponding goodness-of-fit test is applied. For example, the trisomy data originally were available with exact maternal age; the data were then grouped as in Table 11.3 for purposes of testing the goodness of fit of the model (11.16). Another grouping method focuses on the fitted probabilities, $p(\underline{X}_i)$, for each observation. These are ordered in increasing size and then grouped into equal intervals, e.g. quintiles or deciles. The sum of the fitted probabilities in each quintile is compared with the corresponding sum of observed counts Y_i using a multinomial chi squared goodness-of-fit test. See Hosmer and Lemeshow (2000) for further details about this class of tests.

Model-embedding methods require enlarging the class of models so that (11.15) becomes nested within the class as a special case. In the trisomy example, we might introduce quadratic age terms and test whether the coefficients for the quadratic terms are jointly significant. Another model embedding technique is described by Tsiatis (1980). This method involves adding indicator variables to model (11.15) corresponding to d mutually exclusive and exhaustive domains of the space of explanatory factors. A d df log-likelihood-ratio test of the joint significance of the domain indicator coefficients provides the test of goodness of fit. This method works best when there are few explanatory factors, so that the number of domains, d, is not large enough to cause a loss of power to detect model departures.

Table 11.5. *British coal miners classified by age and symptoms of breathlessness and wheeze*

Age Interval	Breathlessness: Wheeze	Present Present	Present Absent	Absent Present	Absent Absent	Total
20–24		9	7	95	1,841	1,952
25–29		23	9	105	1,654	1,791
30–34		54	19	177	1,863	2,113
35–39		121	48	257	2,357	2,783
40–44		169	54	273	1,778	2,274
45–49		269	88	324	1,712	2,393
50–54		404	117	245	1,324	2,090
55–59		406	152	225	967	1,750
60–64		372	106	132	526	1,136
Totals		1,827	600	1,833	14,022	18,282

Source: National Coal Board's Pneumoconiosis Field Research (1957), as reported by Ashford and Sowden (1970).

11.4. POLYTOMOUS LOGISTIC REGRESSION

11.4.1. An Example: The Double Dichotomy

Table 11.5 shows the frequencies of respiratory symptoms among British coal miners aged 20 through 64 in five-year intervals of age. These data are from the (British) National Coal Board's (1957) pneumoconiosis field research reported by Ashford and Sowden (1970) and discussed by several authors, including Grizzle (1971), Mantel and Brown (1973), Fienberg (1980), and Levin and Shrout (1981). Each row of the table contains the cells of a 2×2 table that cross-classifies the presence or absence of symptoms of breathlessness and wheeze for the given age interval. Figure 11.6 plots the log odds on breathlessness among miners without symptoms of wheeze by age group. Note the nearly perfect linear fit and the clear increase in the log odds with age. Figure 11.7 plots the log odds on wheeze among miners without breathlessness. We again find a clear increase in the prevalence of wheeze, although for this symptom there is a slowing of the increase at older ages. Figure 11.8 plots the log odds ratio relating breathlessness and wheeze by age. Note how the association between the two symptoms decreases with age and, again, the striking linearity of the relation.

Polytomous logistic regression offers a parsimonious description of the above relations. Among the several ways to parameterize the four categories of the multinomial sample in each age group, we choose the one most useful for representing the relations of interest. We let $Y = (y_1, y_2)$ be a doubly dichotomous outcome variable denoting breathlessness (present = 1, absent = 0) and wheeze (present = 1, absent = 0). We think of Y as a multinomial

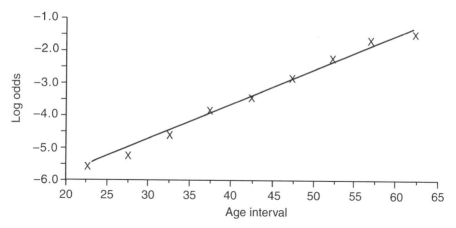

Figure 11.6. Log odds on breathlessness (among miners without wheeze).

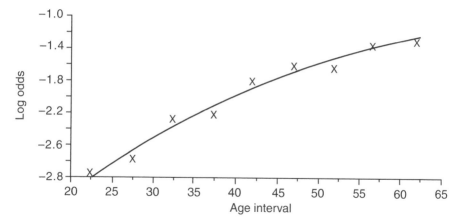

Figure 11.7. Log odds on wheeze (among miners without breathlessness).

response in four categories for each miners symptoms, in this case with the structure of a fourfold table of sample size 1. Thus, each row of Table 11.5 summarizes the sample distribution of Y for miners in the corresponding age group. We then define the following three logistic parameters, which we call *natural parameters*:

$\varphi^{(B)}(x)$ = log odds on breathlessness among miners without wheeze at age x

$$= \ln \frac{P\{Y = (1,0) \mid \text{age} = x\}}{P\{Y = (0,0) \mid \text{age} = x\}} ; \tag{11.25}$$

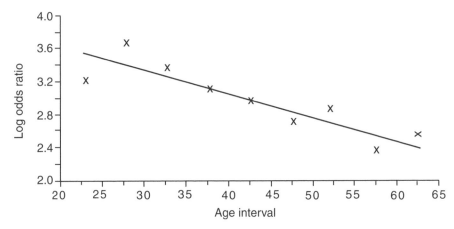

Figure 11.8. Log odds ratio relating breathlessness and wheeze.

$\varphi^{(W)}(x) = $ log odds on wheeze among miners without breathlessness at age x

$$= \ln \frac{P\{Y = (0,1)\,|\,\text{age} = x\}}{P\{Y = (0,0)\,|\,\text{age} = x\}}\,; \qquad (11.26)$$

$\varphi^{(BW)}(x) = $ log odds ratio associating breathlessness and wheeze at age x

$$= \ln \frac{P\{Y = (1,1)\,|\,\text{age} = x\}\,/\,P\{Y = (1,0)\,|\,\text{age} = x\}}{P\{Y = (0,1)\,|\,\text{age} = x\}\,/\,P\{Y = (0,0)\,|\,\text{age} = x\}}\,. \qquad (11.27)$$

These natural parameters allow us to specify the logarithms of the four cell probabilities at any age x as follows:

$$\ln P\{Y = (0,0)\,|\,\text{age} = x\} = -\psi(x), \qquad (11.28)$$

$$\ln P\{Y = (1,0)\,|\,\text{age} = x\} = -\psi(x) + \varphi^{(B)}(x), \qquad (11.29)$$

$$\ln P\{Y = (0,1)\,|\,\text{age} = x\} = -\psi(x) + \varphi^{(W)}(x), \qquad (11.30)$$

$$\ln P\{Y = (1,1)\,|\,\text{age} = x\} = -\psi(x) + \varphi^{(B)}(x) + \varphi^{(W)}(x) + \varphi^{(BW)}(x), \qquad (11.31)$$

where $\psi(x)$ is the logarithm of a normalizing constant to ensure that the four cell probabilities sum to one:

$$\exp\{\psi(x)\} = 1 + \exp\{\varphi^{(B)}(x)\} + \exp\{\varphi^{(W)}(x)\}$$
$$+ \exp\{\varphi^{(B)}(x) + \varphi^{(W)}(x) + \varphi^{(BW)}(x)\}. \qquad (11.32)$$

Thus the cell probabilities can be written

$$P\{Y = (0,0)| \text{age} = x\} = \exp\{-\psi(x)\}$$

$$= \frac{1}{1 + \exp\{\varphi^{(B)}(x)\} + \exp\{\varphi^{(W)}(x)\} + \exp\{\varphi^{(B)}(x) + \varphi^{(W)}(x) + \varphi^{(BW)}(x)\}},$$

$$(11.33)$$

$$P\{Y = (1,0)| \text{age} = x\} = \exp\{-\psi(x) + \varphi^{(B)}(x)\}$$

$$= \frac{\exp\{\varphi^{(B)}(x)\}}{1 + \exp\{\varphi^{(B)}(x)\} + \exp\{\varphi^{(W)}(x)\} + \exp\{\varphi^{(B)}(x) + \varphi^{(W)}(x) + \varphi^{(BW)}(x)\}},$$

$$(11.34)$$

$$P\{Y = (0,1)| \text{age} = x\} = \exp\{-\psi(x) + \varphi^{(W)}(x)\}$$

$$= \frac{\exp\{\varphi^{(W)}(x)\}}{1 + \exp\{\varphi^{(B)}(x)\} + \exp\{\varphi^{(W)}(x)\} + \exp\{\varphi^{(B)}(x) + \varphi^{(W)}(x) + \varphi^{(BW)}(x)\}},$$

$$(11.35)$$

$$P\{Y = (1,1)| \text{age} = x\} = \exp\{-\psi(x) + \varphi^{(B)}(x) + \varphi^{(W)}(x) + \varphi^{(BW)}(x)\}$$

$$= \frac{\exp\{\varphi^{(B)}(x) + \varphi^{(W)}(x) + \varphi^{(BW)}(x)\}}{1 + \exp\{\varphi^{(B)}(x)\} + \exp\{\varphi^{(W)}(x)\} + \exp\{\varphi^{(B)}(x) + \varphi^{(W)}(x) + \varphi^{(BW)}(x)\}}.$$

$$(11.36)$$

The reader may check that the three φ parameters in (11.25)–(11.27) are returned when the appropriate ratios of (11.33)–(11.36) are formed.

We can now state the polytomous logistic regression model that captures the relations displayed in Figures 11.6–11.8:

$$\varphi^{(B)}(x) = \beta_0^{(B)} + \beta_1^{(B)}x^* + \beta_2^{(B)}x^{*2}, \tag{11.37}$$

$$\varphi^{(W)}(x) = \beta_0^{(W)} + \beta_1^{(W)}x^* + \beta_2^{(W)}x^{*2}, \tag{11.38}$$

$$\varphi^{(BW)}(x) = \beta_0^{(BW)} + \beta_1^{(BW)}x^* + \beta_2^{(BW)}x^{*2}, \tag{11.39}$$

where $x^* = (\text{age interval midpoint} - 42.5)/5$ is a linearly transformed version of age, taking values $-4, -3, \ldots, 0, \ldots, +3, +4$. The quadratic term in x^{*2} is used to reflect the nonlinearity in Figure 11.7. Model (11.37)–(11.39) was fitted to the data in Table 11.5 with the results shown in Table 11.6.

The goodness-of-fit statistic for testing model (11.37)–(11.39) as H_0 versus the saturated alternative H_1 of arbitrary probabilities, $P\{Y = (i,j)| \text{age} = x^*\}$, is $G^2(H_0 : H_1) = 17.656$ on $(9 \times 3) - 9 = 18$ df, indicating an excellent fit. The linear terms for $\varphi^{(B)}$ and $\varphi^{(W)}$ are positive and highly significant, reflecting the increasing prevalence of breathlessness and wheeze with age (among miners without wheeze and breathlessness, respectively). The linear term for the log odds ratio $\varphi^{(BW)}$ is negative and highly significant, reflecting the decreasing strength of association with age. Problem 11.7 asks the reader to plot the log odds on breathlessness among miners with wheeze, $\varphi^{(B)}(x) + \varphi^{(BW)}(x)$, against age, and also the log odds on wheeze among miners with breathlessness, $\varphi^{(W)}(x) + \varphi^{(BW)}(x)$. Problem 11.7 also looks at the logarithm of the marginal odds on breathlessness and the logarithm of the marginal odds on wheeze, which are obtained by adding the appropriate terms from the fitted probabilities (11.33)–(11.36) before forming the log odds.

The quadratic term $\hat{\beta}_2^{(W)} = -0.018$ for $\varphi^{(W)}$, which indicates the deceleration of the prevalence of wheeze among miners without breathlessness seen in Figure 11.7, is highly significant [Wald test z-score $= \hat{\beta}_2^{(W)} / \widehat{\text{se}}(\hat{\beta}_2^{(W)}) = -0.018/0.0049 = -3.6$]. However, the estimated quadratic coefficient $\hat{\beta}_2^{(B)}$ for the log odds on breathlessness among miners without wheeze and the quadratic coefficient $\hat{\beta}_2^{(BW)}$ for the log odds ratio are not significantly different from zero. The results of constraining these two coefficients to equal 0 and refitting the model are shown in Table 11.7. The goodness-of-fit statistic for this model, say H_{00}, still indicates a good fit: $G^2(H_{00} : H_1) = 19.824$ on 20 df. The difference in log-likelihood ratio statistics is $G^2(H_{00} : H_1) - G^2(H_0 : H_1) = G^2(H_{00} : H_0) = 19.824 - 17.656 = 2.168$ with 2 df ($p = 0.34$), which indicates that the two quadratic coefficients for $\varphi^{(B)}$ and $\varphi^{(BW)}$ do not significantly improve the fit of the model to the data. The estimated coefficients from the reduced model were entered into (11.37)–(11.39), and Figures 11.6–11.8 show the fitted natural parameters as smooth curves for values of x in the interval [22.5, 62.5]. The figures confirm the good fit of the model.

One might question the use of a quadratic age model on the grounds that for sufficiently old ages, the predicted log odds on wheeze would start to decrease. The objection is moot given the age span in the data set, but one could also use a logarithmic explanatory factor, say ln(age), which would increase monotonically, instead of the quadratic age term. As explained in Section 11.2, this model would be justified by assuming age distributions in the gamma or chi squared family among miners in each of the four categories of respiratory symptoms. The model with linear and logarithmic age terms fits the data about as well as the quadratic model, with virtually identical fitted curves (results not shown).

The reduced model with only seven parameters gives a parsimonious parameterization of the multinomial response model for these data. The elegance of the model compares favorably with the approach using log-linear models for all three variables (breathlessness, wheeze, and age). The latter approach, followed in Gokhale and Kullback (1978), results in a more complicated analysis because of the need to fit parameters for the distributions of age. Restricting the dependent variable to the double dichotomy and conditioning on age as an explanatory factor allows us to focus on the essential relations of the model.

Table 11.6. *Model (11.37)–(11.39) fitted to data of Table 11.5*

Explanatory Factor	$\varphi^{(B)}(x)$				$\varphi^{(W)}(x)$				$\varphi^{(BW)}(x)$			
	mle	se	z	p	mle	se	z	p	mle	se	z	p
Constant	−3.428	0.0648	−52.9	0.000	−1.922	0.0344	−55.8	0.000	2.994	0.0808	37.1	0.000
(Age − 42.5)/5	0.529	0.0303	17.5	0.000	0.202	0.0116	17.4	0.000	−0.143	0.0376	−3.82	0.000
{(Age − 42.5)/5}^{2}	−0.013	0.0101	−1.30	0.194	−0.018	0.0049	−3.60	0.000	0.008	0.0125	0.619	0.535

Goodness-of-fit statistic $G^2(H_0 : H_1) = 17.656$ on 18 df.

Table 11.7. *Results of fitting reduced model (11.37)–(11.39) with quadratic coefficients for $\varphi^{(B)}$ and $\varphi^{(BW)}$ constrained to be zero*

Explanatory Factor	$\varphi^{(B)}(x)$				$\varphi^{(W)}(x)$				$\varphi^{(BW)}(x)$			
	mle	se	z	p	mle	se	z	p	mle	se	z	p
Constant	−3.470	0.0564	−61.5	0.000	−1.916	0.0320	−59.9	0.000	3.019	0.0706	42.8	0.000
(Age − 42.5)/5	0.505	0.0222	22.7	0.000	0.203	0.0116	17.5	0.000	−0.127	0.0289	−4.40	0.000
{(Age − 42.5)/5}^{2}	0	—	—	—	−0.019	0.0041	−4.59	0.000	0	—	—	—

Goodness-of-fit statistic $G^2(H_{00} : H_1) = 19.824$ on 20 df.

11.4.2. A General Framework for Multinomial Responses: The Exponential Family of Distributions

We now consider the general multinomial response model of Bock (1970, 1975), built along lines similar to the prefactor-postfactor multivariate model of Roy (1957). In this section we define the *response structure* for a general polytomous response and consider several examples. The unifying theory is that of the exponential family of distributions (see, e.g., Lehmann, 1997); specifically, all of the examples are discrete linear exponential family distributions. In the next subsection, we allow the natural parameters to be functions of explanatory factors, thus arriving at the general logistic regression model.

Let the discrete outcome variable Y take values in a set Υ with m elements. The elements in Υ can be identified with any set of m labels, such as $\{1, 2, \ldots, m\}$, or any other elements suitable to the application. For example, the double dichotomy considered above takes values in the set $\Upsilon = \{(y_1, y_2): y_i = 0 \text{ or } 1\}$. An *exponential family* of distributions for Y over the outcome space Υ is specified by a collection of s *sufficient statistics*, $t_1(y), \ldots, t_s(y)$, defined for y in Υ; a corresponding set of *natural parameters*, $\varphi_1, \ldots, \varphi_s$; and a set of weights with $a_j \geq 0$ called the *dominating measure*. The family of distributions is defined as

$$P(Y = y) = P(Y = y \mid \varphi_1, \ldots, \varphi_s; a_1, \ldots, a_m)$$

$$= a_y \exp\{-\psi(\varphi_1, \ldots, \varphi_s) + \varphi_1 t_1(y) + \cdots + \varphi_s t_s(y)\} \qquad \text{for } y \in \Upsilon, \tag{11.40}$$

where $\psi = \psi(\varphi_1, \ldots, \varphi_s)$ is a normalizing constant which ensures that the terms in (11.40) sum to 1 over y in Υ:

$$\psi(\varphi_1, \ldots, \varphi_s) = \ln\left[\sum_{y \in \Upsilon} a_y \exp\{\varphi_1 t_1(y) + \cdots + \varphi_s t_s(y)\}\right]. \tag{11.41}$$

A surprisingly large number of problems involving categorical data can be put into exponential family form, depending on the choice of sufficient statistics and dominating measure. We examine some examples below.

The Unordered Multinomial Response

If Y is an unordered categorical response, we identify the outcomes arbitrarily with the elements of $\Upsilon = \{1, \ldots, m\}$, set the dominating measure to be $a_1 = \cdots = a_m = 1$, and define the sufficient statistics $t_1(y), \ldots, t_{m-1}(y)$ as

$$t_j(y) = \begin{cases} 1 & \text{if } y = j, \\ 0 & \text{if } y \neq j \end{cases} \tag{11.42}$$

for $j = 1, \ldots, s$ with $s = m - 1$. This choice of sufficient statistics encodes category m as a reference category and endows the natural parameter φ_j with an interpretation as the logit parameter

$$\varphi_j = \ln \frac{P(Y=j)}{P(Y=m)}. \tag{11.43}$$

To see this, we have from (11.40)

$$\ln P(Y=j) = \ln a_j - \psi(\varphi_1, \ldots, \varphi_{m-1}) + \varphi_1 t_1(j) + \cdots + \varphi_{m-1} t_{m-1}(j)$$
$$= -\psi(\varphi_1, \ldots, \varphi_{m-1}) + \varphi_j$$

and similarly

$$\ln P(Y=m) = -\psi(\varphi_1, \ldots, \varphi_{m-1}),$$

so that, by subtraction, φ_j is given by the logit (11.43). When logit parameters use the same cell probability in their denominators, they are said, in the terminology of generalized linear models, to follow the "canonical link." The specific choice of reference category is arbitrary.

Given a sample $y_1, \ldots, y_N$ of N independent multinomial responses from (11.40), the likelihood function is

$$L(\varphi_1, \ldots, \varphi_{m-1} | y_1, \ldots, y_N)$$
$$= \exp\left(-N\psi(\varphi_1, \ldots, \varphi_{m-1}) + \varphi_1 \sum_{i=1}^{N} t_1(y_i) + \cdots + \varphi_{m-1} \sum_{i=1}^{N} t_{m-1}(y_i) \right). \tag{11.44}$$

The sufficient statistics, now the sums of the t_j's over the sample values $y_1, \ldots, y_N$, are simply the cell frequencies in the multinomial sample, say $n_1, \ldots, n_{m-1}$, with $n_j = \sum_{i=1}^{N} t_j(y_i)$. The reference cell frequency n_m is obtainable by subtraction from N $[n_m = N - (n_1 + \cdots + n_{m-1})]$, so it need not be included in the list of *minimal* sufficient statistics.

The Ordered Multinomial Response

If there is a natural ordering to the m outcomes, we identify $\{1, \ldots, m\}$ with the outcomes in this ordering and again choose the dominating measure to be $a_1 = \cdots = a_m = 1$. Now, let

$$t_j(y) = \begin{cases} 1 & \text{if } y > j, \\ 0 & \text{if } y \le j \end{cases} \qquad \text{for } j = 1, \ldots, s = m - 1. \tag{11.45}$$

This choice encodes category 1 as the reference category, with $\ln P(Y = 1) = -\psi$, and endows the natural parameters with the interpretation as *adjacent logits*,

$$\varphi_j = \ln \frac{P(Y=j+1)}{P(Y=j)} \qquad \text{for } j = 1, \ldots, s = m - 1. \qquad (11.46)$$

To see this, we have from (11.40) $\ln P(Y = 1) = -\psi(\varphi_1, \ldots, \varphi_{m-1})$, and for $j > 1$, $\ln P(Y = j + 1) = -\psi(\varphi_1, \ldots, \varphi_{m-1}) + \varphi_1 + \cdots + \varphi_j$, while $\ln P(Y = j)$ $= -\psi(\varphi_1, \ldots, \varphi_{m-1}) + \varphi_1 + \cdots + \varphi_{j-1}$, so, by subtraction, φ_j is the adjacent logit (11.46).

Given a sample $y_1, \ldots, y_N$ of N independent multinomial responses, the likelihood function is

$$L(\varphi, \ldots, \varphi_{m-1} | y_1, \ldots, y_N) = \exp\{-N\psi(\varphi_1, \ldots, \varphi_{m-1})$$
$$+ \varphi_1(n_2 + \cdots + n_m) + \varphi_2(n_3 + \cdots + n_m) + \cdots + \varphi_{m-1}n_m\}, \quad (11.47)$$

that is, the sufficient statistics $\sum_{i=1}^{N} t_j(y_i)$ are the cumulative cell frequencies $n_{j+1} + \cdots + n_m$ for $j = 1, \ldots, m - 1$.

A parameterization that is not represented by (11.40) is the cumulative logit model of McCullagh (1980) (see Section 9.5). Specifying parameters as cumulative logits as in (9.52) results in a nonlinear exponential family more complex than the linear exponential family considered here. Another parameterization for an ordered categorical outcome uses so-called *conditional log odds*:

$$\ln \frac{P(Y=j)}{P(Y>j)} \qquad \text{for } j = 1, \ldots, m - 1. \qquad (11.48)$$

An advantage of this choice is that estimates of (11.48) based on sample proportions are uncorrelated. Thus, saturated models can be reduced to a sequence of separate binary logistic regression problems. Models imposing parameter constraints lose this simplification, however. Figure 11.9 diagrams various ways to parameterize an ordered multinomial response. The first and last are covered by (11.40).

Instead of comparing $P(Y = j)$ with $P(Y > j)$ using the conditional odds parameterization, one might compare $P(Y = j)$ with an *average* of the probabilities $P(Y = k)$ for $k > j$. In the example of injury severity considered in Chapter 9, one might consider the odds of a response in the lowest category of severity versus an average probability of response in more severe categories; then the odds of a response in the second lowest category of severity versus an average probability of response in categories more severe than that; and so on. If for the "average" probability of response we agree to use the *geometric mean* of the probabilities, then model (11.40) again applies. For

Multinomial Probabilities:

P_1	P_2	P_3	$\cdots$	P_k

1. Adjacent odds model:

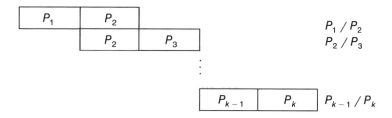

P_1 / P_2
P_2 / P_3

P_{k-1} / P_k

2. Cumulative odds model:

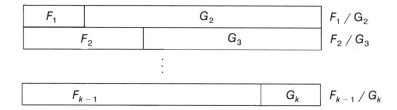

F_1 / G_2
F_2 / G_3

F_{k-1} / G_k

3. Conditional odds model:

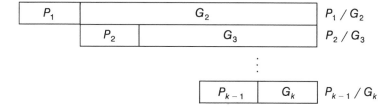

P_1 / G_2
P_2 / G_3

P_{k-1} / G_k

4. Canonical odds model:

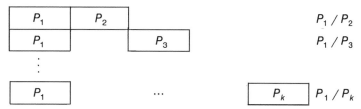

P_1 / P_2
P_1 / P_3

P_1 / P_k

Figure 11.9

example, suppose we define the natural parameters as follows:

$$\varphi_1 = \ln P(Y=1) - \frac{1}{m-1} \sum_{j=2}^{m} \ln P(Y=j) = \ln \frac{P(Y=1)}{\sqrt[m-1]{\prod_{j=2}^{m} P(Y=j)}}$$

$$= \ln \frac{P(Y=1)}{\text{geometric mean of } P(Y=2),\ldots,P(Y=m)},$$

$$\varphi_2 = \ln P(Y=2) - \frac{1}{m-2} \sum_{j=3}^{m} \ln P(Y=j) = \ln \frac{P(Y=2)}{\sqrt[m-2]{\prod_{j=3}^{m} P(Y=j)}}$$

$$= \ln \frac{P(Y=2)}{\text{geometric mean of } P(Y=2),\ldots,P(Y=m)},$$

$$\vdots$$

$$\varphi_{m-1} = \ln P(Y=m-1) - \ln P(Y=m) = \ln \frac{P(Y=m-1)}{P(Y=m)}. \qquad (11.49)$$

The reader is asked to check in Problem 11.8 that these natural parameters can be defined via the sufficient statistics

$$t_j(y) = \begin{cases} \dfrac{1}{m-j+1} & \text{if } y < j, \\ 1 & \text{if } y = j, \\ 0 & \text{if } y > j \end{cases} \qquad \text{for } j = 1,\ldots,m-1. \quad (11.50)$$

Nested Responses

Sometimes response categories are nested hierarchically, as when different questions are asked in an interview depending on responses to a lead-in question. In such cases we can compare an average (read geometric mean) of the response probabilities nested within one set of categories with an average of the response probabilities nested within another set of categories. These cases are conveniently handled using *orthogonal contrasts* of log probabilities.

For example, suppose a "yes" response to the lead-in question results either in response category 1 or 2 to the followup question, while a "no" response to the lead-in results in either response category 3 or 4 to its followup question. Set $\Upsilon = \{1,2,3,4\}$. There are three contrasts of interest: the log odds on response 1 versus 2 (nested within "yes" to the lead-in), the log odds on response 3 versus 4 (nested within "no" to the lead-in), and the log of the ratio of the geometric mean probability of response following "yes" to that following "no":

$$\varphi_1 = \ln P(Y = 1) - \ln P(Y = 2), \quad \varphi_2 = \ln P(Y = 3) - \ln P(Y = 4),$$
$$\varphi_3 = \tfrac{1}{2}\{\ln P(Y = 1) + \ln P(Y = 2)\} \tag{11.51}$$
$$- \tfrac{1}{2}\{\ln P(Y = 3) + \ln P(Y = 4)\}.$$

The reader is asked to check in Problem 11.9 that φ_1, φ_2, φ_3 result from the sufficient statistics

$$
t_1(y) = \begin{cases} \tfrac{1}{2} & \text{if } y = 1, \\ -\tfrac{1}{2} & \text{if } y = 2, \end{cases}
$$

$$
t_2(y) = \begin{cases} \tfrac{1}{2} & \text{if } y = 3, \\ -\tfrac{1}{2} & \text{if } y = 4, \end{cases} \tag{11.52}
$$

$$
t_3(y) = \begin{cases} \tfrac{1}{2} & \text{if } y = 1 \text{ or } 2, \\ -\tfrac{1}{2} & \text{if } y = 3 \text{ or } 4. \end{cases}
$$

Log-Linear Models for Multiway Contingency Tables

In cross-sectional studies with a sample of size N, we may have d categorical variables, say $V_1, \ldots, V_d$, with $I_1, \ldots, I_d$ levels, respectively, cross-classified to produce a d-dimensional $I_1 \times I_2 \times \cdots \times I_d$ multiway contingency table with cell frequencies given by

$$\{ n_{i_1 i_2 \cdots i_d} : i_1 = 1, \ldots, I_1; \ldots; i_d = 1, \ldots, I_d \}. \tag{11.53}$$

To avoid notation with multiple levels of subscripts, consider the case of a three-way, $2 \times 3 \times 4$ table with cell frequencies $\{ n_{ijk} : i = 1, 2, \ j = 1, 2, 3, \ k = 1, 2, 3, 4 \}$ with $\sum_{ijk} n_{ijk} = N$, and call the three variables A, B, and C instead of V_1, V_2, and V_3. The class of log-linear models is represented by (11.40) with $\Upsilon = \{(i, j, k): i = 1, 2, \ j = 1, 2, 3, \text{ and } k = 1, 2, 3, 4\}$ and the following system of sufficient statistics:

One-factor terms:

$$
t_i^{(A)}(y) = \begin{cases} 1 & \text{if } y_1 = i, \\ 0 & \text{if } y_1 \neq i \end{cases} \qquad \text{for } i = 1, \ldots, I_1 - 1 = 1; \tag{11.54a}
$$

$$
t_j^{(B)}(y) = \begin{cases} 1 & \text{if } y_2 = j, \\ 0 & \text{if } y_2 \neq j \end{cases} \qquad \text{for } j = 1, \ldots, I_2 - 1 = 2; \tag{11.54b}
$$

$$
t_k^{(C)}(y) = \begin{cases} 1 & \text{if } y_3 = k, \\ 0 & \text{if } y_3 \neq k \end{cases} \qquad \text{for } k = 1, \ldots, I_3 - 1 = 3. \tag{11.54c}
$$

Two-factor terms:

$$t_{ij}^{(AB)}(y) = t_i^{(A)}(y)t_j^{(B)}(y) = \begin{cases} 1 & \text{if } (y_1, y_2) = (i, j), \\ 0 & \text{if } (y_1, y_2) \neq (i, j) \end{cases}$$

$$\text{for } i = 1, \ldots, I_1 - 1 = 1 \text{ and } j = 1, \ldots, I_2 - 1 = 2; \quad (11.55a)$$

$$t_{ik}^{(AC)}(y) = t_i^{(A)}(y)t_k^{(C)}(y) = \begin{cases} 1 & \text{if } (y_1, y_3) = (i, k), \\ 0 & \text{if } (y_1, y_3) \neq (i, k) \end{cases}$$

$$\text{for } i = 1, \ldots, I_1 - 1 = 1 \text{ and } k = 1, \ldots, I_3 - 1 = 3; \quad (11.55b)$$

$$t_{jk}^{(BC)}(y) = t_j^{(B)}(y)t_k^{(C)}(y) = \begin{cases} 1 & \text{if } (y_2, y_3) = (j, k), \\ 0 & \text{if } (y_2, y_3) \neq (j, k) \end{cases}$$

$$\text{for } j = 1, \ldots, I_2 - 1 = 2 \text{ and } k = 1, \ldots, I_3 - 1 = 3. \quad (11.55c)$$

Three-factor terms:

$$t_{ijk}^{(ABC)}(y) = t_i^{(A)}(y)t_j^{(B)}(y)t_k^{(C)}(y) = \begin{cases} 1 & \text{if } (y_1, y_2, y_3) = (i, j, k), \\ 0 & \text{if } (y_1, y_2, y_3) \neq (i, j, k) \end{cases}$$

$$\text{for } i = 1, \ldots, I_1 - 1 = 1, \ j = 1, \ldots, I_2 - 1 = 2,$$
$$\text{and } k = 1, \ldots, I_3 - 1 = 3. \quad (11.56)$$

The system extends to higher-way tables similarly: for each level l of factors and each choice of variables $V_{i_1}, \ldots, V_{i_l}$, there is a species of sufficient statistic

$$t_{\nu_{i_1} \cdots \nu_{i_l}}^{V_{i_1} \cdots V_{i_l}}(y) = \begin{cases} 1 & \text{if } (y_{i_1}, \ldots, y_{i_l}) = (\nu_{i_1}, \ldots, \nu_{i_l}), \\ 0 & \text{if } (y_{i_1}, \ldots, y_{i_l}) \neq (\nu_{i_1}, \ldots, \nu_{i_l}) \end{cases} \quad (11.57)$$

for indices $\nu_{i_1} = 1, \ldots, I_{i_1} - 1, \ldots, \ \nu_{i_l} = 1, \ldots, I_{i_l} - 1$. This system identifies the cell with all "maximal" subscripts $(I_1, \ldots, I_d)$ as reference category, and creates the following interpretations for the natural parameters, which in this context are called log-linear parameters:

(i) Any natural parameter with a maximal subscript is zero. In the example, these are

$$\varphi_2^{(A)} = \varphi_3^{(B)} = \varphi_4^{(C)} = \varphi_{i3}^{(AB)} = \varphi_{2j}^{(AB)} = \varphi_{i4}^{(AC)} = \varphi_{2k}^{(AC)} = \varphi_{j4}^{(BC)} = \varphi_{3k}^{(BC)}$$

$$= \varphi_{ij4}^{(ABC)} = \varphi_{i3k}^{(ABC)} = \varphi_{2jk}^{(ABC)} = 0$$

for any i, j, and k. In general, $\varphi_{\nu_{i_1}, \ldots, \nu_{i_l}}^{(V_{i_1}, \ldots, V_{i_l})} = 0$ if any subscript $\nu_{i_j} = I_{i_j}$.

(ii) One-factor φ parameters are log odds parameters comparing the cell probability having the given subscript in the named variable with the probability of the reference cell, where all unnamed variables are set equal to their maximal subscript. For example,

$$\varphi_i^{(A)} = \ln \frac{P\{Y = (i, 3, 4)\}}{P\{Y = (2, 3, 4)\}} \qquad \text{for } i = 1,$$

$$\varphi_j^{(B)} = \ln \frac{P\{Y = (2, j, 4)\}}{P\{Y = (2, 3, 4)\}} \qquad \text{for } j = 1, 2, \tag{11.58}$$

$$\varphi_k^{(C)} = \ln \frac{P\{Y = (2, 3, k)\}}{P\{Y = (2, 3, 4)\}} \qquad \text{for } k = 1, 2, 3.$$

(iii) Two-factor φ parameters are log odds ratios for the 2×2 subtable formed from the named subscripts and other cells with maximal subscripts. Thus

$$\varphi_{ij}^{(AB)} = \ln \frac{P\{Y = (i, j, 4)\} \cdot P\{Y = (2, 3, 4)\}}{P\{Y = (i, 3, 4)\} \cdot P\{Y = (2, j, 4)\}} \qquad \text{for } i = 1 \text{ and } j = 1, 2,$$

$$\varphi_{ik}^{(AC)} = \ln \frac{P\{Y = (i, 3, k)\} \cdot P\{Y = (2, 3, 4)\}}{P\{Y = (i, 3, 4)\} \cdot P\{Y = (2, 3, k)\}} \qquad \text{for } i = 1 \text{ and } k = 1, 2, 3,$$

$$\varphi_{jk}^{(BC)} = \ln \frac{P\{Y = (2, j, k)\} \cdot P\{Y = (2, 3, 4)\}}{P\{Y = (2, j, 4)\} \cdot P\{Y = (2, 3, k)\}} \qquad \text{for } j = 1, 2 \text{ and } k = 1, 2, 3.$$

$$\tag{11.59}$$

(iv) Three-factor φ parameters are log ratios of odds ratios, with unnamed variables set to their maximal subscripts. For example,

$$\varphi_{ijk}^{(ABC)} = \ln \left[\frac{P\{Y = (i, j, k)\} \cdot P\{Y = (i, 3, 4)\}}{P\{Y = (i, j, 4)\} \cdot P\{Y = (i, 3, k)\}} \middle/ \frac{P\{Y = (2, j, k)\} \cdot P\{Y = (2, 3, 4)\}}{P\{Y = (2, j, 4)\} \cdot P\{Y = (2, 3, k)\}} \right]$$

$$\text{for } i = 1, \, j = 1, 2, \text{ and } k = 1, 2, 3.$$

$$\tag{11.60}$$

And so on. Higher-order φ parameters are logarithms of ratios of ratios of ... of odds ratios. The reader may check that the sufficient statistics for the likelihood function based on a sample of size N are the *marginal configurations* corresponding to the φ parameters present in the model. Thus the *saturated* model, with all φ parameters present, has sufficient statistics $\{n_{i..}\}$, $\{n_{.j.}\}$, $\{n_{..k}\}$, $\{n_{ij.}\}$, $\{n_{i.k}\}$, $\{n_{.jk}\}$, and $\{n_{ijk}\}$. Since the last set implies the values of all preceding marginal configurations by summing, $\{n_{ijk}\}$ alone is the minimal sufficient statistic.

Parsimony in log-linear models is represented by *unsaturated* models with $s < m - 1$. Most convenient are models that constrain entire species of φ parameters to be zero. For example, the model setting $\varphi_{ijk}^{(ABC)} = 0$ for all (i, j, k), the so-called no-three-factor effect model, is a model of constant odds ratio because, by (11.60), the set of odds ratios involving any two variables at fixed levels of the unnamed variable(s) is constant across all levels of the unnamed variable(s). For the constant-odds-ratio model, the three marginal configurations $\{n_{ij.}\}$, $\{n_{i.k}\}$, and $\{n_{.jk}\}$ constitute the minimal sufficient statistic. There are no closed-form formulas for $P\{Y = (i, j, k)\}$ in terms of marginal probabilities. Maximum likelihood estimates of φ parameters and expected cell frequencies must be obtained by iterative computation.

Another model of interest is $H_{00}: \varphi_{ij}^{(AB)} = \varphi_{ijk}^{(ABC)} = 0$ for all (i, j, k). In this case the model specifies no association between variables A and B given C. That is so because at level 4 of variable C, the log odds ratios between A and B are all equal to 0, since $\varphi_{ij}^{(AB)} = 0$; but because $\varphi_{ijk}^{(ABC)} = 0$, the log odds ratios between A and B at any other level of C are the same, namely, zero. This model may therefore be written succinctly as $A \perp\!\!\!\perp B \,|\, C$, such that, A and B are conditionally independent given C. It follows that

$$P\{Y = (i, j, k)\} = P\{Y = (i, j, k) \,|\, Y_3 = k\} P\{Y_3 = k\}$$
$$= P\{Y_1 = i \,|\, Y_3 = k\} P\{Y_2 = j \,|\, Y_3 = k\} P\{Y_3 = k\}, \quad (11.61)$$

which simplifies calculation of the mle's: from the marginal configurations $\{n_{i.k}\}$ and $\{n_{.jk}\}$, $n_{i.k}/n_{..k}$ is the mle of the first term in (11.61), $n_{.jk}/n_{..k}$ is the mle of the second term, and $n_{..k}/N$ is the mle of the third term. Thus $(n_{i.k} \, n_{.jk})/(Nn_{..k})$ is the mle of $P\{Y = (i, j, k)\}$.

The model $\varphi_{ij}^{(AB)} = \varphi_{ik}^{(AC)} = \varphi_{ijk}^{(ABC)} = 0$ for all (i, j, k) can be identified with the relation $A \perp\!\!\!\perp (B, C)$, that is, variable A is completely independent of the joint variable (B, C), with

$$P\{Y = (i, j, k)\} = P\{Y_1 = i\} P\{(Y_2, Y_3) = (j, k)\}. \quad (11.62)$$

Its mle is $n_{i..} \, n_{.jk}/N^2$.

The model $\varphi_{ij}^{(AB)} = \varphi_{ik}^{(AC)} = \varphi_{jk}^{(BC)} = \varphi_{ijk}^{(ABC)} = 0$ for all (i, j, k), the so-called no-two-factor effect model, specifies the relation of mutual independence, $A \perp\!\!\!\perp B \perp\!\!\!\perp C$, with

$$P\{Y = (i, j, k)\} = P\{Y_1 = i\} P\{Y_2 = j\} P\{Y_3 = k\}. \quad (11.63)$$

Its mle is $n_{i..} \, n_{.j.} \, n_{..k}/N^3$.

As seen from the foregoing, the number of log-linear models one can entertain grows rapidly with the number of cross-classification variables.

Thus, whenever feasible, we prefer to use a logistic regression model for a smaller number of dependent cross-classification variables with other variables serving as explanatory factors, as we did in the coal miner example, rather than treating all variables in a model as dependent.

The Noncentral Multiple Hypergeometric Distribution

Chapter 9 discussed the statistical analysis of several proportions, but deferred discussion of the exact analysis of such data. We touch on that briefly here. Suppose we have M binomial random variables $Y_1, \ldots, Y_M$, with $Y_i \sim \mathrm{Bin}(n_i, P_i)$ for $i = 1, \ldots, M$. The joint conditional distribution of $Y_1, \ldots, Y_M$ with given fixed sum $S = Y_1 + \cdots + Y_M = s$ is said to have the noncentral multiple hypergeometric distribution with odds ratio parameters $\omega_1, \ldots, \omega_{M-1}$, where for $j = 1, \ldots, M-1$ we have $\omega_j = \{P_j/(1 - P_j)\}/\{P_M/(1 - P_M)\}$. As in the case of the univariate noncentral hypergeometric distribution discussed in Chapter 6, the joint conditional distribution depends on the binomial parameters $P_1, \ldots, P_M$ only through the odds ratios $\omega_1, \ldots, \omega_{M-1}$ (see Problem 11.10). The probability function for the noncentral multiple hypergeometric distribution is

$$P(Y_1 = y_1, \ldots, Y_M = y_M \mid S = s, n_1, \ldots, n_M, \omega_1, \ldots, \omega_{M-1})$$

$$= \frac{\binom{n_1}{y_1} \cdots \binom{n_M}{y_M} \omega_1^{y_1} \cdots \omega_{M-1}^{y_{M-1}}}{\sum_{\underline{u}} \binom{n_1}{u_1} \cdots \binom{n_M}{u_M} \omega_1^{u_1} \cdots \omega_{M-1}^{u_{M-1}}}, \tag{11.64}$$

where the sum in the denominator of (11.64) is taken over the set of all integer-valued vectors $\underline{u}$ of length M with $0 \le u_j \le n_j$ and $u_1 + \cdots + u_M = s$. Call this set $D_M(s; n_1, \ldots, n_M)$.

Expression (11.64) can be put into the exponential family form (11.40) as follows. First take $\Upsilon = D_M(s; n_1, \ldots, n_M)$, and enumerate all m vectors $Y = (Y_1, \ldots, Y_M)$ in Υ, identifying these as possible outcomes of a multinomial response in m categories. The number m of such outcomes may be large, but the exact analysis of the $2 \times M$ table is of greatest interest when it is feasible to do the enumeration. The dominating measure is taken as

$$a_y = \binom{n_1}{y_1} \cdots \binom{n_M}{y_M},$$

and the sufficient statistics are simply $t_j(y) = y_j$ for $j = 1, \ldots, M-1$. The natural parameters are the log odds ratios $\varphi_j = \ln \omega_j$ for $j = 1, \ldots, M-1$. With these identifications, (11.40) represents the distribution (11.64), and the entire $2 \times M$ table becomes a single multinomial response from this exponential family.

Table 11.8. *Data of Table 9.2 rearranged*

	Study				
	1	2	3	4	Total
Smokers	83	90	129	70	372
Nonsmokers	3	3	7	12	25
Total	86	93	136	82	397

The exact distribution of test statistics such as chi squared may be calculated with the enumerated distribution. Here we focus on a different aspect of an exact analysis—calculation of conditional maximum likelihood estimates for the log odds ratios. In fact, using software designed to find maximum likelihood estimates of the natural parameters in (11.40), we obtain the *conditional* maximum likelihood estimates of the log odds ratios $\varphi_j = \ln \omega_j$ which maximize the conditional likelihood function given by (11.62).

As an example, consider the data of Table 9.2, which we present in slightly rearranged form in Table 11.8. Let Y_j denote the number of smokers in the jth study ($j = 1, \ldots, 4$). Conditioning on the margins (86, 93, 136, 82) and $s = 372$ of the 2×4 table results in $m = 3{,}276$ possible outcomes for the sufficient statistic (Y_1, Y_2, Y_3) with nonzero dominating measure. The observed table corresponds to the multinomial response with sufficient statistic (83, 96, 129). Maximizing the likelihood (11.40) for this single multinomial response yields the mle's $(\hat{\varphi}_1, \hat{\varphi}_2, \hat{\varphi}_3) = (1.552, 1.633, 1.146)$ with estimated standard errors (0.665, 0.664, 0.497) and Wald test z-scores (2.33, 2.46, 2.30). The conditional mle's of the odds ratios, (4.72, 5.12, 3.15), are close to the unconditional maximum likelihood estimates (4.74, 5.14, 3.16), which are the cross-product ratios for each study compared to study 4. A likelihood ratio test of the hypothesis that $\omega_1 = \omega_2 = \omega_3$, namely, that studies 1, 2, and 3 have the same proportion of smokers, is obtained by subtracting -2 times the multinomial log likelihood, 8.883, for the saturated model (H_1: ω_j arbitrary) from that for the reduced model (H_0: $\omega_1 = \omega_2 = \omega_3 = \omega$), 9.514. Thus $G^2(H_0 : H_1) = 9.514 - 8.883 = 0.631$ on 2 df ($p = 0.73$). We conclude that the three odds ratios underlying studies 1, 2, and 3 are not significantly different. The conditional maximum likelihood estimate of the common odds ratio ω is $\hat{\omega} = \exp(\hat{\varphi}) = \exp(1.3773) = 3.96$ with the estimated standard error of $\hat{\varphi}$ equal to 0.4209.

Conditional maximum likelihood estimation is taken up in greater detail in Chapter 14. The conclusion to be drawn here is that model (11.40) can accommodate conditional distributions quite naturally, and even complicated expressions like (11.64) offer no special theoretical difficulties.

Binomial Goodness of Fit

In Section 9.6.3 we considered whether a sample of N random variables $X_1, \ldots, X_N$ could be accepted as binomial random variables, $X_j \sim \text{Bin}(g, P)$, with constant P, or whether there was random heterogeneity in the parameter P. To do that, we viewed each count X_j as a multinomial response taking values in the set $\Upsilon = \{0, 1, \ldots, g\}$ so that $m = g + 1$. Under the null hypothesis of no heterogeneity, we now write the binomial distribution in exponential family form as

$$P(X_i = j | g, P) = \binom{g}{j} P^j (1 - P)^{g-j} = P(Y = j | g, \varphi)$$

$$= \binom{g}{j} \exp\{-\psi(\varphi) + \varphi j\}, \tag{11.65}$$

where $\psi(\varphi) = \ln\left\{\sum_{j=0}^{g} \binom{g}{j} \exp(\varphi j)\right\}$. Thus the dominating measure is the binomial coefficient $a_j = \binom{g}{j}$, the sufficient statistic is simply $t(y) = y$, and the natural parameter is $\varphi = \ln\{P/(1 - P)\}$. Under the alternative hypothesis, we specify the sufficient statistics for the multinomial response to be (11.45) for $j = 0, \ldots, g - 1$, in which case the natural parameters become the adjacent logit-plus-offset parameters

$$\varphi_j = \ln \frac{P(Y = j + 1) \Big/ \binom{g}{j+1}}{P(Y = j) \Big/ \binom{g}{j}}$$

that played an important role in the general empirical Bayes analysis of Section 9.6.3. In particular, we used the model $\varphi_j = \alpha_g + \beta j$ in (9.83) to test for binomial homogeneity by testing $\beta = 0$.

Many other examples of (11.40) are useful in applications. Levin and Shrout (1981) show generally how to interpret the natural parameters $\varphi_1, \ldots, \varphi_s$ for given sufficient statistics $t_1(y), \ldots, t_s(y)$ in terms of contrasts of log multinomial cell probabilities and, conversely, given an interpretation of $\varphi_1, \ldots, \varphi_s$ as certain desired contrasts of log probabilities, they show how to construct appropriate sufficient statistics $t_1(y), \ldots, t_s(y)$ to accomplish the task. They also consider the use of constrained maximum likelihood estimation and affine transformation of parameters to impose linear constraints on the natural parameters. We used this technique to fit model (9.83).

Next we turn to the modeling of the natural parameters as functions of explanatory factors.

11.4.3.*   General Logistic Regression

In the preceding section, for each multinomial response model examined, we assumed a single sample of data. Here we allow each of the natural parameters $\varphi_1, \ldots, \varphi_s$ to depend on r explanatory factors, say $\underline{X} = (X_1, \ldots, X_r)'$, which vary over n independent samples. This section provides the basic statistical results for a maximum likelihood analysis of the general logistic regression model in this case. It is more challenging because it uses matrices and deals with multivariate concepts.

Notation

As in the coal miner example at (11.37)–(11.39), we assume s linear expressions of the form

$$\varphi_1(\underline{X}) = \beta_{11} X_1 + \cdots + \beta_{r1} X_r,$$
$$\varphi_s(\underline{X}) = \beta_{1s} X_1 + \cdots + \beta_{rs} X_r. \tag{11.66}$$

We assume that we have data from n independent groups of subjects, corresponding to explanatory factors $\underline{X}_{(i)} = (X_{i1}, \ldots, X_{ir})'$ for $i = 1, \ldots, n$, each with a multinomial sample of size $N_i \geq 1$, with cell frequencies $N_{i1}, \ldots, N_{im}$ summing to N_i. We collect the various items of information into the following matrices.

(i) *Sample Design Array.* As in the familiar multiple regression model for continuous dependent variables, the $n \times r$ sample design matrix contains the vectors $\underline{X}_{(i)}$ as rows:

$$\underset{n \times r}{X} = \begin{bmatrix} \underline{X}'_{(1)} \\ \vdots \\ \underline{X}'_{(n)} \end{bmatrix} = \begin{bmatrix} X_{11} & \cdots & X_{1r} \\ \vdots & & \vdots \\ X_{n1} & \cdots & X_{nr} \end{bmatrix}. \tag{11.67}$$

It is conventional to take the first column of X to be the constant 1, in which case $\beta_{11}, \ldots, \beta_{1s}$ are intercepts for the natural parameters.

(ii) *Response Design Array.* The s sufficient statistics $t_1(y), \ldots, t_s(y)$ evaluated at each of the m elements in the response set Υ form an $s \times m$ matrix called the response design array, T:

$$\underset{s \times m}{T} = \begin{bmatrix} t_1(y_1) & \cdots & t_1(y_m) \\ \vdots & & \vdots \\ t_s(y_1) & \cdots & t_s(y_m) \end{bmatrix}. \tag{11.68}$$

The response design array encodes the interpretation of the natural parameters discussed in the previous section.

(iii) *Frequency Data Array.* The multinomial frequencies for each independent group are collected into the $n \times m$ frequency data array, N:

$$\underset{n \times m}{N} = \begin{bmatrix} N_{11} & \cdots & N_{1m} \\ \vdots & & \vdots \\ N_{n1} & \cdots & N_{nm} \end{bmatrix}. \tag{11.69}$$

The rows of N sum to N_i for $i = 1, \ldots, n$. Individual-level multinomial response data correspond to $N_1 = \cdots = N_n = 1$; replicate observations, such as arise with discrete explanatory factors, have sample sizes $N_i \geq 1$.

(iv) *Dominating Measure Array*. The dominating measure weights for each independent sample form an $n \times m$ matrix called the dominating measure array, A:

$$\underset{n \times m}{A} = \begin{bmatrix} a_{11} & \cdots & a_{1m} \\ \vdots & & \vdots \\ a_{n1} & \cdots & a_{nm} \end{bmatrix}. \tag{11.70}$$

Note that the dominating measure may vary from row to row, as is the case with the binomial model (11.65) with $a_{gj} = \binom{g}{j}$ for independent samples of binomial count data with varying indices $g = 1, \ldots, n$. We allow zero values for the dominating measure, e.g., $a_{gj} = \binom{g}{j} = 0$ for $j > g$. It is convenient to write the $n \times m$ array $\ln A = \{\ln a_{ij}\}$, and we shall write $\ln a_{ij}$ even if $a_{ij} = 0$, with the understanding that multinomial outcomes in cells with zero dominating measure do not occur, and so $\ln 0$, though indeterminate, is irrelevant to the statistical analysis.

(v) *Model Cell Probability and Log Probability Arrays*. Define the $n \times m$ matrix of cell probabilities, P:

$$\underset{n \times m}{P} = \begin{bmatrix} P\{Y = 1 \mid \underline{X} = \underline{X}_{(1)}\} & \cdots & P\{Y = m \mid \underline{X} = \underline{X}_{(1)}\} \\ \vdots & & \vdots \\ P\{Y = 1 \mid \underline{X} = \underline{X}_{(n)}\} & \cdots & P\{Y = m \mid \underline{X} = \underline{X}_{(n)}\} \end{bmatrix}, \tag{11.71}$$

and the corresponding matrix of log cell probabilities, L:

$$\underset{n \times m}{L} = \begin{bmatrix} \ln P\{Y = 1 \mid \underline{X} = \underline{X}_{(1)}\} & \cdots & \ln P\{Y = m \mid \underline{X} = \underline{X}_{(1)}\} \\ \vdots & & \vdots \\ \ln P\{Y = 1 \mid \underline{X} = \underline{X}_{(n)}\} & \cdots & \ln P\{Y = m \mid \underline{X} = \underline{X}_{(n)}\} \end{bmatrix}. \tag{11.72}$$

As for the dominating measure array, we interpret $\ln 0$ in components of L as indeterminate but statistically irrelevant.

(vi) *Natural Parameter Array*. The natural parameters vary from group to group due to their dependence on the explanatory factors. We collect these in an $n \times s$ array, Φ:

$$\underset{n \times s}{\Phi} = \begin{bmatrix} \underline{\Phi}'_{(1)} \\ \vdots \\ \underline{\Phi}'_{(n)} \end{bmatrix} = \begin{bmatrix} \varphi_1(\underline{X}_{(1)}) & \cdots & \varphi_s(\underline{X}_{(1)}) \\ \vdots & & \vdots \\ \varphi_1(\underline{X}_{(n)}) & \cdots & \varphi_s(\underline{X}_{(n)}) \end{bmatrix}. \qquad (11.73)$$

(vii) *Logistic Regression Coefficient Array.* The object of the statistical analysis is to draw inferences about the logistic regression coefficients β_{ij}. These are collected in the $r \times s$ logistic regression coefficient array B:

$$\underset{r \times s}{B} = \begin{bmatrix} \beta_{11} & \cdots & \beta_{1s} \\ \vdots & & \vdots \\ \beta_{r1} & \cdots & \beta_{rs} \end{bmatrix}. \qquad (11.74)$$

With these definitions, we can write from the regression part of model (11.66),

$$\underset{1 \times s}{\underline{\Phi}'_{(i)}} = \left[\varphi_i(\underline{X}_{(i)}), \ldots, \varphi_s(\underline{X}_{(i)}) \right] = \underset{1 \times r}{\underline{X}'_{(i)}} \underset{r \times s}{B}, \qquad (11.75)$$

and from the response design part of model (11.40),

$$\underset{1 \times m}{\underline{L}'_{(i)}} = \left[L_{i1} \cdots L_{im} \right]$$

$$= \underset{1 \times m}{[\ln a_{i1}, \ldots, \ln a_{im}]} - \psi\left(\varphi_1(\underline{X}_{(1)}), \ldots, \varphi_s(\underline{X}_{(i)}) \right) \underset{1 \times m}{\underline{1}'_m} + \underset{1 \times s}{\underline{\Phi}'_{(i)}} \underset{s \times m}{T}$$

$$= \underline{(\ln A)}'_{(i)} - \psi\left(\varphi_1(\underline{X}_{(i)}), \ldots, \varphi_s(\underline{X}_{(i)}) \right) \cdot \underline{1}'_m + \underline{X}'_{(i)} BT, \qquad (11.76)$$

where $\underline{1}'_m = (1, \ldots, 1)$ is a row vector of length m consisting of 1's. Putting it all together, the general logistic regression model can be written succinctly as

$$\underset{n \times m}{L} = - \underset{n \times n}{\mathrm{Diag}(\psi_1, \ldots, \psi_n)} \cdot 1_{n \times m} + \underset{n \times r}{X} \underset{r \times s}{B} \underset{s \times m}{T}, \qquad (11.77)$$

where $\mathrm{Diag}(\psi_1, \ldots, \psi_n)$ is an $n \times n$ diagonal matrix with $\psi_i = \psi(\varphi_1(\underline{X}_{(i)}), \ldots, \varphi_s(\underline{X}_{(i)}))$ on the main diagonal, and where $1_{n \times m}$ is an $n \times m$ array of 1's.

To illustrate the notation, consider the simple binary logistic regression model (11.5) with individual-level binary responses $Y_1, \ldots, Y_n$ and explanatory factor observed at values $x_1, \ldots, x_n$. Here $r = 2$, including the constant explanatory factor. The sample design array is

$$\underset{n \times 2}{X} = \begin{bmatrix} 1 & x_1 \\ \vdots & \vdots \\ 1 & x_n \end{bmatrix}, \qquad (11.78)$$

and the response design array for the binary outcome $(m = 2)$ is the 1×2 array

$$T = \begin{bmatrix} 1 & 0 \end{bmatrix}, \tag{11.79}$$

corresponding to the single logit parameter

$$\varphi(x_i) = \ln \frac{P(Y_i = 1 \mid X_i = x_i)}{P(Y_i = 0 \mid X_i = x_i)} = \ln \frac{P_{i1}}{P_{i2}} = L_{i1} - L_{i2}, \tag{11.80}$$

using the identification of outcomes $Y = 1$ or 0 with the elements of the set $\Upsilon = \{1, 2\}$. The frequency data array is the array of 0's and 1's,

$$\underset{n \times 2}{N} = \begin{bmatrix} Y_1 & 1 - Y_1 \\ \vdots & \vdots \\ Y_n & 1 - Y_n \end{bmatrix}, \tag{11.81}$$

and the dominating measure array is the $n \times 2$ matrix of all 1's, $A = 1_{n \times 2}$. The model cell probability array is

$$\underset{n \times 2}{P} = \begin{bmatrix} \dfrac{\exp(\alpha + \beta x_1)}{1 + \exp(\alpha + \beta x_1)} & \dfrac{1}{1 + \exp(\alpha + \beta x_1)} \\ \vdots & \vdots \\ \dfrac{\exp(\alpha + \beta x_n)}{1 + \exp(\alpha + \beta x_n)} & \dfrac{1}{1 + \exp(\alpha + \beta x_n)} \end{bmatrix}, \tag{11.82}$$

with logarithms

$$\underset{n \times 2}{L} = \begin{bmatrix} -\psi_1 + \alpha + \beta x_1 & -\psi_1 \\ \vdots & \vdots \\ -\psi_n + \alpha + \beta x_n & -\psi_n \end{bmatrix}$$

$$= \begin{bmatrix} \alpha + \beta x_1 - \ln\{1 + \exp(\alpha + \beta x_1)\} & -\ln\{1 + \exp(\alpha + \beta x_1)\} \\ \vdots & \vdots \\ \alpha + \beta x_n - \ln\{1 + \exp(\alpha + \beta x_n)\} & -\ln\{1 + \exp(\alpha + \beta x_n)\} \end{bmatrix}. \tag{11.83}$$

The natural parameter array is the $n \times 1$ array

$$
\Phi_{n \times 1} = \begin{bmatrix} \ln \dfrac{P(Y_1 = 1 | X_1 = x_1)}{P(Y_1 = 0 | X_1 = x_1)} \\ \vdots \\ \ln \dfrac{P(Y_n = 1 | X_n = x_n)}{P(Y_n = 0 | X_n = x_n)} \end{bmatrix} = \begin{bmatrix} \alpha + \beta x_1 \\ \vdots \\ \alpha + \beta x_n \end{bmatrix} = X \begin{bmatrix} \alpha \\ \beta \end{bmatrix} = XB, \quad (11.84)
$$

expressing the logits as linear functions of x with coefficients contained in the 2×1 logistic regression coefficient array $B = \begin{bmatrix} \alpha \\ \beta \end{bmatrix}$.

As another illustration, consider the model for the coal miner data. In this case, $m = 4$ for the double dichotomy, $n = 9$ age groups, $r = 3$ for the quadratic age model, and $s = 3$ for the three natural parameters $\varphi^{(B)}$, $\varphi^{(W)}$, and $\varphi^{(BW)}$ given in (11.25)–(11.27). The sample design array is the 9×3 matrix

$$
X = \begin{bmatrix} 1 & -4 & 16 \\ 1 & -3 & 9 \\ 1 & -2 & 4 \\ 1 & -1 & 1 \\ 1 & 0 & 0 \\ 1 & +1 & 1 \\ 1 & +2 & 4 \\ 1 & +3 & 9 \\ 1 & +4 & 16 \end{bmatrix}, \quad (11.85)
$$

and the response design is the 3×4 array

$$
T = \begin{bmatrix} 1 & 1 & 0 & 0 \\ 1 & 0 & 1 & 0 \\ 1 & 0 & 0 & 0 \end{bmatrix}, \quad (11.86)
$$

corresponding to a saturated model for the 2×2 response with log-linear parameters $\varphi^{(B)}$, $\varphi^{(W)}$, $\varphi^{(BW)}$—see (11.54) for the first two rows of T and (11.55) for the third row. The frequency data array N is the 9×4 array given in Table 11.5, and the dominating measure array is again the 9×4 matrix of all 1's, $A = \underline{1}_{9 \times 4}$. The model cell probability array P is the 9×4 array whose rows are given by (11.33)–(11.36), with logarithms L whose rows are given by (11.28)–(11.31), and with $\psi(x) = \ln P\{Y = (0, 0) | \text{coded age} = x = (\text{age} -$

42.5)/5}. The natural parameter array is the 9×3 array

$$
\underset{9 \times 3}{\Phi} = \begin{bmatrix} \varphi^{(B)}(-4) & \varphi^{(W)}(-4) & \varphi^{(BW)}(-4) \\ \vdots & \vdots & \vdots \\ \varphi^{(B)}(+4) & \varphi^{(W)}(+4) & \varphi^{(BW)}(+4) \end{bmatrix}
$$

$$
= \begin{bmatrix} \beta_0^{(B)} - 4\beta_1^{(B)} + 16\beta_2^{(B)} & \beta_0^{(W)} - 4\beta_1^{(W)} + 16\beta_2^{(W)} & \beta_0^{(BW)} - 4\beta_1^{(BW)} + 16\beta_2^{(BW)} \\ \vdots & \vdots & \vdots \\ \beta_0^{(B)} + 4\beta_1^{(B)} + 16\beta_2^{(B)} & \beta_0^{(W)} + 4\beta_1^{(W)} + 16\beta_2^{(W)} & \beta_0^{(BW)} + 4\beta_1^{(BW)} + 16\beta_2^{(BW)} \end{bmatrix}
$$

$$
= X \begin{bmatrix} \beta_0^{(B)} & \beta_0^{(W)} & \beta_0^{(BW)} \\ \beta_1^{(B)} & \beta_1^{(W)} & \beta_1^{(BW)} \\ \beta_2^{(B)} & \beta_2^{(W)} & \beta_2^{(BW)} \end{bmatrix} = XB, \tag{11.87}
$$

expressing the log-linear parameters as the linear functions of x and x^2 given in (11.37)–(11.39) with coefficients contained in the 3×3 logistic regression coefficient array

$$
B = \begin{bmatrix} \beta_0^{(B)} & \beta_0^{(W)} & \beta_0^{(BW)} \\ \beta_1^{(B)} & \beta_1^{(W)} & \beta_1^{(BW)} \\ \beta_2^{(B)} & \beta_2^{(W)} & \beta_2^{(BW)} \end{bmatrix}. \tag{11.88}
$$

Maximum likelihood estimates of the coefficients in B are displayed in the "mle" column of Table 11.6.

Two final bits of matrix notation will be helpful. The first is the *Kronecker product* of two matrices. For any two arrays A ($p \times q$) and B ($r \times s$), the Kronecker product of A and B, denoted by $A \otimes B$, is the $(pr) \times (qs)$ matrix defined by the block diagram

$$
\underset{(pr) \times (qs)}{A \otimes B} = \begin{bmatrix} a_{11} B & \cdots & a_{1p} B \\ \vdots & & \vdots \\ a_{p1} B & \cdots & a_{pq} B \end{bmatrix}. \tag{11.89}
$$

The Kronecker product has the following properties (see Problem 11.11):

(i) The transpose of a Kronecker product is the Kronecker product of the transposes in *original* order,

$$
\underset{(qs) \times (pr)}{(A \otimes B)'} = \underset{q \times p}{A'} \otimes \underset{s \times r}{B'}. \tag{11.90}
$$

(ii) Kronecker multiplication is associative:

$$
(A \otimes B) \otimes C = A \otimes (B \otimes C). \tag{11.91}
$$

(iii) The 1×1 matrix $\{1\}$ serves as an identity matrix:

$$A \otimes \underline{1}_{1 \times 1} = \underline{1}_{1 \times 1} \otimes A = A. \tag{11.92}$$

(iv) Multiplication of two Kronecker products: If A_1 is a $p_1 \times p_2$ matrix and A_2 is a $p_2 \times p_3$ matrix, such that $A_1 A_2$ of dimension $p_1 \times p_3$ is the ordinary matrix product, and if, similarly, B_1 is a $r_1 \times r_2$ matrix and B_2 is a $r_2 \times r_3$ with ordinary matrix product $B_1 B_2$ ($r_1 \times r_3$), then the Kronecker product $A_1 \otimes B_1$ can by multiplied by $A_2 \otimes B_2$ by taking the Kronecker product of $A_1 A_2$ with $B_1 B_2$, which is an array of dimension $(p_1 r_1) \times (p_3 r_3)$:

$$\underset{(p_1 r_1) \times (p_2 r_2)}{(A_1 \otimes B_1)} \cdot \underset{(p_2 r_2) \times (p_3 r_3)}{(A_2 \otimes B_2)} = \underset{p_1 \times p_3}{(A_1 A_2)} \otimes \underset{r_1 \times r_3}{(B_1 B_2)}. \tag{11.93}$$

The last notational convenience is the *vectorization* of a matrix. This operation simply strings out the elements of an $r \times s$ array into a vector of length rs by going down the columns, from left to right. Thus we write the logistic regression coefficient *vector* $\beta = B^V$ as the vectorized logistic regression coefficient array:

$$\underset{(rs) \times 1}{\beta} = B^V = (\beta_{11}, \dots, \beta_{r1}, \beta_{12}, \dots, \beta_{r2}, \dots, \beta_{1s}, \dots, \beta_{rs})'. \tag{11.94}$$

Looking under the Hood

We may now present the elements of a likelihood analysis of the general logistic regression model. The log-likelihood function given the data array N, conditional on the sample design array X, response design array T, and dominating measure array A, is

$$\Lambda(\underline{\beta}) = \sum_{i=1}^{n} \sum_{j=1}^{m} N_{ij} L_{ij} = - \sum_{i=1}^{n} N_i \psi_i + \sum_{i=1}^{n} \sum_{j=1}^{m} N_{ij} \sum_{k=1}^{r} \sum_{l=1}^{s} X_{ik} B_{kl} T_{lj}, \tag{11.95}$$

where ψ_i is the normalizing constant $\psi(\varphi_1(\underline{X}_{(i)}), \dots, \varphi_s(\underline{X}_{(i)}))$ evaluated at the ith sample given $\underline{X}_{(i)}$. The dominating measure array appears implicitly in (11.95); it appears explicitly in the definition of ψ given in (11.41).

The *score function* $U(\beta)$ is the vector of length rs of partial derivatives of $\Lambda(\beta)$ with respect to the components of $\underline{\beta}$:

$$U(\underline{\beta}) = \begin{bmatrix} \dfrac{\partial \Lambda}{\partial \beta_{11}} \\ \vdots \\ \dfrac{\partial \Lambda}{\partial \beta_{rs}} \end{bmatrix} = \sum_{i=1}^{n} N_i (T \otimes \underline{X}_{(i)})(\underline{p}_{(i)} - \underline{P}_{(i)})$$

$$= \sum_{i=1}^{n} N_i T(\underline{p}_{(i)} - \underline{P}_{(i)}) \otimes \underline{X}_{(i)}, \tag{11.96}$$

where $\underline{p}_{(i)} = (N_{i1}/N_i, \ldots, N_{im}/N_i)'$ is the $m \times 1$ vector of sample proportions from the ith sample, and where $\underline{P}_{(i)}$ is the ith row of the model cell probability array P, written as an $m \times 1$ vector. The *likelihood equations* comprise the system of rs equations in the rs unknowns in $\underline{\beta}$ obtained by setting the score function equal to zero. The maximum likelihood estimates $\hat{\underline{\beta}}$ of $\underline{\beta}$ satisfy $U(\hat{\underline{\beta}}) = 0$. Expression (11.96) indicates that at the maximum likelihood estimate, the observed sufficient statistics equal the expected value of the sufficient statistics under the model, $\Sigma_i N_i (T\underline{P}_{(i)}) \otimes \underline{X}_{(i)}$.

The *information matrix*, $I(\underline{\beta})$, is the $(rs) \times (rs)$ matrix of negative second derivatives of $\Lambda(\underline{\beta})$:

$$I(\underline{\beta}) = \left\{ -\frac{\partial^2 \Lambda(\underline{\beta})}{\partial \beta_i \, \partial \beta_j} \right\} = \sum_{i=1}^{n} N_i \{ TW(\underline{P}_{(i)})T' \} \otimes \underline{X}_{(i)} \underline{X}_{(i)}', \quad (11.97)$$

where $W(\underline{P}_{(i)})$ is the $m \times m$ variance-covariance matrix of a single multinomial response evaluated at the model probability for the ith sample:

$$W(\underline{P}_{(i)}) = \text{Diag}\{ P_{i1}, \ldots, P_{im} \} - \underline{P}_{(i)} \underline{P}_{(i)}'. \quad (11.98)$$

In (11.98), the elements on the main diagonal are binary variable variances, $P_{ij}(1 - P_{ij})$; the element off the diagonal in position (j, k) is the multinomial covariance $-P_{ij} P_{ik}$. The information matrix $I(\underline{\beta})$ is both the "observed" information matrix and the "expected" or Fisher information matrix; that is, because the second derivative of the log-likelihood function does not depend on the cell frequency data array, it is a constant (given the explanatory factors). This simplification is a general property of the exponential family of distributions with natural parametrization.

In practice, the information matrix is evaluated at the maximum likelihood estimate, that is, we use the matrix $I(\hat{\underline{\beta}})$, which involves the fitted probabilities $\hat{P}$ and the matrices $W(\hat{\underline{P}}_{(i)})$ evaluated at $\hat{\underline{\beta}}$. The matrix inverse of $I(\hat{\underline{\beta}})$ provides the estimated variance-covariance matrix of the maximum likelihood estimates. Thus the estimated standard error of $\hat{\beta}_j$ is the square root of the jth diagonal element of $I(\hat{\underline{\beta}})^{-1}$, and the estimated covariance between $\hat{\beta}_j$ and $\hat{\beta}_k$ is the element in the jth row and kth column of $I(\hat{\underline{\beta}})^{-1}$.

As an illustration, let us again consider the simple binary logistic regression model represented by (11.78)–(11.84). In this case, $W(\hat{\underline{P}}_{(i)})$ is the 2×2 matrix

$$W(\hat{\underline{P}}_{(i)}) = \begin{bmatrix} \hat{P}_{i1}(1 - \hat{P}_{i1}) & -\hat{P}_{i1}\hat{P}_{i2} \\ -\hat{P}_{i2}\hat{P}_{i1} & \hat{P}_{i2}(1 - \hat{P}_{i2}) \end{bmatrix} = w_i \begin{bmatrix} 1 & -1 \\ -1 & 1 \end{bmatrix}, \quad (11.99)$$

where $w_i = \hat{P}_{i1}(1 - \hat{P}_{i1})$ are the weights used in (11.6)–(11.8). Since the response design matrix is the 1×2 array $T = [1 \quad 0]$, we have $N_i T(\underline{p}_{(i)} - \underline{P}_{(i)}) = N_{i1} - P_{i1} = y_i - P_{i1}$, where $N_{i1} = y_i$ is the binary response for the ith observation. It follows that the score function (11.96) reduces to $\Sigma_i(y_i - P_{i1})x_i$. The likelihood equation defining the maximum likelihood estimates of the intercept coefficient β_1 and the slope coefficient β_2 is $\Sigma_{i=1}^n(N_{i1} - \hat{P}_{i1})x_i = 0$, or, equivalently,

$$\sum_{i=1}^n x_i y_i = \sum_{i=1}^n x_i \hat{P}_{i1}. \tag{11.100}$$

$TW(\hat{\underline{P}}_{(i)})T'$ reduces simply to the 1×1 quantity $w_i = \hat{P}_{i1}(1 - \hat{P}_{i1})$, and so the information matrix at the mle is the 2×2 array

$$\sum_{i=1}^n w_i \otimes \underline{X}_{(i)}\underline{X}'_{(i)} = \begin{bmatrix} \displaystyle\sum_{i=1}^n w_i & \displaystyle\sum_{i=1}^n w_i x_i \\ \displaystyle\sum_{i=1}^n w_i x_i & \displaystyle\sum_{i=1}^n w_i x_i^2 \end{bmatrix}. \tag{11.101}$$

The inverse of (11.101) gives rise to formulas (11.6)–(11.8) for the estimated standard errors of the intercept and slope coefficient mles and their covariance.

The score function and information matrix are used to calculate the maximum likelihood estimates via the *Newton-Raphson* iterative algorithm, a generalization to several dimensions of Newton's method for finding the root of an equation. The algorithm begins with an initial estimate of $\underline{\beta}$, call it $\underline{\beta}^{(0)}$. If $N_i = 1$ for all $i = 1,\ldots,n$, then one usually sets each component of $\underline{\beta}^{(0)}$ equal to zero. If N_i are large and $N_{ij} > 0$ for all i and j, then a more efficient choice of $\underline{\beta}^{(0)}$ in terms of speed of convergence of the algorithm is given by the *weighted least-squares estimate* of $\underline{\beta}$:

$$\tilde{\underline{\beta}} = \left[\sum_{i=1}^n N_i \{TW(\underline{p}_{(i)})T'\} \otimes \underline{X}_{(i)}\underline{X}'_{(i)} \right]^{-1} \sum_{i=1}^n N_i \{TW(\underline{P}_{(i)})\}\{\underline{l}_{(i)} \otimes \underline{X}_{(i)}\}, \tag{11.102}$$

where the matrix $W(\underline{p}_{(i)})$ is evaluated at the sample proportions $\underline{p}_{(i)}$ in the ith sample, and $\underline{l}_{(i)}$ is the $m \times 1$ vector of sample log probabilities, $\underline{l}_{(i)} = (\ln p_{i1},\ldots,\ln p_{im})'$. Note that (11.102) is used only to start the iterations on their way toward the maximum likelihood estimates. Grizzle, Starmer, and Koch (1969) consider inference based on the weighted least-squares estimates rather than maximum likelihood estimates. We generally prefer maximum likelihood estimation because it applies when $N_i = 1$, whereas weighted least-squares estimation requires arbitrary grouping of the data.

After ν stages of the Newton-Raphson iteration, we have the current estimates $\underline{\beta}^{(\nu)}$ ($\nu = 0, 1, \ldots$). The estimates are updated by the adjustment

$$\underline{\beta}^{(\nu+1)} = \underline{\beta}^{(\nu)} + I(\underline{\beta}^{(\nu)})^{-1} U(\underline{\beta}^{(\nu)}). \tag{11.103}$$

As the iteration progresses, the score function approaches zero and the iterates converge to the maximum likelihood estimate. A definite advantage of scheme (11.103) is its rapid convergence: after a few iterations, the errors in the current iterate $\beta_j^{(\nu)} - \hat{\beta}_j$ decrease in proportion to the *square* of the errors of the previous iteration. That means that after the first few iterations, the accuracy in terms of correct decimal places roughly doubles per iteration. In practice, four or five iterations usually suffice to reach convergence with double-precision accuracy (about 13 decimal places). The rapidity of the Newton-Raphson algorithm is an important advantage over other iterative algorithms such as the *iterative proportional fitting* algorithm for log-linear models discussed, for example, in Bishop, Fienberg, and Holland (1975). With modern computers, even a large number *rs* of coefficients can be easily estimated by Newton-Raphson.

Conclusion
The subject of logistic regression has burgeoned since the late 1960s into a versatile tool for many problems involving rates, proportions, counts, and contingency tables. The interested reader may consult the textbooks by Bock (1975), Cox and Snell (1989), and Hosmer and Lemeshow (2000) for additional topics such as logistic regression diagnostics, standardized residuals, indices of high leverage, and overdispersed data.

PROBLEMS

11.1. (a) Let $f_j(x)$ be the normal probability density function with mean μ_j and variance σ_j^2 for $j = 0$ or 1: $f_j(x) = (2\pi\sigma_j^2)^{-1/2} \exp\{-\frac{1}{2}(x - \mu_j)^2/\sigma_j^2\}$. Calculate the log likelihood ratio $l(x) = \ln\{f_1(x)/f_0(x)\}$. Verify that $l(x)$ is of the form $l(x) = \alpha' + \beta x + \gamma x^2$, and find expressions for α', β, and γ in terms of μ_j and σ_j^2.

    (b) Let $f_j(x)$ be the Poisson probability function with mean μ_j: $f_j(x) = \exp(-\mu_j)\mu_j^x/x!$. Calculate the log likelihood ratio $l(x) = \ln\{f_1(x)/f_0(x)\}$. Verify that $l(x)$ is of the form $l(x) = \alpha' + \beta x$, and find expressions for α' and β in terms of μ_j.

    (c) Let $f_j(x)$ be the Gamma probability density function with shape parameter a_j and scale parameter b_j: $f_j(x) = x^{a_j-1}\exp(-x/b_j)/\{\Gamma(a_j)b_j^{a_j}\}$. A chi squared distribution with ν degrees of freedom is in the Gamma family, with shape parameter $\frac{1}{2}\nu$ and scale parameter 2. Calculate the log likelihood ratio $l(x) = \ln\{f_1(x)/f_0(x)\}$. Verify that $l(x)$ is of the form $l(x) = \alpha' + \beta x + \gamma \ln x$, and find expressions for α', β, and γ in terms of a_j and b_j.

11.2. Let $f(x) = e^x/(1 + e^x)$. Find the first derivative $f'(x)$. Use this result in the delta method to derive equation (11.10) for the standard error of the fitted model probability $\hat{P}(x_0)$.

11.3. Verify equations (11.12), (11.13), and (11.14). Check that expression (11.14) in equation (11.7) for the standard error of $\hat{\beta}$ agrees with the familiar formula for the standard error of the log odds ratio in a 2×2 table $\{n_{ij}\}$: $\widehat{\text{se}}(\hat{\beta}) = \sqrt{n_{11}^{-1} + n_{10}^{-1} + n_{01}^{-1} + n_{00}^{-1}}$.

11.4. Let (X_1, X_2) have a bivariate normal distribution with mean (μ_1, μ_2), variances (σ_1^2, σ_2^2), and correlation coefficient ρ. The density function for this distribution is

$$f(x_1, x_2) = \frac{1}{2\pi\sigma_1^2\sigma_2^2(1-\rho)} \exp\left[-\frac{1}{2}\left\{ \frac{(x_1-\mu_1)^2}{\sigma_1^2(1-\rho^2)} \right. \right.$$

$$\left. \left. -\frac{2\rho(x_1-\mu_1)(x_2-\mu_2)}{\sigma_1\sigma_2(1-\rho^2)} + \frac{(x_2-\mu_2)^2}{\sigma_2^2(1-\rho^2)} \right\} \right].$$

Suppose now that given $Y = j$, the mean of (X_1, X_2) is (μ_{j1}, μ_{j2}) for $j = 1$ or 0 but that σ_1^2, σ_2^2, and ρ are the same for $Y = 1$ and 0. Let $f_j(x_1, x_2)$ denote the corresponding densities.

(a) Verify that the log-likelihood ratio function $l(x) = \ln\{f_1(x)/f_0(x)\}$ is of the form $l(x) = \beta_0' + \beta_1 x_1 + \beta_2 x_2$, and find expressions for the coefficients β_0', β_1, β_2 in terms of μ_{11}, μ_{12}, μ_{01}, μ_{02}, σ_1^2, σ_2^2, and ρ.

(b) Given the distributions assumed in this problem, the analysis-of-covariance model $E(X_1|X_2, Y) = \alpha + \beta X_2 + \gamma Y$ is appropriate for explaining variation in X_1 in terms of X_2 and Y. Using the expression for β_1 found in part (a), show that $\beta_1 = \gamma/\sigma_{1.2}^2$, where $\sigma_{1.2}^2 = \sigma_1^2(1 - \rho^2)$ is the residual variance of X_1 given X_2 (within either group $Y = 1$ or 0). Find an analogous relation between β_2 and the coefficient of Y in the analysis-of-covariance model for $E(X_2|X_1, Y)$.

(c) What happens to $l(x)$ in part (a) if the two groups have different variance-covariance structures?

11.5. (a) Verify that $G^2(H_0 : H_1)$ given in (11.18) reduces to $2\{Y \ln 2p + (n - Y)\ln 2q\}$ for testing H_0: $\beta_0 = 0$ (equivalently H_0: $P = \frac{1}{2}$) versus H_1: $\beta_0 \neq 0$ (equivalently H_1: $P \neq \frac{1}{2}$) in the simple binomial model $Y \sim \text{Bin}(n, P)$.

(b) Write $G^2(H_0 : H_1)$ in the form $G^2(H_0 : H_1) = 2nf(p)$, where $f(p) = p \ln 2p + q \ln 2q$. Find expressions for the first two derivatives of $f(p)$ with respect to p, and verify that $f(\frac{1}{2}) = f'(\frac{1}{2}) = 0$ and $f''(\frac{1}{2}) = 4$. Use a Taylor expansion for $f(p)$ about $p = \frac{1}{2}$ to show that $f(p) \approx 2(p - \frac{1}{2})^2$, ignoring terms in third or higher powers of $p - \frac{1}{2}$. Conclude that on ignoring terms of order $1/\sqrt{n}$ or less, $G^2(H_0 : H_1) \approx 4n(p - \frac{1}{2})^2 = X^2$ under H_0.

(c) Use the delta method to show that $\sqrt{n} \ln(p/q)$ is approximately normal with mean 0 and variance $(PQ)^{-1}$, and therefore that $z^2 = \{\ln(p/q)\}^2 npq$ is approximately χ_1^2.

(d) Conclude that under H_0, the three statistics $G^2(H_0 : H_1)$, z^2, and X^2 are all asymptotically equivalent (to chi squared on 1 df).

11.6. For the data in Table 10.1, the saturated model H_2 has maximized log likelihood $L(H_2) = -561.303$, while the model H_1 of constant odds ratio has $L(H_1) = -566.310$. Let H_0 denote the hypothesis of no association between diagnosis and hospital location in any of the $k = 3$ studies.

(a) Find $L(H_0)$. [*Hint.* Under H_0, the maximum likelihood estimate for the common probability in a given study is the sample marginal (or pooled) proportion from that study.]

(b) Calculate $G^2(H_0 : H_2)$ for testing H_0 versus H_2 without the assumption of a common odds ratio. How many degrees of freedom does $G^2(H_0 : H_2)$ have? What is the p-value?

(c) Calculate $G^2(H_0 : H_1)$ for testing H_0 versus H_1. How many degrees of freedom does $G^2(H_0 : H_1)$ have? What is the p-value?

(d) Construct the analysis of information table for these data.

11.7. Plot the log odds on breathlessness among miners with wheeze, and the log odds on wheeze among miners with breathlessness, together with the fitted values from model (11.37)–(11.39). Obtain the fitted probabilities from the model (see Table 11.7), and from these, obtain the marginal proportions $P\{Y_1 = 1 | \text{age} = x\}$ and $P\{Y_2 = 1 | \text{age} = x\}$. Plot the log of the marginal odds on breathlessness against age, and the log of the marginal odds on wheeze against age. Does the log of the marginal odds on breathlessness look as linear as the log odds on breathlessness among miners without wheeze? Does the log of the marginal odds on wheeze look as nonlinear as the log odds on wheeze among miners without breathlessness?

11.8. Demonstrate that sufficient statistics (11.50) give rise to the natural parameters in (11.49), that is, that φ_j is the contrast between $\ln P(Y = j)$ and the average of $\ln P(Y = k)$ for $k > j$.

11.9. Demonstrate that sufficient statistics (11.52) give rise to the natural parameters in (11.51), that is, that φ_1 is the log odds on response 1 versus 2, φ_2 is the log odds on response 3 versus 4, and φ_3 is the difference between the average log probability of responses 1 and 2 and that of responses 3 and 4.

11.10. Let $Y_1, \ldots, Y_m$ be independent binomial random variables with $Y_j \sim$ Bin(n_j, P_j). Show that the joint conditional distribution of $(Y_1, \ldots, Y_m)$ given $Y_1 + \cdots + Y_m = s$ is given by (11.64), with odds ratio parameters $\omega_j = \{P_j/(1 - P_j)\}/\{P_m/(1 - P_m)\}$.

11.11. Demonstrate the algebraic properties of the Kronecker product stated in (11.90)–(11.93).

REFERENCES

Ashford, J. R. and Sowden, R. R. (1970). Multivariate probit analysis. *Biometrics*, **26**, 535–546.

Bishop, Y. M. M. (1969). Full contingency tables, logits, and split contingency tables. *Biometrics*, **25**, 383–399.

Bishop, Y. M. M., Fienberg, S. E., and Holland, P. W. (1975). *Discrete multivariate analysis: Theory and practice*. Cambridge, Mass.: MIT Press.

Bock, R. D. (1970). Estimating multinomial response relations. In R. C. Bose et al. (Eds.), *Essays in probability and statistics*. Chapel Hill: University of North Carolina Press.

Bock, R. D. (1975). *Multivariate statistical methods in behavioral research*. Chapter 8, Multivariate analysis of qualitative data. New York: McGraw-Hill.

Cox, D. R. and Snell, E. J. (1989). *Analysis of binary data*, 2nd ed. Boca Raton, Fla.: Chapman & Hall/CRC Press.

Duncan, O. D. (1979). Constrained parameters in a model for categorical data. *Sociol. Meth. and Res.*, **89**, 57–68.

Fienberg, S. E. (1980). *The analysis of cross-classified categorical data*, 2nd ed. Cambridge, Mass.: MIT Press.

Finney, D. J. (1964). *Statistical method in biological assay*, 2nd ed. New York: Hafner.

Gokhale, D. V. and Kullback, S. (1978). *The information in contingency tables*. New York: Marcel Dekker.

Goodman, L. (1970). The multivariable analysis of qualitative data: Interactions among multiple classifications. *J. Am. Statist. Assoc.*, **65**, 226–256.

Grizzle, J. E. (1971). Multivariate logit analysis. *Biometrics*, **27**, 1057–1062.

Grizzle, J. E., Starmer, C. F., and Koch, G. (1969). Analysis of categorical data by linear models. *Biometrics*, **25**, 489–504.

Hosmer, D. W. and Lemeshow, S. (2000). *Applied logistic regression*, 2nd ed. New York: Wiley.

Kline, J., Levin, B., Shrout, P. E., Stein, Z. A., Susser, M. N., and Warburton, D. (1983). Maternal smoking and trisomy in spontaneously aborted conceptions. *Am. J. Human Genet.*, **35**, 421–431.

Kline, J., Levin, B., Kinney, A., Stein, Z., Susser, M., and Warburton, D. (1995). Cigarette smoking and spontaneous abortion of known karyotype: Precise data but uncertain inferences. *Am. J. Epidemiol.*, **141**, 417–427.

Lehmann, E. L. (1997). *Testing statistical hypotheses*, 2nd ed. New York: Springer.

Levin, B. and Shrout, P. E. (1981). On extending Bock's model of logistic regression in the analysis of categorical data. *Comm. Statist.*, **A10**, 125–147.

Mantel, N. and Brown, C. (1973). A logistic re-analysis of Ashford and Sowden's data on respiratory symptoms in British coal miners. *Biometrics*, **29**, 649–665.

McCullagh, P. (1980). Regression models for ordinal data (with discussion). *J. R. Statist. Soc. B*, **42**, 109–142.

Mosteller, F. (1968). Association and estimation in contingency tables. *J. Am. Statist. Assoc.*, **63**, 1–28.

National Coal Board's Pneumoconiosis Field Research (1975), Great Britain.

Roy, S. N. (1957). *Some aspects of multivariate analysis.* New York: Wiley.

Tsiatis, A. A. (1980). A note on a goodness-of-fit test for the logistic regression model. *Biometrika*, **67**, 250–251.

CHAPTER 12

Poisson Regression

Up to this point we have dealt with statistical methods for proportions. Rates, the other part of the title of this book, are the focus of this chapter. As noted in Section 1.1, the term *rate* attaches a notion of time. A rate, typically the expected number of events in a given population over a given period of time, is expressed in units such as events per thousand person-years. The Poisson distribution is the prototype for assigning probabilities of observing any number of events. In Section 12.1, we introduce Poisson random variables and their properties. Section 12.2 discusses their application in Poisson regression models. Count data often exhibit larger variability than provided for by the Poisson distribution. Such data are said to be *overdispersed*; inference from overdispersed data requires appropriate methods, covered in Section 12.3. We do not cover log-linear models for contingency tables where cell counts are the outcome of Poisson regression models—Bishop, Fienberg, and Holland (1975) and Agresti (1990) thoroughly discuss these models.

12.1. POISSON RANDOM VARIABLES

Named after the French mathematician Siméon Denis Poisson (1791–1840), the Poisson distribution is defined by the probability function

$$P(Y = y \mid \mu) = \frac{e^{-\mu}\mu^{y}}{y!} \qquad \text{for nonnegative integers } y = 0, 1, 2, \dots . \quad (12.1)$$

A random variable having this distribution is called a Poisson random variable, written $Y \sim \text{Poisson}(\mu)$. As demonstrated below, the parameter μ is

Statistical Methods for Rates and Proportions, Third Edition
By Joseph L. Fleiss, Bruce Levin, and Myunghee Cho Paik
ISBN 0-471-52629-0   Copyright © 2003 John Wiley & Sons, Inc.

the mean of Y. For example, let Y be the number of traffic accidents per day in a given geographic region, and suppose Y has the Poisson distribution with mean μ. Then the probability of no accidents on a given day is

$$P(Y=0|\mu) = e^{-\mu}.$$

The probability of exactly one accident that day is $P(Y=1|\mu) = \mu e^{-\mu}$. If the expected number of accidents is $\mu = 1$, these two probabilities are each equal to $P(Y=0|\mu) = P(Y=1|\mu) = e^{-1} \approx 0.368$. When $\mu < 1$, the probabilities in (12.1) decrease steadily for $y = 0, 1, \ldots$. When μ has a noninteger value greater than 1, the probabilities increase for $y < \mu$ and decrease for $y > \mu$: $P(Y=y-1|\mu) < P(Y=y|\mu)$ for $y < \mu$ and $P(Y=y-1|\mu) > P(Y=y|\mu)$ for $y > \mu$; thus $P(Y=y|\mu)$ reaches its maximum at y equal to the greatest integer less than μ. If μ is an integer greater than or equal to 1, then the probabilities are equal for $y = \mu - 1$ and $y = \mu$, increase for $y = 0, \ldots, \mu - 1$, and decrease for $y = \mu, \mu + 1, \ldots$.

Expression (12.1) is a proper probability function, that is, $\sum_{y=0}^{\infty} P(Y=y|\mu) = 1$, because of the power series representation of the exponential function:

$$\sum_{y=0}^{\infty} \frac{\mu^y}{y!} = e^{\mu}.$$

We can also directly verify that the mean of Y is indeed μ:

$$E(Y) = \sum_{y=0}^{\infty} y \frac{e^{-\mu}\mu^y}{y!} = e^{-\mu}\mu \sum_{y=1}^{\infty} \frac{\mu^{y-1}}{(y-1)!} = e^{-\mu}\mu \sum_{y=0}^{\infty} \frac{\mu^y}{y!} = e^{-\mu}\mu e^{\mu} = \mu.$$

Problem 12.1 asks the reader to show that the variance of Y is also μ. Problem 12.2 considers higher-order moments.

Because the Poisson variance is the same as the mean, the sample mean, $\bar{Y}_n$, based on n independent observations $Y_1, \ldots, Y_n$ from (12.1), and the sample variance, $s_n^2 = \sum_{i=1}^{n}(Y_i - \bar{Y}_n)^2/(n-1)$, are both unbiased estimators of the Poisson parameter μ. Under the Poisson assumption, the sample mean is the minimum-variance unbiased estimator of the variance μ, and thus has smaller variance than s_n^2 [see Problem 12.2(h)]. The sample mean is also the maximum likelihood estimate of μ, and thus has the greatest efficiency in large samples among all consistent estimators of μ.

A beautiful relation exists between the cumulative distribution for a Poisson random variable and the upper tail of a chi squared distribution (see Problem 12.3). If $Y \sim \text{Poisson}(\mu)$, then for any integer a, the probability that Y is no greater than a equals the upper tail probability above 2μ of a chi squared distribution with $2(a+1)$ degrees of freedom:

$$P(Y \le a) = P\left(\chi^2_{2(a+1)} \ge 2\mu\right). \tag{12.2}$$

Taking complements, the upper tail of a Poisson distribution can be expressed in terms of the lower tail of a chi squared distribution with $2a$ df:

$$P(Y \geq a) = 1 - P(Y \leq a - 1) = 1 - P(\chi_{2a}^2 \geq 2\mu) = P(\chi_{2a}^2 \leq 2\mu). \quad (12.3)$$

Expressions (12.2) and (12.3) can be used to set an exact confidence interval for μ given an observation of $Y = a$. As in Chapter 2, Section 2.1, the lower and upper bound, μ_L and μ_U, for a 95% confidence interval by the equal-tail method are the values that satisfy the following two equations:

$$P(Y \geq a \mid \mu_L) = 0.025 \qquad\qquad (12.4)$$

and

$$P(Y \leq a \mid \mu_U) = 0.025. \qquad\qquad (12.5)$$

We can use (12.2) and (12.3) to solve these equations. For the upper limit,

$$P(Y \leq a \mid \mu_U) = P(\chi_{2(a+1)}^2 \geq 2\mu_U),$$

so $\mu_U = \frac{1}{2}\chi_{2(a+1);0.025}^2$, that is, the upper limit is one-half the critical value cutting off probability 0.025 in the upper tail of chi squared on $2(a + 1)$ degrees of freedom. For the lower limit,

$$P(Y \geq a \mid \mu_L) = P(\chi_{2a}^2 \leq 2\mu_L)$$

so $\mu_L = \frac{1}{2}\chi_{2a;0.975}^2$, that is, the lower limit is one-half the critical value cutting off probability 0.975 in the upper tail (0.025 in the lower tail) of chi squared on $2a$ df.

For example, suppose we observe the value $Y = 9$. The critical value cutting off 2.5% probability in the upper tail of χ^2 on $2(9 + 1) = 20$ df, from Table A.2, is 34.170, so $\mu_U = 34.170/2 = 17.085$. The critical value cutting off 97.5% probability in the upper tail of χ^2 on $2 \times 9 = 18$ df is 8.231, so $\mu_L = 8.231/2 = 4.115$. Thus the 95% confidence interval is (4.1, 17.1).

There are many other useful properties of the Poisson distribution. One concerns its relation to the normal distribution. As μ increases, $(Y - \mu)/\sqrt{\mu}$ is distributed approximately as a standard normal random variable, $(Y - \mu)/\sqrt{\mu} \sim N(0, 1)$. Thus we may approximate the cumulative distribution function for the Poisson (with continuity correction) by

$$P(Y \leq a) = P(Y < a + \tfrac{1}{2}) = P\left(\frac{Y - \mu}{\sqrt{\mu}} < \frac{a + \frac{1}{2} - \mu}{\sqrt{\mu}}\right) \approx \Phi\left(\frac{a + \frac{1}{2} - \mu}{\sqrt{\mu}}\right),$$

$$(12.6)$$

where $\Phi(z)$ is the cumulative distribution function for the standard normal. $P(Y \leq a)$ can be computed exactly using (12.1) or (12.2), but the difference between $P(Y \leq a)$ and the right-hand side of (12.6) becomes small as μ increases. In technical terms, the difference is of order $1/\sqrt{\mu}$. A better approximation is available, such that the difference is of order $1/\mu$:

$$P(Y \leq a) \approx \Phi(z) - \frac{1}{6\sqrt{\mu}}(z^2 - 1)\varphi(z), \qquad (12.7)$$

where $z = (a + \frac{1}{2} - \mu)/\sqrt{\mu}$, and $\varphi(z) = \Phi'(z)$ is the standard normal density function (Pitman, 1993, p. 225). For example, $P(Y \leq 3 | \mu = 9) = 0.021$ by exact calculation, 0.033 by the normal approximation (12.6) with continuity correction, and 0.024 by (12.7).

Another useful property is closure under addition: if $Y_1, \ldots, Y_n$ are independent Poisson variables with means $\mu_1, \ldots, \mu_n$, respectively, then $S = Y_1 + \cdots + Y_n$ also has a Poisson distribution, with mean $\mu_1 + \cdots + \mu_n$. This property follows directly from the moment generating function found in Problem 12.2(b). Suppose in the example above there were $n = 10$ independent Poisson random variables, each with mean μ, whose total was the observed count $S = 9$. Since S is Poisson with mean 10μ, the exact confidence interval (4.1, 17.1) for 10μ is easily converted to an exact confidence interval for μ by dividing by 10: (0.41, 1.71).

From the central limit theorem we know that $(\bar{Y}_n - \mu)/\sqrt{\mu/n}$ is distributed approximately as a standard normal random variable for large n. Due to (12.6), however, this approximation is accurate for large μ even if n is small. Thus one can construct an approximate 95% confidence interval for μ as follows:

$$\bar{Y}_n - \frac{1}{2n} - 1.96\sqrt{\bar{Y}_n/n} < \mu < \bar{Y}_n + \frac{1}{2n} + 1.96\sqrt{\bar{Y}_n/n}. \qquad (12.8)$$

Applying (12.8) to the example with $n = 10$ and $S = 9$, we obtain $0.9 \pm 0.05 + 1.96\sqrt{0.09} = 0.9 \pm 0.638 = (0.26, 1.54)$. The skewness of the Poisson distribution has caused the normal approximation to be less accurate than it would be for larger μ.

The limiting normal approximation in (12.6) provides the rationale for using the Pearson chi squared statistic for testing goodness-of-fit hypotheses given a sample of independent Poisson random variables Y_i with mean μ_i. The statistic is

$$\chi_P^2 = \sum_{i=1}^{n} \frac{(Y_i - \mu_i)^2}{\mu_i}. \qquad (12.9)$$

The exact expectation of (12.9) is n. Since a sum of n independent squared standard normal random variables is distributed as chi squared with n df, when the μ_i are known and large, χ_P^2 is distributed approximately as chi squared with n df. In practice, μ_i are most often given by a model estimate, say $\hat{\mu}_i$, and we use χ_P^2 as a goodness-of-fit statistic for the given model, replacing μ_i by $\hat{\mu}_i$ in (12.9):

$$\chi_P^2 = \sum_{i=1}^{n} \frac{(Y_i - \hat{\mu}_i)^2}{\hat{\mu}_i}. \tag{12.10}$$

Pearson's χ_P^2 now has an approximate chi squared distribution with $n - p$ degrees of freedom, where p parameters need estimation in order to produce the fitted means $\hat{\mu}_i$. Since the mean of a chi squared random variable is its associated number of degrees of freedom, the Pearson chi squared statistic tends to be close to its number of degrees of freedom when the Poisson assumption is correct and the model for μ_i is correct. The Pearson statistic divided by its degrees of freedom is called the *scaled* Pearson statistic. A value of the scaled Pearson statistic close to one indicates a good fit. Methods for testing goodness of fit when $\hat{\mu}_i$ are small but n is large are considered in Section 12.3.

The following important property allows us to compare two or more Poisson means. Let Y_1 and Y_2 be two independent Poisson random variables, with means μ_1 and μ_2, respectively. Given $S = Y_1 + Y_2 = m$, say, Y_1 is distributed as a binomial random variable with index m and probability parameter $P_1 = \mu_1/(\mu_1 + \mu_2)$; similarly, Y_2 is distributed as a binomial with index m and parameter $P_2 = \mu_2/(\mu_1 + \mu_2)$. See Problem 12.5. For example, let Y_1 and Y_2 represent the numbers of new leukemia patients in equal time periods before and after a nuclear plant accident; we want to test the hypothesis H_0: $\mu_1 = \mu_2$. Since the number of postaccident cases, Y_2, is distributed as a binomial given the total number of cases m, testing $\mu_1 = \mu_2$ reduces to testing the binomial hypothesis H_0: $P_2 = \frac{1}{2}$. This property naturally extends to more than two variables. Let $Y_1, \ldots, Y_n$ be independent Poisson random variables with mean $\mu_1, \ldots, \mu_n$. Given $S = \Sigma_i Y_i = m$, the Y_i's are distributed as a multinomial random vector with sample size m and cell probabilities $(P_1, \ldots, P_n)$, where $P_j = \mu_j/\Sigma_i \mu_i$.

A stochastic process useful in applications is the *Poisson process*. Suppose events occur under the following three assumptions: (i) the numbers of events occurring in nonoverlapping time intervals are statistically independent; (ii) the probability of an event occurring in a short time interval of length h is proportional to h, with a constant of proportionality λ [more precisely, the probability that an event occurs in the time interval $[t, t + h)$ equals $\lambda h + o(h)$, where $o(h)$ is an error term that approaches zero faster than h, i.e., $o(h)/h \to 0$ as $h \to 0$]; and (iii) the probability of two or more events occurring in a short interval of length h is negligible [more precisely, $o(h)$]. Then the events are said to follow a Poisson process with intensity parameter λ. The intensity parameter, a rate parameter, is measured in number of events per unit time interval. It can be shown that the number of events falling in an arbitrary interval of a units of time has a Poisson distribution with mean $\mu = a\lambda$ and that counts falling in disjoint time intervals have independent Poisson distributions. Thus the familiar estimate of number of events divided by person-years of followup is a maximum likelihood estimate of the rate parameter λ. We note that the Poisson process can be defined with units other than time. For example, in spatial models, the unit is often taken as area, with the intensity parameter measured in units of, say, number of gypsy moth infestations per square meter of forest.

In the nuclear accident example, suppose the preaccident period was $a_1 = 5$ years with an observed number of incident leukemia cases $Y_1 = 3$, and $Y_2 = 7$ cases developed after a followup period of $a_2 = 3$ years. Under the assumption of a Poisson process, we have $Y_1 \sim \text{Poisson}(a_1\lambda_1)$ independent of $Y_2 \sim \text{Poisson}(a_2\lambda_2)$, where λ_i is the leukemia event rate per year in the pre- or post-accident period. A test of $H_0: \lambda_1 = \lambda_2$ can be conducted conditionally on $Y_1 + Y_2 = m$, in which case $Y_2 | Y_1 + Y_2 = 10 \sim \text{Bin}(10, P)$ where, under H_0,

$$P = \frac{a_2\lambda_2}{a_1\lambda_1 + a_2\lambda_2} = \frac{a_2}{a_1 + a_2} = \frac{3}{8}. \tag{12.11}$$

Since the binomial upper tail probability for $Y_2 \geq 7$ with $P_2 = 0.375$ is 0.0384, we reject H_0 at the one-tailed 0.05 level.

Note that the binomial parameter in (12.11) depends only on the ratio $R = \lambda_2/\lambda_1$ and on the ratio of the followup times, $\rho = a_2/a_1$:

$$P = \frac{\dfrac{a_2}{a_1}\dfrac{\lambda_2}{\lambda_1}}{1 + \dfrac{a_2}{a_1}\dfrac{\lambda_2}{\lambda_1}} = \frac{\rho R}{1 + \rho R}. \tag{12.12}$$

$R = \lambda_2/\lambda_1$ is the *incidence rate ratio* (or the intensity rate ratio, or hazard rate ratio). An exact confidence interval for R can be obtained by inverting an exact confidence interval for P using (12.12). If $P_L < P < P_U$ is a $100(1 - \alpha)\%$ confidence interval for P using any of the methods of Chapter 2, then

$$\frac{P_L}{1 - P_L}\bigg/\rho < R < \frac{P_U}{1 - P_U}\bigg/\rho \tag{12.13}$$

is a corresponding interval for the intensity rate ratio R. In the example, a 90% two-sided confidence interval for P by the point probability method is (0.398, 0.884). Inverting this using (12.13) with $\rho = 3/5 = 0.6$ gives a lower limit of $0.398/(0.602 \times 0.6) = 1.1$ and an upper limit of $0.884/(0.116 \times 0.6) = 12.7$ for an exact 90% confidence limit for R of (1.1, 12.7).

12.2. POISSON REGRESSION

12.2.1. Simple Poisson Regression

Let Y be a Poisson count associated with given units of observation. Here Y could be the number of cancer patients in a region over a given period of time, the number of defective products in a factory, the number of pixels in a positron emission tomography scan, or a cell count in a contingency table. Consider the case in which the mean of Y varies across levels of exposure to a risk factor X. Denoting the conditional mean of Y given X by $E(Y|X)$, suppose that Y and X are related via the model

$$\ln E(Y|X) = \beta_0 + \beta_1 X, \tag{12.14}$$

or, equivalently,

$$E(Y|X) = \exp(\beta_0 + \beta_1 X) = \exp(\beta_0)\exp(\beta_1 X).$$

This model is called a *multiplicative model*. The intercept β_0 is the log of the mean of Y for a unit with $X = 0$. The slope β_1 is the increase in $\ln E(Y|X)$ per unit increase in X. The interpretation of the coefficient becomes clear in the simple case of single binary covariate X. For the reference group with $X = 0$,

$$\ln E(Y|X=0) = \beta_0,$$

while for the exposed group with $X = 1$,

$$\ln E(Y|X=1) = \beta_0 + \beta_1.$$

By subtraction we obtain

$$\beta_1 = \ln \frac{E(Y|X=1)}{E(Y|X=0)},$$

the log rate ratio. If we assume a linear model instead of (12.14), we have $E(Y|X=0) = \beta_0$ for the reference group and $E(Y|X=1) = \beta_0 + \beta_1$ for the exposed group. By subtraction, $\beta_1 = E(Y|X=1) - E(Y|X=0)$, so β_1 is the rate difference. An advantage of the multiplicative model over the linear model is that the predicted value of μ is always positive, whereas the linear model can yield negative predicted values. Furthermore, the observed Fisher information matrix (see Section 12.2.2) is always nonnegative, greatly simplifying computation of maximum likelihood estimates.

We illustrate these ideas with a subset of data from the study of Doll (1971) concerning cigarette smoking and lung cancer among British physicians, reanalyzed by Frome (1983). Table 12.1 contains the data from Table 1 of Frome (1983) for the group whose number of years of smoking (defined as current age minus 20 years) was 45 to 49. The table shows that the lung cancer rate increases as the number of cigarettes per day increases. Denote the number of lung cancer cases by Y, and number of cigarettes per day by X. To allow for different expectations due to varying numbers of person-years of exposure at any level of smoking, we assume a Poisson process model in

Table 12.1. *Smoking and lung cancer*

Cigarettes/Day*	Person-Years	No. of Cases	Observed Rate	Fitted Rate
0	1421	0	0	0.00079
5.2	927	0	0	0.00117
11.2	988	2	0.0020	0.00182
15.9	849	2	0.0024	0.00261
20.4	1567	9	0.0057	0.00366
27.4	1409	10	0.0071	0.00619
40.8	556	7	0.0126	0.01690

* Mean value within intervals of cigarette consumption.

which the expected number of cases is given by the number of person-years at risk, $a(X)$, multiplied by the lung cancer rate, $\lambda(X)$, given by $\lambda(X) = \exp(\beta_0 + \beta_1 X)$, that is,

$$E(Y|X) = (\text{person-years of exposure at level } X) \times (\text{rate at level } X)$$
$$= a(X) \exp(\beta_0 + \beta_1 X),$$

or, equivalently,

$$\ln E(Y|X) = \ln a(X) + \beta_0 + \beta_1 X.$$

The first term, $\ln a(X)$, is a known quantity called the *offset*. The fitted rates, $\hat{\lambda}(X) = \exp(-7.14 + 0.075X)$, are shown in the final column of Table 12.1. The intercept term $\hat{\beta}_0 = -7.14$ indicates that the predicted lung cancer rate among the nonsmoking population is $\exp(-7.14) = 0.00079$ or 0.79 cases per 1,000 person-years. The slope coefficient $\hat{\beta}_1 = 0.075$ indicates that for each additional cigarette per day, the lung cancer rate increases by a factor of $\exp(0.075) = 1.078$, and for each additional pack of 20 cigarettes per day, the rate increases by a factor of $\exp(20 \times 0.075) = 4.48$. The fit is reasonable, yielding a scaled Pearson chi squared statistic of 0.98. For comparison, we also fit a linear model for $\lambda(X)$, continuing to assume the Poisson process $E(Y|X) = a(X)\lambda(X) = a(X) \cdot (\beta_0 + \beta_1 X)$. The fitted model for the rate is $-0.0025 + 0.0004X$, which produces negative predicted rates for the non-smoking group and the group smoking 5.2 cigarettes per day.

Formulas for the standard errors of the estimates can be obtained from the theory of maximum likelihood. Let $\hat{\beta}_0$ and $\hat{\beta}_1$ be the mle's of β_0 and β_1 in (12.14) based on n units (X_i, Y_i). The formulas for their standard errors are remarkably similar to those for logistic regression coefficient estimates given in (11.6) and (11.7). The only difference is the form of the weights: in Poisson regression, the weight is $w_i = \hat{\mu}_i$ (see Problem 12.5). Denoting the weighted mean of X by $\bar{X}_w = \Sigma_i w_i X_i / \Sigma_i w_i$, and the sum of the weighted squared deviations from the mean by $SS_w = \Sigma_i w_i (X_i - \overline{X}_i)^2$, we have

$$\widehat{se}(\hat{\beta}_0) = \sqrt{\frac{1}{\Sigma_{i=1}^n w_i} + \frac{\overline{X}_w^2}{SS_w}}. \tag{12.15}$$

and

$$\widehat{se}(\hat{\beta}_1) = \frac{1}{\sqrt{SS_w}}. \tag{12.16}$$

The covariance between the estimates $\hat{\beta}_0$ and $\hat{\beta}_1$ is

$$\widehat{Cov}(\hat{\beta}_0, \hat{\beta}_1) = -\frac{\overline{X}_w}{SS_w}. \tag{12.17}$$

The standard error of the linear predictor $\hat{\beta}_0 + \hat{\beta}_1 X$ can be obtained the same way as in (11.9) and, because it refers to the predicted value of $\ln E(Y|X)$, the standard error of the predicted value of $E(Y|X)$ can be derived using the delta method as

$$\widehat{se}\{\hat{E}(Y|X)\} = \hat{E}(Y|X)\,\widehat{se}(\hat{\beta}_0 + \hat{\beta}_1 X).$$

For the smoking and lung cancer data, $\widehat{se}(\hat{\beta}_0) = 0.4540$, $\widehat{se}(\hat{\beta}_1) = 0.0156$, and $\widehat{Cov}(\hat{\beta}_0, \hat{\beta}_1) = -0.006501$. An approximate 95% confidence interval for $\hat{\beta}_1$ is $0.0748 \pm 1.96 \times 0.0156 = (0.0442, 0.1055)$. The slope is highly significant: $z = 0.0748/0.0156 = 4.795$. The standard error of the linear predictor at $X = 5.2$ is $(0.4540^2 - 2 \times 5.2 \times 0.006501 + 5.2^2 \times 0.0156^2)^{1/2} = 0.381$. Using $\hat{E}(Y|X = 5.2) = 1.0853$, the standard error of $\hat{E}(Y|X = 5.2)$ is estimated to be $1.0853 \times 0.381 = 0.4135$.

12.2.2. Multiple Poisson Regression

Poisson regression is widely used. Examples include estimating mortality or morbidity rates in epidemiologic studies (Stevenson and Olson, 1993; Whittemore and Gong, 1991; Vonesh, 1990; Frome and Morris, 1989; Thall, 1988; Whittemore, 1985; Frome, 1983), estimating accident rates (Lindsey, 1997), analyzing imaging data in positron emission tomography (Kay, 1994), and estimating density functions in statistics (Efron and Tibshirani, 1996). An application of Poisson regression for estimating a standardized mortality ratio is given in Chapter 19.

Now consider the case $\underline{X}_i = (1, X_{i1}, X_{i2}, \ldots, X_{i(p-1)})'$, so that $\underline{X}_i$ is a column vector of covariates specific to unit i. Suppose that, given $\underline{X}_i$, Y_i is distributed as a Poisson random variable with mean μ_i, where μ_i is a function of the covariates $\underline{X}_i$. Let $\eta_i = \underline{X}_i' \beta$, where η_i is a linear predictor and β is the regression coefficient of interest. The function that relates η and μ is called the *link function*. The log link and identity link functions were introduced in the previous section. We can rewrite the log link function for a multiple Poisson regression model thus:

$$\eta_i = \ln \mu_i = \beta_0 + \beta_1 X_{i1} + \cdots + \beta_{p-1} X_{i(p-1)} = \underline{X}_i' \beta.$$

As in the simple Poisson regression case, β_0 is the log of the mean of Y when $X_{i1} = \cdots = X_{i(p-1)} = 0$. Now β_j is the log rate ratio per unit increase in X_{ij}, holding all other variables constant. Note that the link function determines the interpretation of β_j. In the case of the identity link,

$$\eta_i = \mu_i = \beta_0 + \beta_1 X_{i1} + \cdots + \beta_{p-1} X_{i(p-1)},$$

β_j is the arithmetic change in rate per unit increase in X_{ij} holding all other variables constant.

In the smoking and lung cancer example, Table 12.1 only shows data for the group of physicians with years of smoking between 45 and 49. The full data set includes eight other groups categorized by varying years of smoking. In Problem 12.6, readers are asked to analyze the full data from Frome (1983). Let $X_1 = $ number of cigarettes/day and $X_2 = $ number of years of smoking, and let $a(\underline{X})$ denote the number of person-years of exposure at given levels of $\underline{X} = (X_1, X_2)'$. Using the full data, we can fit the model

$$\ln E(Y|\underline{X}) = \ln a(\underline{X}) + \beta_0 + \beta_1 X_1 + \beta_2 X_2.$$

Now β_1 is the log rate ratio per unit increase in number of cigarettes per day, adjusted for the number of years of smoking.

Other issues related to multiple Poisson regression are similar to those of multiple logistic regression. The interpretation of the coefficient β_{12} for an interaction term, $X_1 X_2$, remains the same except that β_{12} is the difference not between log odds ratios but between log rate ratios (per unit increase in X_1, say, comparing two values of X_2 differing by one unit). Similarly, the coefficient for a second-order interaction is a difference of differences in log rate ratios. Hypothesis tests using nested models and analysis of information discussed in Section 11.3.4 can be conducted in the same manner. Recall that for logistic regression models, when the log-likelihood ratio goodness-of-fit statistic G^2 is constructed using the saturated model as H_1, the usual likelihood ratio theory does not apply unless there are large samples per independent group. Similarly, the log-likelihood ratio statistic for Poisson regression does not test goodness of fit unless $\mu(\underline{X})$ is large, in which case (12.2) and normal theory assure the asymptotic chi squared distribution of G^2.

Before turning to the next example, we specify the log-likelihood function, the score function, and its derivative for Poisson regression. This discussion lays the groundwork for the quasilikelihood method to be considered in Section 12.3. For convenience we write the $p \times 1$ vector X_i.

The maximized log-likelihood for a multiple Poisson regression model is

$$\ln L(\hat{\beta}) = -\sum_{i=1}^{n} \hat{\mu}_i + \sum_{i=1}^{n} Y_i \ln \hat{\mu}_i - \sum_{i=1}^{n} \ln Y_i!, \tag{12.18}$$

where $\hat{\beta}$ is the maximum likelihood estimate of β, and

$$\hat{\mu}_i = \exp(X_i' \hat{\beta}) = \exp(\hat{\beta}_0 + \hat{\beta}_1 X_{i1} + \cdots + \hat{\beta}_{p-1} X_{i(p-1)}).$$

Expressing the log-likelihood in terms of β explicitly, we have

$$\ln L(\hat{\beta}) = -\sum_{i=1}^{n} \exp(X_i' \hat{\beta}) + \left(\sum_{i=1}^{n} Y_i X_i\right)' \hat{\beta} - \sum_{i=1}^{n} \ln Y_i!.$$

The statistic $\sum_i X_i Y_i$ multiplying $\hat{\beta}$ is the sufficient statistic for β; it is of fundamental importance in drawing inferences about β, both unconditionally as in this chapter, and conditionally as in Section 14.3.

The score function for β for any link function is the $p \times 1$ vector of partial derivatives of $\ln L(\beta)$ with respect to the parameters in β. It has the form

$$U(\beta) = \frac{\partial \ln L(\beta)}{\partial \beta} = \sum_{i=1}^{n} X_i \frac{\partial \mu_i}{\partial \eta_i} V_i^{-1}(Y_i - \mu_i), \tag{12.19}$$

where $V_i = \text{Var}(Y_i | \mu_i)$. This form is actually shared by all regression models for outcomes with exponential family distributions, such as the normal, binomial, Poisson, and Gamma. In each case, V_i is determined by the distribution of Y. Returning to the Poisson case, we have $V_i = \text{Var}(Y_i | \mu_i) = \mu_i$. With the identity link function $\mu_i = \eta_i$, we have $\partial \mu_i / \partial \eta_i = 1$, and the score function is

$$U(\beta) = \sum_{i=1}^{n} X_i \mu_i^{-1}(Y_i - \mu_i).$$

With the log link function $\mu_i = \exp(\eta_i)$, we have $\partial \mu_i / \partial \eta_i = \exp(\eta_i) = \mu_i$, and the score function reduces to

$$U(\beta) = \sum_{i=1}^{n} X_i(Y_i - \mu_i).$$

The variance-covariance matrix of the score function is a $p \times p$ matrix of expected values of the negative derivatives of the components of $U(\beta)$, i.e., the expected values of the negative second derivatives of $\ln L(\beta)$:

$$I(\beta) = E\left(-\frac{\partial^2 \ln L(\beta)}{\partial \beta\, \partial \beta'} \right) = \sum_{i=1}^{n} \mu_i X_i X_i',$$

which is the *Fisher information matrix*. Note that for the log link function, the negative second derivative of the log-likelihood function does not involve the random variables Y_i, and so is equal to its expectation. That is, the observed Fisher information matrix (before taking expectations) and the expected Fisher information matrix are identical, a simplification due to use of the log link function. The solution to the equation $U(\beta) = 0$ is the maximum likelihood estimate, $\hat{\beta}$, and the asymptotic variance of $\hat{\beta}$ is the inverse of the Fisher information matrix:

$$\text{asymptotic Cov}\left(\hat{\beta} \right) = I(\beta)^{-1} = \left(\sum_{i=1}^{n} \mu_i X_i X_i' \right)^{-1}. \qquad (12.20)$$

It is usually estimated at mle(β), so that in practice we use

$$\text{estimated asymptotic Cov}\left(\hat{\beta} \right) = I(\hat{\beta})^{-1} = \left(\sum_{i=1}^{n} \hat{\mu}_i X_i X_i' \right)^{-1}. \qquad (12.21)$$

In the simplest case of inference for a single group, $X_i = 1$ for all i, we have $\mu_i = \mu = \exp(\beta_0)$, and by setting the score function (12.19) equal to zero we obtain the likelihood equation

$$\sum_i Y_i = n \exp\left(\hat{\beta}_0 \right).$$

The maximum likelihood estimate for μ is $\hat{\mu} = \sum_i Y_i / n$ and for β_0 is $\hat{\beta}_0 = \ln(\sum_i Y_i / n)$. The asymptotic variance of $\hat{\beta}_0$ is the inverse of the Fisher information matrix,

$$I(\beta_0)^{-1} = \left(\sum_{i=1}^{n} \mu_i \right)^{-1} = \frac{1}{n\mu}.$$

This agrees with the large-sample variance of $\hat{\beta}_0 = \ln \hat{\mu}$ obtained using the delta method. Since the variance of $\sum_i Y_i / n$ is μ / n,

$$\text{Var}(\ln \hat{\mu}) = \left(\frac{d \ln \mu}{d\mu} \right)^2 \frac{\mu}{n} = \frac{1}{\mu^2} \frac{\mu}{n} = \frac{1}{n\mu}.$$

In the case of simple Poisson regression, the square roots of the diagonal elements of the matrix in (12.21) are exactly (12.15) and (12.16). See also Appendix B.

Example 12.2.1. To illustrate Poisson regression methods, consider the following data on nursing homes, collected by the Department of Health and Social Services of the State of New Mexico, covering $n = 52$ of the 60 licensed nursing facilities in New Mexico in 1988. Detailed descriptions and analyses are given by Smith, Piland, and Fisher (1992). Here we ask whether nursing homes in rural areas tend to have fewer beds per patient population than those in urban areas, adjusting for other factors affecting hospital facilities. The collected variables include the number of beds, annual total patient days, annual total patient care revenue, annual nursing salaries, annual facilities expenditures, and an indicator for rural location. The data appear in Table 12.2.

Let the number of beds be the outcome, Y_i, and assume that the expected number of beds at nursing home i is proportional to the total patient days, $TDAYS_i$:

$$E(BED_i | PCREV_i, NSAL_i, FEXP_i) = TDAYS_i \cdot \lambda_i.$$

Using the log link function, we have

$$\ln E(BED_i | PCREV_i, NSAL_i, FEXP_i) = \ln TDAYS_i + \ln \lambda_i.$$

The first term, $\ln DAYS_i$, is the offset, taken as a known term. We fit the following three models for λ_i:

(M1): $\quad \ln \lambda_i = \beta_0 + \beta_P\, PCREV + \beta_N\, NSAL + \beta_F\, FEXP,$

(M2): $\quad \ln \lambda_i = \beta_0 + \beta_P\, PCREV + \beta_N\, NSAL + \beta_F\, FEXP$

$\qquad\qquad + \beta_{PN} PCREV \cdot NSAL + \beta_{PF}\, PCREV \cdot FEXP$

$\qquad\qquad + \beta_{NF}\, NSAL \cdot FEXP,$

(M3): $\quad \ln \lambda_i = \beta_0 + \beta_P\, PCREV + \beta_N\, NSAL + \beta_F\, FEXP$

$\qquad\qquad + \beta_{PN}\, PCREV \cdot NSAL + \beta_{PF}\, PCREV \cdot FEXP$

$\qquad\qquad + \beta_{NF}\, NSAL \cdot FEXP + \beta_R\, RURAL.$

The results are summarized in Table 12.3. For reference, we also include the saturated model, in which each y_i serves as its own maximum likelihood estimate, that is, $y_i = \hat{\mu}_i$. Twice the difference between the log-likelihood for the saturated model and the log-likelihood for any of the models (M1), (M2), or (M3) produces the deviance for that model.

Table 12.2. *Nursing home data*

Unit	BED	TDAYS	PCREV	NSAL	FEXP	RURAL
1	244	385	2.3521	0.5230	0.5334	0
2	59	203	0.9160	0.2459	0.0493	1
3	120	392	2.1900	0.6304	0.6115	0
4	120	419	2.2354	0.6590	0.6346	0
5	120	363	1.7421	0.5362	0.6225	0
6	65	234	1.0531	0.3622	0.0449	1
7	120	372	2.2147	0.4406	0.4998	1
8	90	305	1.4025	0.4173	0.0966	1
9	96	169	0.8812	0.1955	0.1260	0
10	120	188	1.1729	0.3224	0.6442	1
11	62	192	0.8896	0.2409	0.1236	0
12	120	426	2.0987	0.2066	0.3360	1
13	116	321	1.7655	0.5946	0.4231	0
14	59	164	0.7085	0.1925	0.1280	1
15	80	284	1.3089	0.4166	0.1123	1
16	120	375	2.1453	0.5257	0.5206	1
17	80	133	0.7790	0.1988	0.4443	1
18	100	318	1.8309	0.4156	0.4585	1
19	60	213	0.8872	0.1914	0.1675	1
20	110	280	1.7881	0.5173	0.5686	1
21	120	336	1.7004	0.4630	0.0907	0
22	135	442	2.3829	0.7489	0.3351	0
23	59	191	0.9424	0.2051	0.1756	1
24	60	202	1.2474	0.3803	0.2123	0
25	25	83	0.4078	0.2008	0.4531	1
26	221	776	3.6029	0.1288	0.2543	1
27	64	214	0.8782	0.4729	0.4446	1
28	62	204	0.8951	0.2367	0.1064	0
29	108	366	1.7446	0.5933	0.2987	1
30	62	220	0.6164	0.2782	0.0411	1
31	90	286	0.2853	0.4651	0.4197	0
32	146	375	2.1334	0.6857	0.1198	0
33	62	189	0.8082	0.2143	0.1209	1
34	30	88	0.3948	0.3025	0.0137	1
35	79	278	1.1649	0.2905	0.1279	0
36	44	158	0.7850	0.1498	0.1273	1
37	120	423	2.9035	0.6236	0.3524	0
38	100	300	1.7532	0.3547	0.2561	1
39	49	177	0.8197	0.2810	0.3874	1
40	123	336	2.2555	0.6059	0.6402	1

Table 12.2. (*Continued*)

Unit	BED	TDAYS	PCREV	NSAL	FEXP	RURAL
41	82	136	0.8459	0.1995	0.1911	1
42	58	205	1.0412	0.2245	0.1122	1
43	110	323	1.6661	0.4029	0.3893	1
44	62	222	1.2406	0.2784	0.2212	1
45	86	200	1.1312	0.3720	0.2959	1
46	102	355	1.4499	0.3866	0.3006	1
47	135	471	2.4274	0.7485	0.1344	0
48	78	203	0.9327	0.3672	0.1242	1
49	83	390	1.2362	0.3995	0.1484	1
50	60	213	1.0644	0.2820	0.1154	0
51	54	144	0.7556	0.2088	0.0245	1
52	120	327	2.0182	0.4432	0.6274	0

BED   = number of beds in home,
TDAYS = annual total patient days (in hundreds),
PCREV = annual total patient care revenue (in \$ millions),
NSAL   = annual nursing salaries (in \$ millions),
FEXP   = annual facilities expenditures (in \$ millions),
RURAL= rural (1) or nonrural (0).

Table 12.3. *Log likelihood for the Poisson regression models (M1), (M2), and (M3)*

Model	Added Terms	Log Likelihood*	Deviance	df($= n - p$)	χ^2/df
(M1)	—	17,446.38	245.05	48	5.77
(M2)	$\beta_{PN}, \beta_{PF}, \beta_{NF}$	17,461.07	215.67	45	5.23
(M3)	β_R	17,467.93	201.95	44	4.91
Saturated	All possible	17,568.91	0	0	0

*The constant $\sum_i \ln y_i! = 17,732.35$ has been added to the likelihood in (12.18).

The first model (M1) is the simplest of the three; from there, two-way interaction terms are added in (M2). We first ask whether the two-way interaction terms are necessary, testing

$$H_0: \beta_{PN} = \beta_{PF} = \beta_{NF} = 0.$$

We conduct this test first using the log likelihood ratio statistic and then using the Wald statistic, to compare the two methods.

Most software packages report the log likelihood $\ln L(\hat{\beta})$ for each fitted model as standard output. Therefore, when testing more than one parameter, the likelihood ratio test is easiest to prepare. Note that (M1) and (M2) are nested models, because $\beta_{PN} = \beta_{PF} = \beta_{NF} = 0$ in (M2) reduces to (M1). The log likelihood of (M2) is larger than that of (M1) due to the added two-way interaction terms, suggesting that (M2) fits the data better than (M1). The next question is whether (M2) fits the data significantly better than (M1) or, equivalently, whether the increase in the log likelihood is significant. To answer this question we need to know the distribution of the increase when H_0 is true. As described in Section 11.3.3, when two models are nested, G^2, which is twice the difference between the log-likelihood values of the more inclusive and the less inclusive model, has an approximate chi squared distribution with degrees of freedom equal to the difference between the numbers of unknown parameters in the two models. The log-likelihood ratio statistic is $G^2 = 2 \times (17461.07 - 17446.38) = 29.38$ or, equivalently, the opposite difference between deviances, $245.05 - 215.67 = 29.38$. Referring this to the chi squared distribution with $48 - 45 = 3$ df, the p-value is less than 0.0001. The interaction terms are jointly highly significant.

Computing the Wald statistic requires an extra step. It is given by the quadratic form

$$
W^2 = \left[\, \hat{\beta}_{PN}, \hat{\beta}_{PF}, \hat{\beta}_{NF} \,\right] \left\{ \widehat{\mathrm{Var}} \begin{bmatrix} \hat{\beta}_{PN} \\ \hat{\beta}_{PF} \\ \hat{\beta}_{NF} \end{bmatrix} \right\}^{-1} \begin{bmatrix} \hat{\beta}_{PN} \\ \hat{\beta}_{PF} \\ \hat{\beta}_{NF} \end{bmatrix}.
$$

Most software packages report the maximum likelihood estimates and their standard errors, but the variance-covariance matrix (12.21), also required, may need to be specially requested.

Table 12.4 shows the estimates and their standard errors from (M2) and the estimated variance-covariance matrix of $\hat{\beta}$, $\widehat{\mathrm{Var}}(\hat{\beta}) = I(\hat{\beta})^{-1}$.

Table 12.4. *Maximum likelihood estimates and standard errors of the Poisson regression model (M2)*

Variable	$\hat{\beta}$	Standard Error	p-Value
Intercept	-1.048	0.107	< 0.0001
PCREV	-0.322	0.071	< 0.0001
NSAL	0.017	0.479	0.972
FEXP	1.358	0.280	< 0.0001
PCREV·NSAL	0.372	0.147	0.011
PCREV·FEXP	0.526	0.254	0.038
NSAL·FEXP	-3.653	0.936	< 0.0001

Inverse information matrix $I(\hat{\beta})^{-1}$:

$$
\begin{bmatrix}
0.0115 & -0.00212 & -0.0381 & -0.0107 & 0.0112 & -0.00455 & 0.0400 \\
 & 0.00507 & -0.0101 & 0.00141 & -0.00147 & -0.0143 & 0.0470 \\
 & & 0.2294 & -0.00408 & -0.0586 & 0.0886 & -0.3231 \\
 & & & 0.0786 & 0.0111 & -0.0189 & -0.0842 \\
 & & & & 0.0215 & -0.0159 & 0.0369 \\
 & & & & & 0.0646 & -0.1930 \\
 & & & & & & 0.8766
\end{bmatrix}
$$

Because the inverse information matrix is symmetric, only the upper triangular elements are given. Note that the diagonal elements are equal to the squared standard errors in Table 12.4. Extracting the three coefficient estimates from model (M2) and their variance-covariance estimates (the 3×3 lower right submatrix of the inverse information matrix), we compute the Wald test statistic:

$$W^2 = [0.372 \quad 0.526 \quad -3.653] \begin{bmatrix} 0.0215 & -0.0159 & 0.0369 \\ & 0.0646 & -0.1930 \\ & & 0.8766 \end{bmatrix}^{-1} \begin{bmatrix} 0.372 \\ 0.526 \\ -3.653 \end{bmatrix}$$

$$= 36.28.$$

Comparing 36.28 with the chi squared distribution with 3 df, we see that W^2 is highly significant, with p-value less than 0.0001, agreeing with G^2.

Focusing now on the effect of RURAL, we turn our attention to models (M2) and (M3). Note that the log likelihood for (M2) increases on adding the term RURAL in (M3). The log-likelihood ratio statistic for these two nested models is $2 \times (17467.93 - 17461.07) = 13.72$, and, referring to the chi squared distribution with 1 df, the p-value is 0.0002. RURAL is thus highly significant.

To compute the Wald statistic, we use the estimate of β_R and its standard error from (M3), shown in Table 12.5. Testing H_0: $\beta_R = 0$ involves only one parameter, and the Wald statistic is simply

$$W^2 = \left\{ \frac{\hat{\beta}_R}{\widehat{se}(\hat{\beta}_R)} \right\}^2 = \left(\frac{-0.1331}{0.036} \right)^2 = 13.67,$$

which is close to the log-likelihood ratio statistic $G^2 = 13.72$.

The estimates and standard errors for coefficients other than RURAL are similar to those from (M2). $\hat{\beta}_R = 0.1331$ implies that, adjusting for other factors, rural area hospitals tend to have fewer beds by a factor of $\exp(-0.1331) = 0.875$, with 95% confidence interval (0.816, 0.939).

Table 12.5. *MLEs and standard errors of the Poisson regression model (M3)*

Variable	$\hat{\beta}$	Standard Error	p-Value
Intercept	-0.973	0.109	< 0.0001
PCREV	-0.348	0.071	< 0.0001
NSAL	0.278	0.484	0.565
FEXP	1.468	0.283	< 0.0001
RURAL	-0.133	0.036	0.0002
PCREV·NSAL	0.266	0.150	0.076
PCREV·FEXP	0.709	0.257	0.006
NSAL·FEXP	-4.497	0.955	< 0.0001

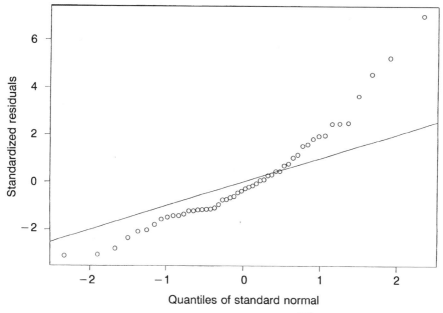

Figure 12.1. Q-Q plot for $(y_i - \hat{\mu}_i)/\sqrt{\hat{\mu}_i}$.

The reader might wonder why we do not fit the model

$$\ln \lambda = \beta_0 + \beta_P \text{ PCREV} + \beta_N \text{ NSAL} + \beta_F \text{ FEXP} + \beta_R \text{ RURAL}$$

and compare it with (M1) in order to calculate the log-likelihood ratio statistic. To do so ignores interaction terms that are clearly important descriptions of the data, in which case the RURAL coefficient is vulnerable to model misspecification bias. In the present case, the RURAL coefficient from the additive model (not shown) is roughly one standard error smaller than in Table 12.5.

As for the goodness of fit, the scaled Pearson chi squared statistic χ_P^2/df for (M3) is 4.91, indicating a rather poor fit. Inclusion of higher-order interaction terms or other possible two-way interaction terms does not improve the goodness of fit. Figure 12.1 shows a Q-Q plot of the standardized residuals, $r_i = (y_i - \text{TDAYS}_i \cdot \hat{\lambda}_i)/(\text{TDAYS}_i \cdot \hat{\lambda}_i)^{1/2}$. Since the number of beds is large, if Y were Poisson-distributed, the standardized residuals would follow the standard normal distribution, approximately. The Q-Q plot clearly indicates that the standardized residuals deviate from the standard normal distribution. The residuals lie on a curve at a steep angle to the straight line of the standard normal, suggesting that their variability is larger than that of standard normal random variables. We address this overdispersion issue in Section 12.3.

12.3.* OVERDISPERSION

Certain integer-valued random variables with mean μ have variance greater than μ. We call such variables *overdispersed* compared to the Poisson case. In this section, we consider methods for handling overdispersion in the context of Poisson regression models.

There are several ways to generate overdispersed variables. One way is to allow random heterogeneity in the underlying Poisson parameters. Suppose that, given Z, Y has a Poisson distribution with mean Z, and that Z itself is a random variable with a Gamma distribution with mean μ and variance μ/α. The density of Z is

$$f(z) = \frac{\alpha^{\mu\alpha} z^{\mu\alpha-1} e^{-\alpha z}}{\Gamma(\mu\alpha)} \qquad \text{for } z > 0. \tag{12.22}$$

Then, marginally, Y has a *negative binomial* distribution with mean μ and variance $\mu(1 + \alpha^{-1})$ (Plackett, 1981, p. 6; McCullagh and Nelder, 1989, p. 199). The probability function for this form of the negative binomial is

$$P(Y=y\,|\,\mu, \alpha) = \frac{1}{y!} \frac{\Gamma(y+\mu\alpha)}{\Gamma(\mu\alpha)} \frac{\alpha^{\mu\alpha}}{(1+\alpha)^{y+\mu\alpha}}$$

$$= \frac{(\mu\alpha + y - 1)(\mu\alpha + y - 2) \cdots (\mu\alpha + 1)(\mu\alpha)}{y(y-1) \times \cdots \times 2 \times 1}$$

$$\times \left(\frac{\alpha}{1+\alpha}\right)^{\mu\alpha} \left(\frac{1}{1+\alpha}\right)^{y}. \tag{12.23}$$

In this case, the variance of Y is larger than μ by the constant factor $\phi = (1 + \alpha^{-1})$, called the *overdispersion parameter*. If we drop the assumption (12.22) of a Gamma distribution, while retaining the two moment assumptions $E(Z) = \mu$ and $\text{Var}(Z) = \mu/\alpha$, the distribution of Y is no longer necessarily negative binomial, but the marginal variance of Y is still $\mu(1 + \alpha^{-1})$:

$$\text{Var}(Y) = E\{\text{Var}(Y|Z)\} + \text{Var}\{E(Y|Z)\} = E\{Z\} + \text{Var}\{Z\}$$

$$= \mu + \mu/\alpha = \mu(1 + \alpha^{-1}).$$

Now consider a slightly different random effects model. Suppose that, given b and μ, Y has a Poisson distribution with mean μb:

$$Y|b \sim \text{Poisson}(\mu b),$$

and $b > 0$ has a Gamma distribution with mean 1 and variance $1/\alpha$, with density function

$$g(b) = \frac{\alpha^\alpha b^{\alpha-1} e^{-\alpha b}}{\Gamma(\alpha)}. \tag{12.24}$$

Then Y has a negative binomial distribution with mean μ and variance $\mu(1 + \mu/\alpha)$, with probability function

$$
\begin{aligned}
P(Y=y) &= \frac{1}{y!} \frac{\Gamma(y+\alpha)}{\Gamma(\alpha)} \frac{(\alpha/\mu)^\alpha}{(1+\alpha/\mu)^{y+\alpha}} \\
&= \frac{(\alpha+y-1)(\alpha+y-2)\cdots(\alpha+1)\alpha}{y(y-1)\times\cdots\times 2\times 1} \left(\frac{\alpha}{\mu+\alpha}\right)^\alpha \left(\frac{\mu}{\mu+\alpha}\right)^y.
\end{aligned}
\tag{12.25}
$$

Note that, in this case, the overdispersion factor $\phi = (1 + \mu/\alpha)$, which depends on μ, could vary from unit to unit in regression settings where $\mu = \mu(X)$. Again, without assuming the functional form (12.24) of $g(b)$, but only that $E(b) = 1$ and $\mathrm{Var}(b) = 1/\alpha$ (or, equivalently, that with $Z = \mu b$, $E(Z) = \mu$ and $\mathrm{Var}(Z) = \mu^2/\alpha$), the same marginal variance of Y results:

$$
\begin{aligned}
\mathrm{Var}(Y) &= E\{\mathrm{Var}(Y|b)\} + \mathrm{Var}\{E(Y|b)\} = E\{\mu b\} + \mathrm{Var}\{\mu b\} \\
&= \mu + \mu^2/\alpha = \mu(1 + \mu/\alpha).
\end{aligned}
$$

Yet another way to generate overdispersed Y is to have events come not one at a time, but in clusters of random size (possibly even empty), where the clusters themselves occur as a Poisson process. Specifically, let $Y = Z_1 + \cdots + Z_N$, where Z_i's are independently and identically distributed integer-valued random variables with mean $E(Z) = 1$ and variance $\mathrm{Var}(Z)$. Z is the number of events per cluster; the Poisson case $Y \sim \mathrm{Poisson}(\mu)$ corresponds to cluster size Z identically equal to 1. Now let the number of clusters N have a Poisson distribution with mean μ (as it would in a Poisson process for clusters over a given time interval). Then the mean of Y is $E(N)E(Z) = \mu$, and the variance of Y is

$$
\begin{aligned}
\mathrm{Var}(Y) &= E\{\mathrm{Var}(Y|N)\} + \mathrm{Var}\{E(Y|N)\} = E\{N \mathrm{Var}(Z)\} + \mathrm{Var}\{NE(Z)\} \\
&= E(N)\mathrm{Var}(Z) + E(N) = \mu\{1 + \mathrm{Var}(Z)\}.
\end{aligned}
$$

If $\mathrm{Var}(Z) > 0$, then Y is overdispersed, with overdispersion parameter $\phi = 1 + \mathrm{Var}(Z)$.

For analysis of overdispersed count data see, for example, Breslow (1984), Brillinger (1986), Lawless (1987), and McCullagh and Nelder (1989, Section 6.2).

Quasi-likelihood

One way to analyze overdispersed count data is to rely on the likelihood function, such as for the Poisson-Gamma mixture given in (12.23) or (12.25). Wedderburn (1974) (see also McCullagh,1983) proposed an alternative method that utilizes assumptions regarding the first two moments of Y only. This quasi-likelihood method is especially convenient when the likelihood function is complicated or unknown, due to uncertainty in the mixing distribution for Z. To describe the quasi-likelihood method, first consider the score equation from the Poisson regression model given in (12.19):

$$U(\beta) = \frac{\partial \ln L(\beta)}{\partial \beta} = \sum_{i=1}^{n} X_i \frac{\partial \mu_i}{\partial \eta_i} V_i^{-1}(Y_i - \mu_i).$$

For overdispersed Y with $V_i = \text{Var}(Y_i) = \phi_i \mu_i$, say, and for the log link with $(\partial \mu_i / \partial \eta_i) = \mu_i$, substitution for V_i and $\partial \mu_i / \partial \eta_i$ in the expression for $U(\beta)$ results in a function we denote by $u(\beta)$:

$$u(\beta) = \sum_{i=1}^{n} X_i \phi_i^{-1}(Y_i - \mu_i). \tag{12.26}$$

Note that $u(\beta)$ is generally *not* the score function, because Y_i are no longer Poisson; we call $u(\beta)$ a *quasi-score function* or an *estimating function*. Although not the score function, it has several of the nice properties of a true score function. The most important property is that its expectation is zero as long as $E(Y_i|X_i) = \mu_i$. Since $u(\beta)$ is a sum of independent random vectors with mean zero, it is, by the central limit theorem, asymptotically distributed as multivariate normal with mean zero. Denote the solution of $u(\beta) = 0$, the *maximum quasi-likelihood estimate* (mqle) of β, by $\tilde{\beta}$. Then $\tilde{\beta} - \beta$ can be expressed approximately as a matrix multiple of the multivariate random vector $u(\beta)$:

$$\tilde{\beta} - \beta \approx \{\Gamma(\beta)\}^{-1} u(\beta),$$

where

$$\Gamma(\beta) = E\left(-\frac{\partial u(\beta)}{\partial \beta'}\right).$$

Therefore $\tilde{\beta} - \beta$ is itself asymptotically multivariate normally distributed. As in the case of the score function and its negative expected derivative $I(\beta)$ (the Fisher information matrix), the negative expected value of the derivative of the estimating function, $\Gamma(\beta)$, turns out to be the variance of $u(\beta)$. For the log link function, the negative derivative does not involve the random variables Y_i, so it equals its expectation:

$$\Gamma(\beta) = E\left(-\frac{\partial u(\beta)}{\partial \beta'}\right) = \sum_{i=1}^{n} \phi_i^{-1}\mu_i X_i X_i',$$

while

$$\text{Var}\{u(\beta)\} = \sum_{i=1}^{n} X_i \phi_i^{-1} \text{Var}(Y_i - \mu_i) \phi_i^{-1} X_i' = \sum_{i=1}^{n} \phi_i^{-1}\mu_i X_i X_i'.$$

Consequently, the asymptotic variance of $\tilde{\beta}$ is $\{\Gamma(\beta)\}^{-1}$:

$$\text{Var}(\tilde{\beta}) = \{\Gamma(\beta)\}^{-1} \text{Var}\{u(\beta)\} \{\Gamma(\beta)\}^{-1} = \{\Gamma(\beta)\}^{-1}.$$

If the overdispersion factor ϕ_i is constant over i, that is, $\phi_i = \phi$ for all i, then ϕ drops out from $u(\beta) = 0$, and the estimating equation becomes

$$u_0(\beta) = \sum_{i=1}^{n} X_i(Y_i - \mu_i)$$

with expected negative derivative

$$E\left(-\frac{\partial u_0(\beta)}{\partial \beta'}\right) = \Gamma_0(\beta) = \sum_{i=1}^{n} \mu_i X_i X_i',$$

where the subscript 0 indicates that the estimating function and the expectation of its derivative are free of the overdispersion parameter. Although $u_0(\beta)$ is identical to the score function for pure Poisson outcomes, $u_0(\beta)$ is not the score function for overdispersed counts. In this constant-overdispersion case,

$$\text{Var}\{u_0(\beta)\} = \sum_{i=1}^{n} X_i \text{Var}(Y_i - \mu_i) X_i' = \phi \sum_{i=1}^{n} \mu_i X_i X_i' = \phi \Gamma_0(\beta), \quad (12.27)$$

$$\tilde{\beta} - \beta \approx \Gamma_0(\beta)^{-1} u_0(\beta), \quad (12.28)$$

and thus

$$\text{Var}(\tilde{\beta}) = \{\Gamma_0(\beta)\}^{-1} \text{Var}\{u_0(\beta)\} \{\Gamma_0(\beta)\}^{-1} = \phi\{\Gamma_0(\beta)\}^{-1}. \quad (12.29)$$

This expression implies that one can fit an ordinary Poisson regression model to overdispersed data as if there were no overdispersion in order to obtain the maximum quasi-likelihood estimate $\tilde{\beta}$. The maximum quasi-likelihood estimate of $\tilde{\beta}$ is consistent and asymptotically normal, but the variance is $\phi\{\Gamma_0(\beta)\}^{-1}$ rather than the usual $\{\Gamma_0(\beta)\}^{-1}$ as in ordinary Poisson regression. Thus, inflating the standard errors by the factor $\phi^{1/2}$ is all that is required for valid analysis in this case.

It is worth pointing out that the quasi-likelihood argument starts from the quasi-score function. If a function is maximized by solving the quasi-score equation $u(\tilde{\beta}) = 0$ and its derivative is $u(\beta)$, we call it a quasi-likelihood function. In general, specification of the mean and variance structure does not guarantee the existence of a quasi-likelihood function. In the case of constant ϕ, there is always a quasi-likelihood function whose logarithm is proportional to the Poisson log-likelihood function. See also Firth (1987).

Estimating the Overdispersion Parameter

Computing standard errors for $\tilde{\beta}$ generally requires estimating the unknown overdispersion parameter. As for the parameter β itself, one could obtain the maximum likelihood estimate for the unknown overdispersion parameter, assuming a parametric form for the marginal distribution of Y, such as (12.23) or (12.25). Alternatively, a consistent estimate can be found based only on the first two moments of Y. Since the estimating methods depend on whether or not the overdispersion is constant, we first consider the constant case.

If ϕ is constant, from the relationship $\sum_i E(Y_i - \mu_i)^2 = \phi \sum_i \mu_i$, a natural estimator of ϕ is

$$\hat{\phi} = \frac{\sum_{i=1}^n (Y_i - \hat{\mu}_i)^2}{\sum_{i=1}^n \hat{\mu}_i}. \tag{12.30}$$

Because estimating β does not require ϕ when ϕ is constant, one can compute $\hat{\mu}_i$ by fitting an ordinary Poisson regression. From the relationship

$$E\left\{ \frac{(Y_i - \mu_i)^2}{\mu_i} \right\} = \phi,$$

another natural estimator is

$$\tilde{\phi} = (n - p)^{-1} \sum_{i=1}^n \frac{(Y_i - \hat{\mu}_i)^2}{\hat{\mu}_i}, \tag{12.31}$$

where p is the number of unknown parameters in β. Note that $\tilde{\phi}$ is the scaled Pearson chi squared statistic, and so is the more common estimator of ϕ.

When the variance of Y_i is $\phi_i \mu_i$, ϕ_i is involved in estimating β. Consider the case in which ϕ_i is of known parametric form, as in $\phi_i = 1 + \mu_i/\alpha$. Setting an initial value for $1/\alpha$ equal to 0, we can fit a regular Poisson regression model and obtain an intermediate estimate $\tilde{\beta}^{(1)}$ of β, from which we compute the predicted values $\hat{\mu}_i^{(1)}$. Then we can consistently estimate $1/\alpha$

given $\tilde{\beta}^{(1)}$ based on the linear regression model

$$E\{(Y_i - \mu_i)^2\} = \gamma_1 \mu_i + \gamma_2 \mu_i^2, \tag{12.32}$$

where $\gamma_1 = 1$ and $\gamma_2 = 1/\alpha$. To do this, enter $(Y_i - \hat{\mu}_i^{(1)})^2$ as an outcome, declare $\hat{\mu}_i^{(1)}$ as an offset with known 0 intercept, declare $\{\hat{\mu}_i^{(1)}\}^2$ as an explanatory factor, and estimate $\gamma_2^{(1)} = 1/\alpha^{(1)}$. Use the new estimate of ϕ_i, namely $\phi_i^{(1)} = 1 + \hat{\mu}_i^{(1)}/\alpha^{(1)}$, as a weight to obtain an updated estimate, $\tilde{\beta}^{(2)}$. Both $\tilde{\beta}^{(1)}$ and $\tilde{\beta}^{(2)}$ are consistent, but the variance of the first estimator is

$$\{\Gamma_0(\beta)\}^{-1} \text{Var}\{u_0(\beta)\} \{\Gamma_0(\beta)\}^{-1} = \{\Gamma_0(\beta)\}^{-1} \left(\sum_i \phi_i \mu_i X_i X_i' \right) \{\Gamma_0(\beta)\}^{-1}$$

(see Problem 12.7), and the variance of the second is $\{\Gamma(\beta)\}^{-1}$. Most software packages report the variance of $\tilde{\beta}^{(2)}$ if ϕ_i is declared as a weight. Model (12.32) can also discriminate between the overdispersion model $\phi_i = 1 + 1/\alpha$ (for which $\gamma_2 = 0$) and the model $\phi_i = 1 + \mu_i/\alpha$ (for which $\gamma_2 > 0$).

For tests concerning the regression parameter β, we construct Wald-like or scorelike statistics based on the properties of $\tilde{\beta}$ and $u(\beta)$. We demonstrate the use of Wald-like statistics in the example to follow.

Testing for Overdispersion
The question remains whether or not overdispersion even exists. When μ_i are large χ_P^2 may be used. Even when μ_i are not large, however, when n is large, one can test for overdispersion by forming a score statistic from a likelihood function such as (12.23) or (12.25). Such score tests are valid and most powerful if the likelihood function is correctly specified. Various statistics derived from this approach have been suggested by Cameron and Trivedi (1990), Collings and Margolin (1985), and Dean and Lawless (1989). Dean (1992) proposed a class of score tests that require specification only of the first two moments of the random effect, which yields several previously proposed statistics as special cases. She shows that when the variance of Y has the form $\mu_i(1 + \mu_i/\alpha)$, as in (12.25), the score statistic for no overdispersion, that is, for zero variance of the random effect, has the form

$$Q_1 = \frac{\sum_{i=1}^n \{(Y_i - \hat{\mu}_i)^2 - Y_i\}}{\sqrt{2\sum_{i=1}^n \hat{\mu}_i^2}}. \tag{12.33}$$

When the variance of Y has the form $\mu_i(1 + 1/\alpha)$, as in (12.23), the score statistic has the form

$$Q_2 = \frac{1}{\sqrt{2n}} \sum_{i=1}^n \frac{(Y_i - \hat{\mu}_i)^2 - Y_i}{\hat{\mu}_i}. \tag{12.34}$$

Table 12.6. *Maximum quasi-likelihood estimates and standard errors of the Poisson regression model (M3) assuming constant ϕ*

Variable	$\tilde{\beta}$	Standard Error	p-Value
Intercept	−0.973	0.234	< 0.0001
PCREV	−0.348	0.152	0.022
NSAL	0.278	1.038	0.789
FEXP	1.468	0.607	0.016
RURAL	−0.133	0.077	0.085
PCREV·NSAL	0.266	0.322	0.408
PCREV·FEXP	0.709	0.551	0.198
NSAL·FEXP	−4.497	2.048	0.028

Both Q_1 and Q_2 are distributed approximately as standard normal random variables when n is large.

Example 12.3.1. We resume the analysis of the nursing home data in Example 12.2.1. The large scaled Pearson chi squared statistic suggests overdispersion. It is not unlikely that the expected number of beds is heterogeneous across the nursing homes, even given patient care revenue, nursing salaries, and facilities expenditures. The formal tests for overdispersion are $Q_1 = 17.01$ from (12.33) and $Q_2 = 16.02$ from (12.34). Both confirm the presence of overdispersion.

Assuming constant overdispersion, the two estimates of ϕ are $\hat{\phi} = 4.60$ from (12.30), and $\tilde{\phi} = 4.91$ from (12.31); see Table 12.3 for $\tilde{\phi}$. In this case, the estimates of β are the same as in Table 12.5, but the standard errors should be multiplied by $\sqrt{\phi}$. Using $\hat{\phi}$, the maximum quasilikelihood estimates and their standard errors are shown in Table 12.6.

Assuming nonconstant overdispersion, from the regression analysis based on (12.32) we obtained the estimate of 0.0354 for $\gamma_2 = 1/\alpha$ with standard error of 0.011. In this case $\tilde{\beta}$ differs from the maximum likelihood estimate

Table 12.7. *Maximum quasi-likelihood estimates and standard errors of the Poisson regression model (M3) assuming nonconstant ϕ*

Variable	$\tilde{\beta}$	Standard Error	p-Value
Intercept	−0.905	0.212	< 0.0001
PCREV	−0.390	0.167	0.020
NSAL	0.149	0.956	0.876
FEXP	1.420	0.544	0.009
RURAL	−0.119	0.075	0.111
PCREV·NSAL	0.334	0.305	0.273
PCREV·FEXP	0.757	0.540	0.160
NSAL·FEXP	−4.558	2.107	0.030

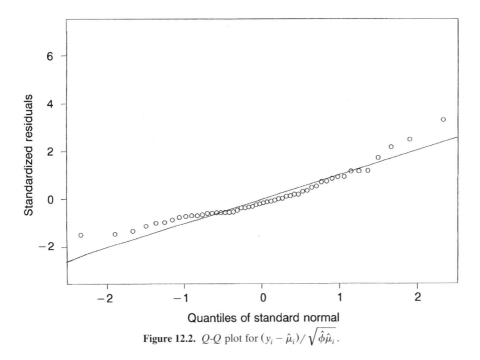

Figure 12.2. *Q-Q* plot for $(y_i - \hat{\mu}_i)/\sqrt{\hat{\phi}\hat{\mu}_i}$.

from the ordinary Poisson regression model. The maximum quasi-likelihood estimates are given in Table 12.7 along with their estimated standard errors.

In both cases the standard errors are substantially larger than in Table 12.4. Clearly, the variability of Y is understated if Y is assumed to be pure Poisson, and consequently the estimated standard errors are understated too. The coefficients estimates, standard errors, and Q-Q plots given in Figures 12.2 and 12.3 from the two overdispersion models are not much different, demonstrating robustness of the results from either model.

Finally, to test the null hypothesis H_0: $\beta_R = 0$, the Wald-like statistics from the two models are $(-0.133/0.0772)^2 = 2.96$ and $(-0.119/0.0747)^2 = 2.54$, respectively. Both are smaller than the critical value from a chi squared distribution with 1 df at the 0.05 level. Using the constant overdispersion model, the estimate of the rate ratio remains the same as before, $\exp(-0.133) = 0.8753$, but a revised 95% confidence interval based on the standard error 0.0772 is (0.7525, 1.0185), which now includes 1. The significant result previously obtained ignoring the substantial overdispersion was overstated.

The reader may also have noticed some *clumping* of BEDS at the value 120 (there are 10 such values in Table 12.2). If not coincidence, such clumping may reflect reporting practices or regulations. Clumping tends to reduce the data's variability. Clumping errors, if present, may introduce systematic bias if, for example, there is a tendency to round the actual value in one direction toward a particular value.

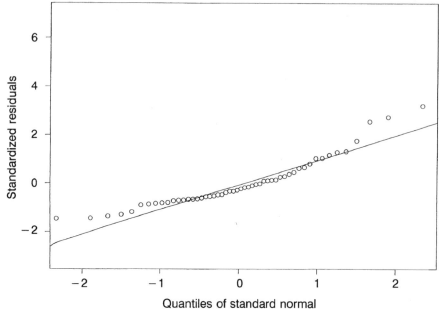

Figure 12.3. Q-Q plot for $(y_i - \hat{\mu}_i)/\sqrt{\hat{\phi}_i \hat{\mu}_i}$.

PROBLEMS

12.1. Show that the variance of a Poisson random variable is μ. [*Hint.* First show $E\{Y(Y - 1)\} = \mu^2$, which leads to $E(Y^2) = \mu^2 + \mu$, and then use $\mathrm{Var}(Y) = E(Y^2) - \{E(Y)\}^2$.]

12.2.* For any integer $r \geq 0$ and any quantity y, let the symbol $y^{(r)}$ denote the rth *descending factorial power of* y, $y^{(r)} = y(y - 1)\cdots(y - r + 1)$, containing r factors, with $y^{(0)} = 1$. For a random variable Y taking integer values, $0, 1, \ldots$, the rth *factorial moment* is defined as $EY^{(r)} = E\{Y(Y - 1)\cdots(Y - r + 1)\}$. Thus $EY = EY^{(1)}$ and $\mathrm{Var}(Y) = EY^{(2)} + EY - (EY)^2$. The *factorial moment generating function* for Y is the function $\zeta_Y(t) = E\{(1 + t)^Y\}$. We consider only random variables for which the expectation exists for all t in a neighborhood of 0. If two random variables have the same factorial moment generating functions, they are identically distributed.

  (a) Show that the factorial moments are generated by differentiating the factorial moment generating function as follows: $EY^{(r)} = d^r\zeta_Y(t)/dt^r|_{t=0}$.

  (b) For a Poisson random variable, $Y \sim \mathrm{Poisson}(\mu)$, show that $\zeta_Y(t) = \exp(t\mu)$, and thus that $E(Y^{(r)}) = \mu^r$. In particular, $E\{Y(Y - 1)\}$

$= \mu^2$. Also, use the factorial moment generating function to demonstrate that the sum of two independent Poisson random variables has a Poisson distribution.

(c) Higher moments of integer-valued random variables are most easily expressed in terms of factorial moments. To this end, demonstrate the following identities:

$$y^2 = y^{(2)} + y, \qquad\qquad EY^2 = EY^{(2)} + EY,$$

$$y^3 = y^{(3)} + 3y^{(2)} + y, \qquad EY^3 = EY^{(3)} + 3EY^{(2)} + EY,$$

$$y^4 = y^{(4)} + 6y^{(3)} + 7y^{(2)} + y, \qquad EY^4 = EY^{(4)} + 6EY^{(3)} + 7EY^{(2)} + EY.$$

(d) For a multivariate random variable $X = (X_1, \ldots, X_n)$, the mixed factorial moment of order $(r_1, \ldots, r_n)$ is defined as $E\{X_1^{(r_1)} \cdots X_n^{(r_n)}\}$, and the factorial moment generating function is defined as $\zeta_X(t) = \zeta_X(t_1, \ldots, t_n) = E\{(1 + X_1)^{t_1} \cdots (1 + X_n)^{t_n}\}$, assumed to exist for t in a neighborhood of 0. Show that

$$E\{X_1^{(r_1)} \cdots X_n^{(r_n)}\} = \left. \frac{\partial^{r_1 + \cdots + r_n} \zeta_X(t)}{\partial t_1^{r_1} \cdots \partial t_n^{r_n}} \right|_{t=0}.$$

(e) Let $X = (X_1, \ldots, X_n)$ have a multinomial distribution in n categories with index m and parameter $P = (P_1, \ldots, P_n)$, denoted by $X \sim \mathrm{Mult}_n(m, P)$. Show that

$$\zeta_X(t) = \left(1 + \sum_{j=1}^{n} P_j t_j \right)^m.$$

Conclude that $E\{X_1^{(r_1)} \cdots X_n^{(r_n)}\} = m^{(r_1 + \cdots + r_n)} P_1^{r_1} \cdots P_n^{r_n}$, where m is raised to a factorial power, and the terms involving P_j are ordinary powers. In particular, the familiar expressions for the means, variances, and covariances of the multinomial distribution are given by $E(X_j) = mP_j$, $E(X_j^{(2)}) = EX_j(X_j - 1) = m(m-1)P_j^2$, $\mathrm{Var}(X_j) = mP_j(1 - P_j)$, and $\mathrm{Cov}(X_i, X_j) = -mP_i P_j$. What is $E\{X_1(X_1 - 1)X_2(X_2 - 1)\}$?

(f) Now let $Y_1, \ldots, Y_n$ be independent and identically distributed Poisson random variables, $Y_i \sim \mathrm{Poisson}(\mu)$, and let the sum be denoted by $S = Y_1 + \cdots + Y_n$. Define

$$T = (n-1)s_n^2 = \sum_{i=1}^{n} \left(Y_i - \bar{Y}_n \right)^2.$$

Use the fact that the conditional distribution of $Y = (Y_1, \ldots, Y_n)$ given $S = m$ is multinomial, $Y \sim \mathrm{Mult}_n(m, P)$ where $P =$

$(1/n, \ldots, 1/n)$, to show that the conditional mean of T given $S = n\bar{Y}_n = m$ is

$$E(T|S = m) = m(n-1)/n.$$

[*Hint.* Write $T = \sum_i Y_i^2 - m^2/n$. Then $E(T|S = m) = nE(Y_1^2|S = m) - m^2/n = nE(X_1^2) - m^2/n$, where $\underline{X} = (X_1, \ldots, X_n) \sim$ Mult$_n(m, (1/n, \ldots, 1/n))$. Use parts (c) and (e) to write $E(X_1^2) = (m^{(2)}/n^2) + (m/n)$, and simplify.]

(g) Continuing, show that the conditional variance of T given $S = m$ is

$$\text{Var}(T|S = m) = \frac{2m^{(2)}}{n^2}(n-1).$$

[*Hint.* $\text{Var}(T|S = m) = \text{Var}(\sum_i Y_i^2|S = m) = \text{Var}(\sum_i X_i^2)$, where, as above, $\underline{X} = (X_1, \ldots, X_n) \sim$ Mult$_n(m, (1/n, \ldots, 1/n))$. Now

$$\text{Var}\left(\sum_i X_i^2\right) = E\left\{\left(\sum_i X_i^2\right)^2\right\} - \left\{E\left(\sum_i X_i^2\right)\right\}^2$$

$$= \sum_{i=1}^n EX_i^4 + 2\sum_{i<j} E(X_i^2 X_j^2) - \sum_{i=1}^n \left(EX_i^2\right)^2 - 2\sum_{i<j} EX_i^2 EX_j^2$$

$$= n\left\{EX_1^4 - \left(EX_1^2\right)^2\right\} + n(n-1)\left\{E(X_1^2 X_2^2) - \left(EX_1^2\right)^2\right\}.$$

Use the results of parts (c) and (e) to express EX_1^4 and $E(X_1^2 X_2^2)$ $= E\{(X_1^{(2)} + X_1)(X_2^{(2)} + X_2)\} = E\{X_1^{(2)} X_2^{(2)}\} + 2E\{X_1 X_2^{(2)}\} + E\{X_1 X_2\}$ in terms of factorial powers of m, and simplify.]

(h) Use the fact that $S = Y_1 + \cdots + Y_n \sim$ Poisson$(n\mu)$ and the identity

$$\text{Var}(T) = E\{\text{Var}(T|S = m)\} + \text{Var}\{E(T|S = m)\}$$

to derive the exact variance of the Poisson sample variance estimator of μ:

$$\text{Var}(s_n^2) = (n-1)^{-2}\text{Var}(T) = \frac{\mu}{n} + \frac{2\mu^2}{n-1} = \frac{\mu}{n}\left(1 + \frac{2\mu n}{n-1}\right).$$

This expression is greater than the variance of the sample mean estimator of μ, namely, μ/n. The relative efficiency of s_n^2 to the sample mean $\bar{Y}_n$, which is the ratio $\text{Var}(\bar{Y}_n)/\text{Var}(s_n^2)$, thus goes to zero as the mean μ becomes large. Note that this result can be obtained in an approximate manner quite simply: for large μ,

$(n - 1)s_n^2/\mu$ is distributed approximately as a chi squared on $n - 1$ df, which has variance $2(n - 1)$. Thus $\text{Var}(s_n^2)$ is approximately $2\mu^2/(n - 1)$. The additional term μ/n in the exact variance formula is relatively small for large μ.

12.3. Let $Y \sim \text{Poisson}(\mu)$, and let U have a Gamma distribution with shape parameter $a + 1$ and scale parameter 1. The density of U is $f_{a+1}(u) = u^a e^{-u}/a!$ for $u \geq 0$. Show that

$$\sum_{y=0}^{a} \frac{e^{-\mu}\mu^y}{y!} = \int_{\mu}^{\infty} f_{a+1}(u)\, du = P(U > \mu).$$

Since $2U$ has a chi squared distribution on $2(a + 1)$ df, conclude that

$$P(Y \leq a) = P\left(\chi^2_{2(a+1)} \geq 2\mu\right).$$

[*Hint.* Verify the equality for the case $\mu = 0$ directly. Then differentiate $\sum_{y=0}^{a} e^{-\mu}\mu^y/y!$ with respect to μ, and show that the derivative is a telescoping series that collapses to the single term $-e^{-\mu}\mu^a/a! = -f_{a+1}(\mu)$. Thus the two functions are identical.]

12.4. Let Y_1 and Y_2 be independent Poisson random variables with means μ_1 and μ_2, respectively. Demonstrate that the conditional distribution of Y_1 given $Y_1 + Y_2 = m$ is $\text{Bin}(m, P)$, where $P = \mu_1/(\mu_1 + \mu_2)$. Generalize to the multinomial case.

12.5. Verify (12.15)–(12.17).

12.6. Table 12.8 shows the full data from Frome (1983). Using these data, fit the following model:

$$\ln E(Y|X) = \ln(\text{person-years}) + \beta_0 + \beta_1 X_1 + \beta_2 X_2,$$

where X_1 is the mean number of cigarettes per day and X_2 is the number of years of smoking. Evaluate whether an interaction term $X_1 X_2$ is necessary for the model to fit the data adequately.

12.7. Verify that the asymptotic variance of $\tilde{\beta}^{(1)}$ is

$$\{\Gamma_0(\beta)\}^{-1}\{\Sigma_i \phi_i \mu_i X_i X_i'\}\{\Gamma_0(\beta)\}^{-1}.$$

[*Hint.* Notice that $\tilde{\beta}^{(1)}$ is the solution of $0 = u_0(\tilde{\beta}^{(1)})$, from which (12.28) follows. But the variance of $u_0(\beta) = \sum_{i=1}^{n} X_i(Y_i - \mu_i)$ is $\text{Var}\{u_0(\beta)\} = \{\Sigma_i \phi_i \mu_i X_i X_i'\}$.]

Table 12.8. *Man-years at risk, number of cases of lung cancer (in parentheses), and fitted values obtained under the product model*

Years of Smoking (Age minus 20 years)	Cigarettes/Day: Mean within Interval	Nonsmokers 0	1–9 5.2	10–14 11.2	15–19 15.9	20–24 20.4	25–34 27.4	35+ 40.8
15–19		10366 (1)	3121	3577	4317	5683	3042	670
20–24		8162	2937	3286 (1)	4214	6385 (1)	4050 (1)	1166
25–29		5969	2288	2546 (1)	3185	5483 (1)	4290 (4)	1482
30–34		4496	2015	2219 (2)	2560 (4)	4687 (6)	4268 (9)	1580 (4)
35–39		3512	1648 (1)	1826	1893	3646 (5)	3529 (9)	1336 (6)
40–44		2201	1310 (2)	1386 (1)	1334 (2)	2411 (12)	2424 (11)	924 (10)
45–49		1421	927	988 (2)	849 (2)	1567 (9)	1409 (10)	556 (7)
50–54		1121	710 (3)	684 (4)	470 (2)	857 (7)	663 (5)	235 (4)
55–59		826 (2)	606	449 (3)	280 (5)	416 (7)	284 (3)	104 (1)

From Frome (1983).

REFERENCES

Agresti, A. (1990). *Categorical data analysis*. New York: Wiley.

Bishop, Y. M. M., Fienberg, S. E., and Holland, P. W. (1975). *Discrete multivariate analysis: Theory and practice*. Cambridge, Mass.: MIT. Press.

Breslow, N. E. (1984). Extra-Poisson variation in log-linear models. *Appl. Statist.*, **33**, 38–44.

Brillinger, D. R. (1986). The natural variability of vital rates and associated statistics. *Biometrics*, **42**, 693–712.

Cameron, A. C. and Trivedi, P. K. (1990). Regression-based tests for overdispersion in the Poisson model. *J. Econometrics*, **46**, 347–364.

Collings, B. J. and Margolin, B. H. (1985). Testing goodness of fit for the Poisson assumption when observations are not identically distributed. *J. Am. Statist. Assoc.*, **80**, 411–418.

Dean, C. B. (1992). Testing for overdispersion in Poisson and binomial regression models. *J. Am. Statist. Assoc.*, **87**, 451–457.

Dean, C. and Lawless, J. F. (1989). Tests for detecting overdispersion in Poisson regression models. *J. Am. Statist. Assoc.*, **84**, 467–472.

Doll, R. (1971). The age distribution of cancer: Implications for models of carcinogenesis (with discussion). *J. R. Statist. Soc. Ser. A*, **134**, 133–166.

Efron, B. and Tibshirani, R. (1996). Using specially designed exponential families for density estimation. *Ann. Statist.*, **24**, 2431–2461.

Firth, D. (1987). On the efficiency of quasi-likelihood estimation. *Biometrika*, **74**, 233–245.

Frome, E. L. (1983). The analysis of rates using Poisson regression models. *Biometrics*, **39**, 665–674.

Frome, E. L. and Morris, M. D. (1989). Evaluating goodness of fit of Poisson regression models in cohort studies. *Am. Statistician*, **43**, 144–147.

Kay, J. (1994). Statistical models for PET and SPECT data. *Statist. Meth. Med. Res.*, **3**, 5–21.

Lawless, J. F. (1987). Regression methods for Poisson process data. *J. Am. Statist. Assoc.*, **82**, 808–815.

Lindsey, J. K. (1997). Parametric multiplicative intensities models fitted to bus motor failure data. *Appl. Statist.*, **46**, 245–252.

McCullagh, P. (1983). Quasi-likelihood functions. *Ann. Statist.*, **11**, 59–67.

McCullagh, P. and Nelder, J. A. (1989). *Generalized linear models*, 2nd ed. London: Chapman and Hall.

Pitman, J. (1993). *Probability*. New York: Springer-Verlag.

Plackett, R. L. (1981). *The analysis of categorical data*. London: Macmillan.

Schall, R. (1991). Estimation in generalized linear models with random effects. *Biometrika*, **78**, 719–727.

Smith, H. L., Piland, N. F., and Fisher, N. (1992). A comparison of financial performance, organizational characteristics, and management strategy among rural and urban nursing facilities. *J. Rural Health*, winter, 27–40.

Stevenson, J. M. and Olson, D. R. (1993). Methods for analysing county-level mortality rates. *Statist in Med.*, **12**, 393–401.

Thall, P. F. (1988). Mixed Poisson likelihood regression models for longitudinal interval count data. *Biometrics*, **44**, 197–209.

Vonesh, E. F. (1990). Modelling peritonitis rates and associated risk factors for individuals on continuous ambulatory peritoneal dialysis. *Statist in Med.*, **9**, 263–271.

Wedderburn, R. W. M. (1974). Quasi-likelihood functions, generalized linear models, and the Gauss-Newton method. *Biometrika*, **61**, 429–437.

Whittemore, A. S. (1985). Analyzing cohort mortality data. *Amer. Statistician*, **39**, 437–441.

Whittemore, A. S. and Gong, G. (1991). Poisson regression with misclassified counts: Application to cervical cancer mortality rates. *Appl. Statist.*, **40**, 81–93.

CHAPTER 13

The Analysis of Data from Matched Samples

A device often employed in controlled trials (sampling method III) is to match subjects on the basis of characteristics that are associated with the response being studied, and to randomize the treatment assignments independently within each matched group. Matched pairs of subjects are used for comparing two treatments, matched triples for comparing three treatments, and in general m-tuples for comparing m treatments. The purpose of matching in controlled trials is to increase the precision of the comparisons among the treatments (Hill, 1962, p. 21).

Matching is also frequently employed in comparative prospective and retrospective studies (sampling method II), but more for increasing the validity of the inferences by controlling for confounding factors than for increasing precision (see Bross, 1969, and Miettinen, 1970a, for a debate on this point). Age and sex, for example, are possible confounding factors in the study of the association between cigarette smoking and lung cancer, because age and sex are associated both with smoking and with the risk of lung cancer. In a retrospective study, therefore, these factors might be controlled by matching each case of lung cancer with a control subject of the same sex and of a similar age. Because the cases and controls would then be similar on sex and age, any difference between the two samples would have to be attributable to other factors. Section 10.5 presents another device for the control of confounding factors.

Sampling method I does not lend itself to matching.

Section 13.1 is devoted to the analysis of data from matched pairs when only a dichotomous (yes-no) outcome is of interest, and Section 13.2 to the analysis of data from matched pairs when more than a dichotomous outcome

Statistical Methods for Rates and Proportions, *Third Edition*
By Joseph L. Fleiss, Bruce Levin, and Myunghee Cho Paik
ISBN 0-471-52629-0   Copyright © 2003 John Wiley & Sons, Inc.

is of interest. Section 13.3 considers the analysis of data resulting from the study of cases matched with multiple controls when the controls all form a single sample. Section 13.4 considers the analysis of data from a study comparing samples from more than two populations when the members of the several samples form matched sets. Section 13.5 concerns sample size determination for matched studies. Some comments on the advantages and disadvantages of matching are made in Section 13.6. Regression analysis for matched samples is discussed in Chapter 14.

13.1. MATCHED PAIRS: DICHOTOMOUS OUTCOME

Suppose that a retrospective study has been conducted in which each case has been matched with a single control and in which the relative frequency of an antecedent factor among the cases is to be compared with that among the controls. Because of the matching of cases with controls, the proper unit of analysis is the matched pair rather than the individual subject. Table 13.1 gives the appropriate means for presenting the resulting data.

Each frequency in Table 13.1 represents a number of *pairs*. Thus there were n pairs studied in all. Of these, a were such that both members (the case and his matched control) had the antecedent factor; b were such that the case had the factor but the control did not; c were such that the control had the factor but the case did not; and d were such that neither member had the factor.

The proportion of controls who had the factor is

$$p_1 = \frac{a+c}{n},$$

and the proportion of cases who had the factor is

$$p_2 = \frac{a+b}{n}.$$

Table 13.1. *Data on two outcomes from matched pairs*

| Cases | Controls | | |
	Factor Present	Factor Absent	Total
Factor present	a	b	$a+b$
Factor absent	c	d	$c+d$
Total	$a+c$	$b+d$	n

The number of pairs in which both the case and the matched control had the factor, a, clearly does not affect the difference between the two proportions,

$$p_2 - p_1 = \frac{b - c}{n}. \tag{13.1}$$

As McNemar (1947) has shown, neither a nor d, the numbers of pairs both of whose members were similar with respect to the antecedent factor, contributes explicitly to the standard error of the difference when the two underlying proportions are equal. In fact, it is estimated by

$$\widehat{se}(p_2 - p_1) = \frac{\sqrt{b + c}}{n}. \tag{13.2}$$

The square of the ratio of (13.1) to (13.2) may, with a correction for continuity, be used to test for the statistical significance of the difference between p_1 and p_2. The correction, due to Edwards (1948), yields the statistic, termed *McNemar's test*,

$$\chi^2 = \left\{ \frac{|p_2 - p_1| - 1/n}{\widehat{se}(p_2 - p_1)} \right\}^2 = \frac{(|b - c| - 1)^2}{b + c}. \tag{13.3}$$

In large samples, the value of χ^2 may be referred to tables of chi squared with 1 df (see McNemar, 1947; Mosteller, 1952; and Stuart, 1957). If χ^2 is large, the inference can be made that the cases and controls differ in the proportion having the antecedent factor. It is noteworthy that only the pairs in which the members differ in the antecedent factor contribute to the test statistic. The power of this test has been studied by Miettinen (1968) and by Bennett and Underwood (1970). The exact distribution of the square root of McNemar's test is derived by Suissa and Schuster (1991).

The test based on (13.3) is illustrated on the hypothetical data of Table 13.2.

The proportion of controls having the factor is $p_1 = 20/100 = 0.20$, and the proportion of cases having the factor is $p_2 = 35/100 = 0.35$. The standard error of the difference [see (13.2)] is $\widehat{se}(p_2 - p_1) = \sqrt{20 + 5}/100 = 5/100 =$

Table 13.2. *Hypothetical data to illustrate McNemar's test*

| | Controls | | |
Cases	Factor Present	Factor Absent	Total
Factor present	15	20	35
Factor absent	5	60	65
Total	20	80	100

0.05, and the test statistic [see (13.3)] has the value

$$\chi^2 = \left(\frac{|0.35 - 0.20| - 0.01}{0.05} \right)^2 = \left(\frac{0.14}{0.05} \right)^2 = 7.84,$$

equal to the value obtained by comparing the numbers of pairs whose members differed on the factor,

$$\chi^2 = \frac{(|20 - 5| - 1)^2}{20 + 5} = \frac{196}{25} = 7.84.$$

Since χ^2 exceeds 6.63, the value needed for significance at the 0.01 level, the conclusion can be drawn that the cases and controls differ in the presence of the antecedent factor.

As pointed out in Chapters 6 and 7, the *odds ratio* (the odds of the disease when the factor is present relative to the odds when the factor is absent) is an important measure of the degree of association between the antecedent factor and the disease. Mantel and Haenszel (1959) and Cornfield and Haenszel (1960) have investigated the proper method for estimating the odds ratio when matched pairs have been studied. When the data are arrayed as in Table 13.1, the estimate obtained by treating each pair as a stratum is simply

$$o = \frac{b}{c}, \tag{13.4}$$

and its standard error is estimated by

$$\widehat{se}(o) = o\sqrt{\frac{1}{b} + \frac{1}{c}} \tag{13.5}$$

(see Ejigou and McHugh, 1977). Formula (13.5) can be obtained using the variance formula for the Mantel-Haenszel log odds ratio given in (10.58). (13.4) is also a conditional maximum likelihood estimator for the common odds ratio underlying each matched pair. For the frequencies of Table 13.2, the estimated odds ratio is $o = 20/5 = 4.0$, and its estimated standard error is

$$\widehat{se}(o) = 4\sqrt{\frac{1}{20} + \frac{1}{5}} = 2.0.$$

An approximate confidence interval for ω, the underlying odds ratio, may be obtained as follows. Define

$$P = \frac{\omega}{\omega + 1}. \tag{13.6}$$

An estimate of P is

$$p = \frac{b}{b+c}.$$ (13.7)

based on a sample size of $b + c$. The methods described in Section 2.4.2 may be applied to find an approximate $100(1 - \alpha)\%$ confidence interval for P, say

$$P_L \leq P \leq P_U,$$ (13.8)

and equation 13.6 inverted to find the desired interval for ω:

$$\frac{P_L}{1 - P_L} \leq \omega \leq \frac{P_U}{1 - P_U}.$$ (13.9)

For the data of Table 13.2, the sample size is $20 + 5 = 25$ and $p = 20/25 = 0.80$. Formulas (2.26) and (2.27) yield

$$0.587 \leq P \leq 0.924$$ (13.10)

as an approximate 95% confidence interval for P, and (13.9) yields

$$1.42 \leq \omega \leq 12.16$$ (13.11)

as an approximate 95% confidence interval for the underlying odds ratio. The simpler approach based on (2.29) yields

$$0.623 \leq P \leq 0.977$$ (13.12)

as an approximate 95% confidence interval for P, and

$$1.65 \leq \omega \leq 42.48$$ (13.13)

as an approximate 95% confidence interval for ω. The lower limits of (13.11) and (13.13) agree well, but the upper limits are greatly different. Because, in this case, $p = 0.80$, which is outside the interval suggested in Section 2.4.2 for close correspondence between the two approaches $(0.3 \leq p \leq 0.7)$, the result given in (13.11) is preferred. Jewell (1984) proposed several bias-corrected estimators for small to moderate sample sizes. One preferred estimator is $o' = b/(c + 1)$, which removes bias of order $1/n$.

So far the analysis of the fourfold table resulting from matched pairs has been presented in the context of a comparative retrospective study. The analysis involving McNemar's test and the estimation of the odds ratio may also be applied to a comparative prospective study with matched pairs. In the analysis of a controlled trial with matched pairs, however, the finding of a significant difference by McNemar's test should be followed by point and

Table 13.3. *Data from a controlled trial with matched pairs*

| New Treatment | Standard Treatment | | Total |
	Recovered	Not Recovered	
Recovered	a	b	$a + b$
Not recovered	c	d	$c + d$
Total	$a + c$	$b + d$	n

interval estimation of either the simple or the relative difference between the two outcome proportions.

Table 13.3 presents the proper means for presenting the data from such a trial, in which we suppose that a new treatment was compared with a standard. As was the case for Table 13.1, each frequency represents a number of pairs.

The proportion of cases who recovered under the standard treatment is

$$p_1 = \frac{a + c}{n},$$

and the proportion who recovered under the new treatment is

$$p_2 = \frac{a + b}{n}.$$

The simple difference between p_2 and p_1 is

$$p_2 - p_1 = \frac{b - c}{n},$$

and an estimate of its standard error appropriate when the two underlying proportions are not hypothesized to be equal is estimated by

$$\widehat{se}(p_2 - p_1) = \frac{\sqrt{n(b + c) - (b - c)^2}}{n\sqrt{n}} = \frac{\sqrt{(a + d)(b + c) + 4bc}}{n\sqrt{n}}. \quad (13.14)$$

An approximate $100(1 - \alpha)\%$ confidence interval for the difference between the two underlying rates of recovery is

$$(p_2 - p_1) - z_{\alpha/2}\,\widehat{se}(p_2 - p_1) - \frac{1}{n} \leq P_2 - P_1$$

$$\leq (p_2 - p_1) + z_{\alpha/2}\,\widehat{se}(p_2 - p_1) + \frac{1}{n}.$$

$$(13.15)$$

Note that all four cell frequencies contribute explicitly to the estimated standard error in (13.14), unlike the standard error in (13.2), which is appropriate only for testing the hypothesis that the underlying proportions are equal.

Under the assumption that the new treatment can benefit only those patients who fail to improve under the standard treatment, the relative value of the new treatment may be estimated by the relative difference,

$$p_e = \frac{p_2 - p_1}{1 - p_1} = \frac{b - c}{b + d}. \tag{13.16}$$

The standard error of the relative difference may be estimated by

$$\widehat{se}(p_e) = \frac{1}{(b + d)^2} \sqrt{(b + c + d)(bc + bd + cd) - bcd}. \tag{13.17}$$

Note that a, the number of pairs both of whose members recovered, contributes neither to the estimation of the relative difference nor to the estimation of its standard error. An approximate $100(1 - \alpha)\%$ confidence interval for the underlying parameter is given by $p_e \pm z_{\alpha/2} \widehat{se}(p_e)$. Alternative confidence intervals are given by Lui (1998). Kuritz and Landis (1988) provide an estimate for attributable risk and its standard error.

Table 13.4 presents some hypothetical data. Of the patients who were given the standard treatment, the proportion who recovered was $p_1 = 50/75 = 0.67$. Of those who were given the new treatment, the proportion who recovered was $p_2 = 65/75 = 0.87$. The value of McNemar's chi squared statistic [see (13.3)] for assessing the significance of the difference between these two proportions is

$$\chi^2 = \frac{(|25 - 10| - 1)^2}{25 + 10} = 5.60.$$

The difference is therefore statistically significant at the 0.05 level.

Table 13.4. Hypothetical data from a controlled trial with matched pairs

New Treatment	Standard Treatment		Total
	Recovered	Not Recovered	
Recovered	40	25	65
Not recovered	10	0	10
Total	50	25	75

The difference between the two proportions is

$$p_2 - p_1 = \frac{25 - 10}{75} = 0.20$$

and an estimate of its standard error is, by (13.14),

$$\widehat{se}(p_2 - p_1) = \frac{1}{75\sqrt{75}} \sqrt{(40 + 0)(25 + 10) + 4 \times 25 \times 10} = 0.08.$$

An approximate 95% confidence interval for $P_2 - P_1$ is, by (13.15),

$$0.20 - 1.96 \times 0.08 - \frac{1}{75} \le P_2 - P_1 \le 0.20 + 1.96 \times 0.08 + \frac{1}{75},$$

or

$$0.03 \le P_2 - P_1 \le 0.37.$$

The value of the relative difference in (13.16) is

$$p_e = \frac{25 - 10}{25} = 0.60,$$

which means that, of every 100 patients who fail to recover under the standard treatment, 60 might be expected to recover under the new treatment. The estimated standard error of the relative difference in (13.17) is

$$\widehat{se}(p_e) = \frac{1}{(25 + 0)^2}$$

$$\times \sqrt{(25 + 10 + 0)(25 \times 10 + 25 \times 0 + 10 \times 0) - 25 \times 10 \times 0}$$

$$= 0.15.$$

An approximate 95% confidence interval for the parameter is $0.60 \pm 1.96 \times 0.15$, or the interval from 0.30 to 0.90.

13.2. MATCHED PAIRS: POLYTOMOUS OUTCOME

Often the response of a subject to treatment or the degree to which he or she possesses a factor may be graded more finely than on the simple presence-absence dichotomy considered in the preceding section. Response to treatment, for example, may be graded as improvement, essentially no change, or worsening. Extent of cigarette smoking, as another example, may be graded as none at all, between 1 and 10 cigarettes per day, between 11 and 20

Table 13.5. *Data from a study of matched pairs with k mutually exclusive outcome categories*

Outcome Category for Cases	Outcome Category for Controls				
	1	2	$\cdots$	k	Total
1	n_{11}	n_{12}	$\cdots$	n_{1k}	$n_{1.}$
2	n_{21}	n_{22}	$\cdots$	n_{2k}	$n_{2.}$
$\vdots$	$\vdots$	$\vdots$		$\vdots$	$\vdots$
k	n_{k1}	n_{k2}	$\cdots$	n_{kk}	$n_{k.}$
Total	$n_{.1}$	$n_{.2}$	$\cdots$	$n_{.k}$	$n_{..}$

cigarettes per day, or 21 or more cigarettes per day. When the samples being compared are not matched, the methods of Chapter 9 may be applied. Here we consider the case of matched pairs, both members of which are classified into one of k (> 2) mutually exclusive categories.

Table 13.5 demonstrates the appropriate presentation of the data. Each entry in the table represents a number of pairs. For example, $n_{..}$ is the total number of matched pairs, $n_{1.}$ is the number of pairs in which the case was in category 1, $n_{.2}$ is the number in which the control was in category 2, and n_{12} is the number in which the case was in category 1 and the control in category 2. The differences between the cases and controls are represented by the k differences $d_1 = (n_{1.} - n_{.1}), d_2 = (n_{2.} - n_{.2}), \ldots, d_k = (n_{k.} - n_{.k})$. Clearly, these differences do not depend on the quantities $n_{11}, n_{22}, \ldots, n_{kk}$, the numbers of pairs both of whose members had outcomes in the same category.

Complicated test statistics for assessing the significance of the k differences $d_1, d_2, \ldots, d_k$ have been proposed by Bhapkar (1966), Grizzle, Starmer, and Koch (1969), and Ireland, Ku, and Kullback (1969). A simpler test statistic, but one that still requires the inversion of a matrix, has been proposed by Stuart (1955) and Maxwell (1970). A simple expression for the Stuart-Maxwell statistic when $k = 3$ has been derived by Fleiss and Everitt (1971).

For $k = 3$, define

$$\bar{n}_{ij} = \frac{n_{ij} + n_{ji}}{2}. \tag{13.18}$$

The statistic

$$\chi^2 = \frac{\bar{n}_{23}d_1^2 + \bar{n}_{13}d_2^2 + \bar{n}_{12}d_3^2}{2(\bar{n}_{12}\bar{n}_{13} + \bar{n}_{12}\bar{n}_{23} + \bar{n}_{13}\bar{n}_{23})} \tag{13.19}$$

may be referred to tables of chi squared with two degrees of freedom. If χ^2 is significantly large, the inference will be made that the distribution across the categories for the cases differs from the distribution for the controls.

Table 13.6. *Hypothetical data to illustrate the Stuart-Maxwell test*

Diagnostician B	Diagnostician A			
	Schizophrenia	Affective	Other	Total
Schizophrenia	35	5	0	40
Affective	15	20	5	40
Other	10	5	5	20
Total	60	30	10	100

Consider the hypothetical data in Table 13.6, in which it is assumed that two diagnositicians independently diagnosed each of a sample of 100 mental patients. The value of the Stuart-Maxwell χ^2 statistic in (13.19) is

$$\chi^2 = \frac{\dfrac{5+5}{2}(40-60)^2 + \dfrac{0+10}{2}(40-30)^2 + \dfrac{5+15}{2}(20-10)^2}{2\left(\dfrac{5+15}{2} \times \dfrac{0+10}{2} + \dfrac{5+15}{2} \times \dfrac{5+5}{2} + \dfrac{0+10}{2} \times \dfrac{5+5}{2}\right)}$$

$$= \frac{3500}{2 \times 125} = 14.00,$$

which, with 2 df, is significant beyond the 0.001 level. It may therefore be concluded that the diagnostic distribution of diagnostician A is different from that of diagnostician B.

When, as in this example, a significant difference is found between the two distributions, the next step in the analysis would be to find those single categories (in the case of more than three categories, possibly those combinations of categories) for which the differences are significant (see Fleiss and Everitt, 1971, for a general discussion). One need only collapse the original table into a 2×2 table and apply McNemar's statistic (13.3). The test for significance, however, must incorporate a control over the fact that the chances of erroneously declaring a difference to be significant increase when a number of tests are applied to the same data. An appropriate control in the case we are considering (see Miller, 1966, Section 6.2) is to refer McNemar's chi squared statistic to the critical value of chi squared with $k - 1$ df.

We illustrate the search for those categories with a significant difference using the data of Table 13.6. To determine whether the proportions who were diagnosed as having schizophrenia by the two diagnosticians were different, we form the 2×2 table in Table 13.7. Sixty percent of the patients were diagnosed as having schizophrenia by A, while only 40% were so diagnosed by B. The value of McNemar's statistic is

$$\chi^2 = \frac{(|5-25|-1)^2}{5+25} = \frac{19^2}{30} = 12.03.$$

Table 13.7. *Two-by-two table for comparing rates of schizophrenia by diagnosticians A and B*

	Diagnostician A		
Diagnostician B	Schizophrenia	Not Schizophrenia	Total
Schizophrenia	35	5	40
Not schizophrenia	25	35	60
Total	60	40	100

Table 13.8. *Hypothetical data to illustrate the analysis of an ordered outcome variable*

	Standard Treatment			
New Treatment	Improved	No Change	Worse	Total
Improved	40	20	10	70
No change	6	6	8	20
Worse	4	4	2	10
Total	50	30	20	100

The critical value of chi squared with two degrees of freedom for a significance level of 0.05 (see Table A.2) is 5.99. Since the obtained value of McNemar's chi squared exceeds 5.99, we may infer that A is more likely to diagnose schizophrenia than B.

Problem 13.1 calls for comparing the proportions of patients diagnosed as affectively ill and diagnosed as having a disorder other than schizophrenia or affective illness by A and B.

If the k outcome categories are ordered (as in the two examples cited at the beginning of this section), the analysis of the data should somehow take the ordering into account. Consider the hypothetical data in Table 13.8, in which it is assumed that the treatments were assigned to the members of each matched pair at random. The value of the Stuart-Maxwell chi squared statistic is significant [see Problem 13.2(a)], so that a more detailed analysis of the data is in order.

The kind of category-by-category analysis illustrated above could be performed, but it would be inefficient in that it would ignore the ordering inherent in grading response to treatment. The following method of analysis is appropriate when interest is in whether one treatment tends to produce more responses than the other treatment at one end of the ordered scale and fewer at the other.

Consider the difference $d_1 - d_3$. If the new treatment is better than the standard in the sense that it has associated with it more improvement (so that d_1 is positive) and less worsening (so that d_3 is negative), $d_1 - d_3$ will be large in the positive direction. If the new treatment is poorer than the standard,

$d_1 - d_3$ will be large in the negative direction. In either case, the hypothesis that the treatments do not differ at the two ends of the scale may be tested by referring the value of

$$\chi^2 = \frac{(d_1 - d_3)^2}{2(\bar{n}_{12} + 4\bar{n}_{13} + \bar{n}_{23})} \tag{13.20}$$

to the chi squared distribution with 1 df if this particular comparison was planned before the data were examined, and to the chi squared distribution with 2 df if the comparison was suggested by the data. This test and the more general one when the number of outcome categories exceeds three were derived by Fleiss and Everitt (1971). Problem 13.2(b) calls for applying it to the data of Table 13.8.

13.3. MULTIPLE MATCHED CONTROLS PER CASE

Occasionally, two matched samples may be generated by matching each case (or each patient given a new treatment) with more than one control (or with more than one patient given a standard treatment). Matching with multiple controls is especially advantageous when the number of potential control subjects is large relative to the number of available cases and when little effort needs to be expended in obtaining the necessary information.

We assume that each subject is characterized by either the presence or the absence of some factor or outcome. A general method of analysis, valid even when the number of controls varies from one case to another, was originally derived by Mantel and Haenszel (1959). An alternative but more complex method of analysis in the general case is due to Cox (1966). Here we assume that each case is matched with the same number, say $m - 1$, of controls, and we consider only the Mantel-Haenszel method.

Suppose that there are a total of N matched sets, each containing one case and $m - 1$ controls. In the ith set ($i = 1, \ldots, N$), let x_i denote the number of controls who had the factor (so that x_i may equal $0, 1, \ldots,$ or $m - 1$), and let n_i denote the total number of subjects—including the case and controls—who had the factor. Thus if the case in the ith set had the factor, then $n_i = x_i + 1$; if he or she did not have the factor, then $n_i = x_i$.

Define

$$A = \sum_{i=1}^{N} x_i, \tag{13.21}$$

the total number of control subjects who had the factor, and define

$$B = \sum_{i=1}^{N} n_i, \tag{13.22}$$

the total number of either kind of subject who had the factor. Note that the total number of cases who had the factor is $B - A$. The rate at which the factor is present among the controls is

$$p_1 = \frac{A}{N(m-1)},$$ (13.23)

and the rate at which it is present among the cases is

$$p_2 = \frac{B - A}{N}.$$ (13.24)

In order to test the significance of the difference between p_1 and p_2, the statistic

$$\chi_u^2 = \left(\frac{p_2 - p_1}{\widehat{se}(p_2 - p_1)}\right)^2 = \frac{[(m-1)B - mA]^2}{mB - \sum_{i=1}^{N} n_i^2}$$ (13.25)

may be referred to tables of chi squared with 1 df (see Miettinen, 1969, and Pike and Morrow, 1970). Miettinen (1969) has studied the power of the test based on (13.25) and has given criteria (in terms of reducing cost) for deciding on an appropriate value for $m - 1$, the number of controls per case.

The data in Table 13.9 are used to illustrate this analysis. Suppose that $N = 10$ matched sets with $m = 3$ were studied, implying $m - 1 = 2$ controls per case. The proportion of controls having the factor [see (13.23)] is

$$p_1 = \frac{7}{10 \times 2} = 0.35,$$

Table 13.9. *Outcome data from matched sets with 1 : 2 matching*

Triple	Case Has Factor*	Number of Controls with Factor ($=x_i$)	Total Having Factor ($=n_i$)	n_i^2
1	1	2	3	9
2	1	1	2	4
3	1	1	2	4
4	1	1	2	4
5	1	1	2	4
6	1	0	1	1
7	1	0	1	1
8	1	0	1	1
9	0	1	1	1
10	0	0	0	0
Total	8 ($= B - A$)	7 ($= A$)	15 ($= B$)	29

*1 = yes, 0 = no.

and the proportion of cases having the factor [see (13.24)] is

$$p_2 = \frac{8}{10} = 0.80.$$

The value of the statistic in (13.25) for testing the significance of the difference between these two proportions is

$$\chi_u^2 = \frac{(2 \times 15 - 3 \times 7)^2}{3 \times 15 - 29} = \frac{9^2}{16} = 5.06.$$

Since this value exceeds 3.84, the value of chi squared with one degree of freedom needed for significance at the 0.05 level, the inference may be drawn that the proportion of cases having the factor is larger than the proportion of controls having it.

Note that χ_u^2 in (13.25) omits the continuity correction. Use of the Mantel-Haenszel 1 df chi squared procedure with continuity correction comes to a slightly different conclusion; from (10.62), $\chi_{cc}^2 = (8 - 5 - \frac{1}{2})^2/1.7778 = 3.516$ ($p = 0.06$). The matter may be settled by the exact two-tailed p-value by the point probability method ($p = 0.054$): a result of borderline significance.

The Mantel-Haenszel estimate of the assumed common odds ratio over the N matched sets (1959, p. 736) is

$$o = \frac{(m-1)(B-A) - \displaystyle\sum_{i=1}^{N} x_i(n_i - x_i)}{A - \displaystyle\sum_{i=1}^{N} x_i(n_i - x_i)}. \tag{13.26}$$

The quantity $\sum_i x_i(n_i - x_i)$ is obtained by restricting attention to sets in which the case had the factor and simply adding the numbers of controls in those sets who had the factor.

For the data of Table 13.9, only the first eight sets had cases with the factor. The total number of controls in those eight sets with the factor is 6 $[= \sum_i x_i(n_i - x_i)]$, so that the estimated odds ratio in (13.26) is

$$o = \frac{2 \times 8 - 6}{7 - 6} = 10.0.$$

An estimate of the variance of the logarithm of the Mantel-Haenszel estimate of the common odds ratio ω was given by (10.58). That expression, a consistent estimate for Var{ln o} in matched samples, can be used to set confidence intervals for ln ω and ω. For the data of Table 13.9, the terms in (10.58), (R_i, S_i, P_i, Q_i), equal $(\frac{1}{3}, 0, \frac{2}{3}, \frac{1}{3})$ for four sets (sets 2 through 5); $(\frac{2}{3}, 0, 1, 0)$ for three sets (sets 6 through 8); and $(0, \frac{1}{3}, \frac{1}{3}, \frac{2}{3})$ for one set (set 9).

Matched sets 1 and 10 are uninformative and may be omitted from the calculations. Then $R = \Sigma_i R_i = \frac{10}{3}$, $S = \Sigma_i S_i = \frac{1}{3}$, and $o = R/S = 10$, as found above. Also $\Sigma_i P_i R_i = 4(\frac{2}{9}) + 3(\frac{2}{3}) = \frac{26}{9}$; $\Sigma_i P_i S_i = \frac{1}{9}$; $\Sigma_i Q_i R_i = 4(\frac{1}{9}) = \frac{4}{9}$; and $\Sigma_i Q_i R_i = \frac{2}{9}$. Thus the estimated variance of ln o from (10.58) is

$$\frac{1}{2}\left\{\frac{26/9}{100/9} + \frac{5/9}{10/9} + \frac{2/9}{1/9}\right\} = 1.38,$$

and the estimated standard error of ln o is $\sqrt{1.38} = 1.1747$. An approximate 95% confidence interval for ln ω is $\ln o \pm 1.96 \times 1.1747 = (0.000, 4.605)$. Exponentiating, an approximate 95% confidence interval for ω is $(\exp 0.000, \exp 4.605) = (1.000, 100.0)$. For comparison, an exact two-sided 95% confidence interval for ω by the point probability method is $(1.000, 194.1)$. The equal-tail method gives $(0.98, 394.1)$. The uncertainty in the upper endpoint reflects the sparse information in the eight informative triplets.

Miettinen (1970b) presents an alternative method for estimating the odds ratio in the case of matched sets by the method of maximum conditional likelihood (see Chapter 14), and gives approximate expressions for the standard error of the estimate. We note that the conditional maximum likelihood estimator agrees with the Mantel-Haenszel estimator for 1-to-1 matching, but not for matched samples with $m > 2$.

The assumption of a common odds ratio across all N matched sets may be tested when $m > 2$. Several tests of odds ratio homogeneity for matched studies have been proposed. See Ejigou and McHugh (1984), Gart (1985), Liang and Self (1985), Zelterman and Chen (1988), Zelterman and Le (1991), and Levin (1992). See also Section 10.9.3. The power of these tests is usually low unless the sample size is greater than 50 matched sets.

Power and sample size calculations for tests of association in matched samples are discussed below in Section 13.5. In brief, the power of the chi squared test based on (13.25) and the precision of the estimated odds ratio in (13.26) both increase as $m - 1$, the number of controls per case, increases. The improvement in power and precision is usually trivial, however, as soon as we get beyond three or four controls per case (Miettinen, 1969; Ury, 1975). The search for five or more controls per case therefore usually represents wasted effort.

13.4. THE COMPARISON OF MATCHED SAMPLES WITH m DISTINCT TYPES

In Section 13.3 we considered the case where the $m - 1$ controls for each case formed a homogeneous group. In this section we consider the comparison of m distinct types of matched subjects, but again restrict attention to the situation where only two outcomes are of interest (see Koch and Reinfurt, 1971, for the general case). We refer to the matched sets as triples ($m = 3$), quadruples ($m = 4$), or, in general, m-tuples.

Table 13.10. *Presentation of data from m matched samples*

	Sample				
m-tuple	1	2	$\cdots$	*m*	Total
1	X_{11}	X_{12}	$\cdots$	X_{1m}	S_1
2	X_{21}	X_{22}	$\cdots$	X_{2m}	S_2
$\vdots$					
N	X_{N1}	X_{N2}	$\cdots$	X_{Nm}	S_N
Total:	T_1	T_2	$\cdots$	T_m	T
Proportion:	p_1	p_2	$\cdots$	p_m	$\bar{p}$

The case being considered would arise in a comparative prospective study in which, for example, a number of quadruples of subjects would be matched on sex and age, under the restriction that one member did not smoke cigarettes, another smoked between 1 and 10 cigarettes per day, a third smoked between 11 and 20 cigarettes per day, and a fourth smoked 21 or more cigarettes per day. The proportions of subjects from the four resulting matched samples who develop a disease would then be compared using the methods of this section. An example of a retrospective study with three matched samples (lung cancer patients, other patients, and community controls) is the study by Doll and Hill (1952).

The methods of this section are also applicable to the results of a controlled trial in which $m > 2$ treatments are compared by grouping together a number of sets of m similar patients each and randomly assigning the treatments to the patients within each matched m-tuple. The methods are applicable, too, when each of a sample of subjects is studied under m different conditions. An example is the comparison of the proportions positive associated with m diagnostic tests, when each test is applied to each patient in the sample.

Table 13.10 illustrates the presentation of the data resulting from the study of m matched samples, with N observations in each sample. In Table 13.10, each X is either 0 (if the response is negative) or 1 (if the response is positive). Thus, for example, S_1 represents the total number of positives from the first m-tuple, T_1 represents the total number of positives from the first sample, and T represents the overall total number of positives.

Define

$$p_j = \frac{T_j}{N}, \tag{13.27}$$

the proportion of subjects from the jth sample who were positive;

$$P_n = \frac{S_n}{m}, \tag{13.28}$$

the proportion of positives in the nth m-tuple; and

$$\bar{p} = \frac{1}{m} \sum_{j=1}^{m} p_j = \frac{1}{N} \sum_{n=1}^{N} P_n = \frac{T}{Nm}, \qquad (13.29)$$

the overall proportion positive. Interest is in whether the proportions $p_1, \ldots, p_m$ differ significantly. The following statistic, due to Cochran (1950), may be used to test for the significance of the differences among the m proportions:

$$Q = \frac{N^2(m-1)}{m} \times \frac{\sum_{j=1}^{m} (p_j - \bar{p})^2}{N\bar{p}(1-\bar{p}) - \sum_{n=1}^{N} (P_n - \bar{p})^2}$$

$$= (m-1) \times \frac{m \sum_{j=1}^{m} T_j^2 - T^2}{mT - \sum_{n=1}^{N} S_n^2}. \qquad (13.30)$$

The value of (13.30) may be referred to tables of chi squared with $m - 1$ df.

Problem 13.5 demonstrates that Q is also the generalized Mantel-Haenszel $(m - 1)$ df chi squared statistic for combining the evidence across the N m-tuples when each m-tuple is viewed as a $2 \times m$ table with column margins of $1, \ldots, 1$ and row margins of S_n and $m - S_n$.

Consider the data of Table 13.11, originally reported by Fleiss (1965a). The proportions p_j of patients judged to have religious preoccupations vary from a low of 0 to a high of 0.375. The value of Q (13.30) for testing whether this variation can be attributed to chance or whether it represents real differences among the raters is

$$Q = 7 \times \frac{8(1^2 + 0^2 + \cdots + 0^2 + 3^2) - 15^2}{8 \times 15 - (0^2 + 1^2 + \cdots + 0^2 + 6^2)} = 14.71.$$

The validity of calculating Q for many ratings on the same subjects has been established by Fleiss (1965b).

Referring to Table A.2 with $m - 1 = 7$ degrees of freedom, we find that Q must exceed 14.07 in order for the variation to be declared significant at the 0.05 level. Since our obtained value of 14.71 exceeds the critical value, we infer that the raters differ in their judgments of religious preoccupation.

Having found significant variation, our next step would be to try to identify those samples or groups of samples (in our example, those raters or groups of raters) that differed. A device that is frequently useful is to *partition* Q into

Table 13.11. *Judgments by eight raters as to presence or absence** *of religious preoccupations in eight patients*

Patient	Rater 1	2	3	4	5	6	7	8	Total $(= S_n)$
1	0	0	0	0	0	0	0	0	0
2	0	0	0	0	1	0	0	0	1
3	0	0	0	0	0	0	0	0	0
4	0	0	0	0	0	0	0	0	0
5	0	0	1	0	0	1	0	1	3
6	0	0	1	1	1	1	0	1	5
7	0	0	0	0	0	0	0	0	0
8	1	0	1	1	1	1	0	1	6
Total $(= T_j)$:	1	0	3	2	3	3	0	3	15 $(= T)$
Proportion $(= p_j)$:	0.125	0	0.375	0.250	0.375	0.375	0	0.375	0.234 $(= \bar{p})$

*1 or 0, respectively.

separate components, each of which measures a specified source of variability. The general method for partitioning a chi squared statistic is described by Everitt (1977, Chapter 3). Here we illustrate the method for the statistic in (13.30).

Suppose that the m samples represent two groups, with m_1 samples in the first group and m_2 in the second. In the first example given at the beginning of the section, one group consists of the single sample of nonsmokers (so that $m_1 = 1$) and the other of the three samples of cigarette smokers (so that $m_2 = 3$). Define

$$U_1 = \sum_{j=1}^{m_1} T_j \qquad (13.31)$$

as the total number of positives in the first group of samples, and

$$U_2 = \sum_{j=m_1+1}^{m} T_j \qquad (13.32)$$

as the total number of positives in the second group. The statistic for testing whether the proportion positive in the first group differs significantly from that in the second is

$$Q_{\text{diff}} = \frac{m-1}{m_1 m_2} \times \frac{(m_2 U_1 - m_1 U_2)^2}{mT - \sum_{n=1}^{N} S_n^2}. \qquad (13.33)$$

The statistic Q_{diff} has 1 df.

Consider again the data of Table 13.11. The first five raters were from New York, and the last three were from Kentucky. They therefore form two natural groups, one containing $m_1 = 5$ raters and the other $m_2 = 3$. It is reasonable to inquire whether the two groups of raters differ in their judgments. The total number of positive ratings by the raters in the first group is

$$U_1 = 1 + 0 + 3 + 2 + 3 = 9,$$

and the total number of positive ratings by those in the second group is

$$U_2 = 3 + 0 + 3 = 6.$$

The value of Q_{diff} (13.33) is

$$Q_{\text{diff}} = \frac{7}{5 \times 3} \times \frac{(3 \times - 5 \times 6)^2}{120 - 71} = 0.09,$$

indicating a negligible difference between the New York raters as a group and the Kentucky raters as a group.

The next step in the analysis would be to compare the m_1 samples within group 1 by means of the statistic

$$Q_{\text{group 1}} = \frac{m(m-1)}{m_1} \times \frac{m_1 \sum\limits_{j=1}^{m_1} T_j^2 - U_1^2}{mT - \sum\limits_{n=1}^{N} S_n^2}, \tag{13.34}$$

and to compare the m_2 samples within group 2 by means of the statistic

$$Q_{\text{group 2}} = \frac{m(m-1)}{m_2} \times \frac{m_2 \sum\limits_{j=m_1+1}^{m} T_j^2 - U_2^2}{mT - \sum\limits_{n=1}^{N} S_n^2}. \tag{13.35}$$

The statistic $Q_{\text{group 1}}$ has $m_1 - 1$ df, and the statistic $Q_{\text{group 2}}$ has $m_2 - 1$. It may be checked that

$$Q = Q_{\text{diff}} + Q_{\text{group 1}} + Q_{\text{group 2}}.$$

In addition, note that the three numbers of degrees of freedom for the Q statistics of (13.33)–(13.35), namely 1, $m_1 - 1$, and $m_2 - 1$, sum to $m_1 + m_2 - 1 = m - 1$, the number of degrees of freedom in the overall Q (13.30).

For the data of Table 13.11, the differences among the five New York raters are assessed by

$$Q_{\text{group 1}} = \frac{8 \times 7}{5} \times \frac{5(1^2 + 0^2 + 3^2 + 2^2 + 3^2) - 9^2}{120 - 71} = 7.77,$$

which with $5 - 1 = 4$ df fails to reach significance at the 0.05 level. The differences among the three Kentucky raters are assessed by

$$Q_{\text{group 2}} = \frac{8 \times 7}{3} \times \frac{3(3^2 + 0^2 + 3^2) - 6^2}{120 - 71} = 6.86,$$

which with $3 - 1 = 2$ df is significant at the 0.05 level. Note that

$$Q_{\text{diff}} + Q_{\text{group 1}} + Q_{\text{group 2}} = 0.09 + 7.77 + 6.86 = 14.72,$$

which equals, except for rounding errors, the overall value of Q, 14.71.

Cochran (1950, p. 265) suggests a slightly different approach to the partitioning of Q. Its effect is to reduce slightly the magnitudes of $Q_{\text{group 1}}$ and of $Q_{\text{group 2}}$ (see also Tate and Brown, 1970). The conclusions for the data of Table 13.11 are the same for both methods of partitioning: there are differences among the judgments of the eight raters, arising essentially from the variability among the three Kentucky raters.

On occasion, the m samples represent m separate levels of a quantitatively ordered variable (e.g., average number of cigarettes smoked per day, as in the example described at the beginning of this section). Let x_j denote the value of this variable for the jth sample $(j = 1, \ldots, m)$, and define

$$b = \frac{\sum\limits_{j=1}^{m} T_j (x_j - \bar{x})}{N \sum\limits_{j=1}^{m} (x_j - \bar{x})^2}, \tag{13.36}$$

where

$$\bar{x} = \frac{1}{m} \sum_{j=1}^{m} x_j, \tag{13.37}$$

the mean value of x for these samples. The statistic b is the slope of the straight line fitted to the data. It describes the average change in the rate of occurrence of the event under study per unit change in x.

The statistical significance of b may be assessed by referring the value of

$$\chi^2_{\text{slope}} = \frac{m(m-1)N^2 \sum\limits_{j=1}^{m}(x_j - \bar{x})^2}{mT - \sum\limits_{n=1}^{N} S_n^2} b^2 \tag{13.38}$$

to the chi squared distribution with 1 df. If b is significant and positive (or negative), the inference would be that the proportions tend to increase (or decrease) with increasing values of x.

Suppose, contrary to fact and purely for illustrative purposes, that the numerals used in Table 13.11 to denote the several raters represent their numbers of years of experience. It might then be of interest to determine whether the likelihood of judging the presence of religious preoccupation varies systematically with length of experience. Note that $\bar{x}$ in Table 13.11 is equal to 4.5, and that $\sum(x_j - \bar{x})^2$ is equal to 42.

The slope of the straight line associating p with x is, by (13.36),

$$b = \frac{7.5}{8 \times 42} = 0.02,$$

indicating an average increase of 0.02 in the likelihood of judging the presence of religious preoccupation for each additional year of experience. The associated value of chi squared from (13.38) is

$$\chi^2_{\text{slope}} = \frac{8 \times 7 \times 64 \times 42}{8 \times 15 - 71}(0.02)^2 = 1.23,$$

which is not significant by any reasonable standard. No tendency for the proportions to vary systematically with length of experience can therefore be asserted.

The test statistics presented in this section, like those presented in the three preceding sections, are unaffected by the deletion of those m-tuples in which either all m responses were positive or all m were negative. Berger and Gold (1973) and Bhapkar and Somes (1977) have shown that the distribution of Q in large samples under the hypothesis of equal underlying probabilities is approximately chi squared with $m - 1$ df only if all pairwise probabilities $P(X_{ni} = 1$ and $X_{nj} = 1)$, $i \neq j$, are equal. Seeger and Gabrielsson (1968) and Tate and Brown (1970) have studied the accuracy of the chi squared approximation to the distribution of Q when this assumption holds and when the sample sizes are small. It seems that the approximation is adequate provided the product of the number of samples $(= m)$ and the number of m-tuples remaining after the deletion of those in which all responses were the same is at least 24. For the data of Table 13.11, four patients (numbers 1, 3, 4, and 7) were such that the ratings were identical. The product of $m = 8$ and the remaining number of patients ($= 4$) is 32, indicating that the approximation was adequate.

A quite different approach from Cochran's (1950) to the comparison of m matched samples is due to Bennett (1967, 1968). The reader is referred to his two papers for the test statistics he derived (more complicated than the Q statistic except when $m = 3$—see Mantel and Fleiss, 1975) and for their powers.

13.5. SAMPLE SIZE DETERMINATION FOR MATCHED SAMPLES

Power and sample size determination in pair-matched studies have been discussed by Schlesselman (1982), Parker and Bregman (1986), Connett, Smith, and McHugh (1987), Dupont (1988), Fleiss and Levin (1988), Lachin (1992), and Ejigou (1996). In this section we follow the development of Fleiss and Levin (1988), who refine the method of Schlesselman and correct an important oversight. The assumed study design is a pair-matched case-control study, although the same formulas apply to prospective or experimental matched pair designs as well. We indicate appropriate modifications at the end of the section for matched sets with $1 : r$ matching.

The determination of the number of matched pairs begins as usual with specification of an odds ratio worth detecting, say ω^*, at given levels of type I error α and power $1 - \beta$. We assume $\omega^* > 1$, and that ω^* is so large that the investigator would want the chance to be at least $1 - \beta$ that the null hypothesis H_0: $\omega = 1$ would be rejected at level α if the true odds ratio ω were ω^* or larger. The next step is to determine the number of discordant pairs, m, that must be obtained, since the power of McNemar's test depends on how many informative pairs enter the analysis. Because that number is not known precisely until after collection of the data, the final step in the sample size determination is to estimate how many subjects pairs, M, to recruit in order to produce the required number of informative pairs. It is important not to overestimate the probability of discordance.

The number of discordant pairs, $m = b + c$, required to achieve power $1 - \beta$ in McNemar's test can be found using the methods of Section 2.5.1 for the single-sample binomial problem because, given m, b has a binomial distribution with index m and probability $P = \omega/(\omega + 1)$. The null hypothesis value of P is $P_0 = \frac{1}{2}$, and the alternative hypothesis value of P at which power is to be $1 - \beta$ is $P^* = \omega^*/(\omega^* + 1)$. An initial value of m (call it m_d) is, ignoring the continuity correction, given by

$$m_d = \frac{\left(z_{\alpha/2}\sqrt{P_0 Q_0} + z_\beta\sqrt{P^* Q^*}\right)^2}{\left(P^* - P_0\right)^2} = \frac{\left\{z_{\alpha/2}(1 + \omega^*) + 2z_\beta\sqrt{\omega^*}\right\}^2}{\left(\omega^* - 1\right)^2}. \quad (13.39)$$

McNemar's test with continuity correction requires augmenting m_d to

$$m_d^* = \frac{m_d}{4}\left\{1 + \sqrt{1 + \frac{4(\omega^* + 1)}{m_d(\omega^* - 1)}}\right\}^2. \qquad (13.40)$$

A simple and excellent approximation is

$$m_d^* \approx m_d + \frac{2(\omega^* + 1)}{\omega^* - 1}. \qquad (13.41)$$

We illustrate with an example discussed by Schlesselman (1982, p. 162), in which it is required to achieve a power of $1 - \beta = 0.90$ (so that $z_\beta = 1.282$ when $\omega^* = 2$) for a two-tailed McNemar test with a significance level of $\alpha = 0.05$ (so that $z_{\alpha/2} = 1.96$). Formula (13.39) yields $m_d = 90.26$ as the required number of discordant pairs, without continuity correction, and (13.40) yields $m_d^* = 96.17$, close to the value $m_d^* = 96.26$ produced by the simpler formula (13.41). Thus we need 97 discordant pairs. So far, so good.

Let the probability that a matched pair will be discordant be denoted by p_d. If p_d were known, then the total number of pairs to be recruited would be $M^* = m_d^*/p_d$, with the expectation that the number of discordant pairs will be $M^* p_d = m_d^*$ on average. In practice, one ought to augment M^* in order to increase the likelihood that m will be at least m_d. For example, to insure adequate power, one might augment M^* by the multiplicative factor $1 + 0.842\{(1 - p_d)/m_d^*\}^{1/2}$, which allows an 80% chance that the number of discordant pairs m would exceed m_d^* (see Problem 13.6). For simplicity, we will just use $M^* = m_d^*/p_d$ in the discussion below.

The probability of discordance p_d depends fundamentally on the prevalence of exposure, the odds ratio ω, *and the strength of the unconditional association of the exposure status of a case with the exposure status of his or her matched control.* To be precise, let us introduce the following notation. Let p_0 denote the marginal or overall proportion of control subjects expected to have been exposed to the risk factor under study, and let p_1 denote the marginal proportion of case subjects exposed. First suppose that the value of p_0 can be specified. Now assume for the moment that there is no association at all between the matching factors and exposure. Then p_0 is also the constant within-pair probability of exposure for controls. The within-pair proportion of cases exposed to the risk factor is also constant (assuming the common odds ratio ω), equal to p_1, and would equal, say,

$$p_1^* = \frac{\omega p_0}{1 + (\omega - 1)p_0}. \qquad (13.42)$$

Then the the probability of discordance would be

$$p_d^* = p_0(1 - p_1^*) + p_1^*(1 - p_0) = \frac{(\omega + 1)p_0(1 - p_0)}{1 + (\omega - 1)p_0}. \qquad (13.43)$$

However, if the matching has been effective, in the sense that the matching variables are associated with exposure, as they ought to be as confounders, then the within-pair probabilities of exposure vary, the overall proportion of exposed cases is no longer equal to p_1^*, and the use of p_d^* for p_d results in an underestimation of the required sample size M, no matter what the true value of ω is (Parker and Bregman, 1986). Variation in the within-pair probabilities of exposure will be manifest in the marginal association of the case exposures with the exposures of their matched controls; we need to assess the strength of that association.

Let the marginal (overall) probabilities of exposure for the members of the matched pairs in the underlying population be as follows:

| | Status of Control | | | |
Status of Case	Exposed	Not Exposed	Total	
Exposed	u	v	p_1	
Not exposed	w	x	$1 - p_1$	(13.44)
Total	p_0	$1 - p_0$	1	

A natural measure of the strength of association between the exposure status of cases with matching controls is the odds ratio,

$$\psi = \frac{ux}{vw}. \qquad (13.45)$$

It is important to understand the difference between the two odds ratios ω and ψ. The former measures the association between exposure status on the one hand and disease development on the other. It is the parameter about which the study is intended to provide information. The latter measures the association between cases' and matched controls' exposure status. It reflects the variation of exposure probabilities across matched pairs, i.e., how successful the matching has been, and is thus a characteristic of the study design.

In the notation of (13.44), the probability of discordance is $p_d = v + w$, the marginal probability of control exposure is $p_0 = u + w$, the marginal probability of case exposure is $p_1 = u + v$, and the common odds ratio is $\omega = v/w$ (see Problem 13.7). With values of $\psi \geq 1$, the discordance probability is given by

$$p_d = p_d^* \frac{\sqrt{1 + 4(\psi - 1)p_1^* q_1^*} - 1}{2(\psi - 1)p_1^* q_1^*}, \qquad (13.46)$$

where p_1^* is given by (13.42) and p_d^* is given by (13.43). When the value of ψ is close to 1, the value of p_d will be close to that of p_d^*. For stronger association $\psi > 1$, p_d can be substantially smaller than p_d^*. Then (13.46) should be used in place of p_d^* in determining the required number of matched pairs: $M^* = m_d^*/p_d$.

Expressions (13.43) and (13.46) may be applied when the value of p_0, the marginal probability that a control is exposed, can be specified. When instead the investigator can specify the value of p_1, the marginal probability that a case is exposed, the value of p_d corresponding to the odds ratio $\psi > 1$ is

$$p_d = p_d^{**} \frac{\sqrt{1 + 4(\psi - 1)p_0^* q_0^*} - 1}{2(\psi - 1)p_0^* q_0^*}, \tag{13.47}$$

where

$$p_0^* = \frac{p_1}{1 + q_1(\omega - 1)} \tag{13.48}$$

and

$$p_d^{**} = \frac{(\omega + 1)p_1 q_1}{1 + q_1(\omega - 1)}. \tag{13.49}$$

Formulas (13.46) and (13.47) require a value for ψ. The best estimates derive from prior evidence, of course. When such information is lacking, however, one may use a conservative (high) value of ψ. A far from exhaustive examination of the literature led Fleiss and Levin (1988) to suggest that $\psi = 2.5$ was among the largest odds ratios induced by matching in actual case control studies; ψ rarely exceeded 3.

Continuing with the example, Schlesselman (1982) used $m_d = 90.26$ and assumed a marginal exposure probability for controls of $p_0 = 0.3$, so that $p_1^* = \frac{6}{13}$. He then assumed, in effect, that $\psi = 1$, obtaining $p_d^* = 0.484$ as the discordance probability. Dividing p_d^* into m_d, he obtained the value $M = 90.26/0.4846 = 186.3$, or 187 matched pairs. This value could be too small. Assume that matching is on a set of strong confounders, such that the induced odds ratio is $\psi = 2.5$. Then (13.46) with $\omega = \omega^* = 2$ yields the value $p_d = 0.3759$ as the probability of discordance; dividing this into m_d yields $M = 90.26/0.3759 = 240.1$, or 241, almost 30% larger than Schlesselman's value. Using the continuity correction yields $M^* = m_d^*/p_d = 96.26/0.3759 = 256$ as the required number of matched pairs, more than $\frac{1}{3}$ greater than 187.

For studies with $1:r$ matching of one case to r controls, Parker and Bregman (1986) have shown that to an excellent approximation, the required number N of matched sets can be obtained from M^* as

$$N = \frac{r + 1}{2r} M^*. \tag{13.50}$$

The Mantel-Haenszel procedure would now be the test statistic.

In the example, suppose that $r = 3$ controls are to be matched to each case. Then the total number of matched sets required (and therefore the total number of cases) is

$$N = \frac{3 + 1}{2 \times 3} 255.8 \approx 171,$$

or $N = 171$ cases and $3N = 513$ controls. The number of cases is reduced by one-third, from 256 to 171, but the total sample size is increased also by about one-third, from $2 \times 256 = 512$ to $4 \times 171 = 684$.

13.6. ADVANTAGES AND DISADVANTAGES OF MATCHING

In comparative prospective and retrospective studies, the matching of subjects is usually employed to assure that the samples being contrasted are similar with respect to characteristics associated with the factors being studied (see, e.g., Billewicz, 1965, and Miettinen, 1970a). The possible gain in efficiency due to the study of matched samples (i.e., increase in the power of the test of significance and increase in the precision of the estimated degree of association) therefore assumes lesser importance, but some results are available.

Cochran (1950) and Worcester (1964) have shown that matching is not guaranteed to increase efficiency. It can be expected to do so only when the characteristics being matched on are strongly associated with the factors under study. When the characteristics used for matching are only slightly or not at all associated with the factors under study, Youkeles (1963) has shown that efficiency may even be lost. When the number of matched sets exceeds 30, however, matching on irrelevant characteristics seems not to affect efficiency.

In the context of controlled comparative trials with random assignment of treatments to subjects, on the other hand, the purpose of matching is mainly the increase of efficiency. Chase (1968) has shown that matching is at least as efficient as no matching except for small sample sizes. Billewicz (1964, 1965), however, has indicated that the increase in efficiency is frequently small and may not be worth the effort involved in securing adequate matches.

He has shown how the length of time required to complete a study increases either as the number of matching characteristics increases or as the relative frequencies of some categories of the matching characteristics decrease. With too many matching characteristics, or with only a few but some containing too many categories, the investigator may find a large proportion of subjects left unmatched at the end of the study.

In view of the need to assure comparability in comparative prospective and retrospective studies, matching or some other method of control for biasing factors in these contexts is often necessary. In addition to matching, control may be effected by means of stratification or regression techniques (Cochran, 1968; Rubin, 1973; McKinlay, 1975a). When stratification is the method adopted, the techniques presented in Chapter 10 are applicable.

McKinlay (1977) has critically analyzed matching for the control of unwanted sources of variation and cites as its major advantages its easy understandability and the relative simplicity of the analysis of the resulting data. Its major disadvantages include the possibly excessive costs associated both with finding matches and with discarding subjects who could not be matched, and the likely failure to detect *interaction*, the phenomenon in which the magnitude of the difference or association varies across different subgroups. McKinlay (1975b, 1977) also points out that whereas matching may well yield greater precision than designs that do not control for sources of bias, it does not necessarily yield greater precision than other designs in which control is attempted. Rosenbaum (1987, 1991) considers sensitivity analyses for matched case-control studies and examines the influence of an unobserved confounder on inference.

It may be that an investigator nevertheless decides to employ matching instead of another method for control of biasing factors in a comparative prospective or retrospective study. In studies of hospitalized patients, for example, matching on the date of hospitalization is probably the best method for control of the effect of an epidemic. Matching should, however, be on a small number of characteristics (rarely more than four and preferably no more than two), with each defined by a small number of categories (with respect to age, e.g., matching by 10-year intervals should frequently suffice). If the investigator insists on controlling for a large number of biasing factors simultaneously, multivariate methods such as those proposed by Althouser and Rubin (1970) and Rosenbaum and Rubin (1983, 1984, 1985a, and 1985b) may have to be used.

Once matching is employed in the design of a study, it should be taken into account in the analysis (Breslow and Day, 1980). If the matching is ignored in a matched pairs study with binary outcomes, and the odds ratio estimated from the pooled fourfold table, serious bias may result unless $\omega = 1$. Liang and Zeger (1988) and Kalish (1990) proposed estimators that are weighted averages of the pooled odds ratio and the Mantel-Haenszel estimator, in an attempt to reduce the overall mean squared error. Levin (1997) provides a lower bound for the Mantel-Haenszel chi squared statistic based on the pooled chi squared statistic in 1-to-r matched samples. This is useful when the proper presentation of the matched sample data is unavailable. Specifically, Levin shows that

$$\chi^2_{MH} \geq \frac{r}{r+1} \chi^2_{pooled},$$

where χ^2_{MH} is the proper Mantel-Haenszel statistic to use for one case matched to $r = m - 1$ controls, and where χ^2_{pooled} is the ordinary chi squared statistic one would use if the data were collapsed into a single 2×2 table cross-classifying case-control status by exposure status (an incorrect statistic to use for matched sets). Thus if χ^2_{pooled} is at least $(r+1)/r = m/(m-1)$ times the required critical value to declare significance at any given level, then the appropriate χ^2_{MH} would also reject H_0.

PROBLEMS

13.1. Consider the hypothetical data of Table 13.6. Do the two diagnosticians differ significantly in the proportions of patients they diagnose as affectively ill? as other? [*Hint*. Be sure to refer the value of McNemar's statistic to the critical value of chi squared with 2 df.]

13.2. Consider the hypothetical data of Table 13.8.

(a) What is the value of the Stuart-Maxwell statistic given in (13.19)? Does the outcome distribution of patients given the new treatment differ significantly from that of patients given the standard treatment?

(b) What are the values of d_1, d_3, and $d_1 - d_3$? What does the sign of $d_1 - d_3$ suggest about the direction of the difference between the two treatments? What is the value of the test statistic in (13.20)? Is the new treatment significantly better than the standard?

13.3. When not corrected for continuity, McNemar's chi squared statistic is given by

$$\chi^2_u = \frac{(b-c)^2}{b+c}.$$

Prove that, when $m = 2$, the expression for χ^2_u given by (13.25) is equal to that of χ^2_u above. [*Hint*. Refer to Table 13.1 for notation. Prove that, when $m = 2$, A (13.21) equals $a + b$, B (13.22) equals $2a + b + c$, and $\sum_i n_i^2$ equals $4a + b + c$.]

13.4. Prove that, when $m = 2$, the value of Q given by (13.30) is equal to that of χ^2_u. [*Hint*. Prove that, when $m = 2$, one has $T_1 = a + c$, $T_2 = a + b$, $T = 2a + b + c$, and $\sum_n S_n^2 = 4a + b + c$.]

13.5. Each row of Table 13.10 represents the first row of a $2 \times m$ table with column margins equal to 1. For example, patient 8 in Table 13.11

represents the 2×8 table

						Rater				
		1	2	3	4	5	6	7	8	Total
Religious	Present	1	0	1	1	1	1	0	1	6
preoccupation	Absent	0	1	0	0	0	0	1	0	2
	Total	1	1	1	1	1	1	1	1	8

The *generalized Mantel-Haenszel* procedure is used to combine the evidence across the N $2 \times m$ tables. The basic idea is to sum the multiple hypergeometric vectors $\underline{X}_n = (X_{n1}, \ldots, X_{nm})'$ for $n = 1, \ldots, N$, subtract the sum of their conditional expectations given all margins fixed under H_0, $(S_n/m, \ldots, S_n/m)'$, and note that the resulting vector

$$\left(\sum_{n=1}^{N} \left(X_{n1} - \frac{S_n}{m} \right), \ldots, \sum_{n=1}^{N} \left(X_{nm} - \frac{S_n}{m} \right) \right)' = \left(T_1 - \frac{T}{m}, \ldots, T_m - \frac{T}{m} \right)'$$

is distributed approximately as a multivariate normal vector with mean $(0, \ldots, 0)'$ and covariance matrix

$$\sum_{n=1}^{N} \frac{S_n(m - S_n)}{m - 1} \left\{ \text{Diag}(\tfrac{1}{m}, \cdots, \tfrac{1}{m}) - \begin{bmatrix} \frac{1}{m} \\ \vdots \\ \frac{1}{m} \end{bmatrix} [\tfrac{1}{m}, \cdots, \tfrac{1}{m}] \right\}.$$

Equivalently, the vector

$$U = \sqrt{\frac{m(m-1)}{\sum_{n=1}^{N} S_n(m - S_n)}} \left(T_1 - \frac{T}{m}, \ldots, T_m - \frac{T}{m} \right)'$$

has an approximately normal distribution with mean $(0, \ldots, 0)'$ and covariance matrix

$$\text{Cov}(U) = I - \sqrt{\underline{p}} \sqrt{\underline{p}'},$$

where I is the $m \times m$ identity matrix, $\underline{p} = (1/m, \ldots, 1/m)'$, and $\sqrt{\underline{p}} = (1/\sqrt{m}, \ldots, 1/\sqrt{m})'$.

(a) Show that if $\underline{p}$ is any nonnegative vector with $\sum_i p_i = 1$ and $\sqrt{\underline{p}} = (\sqrt{p_1}, \ldots, \sqrt{p_m})'$ and U has a multivariate normal distribution with mean $\underline{0}$ and covariance matrix $I - \sqrt{\underline{p}} \sqrt{\underline{p}'}$, $U \sim N_m(\underline{0}, I - \sqrt{\underline{p}} \sqrt{\underline{p}'})$, then $U'U = \sum_i U_i^2 \sim \chi_{m-1}^2$, the chi squared distribution with $m - 1$ df.

(b) Show that with $p = (1/m, \ldots, 1/m)'$, one has $U'U = \Sigma_i U_i^2 = Q$.
[*Hint*:

$$U'U = m(m-1) \frac{\displaystyle\sum_{j=1}^{m} \left(T_j - \frac{T}{m}\right)^2}{\displaystyle\sum_{n=1}^{N} S_n(m - S_n)} = (m-1) \frac{m \displaystyle\sum_{j=1}^{m} T_j^2 - T^2}{mT - \displaystyle\sum_{n=1}^{N} S_n^2} = Q.]$$

13.6. Let $m \sim \text{Bin}(M^*, p_d)$. Show that for the event $[m \geq m_d]$ to occur with probability at least $1 - \beta$, M^* should be chosen to satisfy the inequality (ignoring continuity correction)

$$M^* p_d - z_\beta (M^* p_d q_d)^{1/2} \geq m_d.$$

This is a quadratic equation in $(M^*)^{1/2}$, whose solution is

$$M^* \geq \frac{z_\beta^2}{4} \frac{q_d}{p_d} \left(1 + \sqrt{1 + \frac{4m_d}{q_d z_\beta^2}}\right)^2.$$

Expand the square and ignore terms of order smaller than $m_d^{1/2}$ to derive the augmented number of pairs $(m_d^*/p_d)\{1 + z_\beta(q_d/m_d)^{1/2}\}$ that will give at least m_d discordant pairs with probability $1 - \beta$.

13.7. Suppose that given probabilities (P_{i1}, P_{i0}), a case exposure has probability P_{i1}, namely, $X_{i1} \sim \text{Bin}(1, P_{i1})$, the matched control exposure has probability P_{i0}, such that, $X_{i0} \sim \text{Bin}(1, P_{i0})$, and that given (P_{i1}, P_{i0}), X_{i1} and X_{i0} are conditionally independent. Assume that the probabilities have a constant odds ratio with $(P_{i1}/Q_{i1})/(P_{i0}/Q_{i0}) = \omega$, but that P_{i0} has an arbitrary and unknown distribution in the population of controls. Prove the following assertions:

(a) The marginal covariance of X_{i1} and X_{i0} equals the covariance between P_{i1} and P_{i0}. [*Hint*. Use the identity $\text{Cov}(X_{i1}, X_{i0}) = E\{\text{Cov}(X_{i1}, X_{i0} | P_{i1}, P_{i0})\} + \text{Cov}\{E(X_{i1} | P_{i1}), E(X_{i0} | P_{i0})\}$.]

(b) The odds ratio ω equals the quantity v/w, where $v = P(X_{i1} = 1, X_{i0} = 0)$ is the marginal proportion of matched pairs with exposed case and unexposed control, and where $w = P(X_{i1} = 0, X_{i0} = 1)$ is the marginal proportion of matched pairs with unexposed case and exposed control. This result gives another proof of the consistency of the odds ratio estimator b/c for matched pairs. [*Hint*. In general, for any joint distribution of two random probabilities (P_1, P_0), show that the conditional expected value of the odds ratio $(P_1/Q_1)/(P_0/Q_0)$ given that $(X_1, X_0) = (0, 1)$ is equal to the ratio v/w. Under the assumption of a constant odds ratio ω, the conditional expectation in the subgroup with $(X_1, X_0) = (0, 1)$ is still ω.]

REFERENCES

Althouser, R. P. and Rubin, D. B. (1970). The computerized construction of a matched sample. *Am. J. Sociol.*, **76**, 325–346.

Bennett, B. M. (1967). Tests of hypotheses concerning matched samples. *J. R. Stat. Soc.*, *Ser. B*, **29**, 468–474.

Bennett, B. M. (1968). Note on X^2 tests for matched samples. *J. R. Stat. Soc.*, *Ser. B*, **30**, 368–370.

Bennett, B. M. and Underwood, R. E. (1970). On McNemar's test for the 2×2 table and its power function. *Biometrics*, **26**, 339–343.

Berger, A. and Gold, R. Z. (1973). Note on Cochran's Q-test for the comparison of correlated proportions. *J. Am. Statist. Assoc.*, **68**, 989–993.

Bhapkar, V. P. (1966). A note on the equivalence of two test criteria for hypotheses in categorical data. *J. Am. Statist. Assoc.*, **61**, 228–235.

Bhapkar, V. P. and Somes, G. W. (1977). Distribution of Q when testing equality of matched proportions. *J. Am. Statist. Assoc.*, **72**, 658–661.

Billewicz, W. Z. (1964). Matched samples in medical investigations. *Brit. J. Prev. Soc. Med.*, **18**, 167–173.

Billewicz, W. Z. (1965). The efficiency of matched samples: An empirical investigation. *Biometrics*, **21**, 623–644.

Bross, I. D. J. (1969). How case-for-case matching can improve design efficiency. *Am. J. Epidemiol.*, **89**, 359–363.

Chase, G. R. (1968). On the efficiency of matched pairs in Bernoulli trials. *Biometrika*, **55**, 365–369.

Cochran, W. G. (1950). The comparison of percentages in matched samples. *Biometrika*, **37**, 256–266.

Cochran, W. G. (1968). The effectiveness of subclassification in removing bias in observational studies. *Biometrics*, **24**, 295–313.

Connett, J. E., Smith, J. A., and McHugh, R. B. (1987). Sample size and power for pair-matched case-control studies. *Statist. in Med.*, **6**, 53–59.

Cornfield, J. and Haenszel, W. (1960). Some aspects of retrospective studies. *J. Chronic Dis.*, **11**, 523–534.

Cox, D. R. (1966). A simple example of a comparison involving quantal data. *Biometrika*, **53**, 215–220.

Doll, R. and Hill, A. B. (1952). A study of the etiology of carcinoma of the lung. *Brit. Med. J.*, **2**, 1271–1286.

Dupont, W. D. (1988). Power calculations for matched case-control studies. *Biometrics*, **44**, 1157–1168.

Edwards, A. L. (1948). Note on the "correction for continuity" in testing the significance of the difference between correlated proportions. *Psychometrika*, **13**, 185–187.

Ejigou, A. (1996). Power and sample size for matched case-control studies. *Biometrics*, **52**, 925–933.

Ejigou, A. and McHugh, R. (1977). Estimation of relative risk from matched pairs in epidemiologic research. *Biometrics*, **33**, 552–556.

Ejigou, A. and McHugh, R. (1984). Testing the homogeneity of the relative risk under multiple matching. *Biometrika*, **71**, 408–411.

Everitt, B. S. (1977). *The analysis of contingency tables*. London: Chapman and Hall.

Fleiss, J. L. (1965a). Estimating the accuracy of dichotomous judgments. *Psychometrika*, **30**, 469–479.

Fleiss, J. L. (1965b). A note on Cochran's Q test. *Biometrics*, **21**, 1008–1010.

Fleiss, J. L. and Everitt, B. S. (1971). Comparing the marginal totals of square contingency tables. *Brit. J. Math. Stat. Psychol.*, **24**, 117–123.

Fleiss, J. L. and Levin, B. (1988). Sample size determination in studies with matched pairs. *J. Clin. Epidemiol.*, **41**, 727–730.

Gart, J. J. (1985). Testing for interaction in multiply-matched case-control studies. *Biometrika*, **72**, 468–470.

Grizzle, J. E., Starmer, C. F., and Koch, G. G. (1969). Analysis of categorical data by linear models. *Biometrics*, **25**, 489–504.

Hill, A. B. (1962). *Statistical methods in clinical and preventive medicine*. New York: Oxford University Press.

Ireland, C. T., Ku, H. H., and Kullback, S. (1969). Symmetry and marginal homogeneity of an $r \times r$ contingency table. *J. Am. Statist. Assoc.*, **64**, 1323–1341.

Jewell, N. P. (1984). Small-sample bias of point estimators of the odds ratio from matched sets. *Biometrics*, **40**, 421–435.

Kalish, L. A. (1990). Reducing mean squared error in the analysis of pair-matched case-control studies. *Biometrics*, **46**, 493–499.

Koch, G. G. and Reinfurt, D. W. (1971). The analysis of categorical data from mixed models. *Biometrics*, **27**, 157–173.

Kuritz, S. J. and Landis, J. R. (1988). Attributable risk estimation from matched case-control data. *Biometrics*, **44**, 355–367.

Lachin, J. M. (1992). Power and sample size evaluation for the McNemar test with application to matched case-control studies. *Statist. in Med.*, **11**, 1239–1251.

Levin, B. (1992). Tests of odds ratio homogeneity with improved power in sparse fourfold tables. *Comm. Statist.—Theory Meth.*, **21**, 1469–1500.

Levin, B. (1997). A lower bound for the Mantel-Haenszel one degree of freedom chi-squared statistic in $1 : m$ matched samples. *Am. Statistician*, **51**, 318–320.

Liang, K.-Y. and Self, S. G. (1985). Tests for homogeneity of odds ratio when the data are sparse. *Biometrika*, **72**, 353–358.

Liang, K.-Y. and Zeger, S. L. (1988). On the use of concordant pairs in matched case-control studies. *Biometrics*, **44**, 1145–1156.

Lui, K.-J. (1998). A note on interval estimation of the relative difference in data with matched pairs. *Statist. in Med.*, **17**, 1509–1515.

Mantel, N. and Fleiss, J. L. (1975). The equivalence of the generalized McNemar tests for marginal homogeneity in 2^3 and 3^2 tables. *Biometrics*, **31**, 727–729.

Mantel, N. and Haenszel, W. (1959). Statistical aspects of the analysis of data from retrospective studies of disease. *J. Natl. Cancer Inst.*, **22**, 719–748.

Maxwell, A. E. (1970). Comparing the classification of subjects by two independent judges. *Brit. J. Psychiatry*, **116**, 651–655.

McKinlay, S. M. (1975a). The design and analysis of the observational study: A review. *J. Am. Statist. Assoc.*, **70**, 503–520.

McKinlay, S. M. (1975b). A note on the chi-square test for pair-matched samples. *Biometrics*, **31**, 731–735.

McKinlay, S. M. (1977). Pair-matching: A reappraisal of a popular technique. *Biometrics*, **33**, 725–735.

McNemar, Q. (1947). Note on the sampling error of the difference between correlated proportions or percentages. *Psychometrika*, **12**, 153–157.

Miettinen, O. S. (1968). The matched pairs design in the case of all-or-none responses. *Biometrics*, **24**, 339–352.

Miettinen, O. S. (1969). Individual matching with controls in the case of all-or-none responses. *Biometrics*, **25**, 339–355.

Miettinen, O. S. (1970a). Matching and design efficiency in retrospective studies. *Am. J. Epidemiol.*, **91**, 111–118.

Miettinen, O. S. (1970b). Estimation of relative risk from individually matched series. *Biometrics*, **26**, 75–86.

Miller, R. G. (1966). *Simultaneous statistical inference*. New York: McGraw-Hill.

Mosteller, F. (1952). Some statistical problems in measuring the subjective response to drugs. *Biometrics*, **8**, 220–226.

Parker, R. A. and Bregman, D. J. (1986). Sample size for individually matched case-control studies. *Biometrics*, **42**, 919–926.

Pike, M. C. and Morrow, R. H. (1970). Statistical analysis of patient-control studies in epidemiology: Factor under investigation an all-or-none variable. *Brit. J. Prev. Soc. Med.*, **24**, 42–44.

Rosenbaum, P. R. (1987). Sensitivity analysis for certain permutation inferences in matched observational studies. *Biometrika*, **74**, 13–26 (Correction, **75**, 396).

Rosenbaum, P. R. (1991). Sensitivity analysis for matched case-control studies. *Biometrics*, **47**, 87–100.

Rosenbaum, P. R. and Rubin, D. B. (1983). The central role of the propensity score in observational studies for causal effects. *Biometrika*, **70**, 41–55.

Rosenbaum, P. R. and Rubin, D. B. (1984). Reducing bias in observational studies using subclassification on the propensity score. *Am. Statist. Assoc.*, **79**, 516–524.

Rosenbaum, P. R. and Rubin, D. B. (1985a). Constructing a control group using multivariate matched sampling methods that incorporate the propensity score. *Am. Statistician*, **39**, 33–38.

Rosenbaum, P. R. and Rubin, D. B. (1985b). The bias due to incomplete matching. *Biometrics*, **41**, 103–116.

Rubin, D. B. (1973). The use of matched sampling and regression adjustment to remove bias in observational studies. *Biometrics*, **29**, 185–203.

Schlesselman, J. J. (1982). *Case-control studies: Design, conduct, analysis*. London: Oxford Univ. Press.

Seeger, P. and Gabrielsson, A. (1968). Applicability of the Cochran Q test and the F test for statistical analysis of dichotomous data for dependent samples. *Psychol. Bull.*, **69**, 269–277.

Stuart, A. (1955). A test for homogeneity of the marginal distribution in a two-way classification. *Biometrika*, **42**, 412–416.

Stuart, A. (1957). The comparison of frequencies in matched samples. *Brit. J. Statist. Psychol.*, **10**, 29–32.

Suissa, S. and Schuster, J. J. (1991). The 2×2 matched-pairs trial: Exact unconditional design and analysis. *Biometrics*, **47**, 361–372.

Tate, M. W. and Brown, S. M. (1970). Note on the Cochran Q test. *J. Am. Statist. Assoc.*, **65**, 155–160.

Ury, H. K. (1975). Efficiency of case-control studies with multiple controls per case: Continuous or dichotomous data. *Biometrics*, **31**, 643–649.

Worcester, J. (1964). Matched samples in epidemiologic studies. *Biometrics*, **20**, 840–848.

Youkeles, L. H. (1963). Loss of power through ineffective pairing of observations in small two-treatment all-or-none experiments. *Biometrics*, **19**, 175–180.

Zelterman, D. and Chen, C.-F. (1988). Homogeneity tests against central-mixture alternatives. *J. Am. Statist. Assoc.*, **83**, 179–182 (Correction, **86**, 837).

Zelterman, D. and Le, C. T. (1991). Tests of homogeneity for the relative risk in multiply-matched case-control studies. *Biometrics*, **47**, 751–755.

CHAPTER 14

Regression Models for Matched Samples

The previous chapter presented the analysis of matched data in the case of a single risk factor. This chapter presents analytic methods for matched studies with multiple risk factors of interest. We consider matched sample designs of two types, prospective (cohort or randomized) and retrospective (case-control) studies. In the simplest nontrivial case, we have a single binary exposure variable, X, a single binary disease indicator, Y, and a potent confounder, Z, such as age, upon which the samples are matched. In pair-matched prospective studies, we match one exposed subject ($X = 1$) and one unexposed subject ($X = 0$) on Z, and then follow them to observe Y. In pair-matched case-control studies, we match one case ($Y = 1$) and one control ($Y = 0$) on Z, and then observe the antecedent risk factor X. Matching guarantees balance in Z between exposed and unexposed in prospective studies, and between cases and controls in retrospective studies.

When there are multiple risk factors $X = (X_1, X_2, X_3, \ldots)$, we must decide how many exposure groups will be matched in a prospective study, and which factors will remain uncontrolled. For example, with two binary risk factors, $X = (X_1, X_2)$, a prospective study could match pairs of subjects exposed or unexposed to X_1 on Z, leaving X_2 to covary in an uncontrolled manner with X_1 and Z. (This is essentially the strategy of a randomized trial with randomization within matched pairs.) To gain more detailed information, the prospective study could be designed to match four samples—$(X_1, X_2) = (1, 1)$, $(1, 0)$, $(0, 1)$, and $(0, 0)$—on Z and then use the methods of Section 13.4 for quadruplet data. In retrospective studies, we do not have to decide which exposure variables will be matched on Z (because none are),

Statistical Methods for Rates and Proportions, Third Edition
By Joseph L. Fleiss, Bruce Levin, and Myunghee Cho Paik
ISBN 0-471-52629-0   Copyright © 2003 John Wiley & Sons, Inc.

but we must deal with the multivariate response variable X and its relationship to Y. When there are polytomous disease states $Y = (Y_1, Y_2, Y_3, \ldots)$, the design and analysis considerations become more complex because the relations between $(X_1, X_2, X_3, \ldots)$ and $(Y_1, Y_2, Y_3, \ldots)$ multiply.

Regardless of the number of elements in X and Y, some general remarks hold true. Prospective studies provide direct estimates of $P(Y|X, Z)$, the joint conditional distribution of disease status Y given risk factors X and matching factors Z; the effect of Z on X cannot be estimated. Retrospective studies provide direct estimates of $P(X|Y, Z)$, the joint distribution of the risk factors given disease status and matching factors; the effect of Z on Y cannot be estimated.

In a prospective matched-sample study, we can occasionally model $P(Y|X, Z)$ parametrically by accounting explicitly for the effect of Z on Y in a logistic regression model. In this case, the analytic methods of Chapter 11 apply. When matching variables are not readily quantifiable, explicit parametric modeling is not feasible. Examples include matching on identical twins reared separately or matching on self (e.g., pre- and posttreatment observations on the same individual), wherein the matching device controls a large number of factors. If we try to model the dependence of Y on Z nonparametrically, by estimating separate parameters for each matched set, then the number of unknown parameters increases in proportion to the sample size, rendering maximum likelihood estimation inconsistent (Andersen, 1970, 1973; Neyman and Scott, 1948). *Conditional logistic regression*, the primary focus of this chapter, provides a solution to this dilemma: conditioning eliminates the nuisance parameters for both quantifiable and unquantifiable matching factors from the likelihood function, so that estimation of the odds ratio of interest becomes consistent.

In a retrospective matched-sample study, we can occasionally model $P(X|Y, Z)$ parametrically by accounting explicitly for the effect of Z on X. When X is a single binary exposure variable of primary interest, we can fit a logistic regression model for X, using the case-control indicator Y as an explanatory factor, together with the matching factors and other covariates. This approach is discussed by Prentice (1976). As long as the model for X is correctly specified, the coefficient of Y is a consistent estimate of the disease-exposure log odds ratio, thanks to the invariance property of the odds ratio. Multiple exposure variables require multivariate regression models to fit the vector X as dependent variables. (See also Section 15.5.) If a parametric model for the matching variables is unavailable, we can specify nonparametric indicators for the matched sets. Neyman-Scott inconsistency of the unconditional maximum likelihood estimates leads again to the use of conditional logistic regression. This approach was popularized for case-control studies by Holford, White, and Kelsey (1978), Pike, Hill, and Smith (1980), and Breslow and Day (1980).

Additional biases arise from attempts to use parametric logistic regression models for $P(Y|X, Z)$ with data collected retrospectively in matched samples, or for $P(X|Y,Z)$ with data collected prospectively in matched samples. These issues are discussed in Section 14.1. Section 14.2 describes conditional likelihood analysis for $1:1$ or $1:k$ matched samples, and Section 14.3 describes the general case for matched samples including polytomous outcomes. An illustration of matched-sample case-control analysis is presented in Section 14.4, and further topics are discussed in Section 14.5.

14.1. DIRECT AND INDIRECT PARAMETRIC MODELING OF MATCHED-SAMPLE DATA

To motivate the discussion of this section, we pose the following question: Is it valid to analyze data from a matched case-control study as if they had been collected prospectively, that is, to ignore the retrospective design and to fit a parametric logistic regression model for $P(Y|X,Z)$ to estimate the disease-exposure log odds ratio? There is strong interest in doing so, because it is natural to think about disease etiology in terms of the parameters of a model for $P(Y|X,Z)$. Also, as indicated above, models for $P(X|Y,Z)$, the directly estimable quantity from a retrospective study, require multivariate methods for risk factors in several dimensions and formats, so it is generally much simpler to fit a single multiple logistic regression model with a prospective specification, using the case-control indicator Y as if it were the observed outcome.

In *unmatched* case-control studies, Prentice and Pyke (1979), Farewell (1979), Carroll, Wang, and Wang (1995), and others have shown that using logistic regression as if the data had been collected prospectively provides consistent estimates of, and standard errors for, all coefficients except the intercept term, assuming a correctly specified population disease prevalence model and unbiased sampling for cases and controls. It is surprising to learn, therefore, that no such justification holds for pair-matched case-control studies, where the intention is to model the case-control indicator logistically as an explicit, parametric function of the risk factors X and the matching factors Z, *even if the chosen model is a correct specification of true disease prevalence in the population.* Levin and Paik (2001) show that such an analysis may lead to biased log odds ratio estimates and, worse, grossly misleading coefficients for other terms in the model. They also map out situations where the bias is negligible or extreme. We discuss this problem in more detail in the rest of this section. We hasten to add that the conditional logistic regression methods discussed in Section 14.2 do not suffer from this potential bias, a strong recommendation for their use.

In matched-sample prospective studies, we observe disease outcome Y for given instances of X and Z, so we can directly estimate $P(Y|X,Z)$. Henceforth we assume that the linear logistic disease prevalence model,

$$\ln\frac{P(Y=1|X,Z)}{P(Y=0|X,Z)} = \beta X + g(Z), \tag{14.1}$$

is valid in the population from which cases and controls are drawn. When $g(Z)$ is of a known functional form, for example, $g(Z) = \alpha + \gamma Z$, a standard logistic regression model estimates β consistently using the methods of Chapter 11. Lynn and McCulloch (1992) discuss the bias introduced by partially omitting relevant matching factors from a logistic regression model in the context of a prospective matched-pairs study. When the matching factors are quantifiable but $g(Z)$ is of unknown functional form, Hastie and Tibshirani (1990) and Severini and Staniswalis (1994) consider semiparametric regression models. Direct modeling approaches apply to both matched and unmatched designs, so no distinction need be made between them.

To avoid biased sampling in a matched-sample prospective study, the probability of selection into the study, either as an exposed or as an unexposed participant, must not depend on Y given X and Z. Often selection occurs even before outcome Y can be observed. Bias can occur if subjects with markers that correlate with future Y are differentially sampled from those exposed versus unexposed. Randomization in experimental studies avoids biased sampling.

In matched-sample retrospective studies, we observe antecedent risk factors X for given instances of Y and Z. We now make the role of selection explicit by introducing the *selection indicator* S: the event $[S = 1]$ denotes selection and inclusion in the case-control study. We make S explicit because cases and controls are not selected by random sampling from (14.1) as in the prospective design. The proper likelihood function for the retrospective design is a product of conditional densities for X given Y, Z, and $S = 1$, denoted by $f(X|Y, Z, S = 1)$. To avoid biased sampling, the selection indicator must be conditionally independent of X given Y and Z, that is,

$$P(S = 1|X, Y, Z) = P(S = 1|Y, Z). \tag{14.2}$$

For example, if subjects having the same Y and Z are equally likely to be selected into the case-control sample, the sampling is unbiased. With unbiased sampling, we have, by Bayes' theorem,

$$f(X|Y, Z, S = 1) = \frac{P(S = 1|X, Y, Z) \cdot f(X|Y, Z)}{P(S = 1|Y, Z)} = f(X|Y, Z). \tag{14.3}$$

In particular, if X is a single binary variable, by the invariance of the odds ratio,

$$\frac{f(X = 1|Y = 1, Z)/f(X = 0|Y = 1, Z)}{f(X = 1|Y = 0, Z)/f(X = 0|Y = 0, Z)}$$

$$= \frac{P(Y = 1|X = 1, Z)/P(Y = 0|X = 1, Z)}{P(Y = 1|X = 0, Z)/P(Y = 0|X = 0, Z)}, \tag{14.4}$$

so it is possible to estimate the odds ratio of interest on the right-hand side of (14.4) by modeling $f(X|Y, Z, S = 1) = f(X|Y, Z)$ (Prentice, 1976). For example, if we assume the model

$$\ln \frac{f(X = 1|Y, Z)}{f(X = 0|Y, Z)} = \beta' Y + h(Z)$$

for some function $h(Z)$, then (14.4) implies $\beta' = \beta$ in (14.1). Note, however, that if $g(Z)$ in (14.1) is linear and Z is continuous, $h(Z)$ will generally be nonlinear, and conversely. Only if Z is discrete and $h(Z)$ is saturated with parameters will the two models be mutually consistent. See Section 15.5 for cases in which X is a vector of binary exposure variables or a vector of continuous and categorical variables.

As an alternative to direct modeling, we can express the likelihood function in terms of the disease prevalence model (14.1) via

$$f(X|Y, Z, S = 1) = \frac{P(Y|X, Z, S = 1) f(X|Z, S = 1)}{P(Y|Z, S = 1)}. \qquad (14.5)$$

In (14.5), $f(X|Z, S = 1)$ denotes the marginal distribution *in the sample* of the risk factors X for given matching factors Z. It can be estimated empirically from the data in the sample, without reference to any model, and, as Prentice and Pyke (1979) demonstrate for unmatched samples, estimating $f(X|Z, S = 1)$ from the empirical distribution without any constraints independently maximizes that portion of the likelihood function based on products of $f(X|Y, Z, S = 1)$. The term in the denominator of (14.5) is a constant depending on the matched-sample design, for example, $P(Y|Z, S = 1) = \frac{1}{2}$ for matched pairs. Therefore, instead of modeling the left-hand side of (14.5), one could choose to model $P(Y|X, Z, S = 1)$ on the right-hand side of (14.5), which we call *indirect modeling with prospective analysis*, or simply *prospective analysis*, for the retrospective design. Whatever parameters maximize the likelihood function based on products of $P(Y|X, Z, S = 1)$ also maximize the likelihood function based on products of (14.5).

One should note that while (14.3) is true, generally $P(Y|X, Z, S = 1) \neq P(Y|X, Z)$. $P(Y = 1|X, Z, S = 1)$ is the probability that a given subject *in the sample* with (X, Z) is a case. With indirect modeling, we can estimate the parameters of $P(Y|X, Z, S = 1)$, but model (14.1) for $P(Y|X, Z)$ is the object of interest. The difference between the two will become apparent below.

Suppose, for a single risk factor X and single quantitative matching factor Z, that the following linear logistic disease prevalence model is valid in the population from which cases and controls are drawn:

$$\ln \frac{P(Y = 1|X, Z)}{P(Y = 0|X, Z)} = \alpha + \beta X + \gamma Z, \qquad (14.6)$$

so that $g(Z) = \alpha + \gamma Z$. Coefficient γ provides the increase in log odds on disease per unit increment in Z. We emphasize that, because we are assuming model (14.6) is valid, any inconsistency in the estimation of β demonstrated below does not arise from misspecification of the true model for disease prevalence. The relation between $P(Y|X, Z, S = 1)$ and $P(Y|X, Z)$ is given by

$$\ln\frac{P(Y=1|X,Z,S=1)}{P(Y=0|X,Z,S=1)} = \ln\frac{P(Y=1|X,Z)}{P(Y=0|X,Z)} + \ln\frac{P(S=1|Y=1,Z)}{P(S=1|Y=0,Z)}$$

$$= \ln\frac{P(Y=1|X,Z)}{P(Y=0|X,Z)} - \ln\frac{P(Y=1|Z)}{P(Y=0|Z)},$$

where the last equality follows because $P(Y = 1|Z, S = 1) = P(Y = 0|Z, S = 1) = \frac{1}{2}$ in the pair-matched design (see Problem 14.3). To simplify the notation, denote the logarithm of the ratio of selection probabilities for cases and controls by

$$\alpha^*(Z) = \ln\frac{P(S=1|Y=1,Z)}{P(S=1|Y=0,Z)} = -\ln\frac{P(Y=1|Z)}{P(Y=0|Z)},$$

and let

$$g^*(Z) = \alpha + \gamma Z + \alpha^*(Z).$$

Then we have

$$\ln\frac{P(Y=1|X,Z,S=1)}{P(Y=0|X,Z,S=1)} = a + \beta X + \gamma Z + \alpha^*(Z) = \beta X + g^*(Z). \quad (14.7)$$

Note that the logit of $P(Y|X, Z, S = 1)$ is still linear in X, but the functional forms of $g(Z)$ in (14.6) and $g^*(Z)$ in (14.7) are different. Even though $g(Z) = \alpha + \beta Z$ is linear, $g^*(Z)$ is generally nonlinear because the marginal probabilities $P(Y|Z)$ involved in $\alpha^*(Z)$ [which are obtained by integrating $P(Y|X, Z)$ from (14.6) with respect to the marginal distribution of X given Z] do not preserve the linear logistic form. Consequently, if we use a linear prospective specification for $g^*(Z)$, such as $g^*(Z) = \alpha' + \gamma' Z$, the coefficients, including β, are estimated with bias because the indirect model (14.7) is misspecified in Z.

We can be more explicit when X is a binary risk factor. In that case we have

$$g^*(Z) = \ln\frac{P(X=0|Y=1,Z)}{P(X=0|Y=0,Z)} = \ln\frac{1 + e^{\beta+g(Z)} + e^{d(Z)}\{1 + e^{g(Z)}\}}{1 + e^{\beta+g(Z)} + e^{\beta+d(Z)}\{1 + e^{g(Z)}\}},$$

where $d(Z) = \ln\{P(X=1|Z)/P(X=0|Z)\}$ is the population log odds on exposure given Z (see Problem 14.4). Even if $g(Z)$ and $d(Z)$ are both linear functions, $g^*(Z)$ generally is not, so β will not be estimated consistently. Note that by (14.7), when one models $\ln\{P(Y=1|X, Z, S=1)/P(Y= 0|X, Z, S=1)\}$ as a function of X and Z, to avoid bias we must essentially model the log-likelihood ratio for $X=0$ comparing $Y=1$ with $Y=0$ as a nonlinear function of Z.

In unmatched retrospective studies, because $P(Y|X)$ and $P(Y|X, S=1)$ differ only by the constant $\alpha^* = \ln\{P(S=1|Y=1)/P(S=1|Y=0)\}$, model misspecification does not occur. That is why the estimate of β by indirect modeling with prospective analysis is consistent in unmatched case-control studies. Misspecification, however, is the key reason that prospective modeling for matched case-control studies provides inconsistent estimates. The regression coefficient γ for Z in (14.6) cannot be estimated sensibly in a matched-pairs design, so the coefficient γ' estimated in the misspecified model $\beta X + g^*(Z) = \alpha' + \beta'X + \gamma'Z$ leads to misinterpretation. It is typical for the estimate of γ' to be of the wrong magnitude and even the wrong sign. Gail, Wieand, and Piantadosi (1984) study the general biasing effects of model misspecification on logistic regression coefficients.

As an illustration, consider the hypothetical data in Table 14.1 from a case-control study with close pair matching on age, assumed to be a strong confounding factor for the association between binary risk factor X and disease Y. Large sample sizes have been chosen to distance the discussion from issues of sampling variation. The data were constructed according to the following assumptions:

(i) The sample design calls for matched case-control pairs of equal sample sizes from four age groups, 30, 40, 60, and 70 years of age; defining $Z = (\text{age} - 50)/10$, Z takes on the four values -2, -1, $+1$, and $+2$. We omit the central age group $Z = 0$ in order to make a point below.

(ii) In the population, the risk factor X is strongly correlated with Z according to the logistic model

$$\ln\frac{P(X=1|Z)}{P(X=0|Z)} = 3Z.$$

Thus, in the population, the prevalence of X at ages 30, 40, 60, and 70 is 0.25%, 4.74%, 95.26%, and 99.75%, respectively.

(iii) The prevalence of disease in the population given coded age Z and exposure to X follows the logistic model

$$\ln\frac{P(Y=1|X, Z)}{P(Y=0|X, Z)} = X + 3Z,$$

with true coefficients $\alpha = 0$, $\beta = 1$, and $\gamma = 3$ in (14.6). The disease prevalence in the population among the unexposed in the four age groups is

Table 14.1. *Hypothetical data from a matched-pairs case-control study*
[*The left-hand panel reports data in the standard format for matched pairs.*
The right-hand panel reports data in a format suitable for input to the
prospective logistic regression model (14.6)]

Age (years)						Z	X	Number $Y=1$	$Y=0$	Total
30			Control							
			Exp'd	Unexp'd	Total					
	Case	Exp'd	0	7	7	-2	1	7	2	9
		Unexp'd	2	991	993	-2	0	993	998	1991
		Total	2	998	1000			1000	1000	2000
40			Control							
			Exp'd	Unexp'd	Total					
	Case	Exp'd	4	106	110	-1	1	110	44	154
		Unexp'd	40	850	890	-1	0	890	956	1846
		Total	44	956	1000			1000	1000	2000
60			Control							
			Exp'd	Unexp'd	Total					
	Case	Exp'd	843	111	954	$+1$	1	954	884	1838
		Unexp'd	41	5	46	$+1$	0	46	116	162
		Total	884	116	1000			1000	1000	2000
70			Control							
			Exp'd	Unexp'd	Total					
	Case	Exp'd	991	7	998	$+2$	1	998	993	1991
		Unexp'd	2	0	2	$+2$	0	2	7	9
		Total	993	7	1000			1000	1000	2000

$b = 231$, $c = 85$, $b/c = 2.718$, $\ln(b/c) = 1.000$, $\widehat{\text{se}}\{\ln(b/c)\} = 0.127$.

0.25%, 4.74%, 95.26%, and 99.75%, respectively (the same as the marginal prevalence of X only because the two models happen to be the same); among the exposed, the disease prevalence is 0.67%, 11.92%, 98.20%, and 99.91%. The odds ratio on disease versus no disease comparing exposed and unexposed is equal to $e^\beta = 2.718$ for each age group.

Assumptions (ii) and (iii) completely determine the joint distribution of X and Y in the population at each age. The joint probabilities of exposure in the matched case-control pairs for the example were then obtained under conditional independence of the case and control exposures within matched pairs,

$$P(X_1, X_2 | Y_1 = 1, Y_2 = 0, Z) = P(X_1 | Y_1 = 1, Z) \cdot P(X_2 | Y_2 = 0, Z),$$

and, by Bayes' theorem, the individual factors are obtained from

$$\ln \frac{P(X_2 = 1 | Y_2 = 0, Z)}{P(X_2 = 0 | Y_2 = 0, Z)} = \ln \frac{P(Y_2 = 0 | X_2 = 1, Z)}{P(Y_2 = 0 | X_2 = 0, Z)} + \ln \frac{P(X_2 = 1 | Z)}{P(X_2 = 0 | Z)}$$

$$= \ln \left\{ \frac{1 + \exp(3Z)}{1 + \exp(1 + 3Z)} \right\} + 3Z$$

and, by invariance of the odds ratio, from

$$\ln \frac{P(X_1 = 1 | Y_1 = 1, Z)}{P(X_1 = 0 | Y_1 = 1, Z)} = \ln \frac{P(X = 1 | Y = 0, Z)}{P(X = 0 | Y = 0, Z)} + \beta$$

$$= \ln \left\{ \frac{1 + \exp(3Z)}{1 + \exp(1 + 3Z)} \right\} + 3Z + 1$$

(see Problem 14.4). For cases, the equation yields probabilities $P(X = 1 | Y = 1, Z) = 0.0067$, 0.1112, 0.9539, and 0.9975 for $Z = -2$, -1, $+1$, and $+2$, respectively, and $P(X = 1 | Y = 0, Z) = 0.0025$, 0.0440, 0.8840, and 0.9933, respectively, for controls. The frequency of outcomes $(X_1, X_2) = (1,1)$, (1,0), (0,1), and (0,0) at each age were set approximately equal to their expectations in samples of size 1000 pairs per age group, namely, 1000 times $P(X_1 = x_1, X_2 = x_2 | Y_1 = 1, Y_2 = 0, Z)$.

The left-hand panel of Table 14.1 allows the data to be analyzed in the correct (conditional) way. There are $b = 231$ pairs in which the case is exposed but not the control, and $c = 85$ pairs in which the control is exposed but not the case. For matched pairs, the conditional maximum likelihood estimate (cmle) of $\exp(\beta)$ is the same as the Mantel-Haenszel estimate of the odds ratio, and equals $b/c = 231/85 = 2.718$, with $\ln(b/c) = 1.000$, in perfect agreement with the correct parameter value $\beta = 1$.

The right-hand panel of Table 14.1 reports data in a format suitable for input to a prospective logistic regression analysis using model (14.6). The results of fitting the prospective model are given in Table 14.2. The prospec-

Table 14.2. Results of fitting the logistic regression model logit
$P(Y | X, Z, S = 1) = \alpha' + \beta' X + \gamma' Z$ **to the data of Table 14.1**
from a matched-pairs case-control study

Variable	Coeff.	mle	se	Z
Constant	α'	−0.3656	0.0555	−6.58
X = exposure	β'	0.7327	0.1018	7.20
Z = (age − 50)/10	γ'	−0.2072	0.0321	−6.45

tive-analysis estimate of β (0.7327) is seriously biased (the true value equals 1), and the estimate of γ (-0.2072) is of the wrong magnitude and sign (the true value equals $+3.0$). The estimated standard error of the cmle, 0.127, is slightly larger than the standard error of the prospective estimate of β, 0.102, but, of course, the bias in the prospective estimate precludes its use.

Prospective analyses of pair-matched case-control data are published from time to time in leading medical journals (Jacobs et al., 1999; Marshall et al., 1997; Nuako et al., 1998; London et al., 1992). Ironically, prospective modeling in retrospective matched designs often produces estimates for the disease-exposure odds ratio β that are numerically close to the cmle's (Marshall et al., 1997; London et al., 1992). Breslow and Day (1980, p. 270) deemed this phenomenon "of considerable theoretical interest." Levin and Paik (2001) quantify the bias of prospective analysis for matched pairs of cases and controls, identify situations in which the bias is large, and explain the "unreasonable effectiveness" of the method in cases where the bias is small. In the illustration, for example, they show that if the design calls for three groups at ages $Z = -1, 0$, and $+1$, with equal sample sizes of matched pairs, as the sample size grows the limiting mle of β is 0.9986—bias is negligible. With five groups of equal size at ages $Z = -2, -1, 0, +1$, and $+2$, the limiting mle of β is 0.8770—bias is moderate. With seven groups of equal size at ages $Z = -3, -2, -1, 0, +1, +2, +3$, the limiting mle of β is 0.7305. Omitting the central age group in the last scenario produces a limiting mle of 0.5065 with severe bias. The shape of the distribution of age in the design also affects the bias: a U-shaped distribution for Z increases bias, relative to a uniform distribution (which was why we omitted $Z = 0$ in the starting illustration), while a unimodal distribution tends to decrease bias. All these assertions can be explained by the approximate linearity or nonlinearity of $g^*(Z)$. In the starting example, $g^*(Z)$ is markedly nonlinear. If Z has a normal distribution, results of Zeger et al. (1988) show that $g^*(Z)$ is approximately linear.

Because of the potential for bias and the monstrous distortion of the coefficients of the matching variables, prospective modeling for matched retrospective designs should be avoided. Conditional likelihood methods provide the analyses of choice, and we turn to these next.

14.2. CONDITIONAL LOGISTIC REGRESSION

14.2.1. Matched Case-Control Studies: One Case Matched to One or More Controls

In this section we focus on conditional logistic regression in matched case-control studies. The method for matched prospective studies, outlined in Section 14.2.2, is similar. The main idea of conditional likelihood is illustrated by the simplest case of the pair-matched case-control study. The design fixes the first subject as a case, say, and the second subject as a control. Suppose, however, their exposure vectors, X_1 and X_2, are known only in terms of their values, not their owners. Then we can condition on the number of cases and controls per pair (or, as we shall say in general, per *stratum*) and on the unordered set of exposure vectors $\{X_1, X_2\}$. As there are only two subjects per stratum, only two scenarios are possible: (A) X_1 belongs to the case and X_2 belongs to the control (as observed); or (B) X_2 belongs to the case and X_1 belongs to the control. The conditional probability that scenario (A) occurs, given that either (A) or (B) occurs, is, using the notation of the previous section,

$$\frac{P(X_1|Y_1=1,Z,S=1)P(X_2|Y_2=0,Z,S=1)}{\{P(X_1|Y_1=1,Z,S=1)P(X_2|Y_2=0,Z,S=1) + P(X_2|Y_1=1,Z,S=1)P(X_1|Y_2=0,Z,S=1)\}}.$$

Using (14.5) and canceling terms, this conditional probability can be written as

$$\frac{\dfrac{P(Y_1=1|X_1,Z,S=1)}{P(Y_1=0|X_1,Z,S=1)}}{\dfrac{P(Y_1=1|X_1,Z,S=1)}{P(Y_1=0|X_1,Z,S=1)} + \dfrac{P(Y_2=1|X_2,Z,S=1)}{P(Y_2=0|X_2,Z,S=1)}}.$$

When the prevalence model has the form (14.1), relation (14.7) holds and the conditional probability reduces to

$$\frac{\exp\{\beta'X_1+g^*(Z)\}}{\exp\{\beta'X_1+g^*(Z)\}+\exp\{\beta'X_2+g^*(Z)\}} = \frac{\exp(\beta'X_1)}{\exp(\beta'X_1)+\exp(\beta'X_2)}.$$

Note that $g^*(Z)$ cancels out because it is common to each subject in the stratum. Since the conditioning effectively eliminates $g^*(Z)$, we do not have to assume any functional form for $g(Z)$ in (14.1). The conditional likelihood is the product of these conditional probabilities over all strata. It is clear that if both the case and the control in a given pair have identical X's, then the stratum is not informative. When each case has k controls, the conditional likelihood is obtained similarly as a product of conditional probabilities that one scenario occurred out of $k+1$ possible scenarios. We formalize these ideas next.

Conditional Likelihood—Formal Definition for One Case Matched to Any Number of Controls

Let Y_{ij} be the case indicator for the jth subject, $j=0,\ldots,k(i)$, in the ith matched set, $i=1,\ldots,n$. Arrange the data so that $j=0$ corresponds to the case, that is, $Y_{i0}=1$, $Y_{i1}=\cdots=Y_{ik(i)}=0$, where $k(i)$ is the number of controls for matched set i. Similarly, let X_{ij} be the vector of exposure variables, of order r, say, for this subject. We denote the matching variables for matched set i by Z_i.

Assume the logit model (14.1) for disease prevalence holds in the population; coefficient β is the log odds ratio parameter of primary interest. As in the previous section, let $f_{ij}(y) = f(X_{ij}|Y_{ij}=y, Z_i, S_{ij}=1) = f(X_{ij}|Y_{ij}=y, Z_i)$ denote the sampling density of X_{ij} given $Y_{ij}=y$ and Z_i under unbiased retrospective sampling. Then the proper likelihood function for the matched case-control study is given by

$$L = \prod_{i=1}^{n} \prod_{j=0}^{k(i)} f_{ij}(Y_{ij}),$$

which can be expressed as a product of two parts:

$$L = \prod_{i=1}^{n} \left[\frac{\prod_{j=0}^{k(i)} f_{ij}(Y_{ij})}{\sum_{j=0}^{k(i)} \left\{ f_{ij}(1) \prod_{k \neq j} f_{ik}(0) \right\}} \right] \sum_{j=0}^{k(i)} \left\{ f_{iy}(1) \prod_{k \neq j} f_{ik}(0) \right\}.$$

The first factor in each term is the conditional probability that the X_{ij}'s belong to the case and controls as in fact they do, given the $k(i)+1$ ways the risk factor vectors might belong to the case and controls in stratum i. Conditional likelihood methods draw inferences by maximizing only the product of the first factors, called the *conditional likelihood, L_c*. The conditional likelihood can be reexpressed as

$$L_c = \prod_{i=1}^{n} \frac{f_{i0}(1) \prod_{k \neq 0} f_{ik}(0)}{\sum_{j=0}^{k(i)} \left\{ f_{ij}(1) \prod_{k \neq j} f_{ik}(0) \right\}} = \prod_{i=1}^{n} \frac{\dfrac{f_{i0}(1)}{f_{i0}(0)}}{\sum_{j=0}^{k(i)} \dfrac{f_{ij}(1)}{f_{ij}(0)}}$$

upon division of each numerator and denominator in the product by $\prod_{j=0}^{k(i)} f_{ij}(0)$. Furthermore, from Bayes' theorem and Problem 14.3,

$$\frac{f(1)}{f(0)} = \frac{\dfrac{P(Y=1|X, Z)}{P(Y=0|X, Z)}}{\dfrac{P(Y=1|Z)}{P(Y=0|Z)}}. \tag{14.8}$$

The ratio in the denominator, $P(Y=1|Z)/P(Y=0|Z)$, which is common to all subjects in a stratum, cancels out in the conditional likelihood. Thus

$L_c = L_c(\beta)$ depends only on β:

$$L_c(\beta) = \prod_{i=1}^{n} \frac{\exp(\beta'X_{i0})}{\sum_{j=0}^{k(i)} \exp(\beta'X_{ij})}. \tag{14.9}$$

To repeat, $L_c(\beta)$ is a product of conditional probabilities that X_{i0} is the risk factor vector belonging to the case among all $k(i) + 1$ possibilities in $\{X_{i0}, X_{i1}, \ldots, X_{ik(i)}\}$, viewing these as fixed, and given that there is one case in stratum i.

Whether use of L_c to draw inferences about β instead of the full likelihood L results in a noticeable loss of efficiency depends on circumstances. The product of second factors in L,

$$\frac{L}{L_c} = \prod_{i=1}^{n} \sum_{j=0}^{k(i)} \left\{ f_{ij}(1) \prod_{k \neq j} f_{ik}(0) \right\}.$$

may contain only a small amount of information about β; it certainly does not depend on the cases' identities. When there is little information about β in L/L_c and few sets are noninformative, L_c results in near-efficient estimation compared to use of L. However, a parametric analysis based on L could be much more efficient, especially when there are many noninformative sets.

In the special case of $1:1$ matching, the conditional likelihood reduces to

$$L_c(\beta) = \prod_{i=1}^{n} \frac{\exp(\beta'X_{i0})}{\exp(\beta'X_{i0}) + \exp(\beta'X_{i1})} = \prod_{i=1}^{n} \frac{\exp\{\beta'(X_{i0} - X_{i1})\}}{1 + \exp\{\beta'(X_{i0} - X_{i1})\}}.$$

This has the form of a likelihood function of standard logistic regression where the sample size is the number n of matched sets, the outcomes are all equal to 1, the covariate is $X_{i0} - X_{i1}$, and the intercept term is 0. The conditional maximum likelihood estimator, $\hat{\beta}_c$, can be obtained in this case from an ordinary (unconditional) logistic regression program.

In the general setting, the conditional score function is

$$U_c(\beta) = \frac{\partial \ln L_c(\beta)}{\partial \beta} = \sum_{i=1}^{n} \left\{ X_{i0} - \frac{\sum_{j=0}^{k(i)} X_{ij} \exp(\beta'X_{ij})}{\sum_{j=0}^{k(i)} \exp(\beta'X_{ij})} \right\}$$

$$= \sum_{i=1}^{n} \left\{ X_{i0} - \sum_{j=0}^{k(i)} p_{ij}(\beta) X_{ij} \right\} = \sum_{i=1}^{n} \{ X_{i0} - E_c(X_i|\beta) \},$$

where we have written $\rho_{ij}(\beta) = \exp(\beta' X_{ij})/\sum_{k=0}^{k(i)} \exp(\beta' X_{ik})$ and $E_c(X_i|\beta)$ $= \sum_{j=0}^{k(i)} \rho_{ij}(\beta) X_{ij}$. In words, the score function has the familiar "observed minus expected" form, where "observed" is the observed covariate of the case and "expected" is the expected covariate of the case given the $k(i) + 1$ values of the covariates. For given β, the expected covariate $E_c(X_i|\beta)$ is a weighted average of all the covariates in the stratum with weights $\rho_{ij}(\beta)$ proportional to $\exp(\beta' X_{ij})$. The conditional likelihood equation sets $U_c(\beta)$ equal to 0, and the solution is the conditional maximum likelihood estimator, $\hat{\beta}_c$. Denoting the true value of β by β_0, for large n, $\sqrt{n}(\hat{\beta}_c - \beta_0)$ is distributed approximately as a multivariate normal with mean 0 and variance $n I_c(\beta)^{-1}$, where $I_c(\beta)$ is the conditional information matrix,

$$I_c(\beta) = -\frac{\partial U_c(\beta)}{\partial \beta} = -\frac{\partial^2 \ln L_c(\beta)}{\partial \beta\, \partial \beta'}$$

$$= \sum_{i=1}^{n} \sum_{j=0}^{k(i)} \rho_{ij}(\beta)\{X_{ij} - E_c(X_{ij}|\beta)\}\{X_{ij} - E_c(X_{ij}|\beta)\}'.$$

$I_c(\beta)$ thus has the form of a sum of variance-covariance matrices of the exposure vectors with respect to the conditional distribution specified by $\rho_{ij}(\beta)$.

Levin (1990) gives a useful double saddlepoint approximation to $L_c(\beta)$, $U_c(\beta)$, and $W_c(\beta)$. The approximation, accurate even for small strata, facilitates computation of the conditional maximum likelihood estimate, especially when large strata cause exact computation to be time-consuming or not feasible. Exact computation of $L_c(\beta)$, $U_c(\beta)$, $W_c(\beta)$, and $\hat{\beta}_c$ is discussed in Levin (1987). Exact inference is considered by Hirji, Mehta, and Patel (1988) and is compared with asymptotic inference by Hirji et al. (1988).

Illustration

Consider the data of Table 13.9. The conditional likelihood function (14.9) is

$$L_c(\beta) = \left(\frac{e^\beta}{e^\beta + e^\beta + 1}\right)^4 \left(\frac{e^\beta}{e^\beta + 1 + 1}\right)^3 \left(\frac{1}{1 + e^\beta + 1}\right)^1$$

$$= \frac{e^{7\beta}}{(2e^\beta + 1)^4(e^\beta + 2)^4}.$$

$L_c(\beta)$ is maximized [and $U_c(\beta)$ equals zero] at the cmle $\hat{\beta}_c = 2.121$, corresponding to an odds ratio of 8.34. The conditional information at $\hat{\beta}_c$ is $I_c(\hat{\beta}_c) = 0.8375$. Thus the asymptotic standard error of $\hat{\beta}_c$ is estimated to be $I_c(\hat{\beta}_c)^{-1/2} = 1.0927$. An approximate 95% confidence interval for $\hat{\beta}_c$ is $2.121 \pm 1.96 \times 1.0927 = (-0.021, 4.26)$, corresponding to the interval $(0.980,$

71.0) for the odds ratio. These results should be compared with the Mantel-Haenszel estimate of 10.0 for the odds ratio, with approximate 95% confidence interval (1.000, 100.0) and exact two-sided 95% confidence interval by the equal-tail method of (0.98, 394.1) (see Section 13.3).

Goodness of Fit
Several authors have considered diagnostic statistics to evaluate model goodness of fit for matched case-control studies. Pregibon (1984), viewing Y as an outcome, forms residuals for each subject as a unit. Here we present a diagnostic statistic with each stratum as a unit; this statistic is asymptotically equivalent to a statistic suggested by Moolgavkar, Lustbader, and Vanzon (1985). Bedrick and Hill (1996) proposed an exact method for checking goodness of fit.

Model checking requires three steps: (i) identify a statistic with which to examine observed values versus expected values under the model assumption; (ii) find the distribution of the statistic when the model is correct; and (iii) assess the deviation of observed versus expected according to the distribution.

Now let

$$u_i(\beta) = X_{i0} - E_c(X_i|\beta).$$

Note that $u_i(\beta)$, the contribution of the ith stratum to the conditional score function $U_c(\beta)$, has the desired "observed minus expected" form. The $u_i(\beta)$ may serve as residuals, but they are r-variate vectors. So consider the following quadratic function of $u_i(\beta)$:

$$e_i(\beta) = u_i(\beta)'I_c(\beta)^{-1}u_i(\beta).$$

which, when evaluated at $\hat{\beta}_c$, produces the one-dimensional diagnostic statistic $e_i(\hat{\beta}_c)$. Because $\hat{\beta}_c$ is the solution of $\sum_i u_i(\beta) = 0$, we have

$$u_i(\hat{\beta}_c) = -\sum_{j \neq i} u_j(\hat{\beta}_c).$$

Denote by $\hat{\beta}_{-i}$ the estimate of β obtained after deleting the ith stratum. Then, by a Taylor expansion of $0 = \sum_{j \neq i} u_j(\hat{\beta}_{-i})$ about $\hat{\beta}_c$, and ignoring terms of order $1/n$, we find

$$\hat{\beta}_{-i} - \hat{\beta}_c \approx I_c(\hat{\beta}_c)^{-1}\left\{\sum_{j \neq i} u_j(\hat{\beta}_c)\right\} = -I_c(\hat{\beta}_c)^{-1}u_i(\hat{\beta}_c).$$

This leads to the interpretation of $e_i(\hat{\beta}_c)$ as approximately equal to

$$\left(\hat{\beta}_{-i} - \hat{\beta}_c\right)' I_c\left(\hat{\beta}_c\right)\left(\hat{\beta}_{-i} - \hat{\beta}_c\right).$$

This statistic, called Cook's distance, measures the sensitivity of $\hat{\beta}_c$ to deletions of single strata. Now that we have identified the diagnostic statistic $e_i(\hat{\beta}_c)$ to examine, the next step is to find its distribution when the model is correct. We generate a reference distribution for $e_i(\hat{\beta}_c)$ as follows:

(1) For every i, pick one vector from $\{X_{i0}, \ldots, X_{ik(i)}\}$ with selection probabilities $\{p_{i0}(\hat{\beta}_c), \ldots, p_{ik(i)}(\hat{\beta}_c)\}$. Call the selected covariate X_{i0}^*.

(2) Pretend that X_{i0}^* is the observed covariate for the case, and solve the likelihood equation

$$\sum_{i=1}^{n} \{X_{i0}^* - E_c(X_i|\beta)\} = 0.$$

for β. Denote the solution by $\hat{\beta}^*$.

(3) Calculate $e_i(\hat{\beta}^*)$ for $i = 1, \ldots, n$.

(4) Repeat (1)–(3) m times, where m is a large number, e.g., $m = 1,000$.

The m generated values of $e_i(\hat{\beta}^*)$ form a reference distribution for $e_i(\hat{\beta}_c)$. For each $e_i(\hat{\beta}_c)$ we can form a 95% confidence interval from the $(0.025m)$th smallest and largest $e_i(\hat{\beta}^*)$ values. Figure 14.1 in Section 14.4 shows a plot of $e_i(\hat{\beta}_c)$ and their 95% confidence limits obtained from a conditional logistic regression analysis for the stroke study discussed below.

Computation

Software packages such as EGRET® or STATA® (procedure CLOGIT) have routines to compute conditional maximum likelihood estimates and standard errors. Software for fitting the Cox proportional hazards model can also be used to compute cmle's. The conditional likelihood function $L_c(\beta)$ is formally equivalent to the partial likelihood function $L_p(\beta)$ for the Cox model. The only differences are that β in $L_p(\beta)$ refers to the proportional hazards constant and that the partial likelihood conditions on risk sets from a survival study (whereas conditional likelihood conditions on strata from a matched sample study). The SAS® procedure PHREG, the SPSS® procedure COXREG, or the Splus® procedure COXREG for survival analysis can be used to compute the conditional maximum likelihood estimate and its standard error when there is only one case per stratum. When there are multiple cases, which is equivalent to having tied failure times in the Cox model, SAS® constructs the proper likelihood function upon specifying ties= discrete. SPSS® currently does not handle ties appropriately for construction of the conditional likelihood function. Code for a SAS® procedure to fit a conditional logistic regression model is given in Table 14.5 for the stroke study discussed in Section 14.4.

14.2.2. Matched Prospective Studies

Consider a pair-matched prospective study with a single binary risk factor X. For matched set i with matching variable Z_i, label the subjects so that $X_{i1} = 1$, and $X_{i2} = 0$; we observe Y_{ij}, $j = 1, 2$. We continue to assume the linear logistic disease prevalence model (14.1). The full likelihood function is

$$L = \prod_{i=1}^{n} \prod_{j=1}^{2} P\left(Y_{ij} = 1 | X_{ij}, Z_i\right)^{Y_{ij}} P\left(Y_{ij} = 0 | X_{ij}, Z_i\right)^{1-Y_{ij}}.$$

Let

$$p_{ij}(x) = P\left(Y_{ij} = 1 | X_{ij} = x, Z_i\right) = 1 - q_{ij}(x).$$

The conditional likelihood function is obtained by conditioning on the design features, which are the risk factors, $X_{i1} = 1$ and $X_{i2} = 0$, and the unordered set of observed outcomes, $\{Y_{i1}, Y_{i2}\}$. The outcomes correspond to subjects 1 and 2 as (Y_{i1}, Y_{i2}) or as (Y_{i2}, Y_{i1}). The conditional probability of observing (Y_{i1}, Y_{i2}) given either (Y_{i1}, Y_{i2}) or (Y_{i2}, Y_{i1}) is

$$
\frac{p_{i1}(1)^{Y_{i1}} q_{i1}(1)^{1-Y_{i1}} p_{i2}(0)^{Y_{i2}} q_{i2}(0)^{1-Y_{i2}}}{p_{i1}(1)^{Y_{i1}} q_{i1}(1)^{1-Y_{i1}} p_{i2}(0)^{Y_{i2}} q_{i2}(0)^{1-Y_{i2}} + p_{i1}(1)^{Y_{i2}} q_{i1}(1)^{1-Y_{i2}} p_{i2}(0)^{Y_{i1}} q_{i2}(0)^{1-Y_{i1}}}
$$

$$
= \frac{\{p_{i1}(1)/q_{i1}(1)\}^{Y_{i1}} \{p_{i2}(0)/q_{i2}(0)\}^{Y_{i2}}}{\{p_{i1}(1)/q_{i1}(1)\}^{Y_{i1}} \{p_{i2}(0)/q_{i2}(0)\}^{Y_{i2}} + \{p_{i1}(1)/q_{i1}(1)\}^{Y_{i2}} \{p_{i2}(0)/q_{i2}(0)\}^{Y_{i1}}}
$$

$$
= \frac{\exp[Y_{i1}\{\beta + g(Z_i)\} + Y_{i2} g(Z_i)]}{\exp[Y_{i1}\{\beta + g(Z_i)\} + Y_{i2} g(Z_i)] + \exp[Y_{i2}\{\beta + g(Z_i)\} + Y_{i1} g(Z_i)]}
$$

$$
= \frac{\exp(\beta Y_{i1})}{\exp(\beta Y_{i1}) + \exp(\beta Y_{i2})}. \tag{14.10}
$$

The conditional likelihood thus reduces to

$$L_c(\beta) = \prod_{i=1}^{n} \frac{\exp(\beta Y_{i1})}{\exp(\beta Y_{i1}) + \exp(\beta Y_{i2})}. \tag{14.11}$$

Suppose that another risk factor W, observed at baseline but not controlled in the design, is potentially confounding, such that the correct disease prevalence model is not (14.1) but instead

$$\ln\frac{P(Y=1|X,W,Z)}{P(Y=0|X,W,Z)} = \beta X + \gamma W + g(Z). \tag{14.12}$$

In that case we condition on the risk factor *vectors*

$$\begin{pmatrix} X_{i1} \\ W_{i1} \end{pmatrix} = \begin{pmatrix} 1 \\ W_{i1} \end{pmatrix} \quad \text{and} \quad \begin{pmatrix} X_{i2} \\ W_{i2} \end{pmatrix} = \begin{pmatrix} 0 \\ W_{i2} \end{pmatrix}$$

and the unordered set of outcomes $\{Y_{i1}, Y_{i2}\}$. Repeating the argument above, the conditional probability of observing (Y_{i1}, Y_{i2}) given either (Y_{i1}, Y_{i2}) or (Y_{i2}, Y_{i1}) is, instead of (14.10),

$$\frac{\exp[Y_{i1}\{\beta + \gamma W_{i1} + g(Z_i)\} + Y_{i2}\{\gamma W_{i2} + g(Z_i)\}]}{\left\{\begin{matrix}\exp[Y_{i1}\{\beta + \gamma W_{i1} + g(Z_i)\} + Y_{i2}\{\gamma W_{i2} + g(Z_i)\}] \\ + \exp[Y_{i2}\{\beta + \gamma W_{i1} + g(Z_1)\} + Y_{i1}\{\gamma W_{i2} + g(Z_i)\}]\end{matrix}\right\}}.$$

Dividing numerator and denominator by $\exp[(Y_{i1} + Y_{i2})\{\gamma W_{i2} + g(Z_i)\}]$ yields

$$\frac{\exp[Y_{i1}\{\beta + \gamma(W_{i1} - W_{i2})\}]}{\exp[Y_{i1}\{\beta + \gamma(W_{i1} - W_{i2})\}] + \exp[Y_{i2}\{\beta + \gamma(W_{i1} - W_{i2})\}]},$$

whence the conditional likelihood function is

$$L_c(\beta, \gamma) = \prod_{i=1}^{n} \frac{\exp[Y_{i1}\{\beta + \gamma(W_{i1} - W_{i2})\}]}{\exp[Y_{i1}\{\beta + \gamma(W_{i1} - W_{i2})\}] + \exp[Y_{i2}\{\beta + \gamma(W_{i1} - W_{i2})\}]}. \tag{14.13}$$

Note that the only informative terms in (14.13) occur when (Y_{i1}, Y_{i2}) are discordant—$(1, 0)$ or $(0, 1)$—in which case the factors reduce to either

$$\frac{\exp\{\beta + \gamma(W_{i1} - W_{i2})\}}{1 + \exp\{\beta + \gamma(W_{i1} + W_{i2})\}}$$

or its complement

$$\frac{1}{1 + \exp\{\beta + \gamma(W_{i1} + W_{i2})\}}.$$

This is an ordinary binary logistic regression with $Y_i = 1$ corresponding to $(Y_{i1}, Y_{i2}) = (1, 0)$ and $Y_i = 0$ to $(Y_{i1}, Y_{i2}) = (0, 1)$, and explanatory factor $W_{i1} - W_{i2}$. The intercept term is β, the log odds ratio of interest adjusted for the effect of W, and the slope coefficient is γ. Generalization to the case of multiple risk factors is straightforward.

A final point: Suppose we ask what the conditional likelihood would be if, instead of (14.12), one posited a retrospective model for X where, say, $P(X|Y,W,Z)$ is of linear logistic form,

$$\ln \frac{P(X=1|Y,W,Z)}{P(X=0|Y,W,Z)} = \beta'Y + \gamma'W + h(Z).$$

This situation is formally the reverse of that considered in Section 14.2.1, so we find the conditional likelihood to be

$$L_c(\beta',\gamma') = \prod_{i=1}^{n} \frac{\exp(\beta'Y_{i1} + \gamma'W_{i1})}{\exp(\beta'Y_{i1} + \gamma'W_{i1}) + \exp(\beta'Y_{i2} + \gamma'W_{i2})}.$$

By invariance of the odds ratio, the regression coefficient for Y would be the same as β in (14.12), that is, $\beta = \beta'$, but the coefficient for W would measure the effect of W on X, not the effect of W on Y, such that, $\gamma \neq \gamma'$.

Illustration
Consider Table 13.11 on judgments by eight raters on the presence or absence of a psychiatric symptom in eight patients. We can view this study as a prospective matched design with $n_i = 8$ dichotomous ratings ($Y = 1$ for symptoms present or positive, $Y = 0$ for symptoms absent or negative) matched on patient Z under eight different conditions (raters), identified by the seven vectors $X_{i1} = (1, 0, 0, 0, 0, 0, 0)'$, $X_{i2} = (0, 1, 0, 0, 0, 0, 0)$, ..., $X_{i7} = (0, 0, 0, 0, 0, 0, 1)$, each with seven components. Rater 8, the reference rater, is identified by the zero vector $X_{i8} = (0, 0, 0, 0, 0, 0, 0)$. We consider the logit model

$$\ln \frac{P(Y=1|X,Z)}{P(Y=0|X,Z)} = \beta'X + g(Z),$$

where $\beta = (\beta_1, \ldots, \beta_7)'$. β_j gives the log odds ratio comparing the odds on a positive rating for a given patient by rater j with the odds on a positive rating for the same patient by the reference rater. The conditional likelihood function is

$$L_c(\beta) = \prod_{i=1}^{n} \frac{p_{i1}(X_{i1})^{Y_{i1}} q_{i1}(X_{i1})^{1-Y_{i1}} \cdots p_{i8}(X_{i8})^{Y_{i8}} q_{i8}(X_{i8})^{1-Y_{i8}}}{\sum_\sigma p_{i\sigma(0)}(X_{i\sigma(1)})^{Y_{i\sigma(1)}} q_{i\sigma(1)}(X_{i\sigma(1)})^{1-Y_{i\sigma(1)}} \cdots p_{i\sigma(8)}(X_{i\sigma(8)})^{Y_{i\sigma(8)}} q_{i\sigma(8)}(X_{i\sigma(8)})^{1-Y_{i\sigma(8)}}},$$

where the sum is over all permutations of the outcomes $\{Y_{i1}, \ldots, Y_{i8}\}$. For patient i, let $m_i = \sum_j Y_{ij}$ be the total number of positive diagnoses (this was denoted by S_i in the notation of Table 13.10). Let $\pi^{(i)}$ denote any one of the $\binom{8}{m_i}$ ways to assign m_i positive and $8 - m_i$ negative ratings from the eight raters, and let $S_i(\pi^{(i)})$ be the sum of the X vectors corresponding to the positive ratings. Then $L_c(\beta)$ is equivalent to

$$
L_c(\beta) = \prod_{i=1}^{n} \frac{\exp\{\beta'S_i(\pi_{\text{obs}}^{(i)})\}}{\sum_{\pi^{(i)}} \exp\{\beta'S_i(\pi^{(i)})\}},
$$

where $S_i(\pi_{\text{obs}}^{(i)})$ is the sum of the X vectors for patients with positive diagnoses, that is, a vector with a one in position j if rater j gave a positive rating for $j = 1, \ldots, 7$. For example, patient 5 in Table 13.11 had $m_5 = 3$ positive ratings, from raters 3, 6, and 8. The contribution to the conditional likelihood function for this patient is

$$
\frac{\exp\{\beta'(X_{5,3} + X_{5,6} + X_{5,8})\}}{\sum_{\pi^{(5)}} \exp\{\beta'S_5(\pi^{(5)})\}}
$$

$$
= \frac{e^{\beta_3 + \beta_6}}{e^{\beta_1 + \beta_2 + \beta_3} + e^{\beta_1 + \beta_2 + \beta_4} + \cdots + e^{\beta_5 + \beta_7} + e^{\beta_6 + \beta_7}},
$$

where the sum in the denominator is over all $\binom{8}{3} = 56$ ways of choosing three X vectors; equivalently, the denominator is the sum over all ways of writing the exponential of a sum of three terms from among $\{\beta_1, \ldots, \beta_7, 0\}$.

Differentiating $\ln L_c(\beta)$ with respect to β and evaluating at $\beta = 0$ gives the score statistic

$$
U_c(0) = \sum_{i=1}^{n} \{S_i(\pi_{\text{obs}}^{(i)}) - E_c(S_i | \beta = 0)\} = \begin{bmatrix} T_1 - T/8 \\ \vdots \\ T_7 - T/8 \end{bmatrix}
$$

in the notation of Table 13.10. The information matrix is

$$
I_c(0) = \sum_{i=1}^{n} \frac{S_i(8 - S_i)}{7} \left\{ \text{Diag}(\tfrac{1}{8}, \ldots, \tfrac{1}{8}) - \begin{bmatrix} \tfrac{1}{8} \\ \vdots \\ \tfrac{1}{8} \end{bmatrix} [\tfrac{1}{8}, \ldots, \tfrac{1}{8}] \right\}
$$

(see Problem 13.5). It follows that the score test statistic $U_c(0)'I_c(0)^{-1}U_c(0)$ is equal to Cochran's Q statistic (13.30).

It is remarkable that this score test statistic is informative at all, because there is very little information contained in the data about the individual log odds ratio components of β. Note first that patients 1, 3, 4, and 7, who received no positive ratings, are conditionally uninformative about β. Furthermore, raters 2 and 7 gave no positive ratings, so that calculation of the cmle of β does not converge, due to the singularity at $\hat{\beta}_2 = \hat{\beta}_7 = -\infty$. The singularity merely indicates that any arbitrarily small value of β_2 or β_7 is consistent with the data, a reflection of lack of information. If we omit raters 2 and 7 from the analysis, patient number 8, now with all positive ratings, becomes conditionally uninformative about the odds ratios among the six other raters. For the three remaining patients—2, 5, and 6—there is insufficient information to estimate the remaining five parameters. This example illustrates an advantage of the score statistic over the Wald statistic for testing the hypothesis H_0: $\beta = 0$: the score statistic is calculated under the null hypothesis, so that singularities in the cmle do not pose a problem.

14.3. EXTENSIONS

14.3.1. Matched Studies with Varying Numbers of Cases and Controls

Sometimes a study is planned for $1:1$ or $1:2$ matching, but eligible controls (or cases) are not available for some cases (or controls). In this situation, it may be possible to merge a lone case or control into an appropriate stratum, i.e., with the same matching variables. In fact, Brookmeyer, Liang, and Linet (1986) showed that this approach can increase efficiency. Such merging creates variable numbers of cases and controls per stratum. Another example arises when one stratifies data post hoc, creating many strata with varying numbers of cases and controls. In this section we consider retrospective matched samples with m_i cases and $n_i - m_i$ controls in stratum i.

The principle of conditional likelihood, suitably generalized, is the same as that for $1:k$ matching described in Section 14.2. Let Y_{ij}, $j = 1, \ldots, n_i$ be the case indicator for the jth subject in the ith stratum. We assign the cases to the index $j = 1, \ldots, m_i$ and controls to $j = m_i + 1, \ldots, n_i$, so that $Y_{i1} = \cdots = Y_{im_i} = 1$ and $Y_{im_i+1} = \cdots = Y_{in_i} = 0$. There are $\binom{n_i}{m_i}$ possible ways of partitioning the set of n_i exposure vectors into two groups: one of size m_i associated with the cases, and the other of size $n_i - m_i$ associated with the controls. For each of these ways, let the index of the vectors assigned to the cases be $\sigma(1), \ldots, \sigma(m_i)$, and let the index of the vectors assigned to the controls be $\sigma(m_i + 1), \ldots, \sigma(n_i)$, where σ is an appropriate permutation of $\{1, \ldots, n_i\}$. We call σ a partition of $\{1, \ldots, n_i\}$. The conditional likelihood is the product over all strata of the conditional probabilities that the first m_i exposure vectors belong to the cases, given that some such partition occurs.

Again writing the density of the exposure vectors as $f_{ij}(y) = f(X_{ij}|Y_{ij} = y, Z_i)$ $= f(X_{ij}|Y_{ij} = y, Z_i, S_{ij} = 1)$, the conditional likelihood is

$$L_c(\beta) = \prod_{i=1}^{n} \frac{\prod_{j=1}^{m_i} f_{ij}(1) \prod_{j=m_i+1}^{n_i} f_{ij}(0)}{\sum_{\sigma} \prod_{j=1}^{m_i} f_{i\sigma(j)}(1) \prod_{j=m_i+1}^{n_i} f_{i\sigma(j)}(0)} = \prod_{i=1}^{n} \frac{\prod_{j=1}^{m_i} \exp(\beta' X_{ij})}{\sum_{\sigma} \prod_{j=1}^{m_i} \exp\{\beta' X_{i\sigma(j)}\}}$$

$$= \prod_{i=1}^{n} \frac{\exp(\beta' S_i)}{\sum_{\sigma} \exp\{\beta' S_i(\sigma)\}},$$

where the summation is over the $\binom{n_i}{m_i}$ distinct partitions σ of $\{1, \dots, n_i\}$, and where we have written $S_i = X_{i1} + \cdots + X_{im_i}$ for the observed partition $\sigma(j) = j$, and $S_i(\sigma) = X_{i\sigma(1)} + \cdots + X_{i\sigma(m_i)}$ for an arbitrary partition σ. The resulting score equation is

$$U_c(\beta) = \sum_{i=1}^{n} \{S_i - E_c(S_i|\beta)\} = \sum_{i=1}^{n} \left\{S_i - \sum_{\sigma} \rho_{i\sigma}(\beta) S_i(\sigma)\right\} = 0,$$

where for each partition σ of $\{1, \dots, n_i\}$, $\rho_{i\sigma}(\beta) = \exp\{\beta' S_i(\sigma)\} / \sum_{\sigma} \exp\{\beta' S_i(\sigma)\}$. The information matrix is

$$I_c(\beta) = -\frac{\partial U_c(\beta)}{\partial \beta} = -\frac{\partial^2 \ln L_c(\beta)}{\partial \beta \, \partial \beta'}$$

$$= \sum_{i=1}^{n} \sum_{\sigma} \rho_{i\sigma}(\beta)\{S_i(\sigma) - E_c(S_i|\beta)\}\{S_i(\sigma) - E_c(X_{ij}|\beta)\}'.$$

14.3.2. Matched Studies with Polytomous Outcomes

In some studies, there are more than two kinds of outcome. For example, Y may take values 0, 1, or 2, labeling three disease states of none, mild, and severe. Another example is the matched triplet retrospective study, matching, say, a case, a community control, and a hospital control on Z, with an exposure vector X observed on each. We assume that Y has a multinomial distribution given X and Z. Multinomial regression models for unmatched data are described in Chapter 11 and also in the literature (e.g., McCullagh and Nelder, 1989). For matched studies, Levin (1987) and Liang and Stewart (1987, correction by Levin, 1988) proposed conditional polytomous logistic regression models.

There are several ways to contrast multinomial probabilities, as depicted in Figure 11.9, but here we consider only the canonical contrasts of each cell probability to that of the reference category, $Y = 0$. The polytomous logistic regression model we assume is

$$\ln\frac{P(Y=1|X,Z)}{P(Y=0|X,Z)} = \beta'X + g_1(Z),$$

$$\ln\frac{P(Y=2|X,Z)}{P(Y=0|X,Z)} = \gamma'X + g_2(Z).$$

(14.14)

In a matched triplet stratum, suppose we arrange the notation so that the first subject has $Y = 0$, the second has $Y = 1$, and the third has $Y = 2$. The contribution of this stratum to the conditional likelihood function is the conditional probability that the first subject has exposure vector $X = X_1$, the second has $X = X_2$, and the third has $X = X_3$, given that the study design fixes $(Y_1, Y_2, Y_3) = (0, 1, 2)$ and that some permutation of $\{X_1, X_2, X_3\}$ corresponds to the members of the triplet. There are six ways to assign the three subscripts $\{1, 2, 3\}$ of X to the matched triplet: $(1, 2, 3)$, $(1, 3, 2)$, $(2, 1, 3)$, $(2, 3, 1)$, $(3, 1, 2)$, and $(3, 2, 1)$. We denote these permutations generically by σ. The conditional probability is

$$\frac{p_0(X_1)p_1(X_2)p_2(X_3)}{\sum_\sigma p_0(X_{\sigma(1)})p_1(X_{\sigma(2)})p_2(X_{\sigma(3)})},$$

where the summation is over the above six permutations and $p_j(X) = P(Y = j|X, Z)$. After dividing numerator and denominator by $p_0(X_1)p_0(X_2)p_0(X_3)$, the conditional likelihood simplifies to

$$\frac{\exp\{\beta'X_{i2} + g_1(Z_i)\}\exp\{\gamma'X_{i3} + g_2(Z)\}}{\sum_\sigma \exp\{\beta'X_{i\sigma(2)} + g_1(Z_i)\}\exp\{\gamma'X_{i\sigma(3)} + g_2(Z_i)\}}$$

$$= \frac{\exp(\beta'X_{i2} + \gamma'X_{i3})}{\sum_\sigma \exp(\beta'X_{i\sigma(2)} + \gamma'X_{i\sigma(3)})}$$

Note that elimination of $g_1(Z_i)$ and $g_2(Z_i)$ follows from the choice of logit parameterization (14.14). If cumulative probabilities are assumed to be linear in the logit scale, $g_1(Z_i)$ and $g_2(Z_i)$ do not cancel out of the conditional likelihood.

The General Case
Given $t + 1$ disease states labeled $Y = 0, 1, \ldots, t$, with $\underline{m} = (m_0, m_1, \ldots, m_t)$ subjects of each kind, the conditional likelihood function is most easily specified in terms of *ordered partitions* of the set of exposure vectors, $\xi^{(i)} = \{X_{i1}, \ldots, X_{in_i}\}$, *consistent with the frequencies* $\underline{m}$. An ordered partition is a list of subsets, $\pi = (D_0, D_1, \ldots, D_t)$, such that there are m_j exposure

vectors in D_j, the component D_j's are mutually disjoint, and their union is all of $\xi^{(i)}$. An ordered partition represents one of the $n_i!/m_{i0}! \cdots m_{it}!$ ways the exposure vectors might have been associated with the m_{ij} cases of type $Y=j$ for $j=0,1,\ldots,t$. The conditional likelihood function is the product over the n strata of the conditional probability of occurrence of the observed partition, $\pi_{\text{obs}}^{(i)} = (\{X_{ik}: Y_{ik}=0\},\ldots,\{X_{ik}: Y_{ik}=t\})$, given that any of the $n_i!/(m_{i0}! \cdots m_{it}!)$ ordered partitions $\pi^{(i)}$ of $\xi^{(i)}$ might have been so associated. Let $S^{(i)}(\pi^{(i)})$ denote the vector of length rt given by stringing together the individual sums of exposure vectors:

$$S^{(i)}(\pi^{(i)}) = \begin{bmatrix} \sum_{X_{ik}\in D_1} X_{ik} \\ \vdots \\ \sum_{X_{ik}\in D_t} X_{ik} \end{bmatrix} \quad \text{for ordered partition } \pi^{(i)} = (D_0,\ldots,D_t) \text{ of } \xi^{(i)}.$$

Note that $S^{(i)}(\pi^{(i)})$ does not include the vectors in the reference component D_0 of $\pi^{(i)}$. Also, assume the t logit equations

$$\ln \frac{P(Y=j|X,Z)}{P(Y=0|X,Z)} = \beta_j'X + g_j(Z), \quad \text{for } j=1,\ldots,t.$$

String the coefficient vectors together into one vector of length rt, $\beta = (\beta_1',\ldots,\beta_t')'$. Then the conditional likelihood function is given by

$$L_c(\beta) = \prod_{i=1}^n \frac{\exp\{\beta'S^{(i)}(\pi_{\text{obs}}^{(i)})\}}{\sum_{\pi^{(i)}} \exp\{\beta'S^{(i)}(\pi^{(i)})\}},$$

where the sum is taken over all ordered partitions $\pi^{(i)}$ of $\xi^{(i)}$ consistent with $\underline{m}^{(i)}$. The score function is

$$U_c(\beta) = \sum_{i=1}^n \left\{ S^{(i)}(\pi_{\text{obs}}^{(i)}) - E_c(S^{(i)}|\beta) \right\}$$

$$= \sum_{i=1}^n \left\{ S^{(i)}(\pi_{\text{obs}}^{(i)}) - \sum_{\pi^{(i)}} P_{i\pi^{(i)}}(\beta)S^{(i)}(\pi^{(i)}) \right\},$$

where, for each ordered partition $\pi^{(i)}$ of $\xi^{(i)}$ consistent with $\underline{m}^{(i)}$, we have

$$P_{i\pi^{(i)}}(\beta) = \frac{\exp\{\beta'S^{(i)}(\pi^{(i)})\}}{\sum_{\pi^{(i)}} \exp\{\beta'S^{(i)}(\pi^{(i)})\}}.$$

The information matrix is

$$
I_c(\beta) = -\frac{\partial U_c(\beta)}{\partial \beta} = -\frac{\partial^2 \ln L_c(\beta)}{\partial \beta \, \partial \beta'}
$$

$$
= \sum_{i=1}^{n} \sum_{\pi^{(i)}} \rho_{i\pi^{(i)}}(\beta) \left\{ S^{(i)}\left(\pi_{\mathrm{obs}}^{(i)}\right) - E_c\left(S^{(i)} | \beta\right) \right\} \left\{ S^{(i)}\left(\pi_{\mathrm{obs}}^{(i)}\right) - E_c\left(S^{(i)} | \beta\right) \right\}'.
$$

The computations required to evaluate $L_c(\beta)$, $U_c(\beta)$, and $I_c(\beta)$ are nontrivial in the polytomous case. Levin (1987) gives an efficient recursive algorithm for exact computation of these quantities, and Levin (1990) gives a highly accurate double saddlepoint approximation.

14.4. AN EXAMPLE

The Northern Manhattan Stroke Study (NOMASS) is a population-based study to determine stroke incidence, risk factors, and prognosis in a multiethnic, urban population. The initial phase of NOMASS was an incidence study. The study was extended to a case-control study described in Sacco et al. (1999); later phases followed subjects in a cohort design. The case-control data used in this example are the complete records from Paik and Sacco (2000).

In the case-control portion of NOMASS, the cases were northern Manhattan area residents with an incident ischemic stroke. Two controls were matched to each case on age, gender, and ethnicity. Controls were sampled in two stages: first, candidate controls were sampled from northern Manhattan via random digit dialing; second, two controls were randomly selected from among all matching candidate controls. For 71 cases, only one control was available. For the 237 cases and 403 controls, there were 166 strata with 1:2 matching and 71 strata with 1:1 matching.

The mean age of the stroke cases was 68.3. Of the cases, 57.3% were women; 16.3% were non-Hispanic white, 29.7% non-Hispanic black, 53.1% Hispanic (black or nonblack), and 0.9% other. Cases were more likely than controls to have hypertension, cardiac disease, or diabetes mellitus. Controls were more likely to have at least a high school education (see Table 14.3).

Results of three conditional logistic regression models are shown in Table 14.4. Model 1 includes an indicator for level of physical activity and an indicator for winter season at the time of the case's or controls' interview. The latter indicator is intended to adjust for the effect of season on physical activity. Model 2 includes conventional risk factors for stroke, such as hypertension, diabetes, cardiac disease, current smoking, low education level, and obesity. Model 3 combines the variables of the other two. Table 14.5 provides SAS® code for fitting the third model.

Table 14.3. *Northern Manhattan Stroke Study: Marginal frequencies of risk factors*

	Cases			Controls		
Variable	Yes	No	% Yes	Yes	No	% Yes
ACT	121	116	51.1	306	97	75.9
WIN	56	181	23.6	53	350	13.2
EDU	74	163	31.2	184	219	45.7
HTN	169	68	71.3	233	170	66.6
DIAB	88	149	37.1	78	325	19.4
PVD	58	179	24.5	57	346	14.1
CARD	85	152	35.9	87	316	21.6
CIG	56	181	23.6	83	320	20.6
BMI	96	141	40.5	170	233	42.2
ALC	24	213	10.1	30	373	7.4

All variables are dichotomies, with 1 = yes, 0 = no:

ACT   Physically active
WIN   Winter at time of case's stroke or control's interview
EDU   High school graduation
HTN   History of hypertension
DIAB   History of diabetes
PVD   History of peripheral vascular disease
CARD History of cardiovascular disease
CIG   Current cigarette smoking
BMI   Obesity: BMI > 30
ALC   14 + alcoholic drinks per week

Table 14.4. *Northern Manhattan Stroke Study: Conditional logistic regression coefficient estimates and standard errors for the matched case-control data*

	Model 1		Model 2		Model 3	
Variable	CMLE	SE	CMLE	SE	CMLE	SE
ACT	−1.300	0.211	—	—	−1.130	0.226
WIN	0.733	0.249	—	—	0.716	0.271
EDU	—	—	−0.884	0.226	−0.813	0.241
HTN	—	—	0.528	0.206	0.394	0.218
DIAB	—	—	0.761	0.200	0.648	0.206
PVD	—	—	0.280	0.254	0.233	0.265
CARD	—	—	0.544	0.206	0.568	0.217
CIG	—	—	0.132	0.236	0.147	0.250
BMI	—	—	−0.246	0.201	−0.278	0.210
ALC	—	—	0.301	0.349	0.259	0.367

Table 14.5. *SAS* ® *code to fit conditional logistic regression model 3*

```
proc phreg data=casect12 outest=beta noprint;
model time*case(0)=ACTS WINTER HTN DIABET PVD CIGCUR CARDIO
OBESE ETHVY EDU / ties=discrete;
strata id;
```

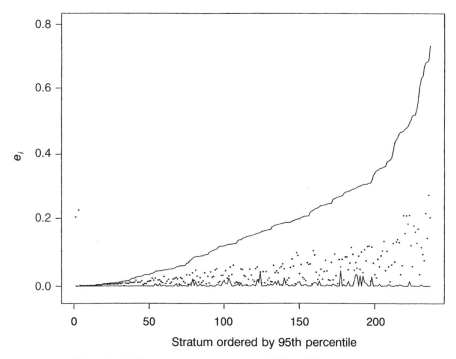

Figure 14.1. Diagnostic statistics and their 95% confidence intervals.

Model 1 suggests that physically active subjects have a significantly smaller odds on ischemic stroke than sedentary subjects [OR = exp(-1.3) = 0.273, $p < 0.05$]. This protective effect persists even after adjustment for conventional risk factors for stroke, showing a significant odds ratio in model 3 [OR = exp(-1.13) = 0.323, $p < 0.05$]. Figure 14.1 shows $e_i(\hat{\beta}_c)$ and their 95% confidence limits, obtained by the method described in Section 14.2.1. All but two diagnostic statistics lie inside the 95% confidence interval. Figure 14.2 shows a plot of $\hat{\beta}_{-i}$ for physical activity versus stratum i. No single stratum has a major effect on the cmle for this coefficient.

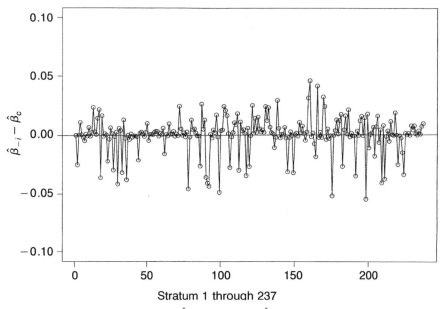

Figure 14.2. Difference between $\hat{\beta}_{-i}$ for ACT and $\hat{\beta}_c$ for ACT against stratum index.

14.5. OTHER ISSUES

Missing Covariates

It is not uncommon for covariates to be missing, but in matched-sample analyses the effect can be greater than in other analyses. To illustrate the point, let W and X denote a completely and a partially observed covariate, respectively. Consider a missing-at-random (MAR) mechanism, for which the probability that a covariate is missing may depend on the observed data, (Y, W, Z), but not on X:

$$P\{R_i(j) = 1 \,|\, X_{ij}, W_{ij}, Y_{ij}, Z_i\} = P\{R_i(j) = 1 \,|\, W_{ij}, Y_{ij}, Z_i\},$$

where $R_i(j)$ denotes the observation indicator for X_{ij}: $R_i(j) = 1$ if X_{ij} is observed, and $R_i(j) = 0$ if X_{ij} is missing ($j = 0, \ldots, k_i$). (See Chapter 16 for a detailed exposition of missing-data mechanisms.) In complete-record analysis for a single case matched to k_i controls, the estimating function for $\beta = (\beta_1', \beta_2')'$ becomes

$$\sum_{i=1}^{n} R_i(0) \begin{pmatrix} W_{i0} - \overline{W} \\ X_{i0} - \overline{X}_i \end{pmatrix},$$

where

$$
\begin{pmatrix} \overline{W}_i \\ \overline{X}_i \end{pmatrix} = \frac{\displaystyle\sum_{j=0}^{k_i} R_i(j) \begin{pmatrix} W_{ij} \\ X_{ij} \end{pmatrix} \exp\left(\beta_1' W_{ij} + \beta_2' X_{ij} \right)}{\displaystyle\sum_{j=0}^{k_i} R_i(j) \exp\left(\beta_1' W_{ij} + \beta_2' X_{ij} \right)}.
$$

If the case in stratum i is not completely observed, $R_i(0) = 0$, so the ith stratum does not contribute to the estimating function. Also, if the case is the only completely observed subject, $R_i(0) = 1$, $R_i(j) = 0$, $j > 0$, then the mean vector equals the case vector, and the contribution is again zero.

Complete-record analysis thus discards not only incompletely observed subjects but also completely observed subjects if no matching case or controls are completely observed. More important, if the missingness mechanism is not missing completely at random (MCAR), complete-record analysis yields biased estimates.

To utilize completely observed but discarded subjects, we can use the method of Brookmeyer, Liang, and Linet (1986) to merge "neighboring" strata if values of the matching variables are close. This analysis, valid under MCAR, increases efficiency by rescuing completely observed records. Gibbons and Hosmer (1991) propose imputing expected values of X from regression models for the missing covariate given other observed variables. The resulting estimates generally have reduced bias, but are still biased. Lipsitz, Parzen, and Ewell (1998) use a weighting method for conditional likelihood functions. This method, which uses completely observed records weighted by the reciprocal of the probability of observation, is valid under MAR. Efficiency may still suffer because, as in complete-record analysis, some completely observed records must be dropped. Paik and Sacco (2000) propose an imputation method, valid under MAR, in which a missing covariate is replaced by a weighted average of the predicted values from a regression model for cases and controls. Satten and Carroll (2000) propose a likelihood method valid under MAR. Their approach, maximization of the conditional likelihood based on $P(Y|W, Z)$, is asymptotically most efficient if the models are correctly specified.

Selection Bias

Another issue in analyzing case-control data is selection bias. The selection process is biased if $P(S = 1|Y, X, Z) \neq P(S = 1|Y, Z)$. Then the log odds of $P(Y = 1|X, Z, S = 1)$ is

$$
\ln \frac{P(Y = 1|X, Z, S = 1)}{P(Y = 0|X, Z, S = 1)} = \ln \frac{P(Y = 1|X, Z)}{P(Y = 0|X, Z)} + \ln \frac{P(S = 1|Y = 1, X, Z)}{P(S = 1|Y = 0, X, Z)}.
$$

The last term, now a function of X and Z, does not cancel out in the conditional likelihood. Therefore, the maximum conditional likelihood estimator obtained ignoring the selection bias is inconsistent. Bias in the estimate of the odds ratio depends on the probability of being selected given disease status, exposure status, and the matching factors. Kleinbaum, Morganstern, and Kupper (1981) propose a bias-corrected estimator of the odds ratio for a classical 2×2 table assuming that the selection probabilities are known. Maclure and Hankinson (1990) consider the case in which the selection probability can be estimated by logistic regression, but their variance estimate of the bias-corrected odds ratio does not take account of variation introduced by estimating the selection probabilities. In the regression context, Weinberg and Wacholder (1990) estimate a bias-corrected odds ratio assuming the selection probability is known by design. When selection probabilities are unknown, Lin and Paik (2001) provide a consistent method for avoiding selection bias in unmatched or matched case-control studies that takes account of the variation introduced by estimating the selection probabilities.

PROBLEMS

14.1. When X is a binary variable and there is only one covariate in (14.1), obtain an explicit estimator of $\exp(\beta)$ by solving $U_c(\beta) = 0$.

14.2. Under unbiased sampling as defined in (14.2), verify by a simple example that $P(Y|X, Z, S = 1) \neq P(Y|X, Z)$.

14.3. Verify the following relationships:

$$\ln \frac{P(Y=1|X, Z, S=1)}{P(Y=0|X, Z, S=1)} = \ln \frac{P(Y=1|X, Z)}{P(Y=0|X, Z)} + \ln \frac{P(S=1|Y=1, Z)}{P(S=1|Y=0, Z)}$$

and

$$\ln \frac{P(S=1|Y=1, Z)}{P(S=1|Y=0, Z)} = -\ln \frac{P(Y=1|Z)}{P(Y=0|Z)}.$$

14.4. Let $\ln\{P(Y=1|X, Z)/P(Y=0|X, Z)\} = \beta X + g(Z)$, where X is a binary risk factor, and let

$$\ln \frac{P(X=1|Z)}{P(X=0|Z)} = d(Z)$$

for some function $d(Z)$.

(a) Show that

$$\ln \frac{P(Y=1|X, Z)}{P(Y=0|X, Z)} - \ln \frac{P(Y=1|Z)}{P(Y=0|Z)} = \ln \frac{P(X|Y=1, Z)}{P(X|Y=0, Z)}.$$

Conclude that

$$\ln\frac{P(Y=1|X,Z,S=1)}{P(Y=0|X,Z,S=1)} = \beta X + \ln\frac{P(X=0|Y=1,Z)}{P(X=0|Y=1,Z)},$$

namely, that

$$g^*(Z) = \ln\frac{P(X=0|Y=1,Z)}{P(X=0|Y=1,Z)}.$$

[*Hint*. Use Bayes' theorem.]

(b) Show that

$$\ln\frac{P(X=1|Y=0,Z)}{P(X=0|Y=0,Z)} = \ln\frac{P(Y=0|X=1,Z)}{P(Y=0|X=0,Z)} + d(Z)$$

$$= \ln\left\{\frac{1+e^{g(Z)}}{1+e^{\beta+g(Z)}}\right\} + d(Z)$$

and that

$$\ln\frac{P(X=1|Y=1,Z)}{P(X=0|Y=1,Z)} = \ln\left\{\frac{1+e^{g(Z)}}{1+e^{\beta+g(Z)}}\right\} + \beta + d(Z).$$

[*Hint*. Use Bayes' theorem and invariance of the odds ratio.]

(c) Conclude that

$$P(X=0|Y=0,Z) = \frac{1+e^{\beta+g(Z)}}{1+e^{\beta+g(Z)}+e^{d(Z)}\{1+e^{g(Z)}\}},$$

$$P(X=0|Y=1,Z) = \frac{1+e^{\beta+g(Z)}}{1+e^{\beta+g(Z)}+e^{\beta+d(Z)}\{1+e^{g(Z)}\}}$$

and thus that

$$g^*(Z) = \ln\left\{\frac{1+e^{\beta+g(Z)}+e^{d(Z)}\{1+e^{g(Z)}\}}{1+e^{\beta+g(Z)}+e^{\beta+d(Z)}\{1+e^{g(Z)}\}}\right\}.$$

Plot $g^*(Z)$ for Z varying between -2 and $+2$ with $g(Z)=d(Z)=3Z$ and $\beta=1$.

REFERENCES

Andersen, E. B. (1970). Asymptotic properties of conditional maximum likelihood estimators. *J. R. Statist. Soc., Ser. B*, **32**, 283–301.

Andersen, E. B. (1973). *Conditional inference and models for measuring*. Copenhagen: Mental Hygienisk Forlag., p. 69.

Bedrick, E. J. and Hill, J. R. (1996). Assessing the fit of the logistic regression model to individual matched sets of case-control data. *Biometrics*, **52**, 1–9.

Breslow, N. E. and Day, N. E. (1980). *Statistical methods in cancer research, Vol. 1: The analysis of case-control studies*. IARC Scientific Publications No. 32. Lyon, France: International Agency for Research on Cancer.

Brookmeyer, R., Liang, K.-Y., and Linet, M. (1986). Matched case-control designs and over-matched analyses. *Am. J. Epidemiol.*, **124**, 693–701.

Carroll, R. J., Wang, S., and Wang, C.-Y. (1995). Prospective analysis of logistic case-control studies. *J. Am. Statist. Assoc.*, **90**, 157–169.

Farewell, V. T. (1979). Some results on the estimation of logistic models based on retrospective data. *Biometrika*, **66**, 27–32.

Gail, M. H., Wieand, S., and Piantadosi, S. (1984). Biased estimates of treatment effect in randomized experiments with nonlinear regressions and omitted covariates. *Biometrika*, **71**, 431–444.

Gibbons, L. E. and Hosmer, D. W. (1991). Conditional logistic regression with missing data. *Comm. Statist—Simul. Comp.*, **20**, 109–120.

Hastie, T. A. and Tibshirani, R. J. (1990). *Generalized additive models*. London: Chapman and Hall.

Hirji, K. F., Elashoff, R. M., Moore, D. H., and Bennett, D. E. (1988). Exact versus asymptotic analysis for a matched case-control study. *Statist. in Med.*, **7**, 765–772.

Hirji, K. F., Mehta, C. R., and Patel, N. R. (1988). Exact inference for matched case-control studies. *Biometrics*, **44**, 803–814.

Holford, T. R., White, C., and Kelsey, J. L. (1978). Multivariate analysis for matched case-control studies. *Am. J. Epidemiol.*, **107**, 245–256.

Jacobs, T. W., Byrne, C., Colditz, G. A., Connolly, J. L., and Schnitt, S. J. (1999). Radial scars in benign breast-biopsy specimens and the risk of breast cancer. *N. Engl. J. Med.*, **340**, 430–436.

Kleinbaum, D. G., Morgenstern, H., and Kupper, L. L. (1981). Selection bias in epidemiologic studies. *Am. J. Epidemiol.*, **113**, 452–463.

Levin, B. (1987). Conditional likelihood analysis in stratum-matched retrospective studies with polytomous disease states. *Comm. Statist.*, **B16**, 699718.

Levin, B. (1988). Re: "Polychotomous logistic regression methods for matched case-control studies with multiple case or control groups." *Am. J. Epidemiol*, **128**, 446.

Levin, B. (1990). The saddlepoint correction in conditional logistic likelihood analysis. *Biometrika*, **77**, 275–285.

Levin, B. and Paik, M. C. (2001). The unreasonable effectiveness of a biased logistic regression procedure in the analysis of pair-matched case-control studies. *J. Statist. Plann. Inference*, **96**, 371–385.

Liang, K. Y. and Stewart, W. F. (1987). Polychotomous logistic regression methods for matched case-control studies with multiple case or control groups. *Am. J. Epidemiol.*, **125**, 720–730.

Lin, I.-F. and Paik, M. C. (2001). Matched case-control data analysis with selection bias. *Biometrics*, **57**, 1106–1112.

Lipsitz, S. R., Parzen, M., and Ewell, M. (1998). Inference using conditional logistic regression with missing covariates. *Biometrics*, **54**, 295–303.

London, S. J., Connolly, J. L., Schnitt, S. J., and Colditz, G. A. (1992). A prospective study of benign breast disease and the risk of breast cancer. *J. Am. Med. Assoc.*, **267**, 941–944.

Lynn, H. S. and McCulloch, C. E. (1992). When does it pay to break the matches for analysis of a matched-pairs design? *Biometrics*, **48**, 397–409.

Maclure, M. and Hankinson, S. (1990). Analysis of selection bias in a case-control study of renal adenocarcinoma. *Epidemiology*, **1**, 441–447.

Marshall, L. M., Hunter, D., Connolly, J. L., Schnitt, S. J., Byrne, C., London, S. J., and Colditz, G. A. (1997). Risk of breast cancer associated with atypical hyperplasia of lobular and ductal types. *Cancer Epidemiol. Biomarkers Prevention*, **6**, 207–301.

McCullagh, P. and Nelder, J. A. (1989). *Generalized linear models*, 2nd ed. London: Chapman and Hall.

Moolgavkar, S., Lustbader, E., and Vanzon, D. J. (1985). Assessing the adequacy of the logistic regression model for matched case-control studies. *Statist. in Med.*, **42**, 147–156.

Neymann, J. and Scott, E. L. (1948). Consistent estimates based on partially consistent observations. *Econometrica*, **16**, 1–32.

Nuako, K. W., Ahlquist, D. A., Mahoney, D. W., Shaid, D. J., Siems, D. M., and Lindor, N. M. (1998). Familial predisposition for colorectal cancer in chronic ulcerative colitis: A case-control study. *Gastroenterology*, **115**, 1079–1083.

Paik, M. C. and Sacco, R. L. (2000). Matched case-control data analyses with missing covariates. *Appl. Statist.*, **49**, 145–156.

Pike, M. C., Hill, A. P., and Smith, P. G. (1980). Bias and efficiency in logistic analyses of stratified case-control studies. *Int. J. Epidemiol.*, **9**, 89–95.

Pregibon, D. (1984). Data analytic methods for matched case-control studies. *Biometrics*, **40**, 639–651.

Prentice, R. (1976). Use of the logistic model in retrospective studies. *Biometrics*, **32**, 599–606.

Prentice, R. and Pyke, R. (1979). Logistic disease incidence models and case-control studies. *Biometrika*, **65**, 153–158.

Sacco, R. L., Elking, M., Boden-Albala, B., Lin, I.-F., Kargman, D. E., Hauser, W. A., Shea, S., and Paik, M. C. (1999). The protective effect of moderate alcohol consumption on ischemic stroke. *J. Am. Med. Assoc.*, **281**, 53–60.

Satten, G. A. and Carroll, R. J. (2000). Conditional and unconditional categorical regression models with missing covariates. *Biometrics*, **56**(2), 384–388.

Severini, T. A. and Staniswalis, J. G. (1994). Quasi-likelihood estimation in semiparametric models. *J. Am. Statist. Assoc.*, **89**, 501–511.

Weinberg, C. R. and Wacholder, S. (1990). The design and analysis of case-control studies with biased sampling. *Biometrics*, **46**, 953–975.

Zeger, S. L., Liang, K.-Y., and Albert, P. S. (1988). Models for longitudinal data: A generalized estimating equation approach. *Biometrics*, **44**, 1049–1060.

CHAPTER 15

Analysis of Correlated Binary Data

An important assumption in the analysis of binary data is that the binary outcomes are statistically independent. This assumption is typically violated if the units of measurement are clustered. In longitudinal or panel studies, for example, measurements are taken at multiple time points for the same individual. Repeated measurements from the same individual are correlated when one outcome affects the probability of occurrence of the next. Even if uncorrelated within subjects, however, repeated measurements will appear correlated when there is substantial person-to-person variability in the probability of outcomes. In family studies, measurements from members of the same family are typically more similar than measurements from members of different families, and are thus correlated. In periodontal research, correlated measurements are taken from multiple sites in the mouth. Other examples arise in surveys conducted with cluster sampling, in data from ophthalmological or otolaryngological studies (with two eyes or two ears per person), in group-randomized behavioral intervention trials, and in hospital utilization studies where patients are clustered within treating physicians and physicians are clustered within hospitals. In each of these examples, the statistically independent sampling units have subunits which furnish the measurements and which are the natural units of analysis. If the analysis ignores the correlation between subunit measurements, point estimates may be valid, but naively estimated standard errors will not, leading to invalid p-values and confidence intervals and to poorly designed future studies. In this chapter we explain how to analyze correlated binary data properly. Section 15.1 presents methods for a single sample prevalence study. Section 15.2 covers inference for two correlated proportions, and Section 15.3 makes

Statistical Methods for Rates and Proportions, Third Edition
By Joseph L. Fleiss, Bruce Levin, and Myunghee Cho Paik
ISBN 0-471-52629-0 Copyright © 2003 John Wiley & Sons, Inc.

some design recommendations. Section 15.4 discusses problems that arise from a pair of fourfold tables which have clustered or correlated data. Section 15.5 contains material for the more advanced reader. It covers extensions of logistic regression methods for correlated outcomes, including generalized estimating equations, methods for random effects models, and likelihood-based methods.

15.1. INFERENCE FOR A SINGLE PROPORTION

To illustrate the effect of clustering on inference, we first consider estimation of a single proportion, as in a prevalence study. Let Y_{ij} be a binary outcome for independent unit i ($i = 1, \ldots, K$) and subunit ($j = 1, \ldots, n_i$). In a random sample of K families, for example, Y_{ij} could represent the presence or absence of some disease or condition for the jth member of the ith family, with varying numbers n_i of family members. Let the total number of subjects in the study be $N = n_1 + \cdots + n_K$, and the number of diseased members in family i be $Y_{i+} = Y_{i1} + \cdots + Y_{in_i}$. The proportion with disease in family i is Y_{i+}/n_i. An estimator of the proportion P of diseased individuals in the population, say p, is the total number of diseased subjects divided by N, which is also a weighted average of the family-specific proportions with disease, with weights proportional to family size:

$$p = \sum_{i=1}^{K} \sum_{j=1}^{n_i} \frac{Y_{ij}}{N} = \sum_{i=1}^{K} \frac{n_i}{N} \frac{Y_{i+}}{n_i}.$$

If the disease indicators from all subjects were independent, p would be asymptotically normally distributed with mean P and variance $P(1 - P)/N = PQ/N$. Suppose, though, that the disease indicators among family members are correlated, with $\text{Cov}(Y_{ij}, Y_{ik}) = PQ\rho$ for $j \neq k$, where $\rho = \text{Corr}(Y_{ij}, Y_{ik})$ is the correlation between outcomes for subjects in the same family. This type of correlation structure is called *intraclass correlation*, wherein any two measurements from the same cluster have the same correlation. Then p is asymptotically normally distributed with mean P and variance

$$\text{Var}(p) = \sum_{i=1}^{K} \frac{n_i PQ\{1 + (n_i - 1)\rho\}}{N^2} = \frac{PQ}{N}\{1 + (\bar{n}_w - 1)\rho\}, \quad (15.1)$$

where $\bar{n}_w = \sum_{i=1}^{K} n_i^2 / \sum_{i=1}^{K} n_i = \sum_{i=1}^{K}(n_i/N)n_i$ is the cluster-size-weighted average cluster size. Thus the variance of p is PQ/N times a *variance inflation factor*, or VIF (see also Section 9.6). Re-expressing the sum of squared cluster sizes in $\bar{n}_w$ in terms of the arithmetic mean cluster size $\bar{n}_a = \sum_{i=1}^{K} n_i/K$ and the finite-population variance of the cluster sizes, $s^2 = \sum_{i=1}^{K}(n_i - \bar{n}_a)^2/K$, we have

$$\text{VIF} = 1 + (\bar{n}_w - 1)\rho = 1 + \left\{(s^2/\bar{n}_a) + (\bar{n}_a - 1)\right\}\rho. \qquad (15.2)$$

When VIF > 1, we say the data are *overdispersed*.

The variance of p can be estimated by

$$\widehat{\text{Var}}(p) = \frac{pq}{N}\widehat{\text{VIF}} = \frac{pq}{N}\left[1 + \left\{(s^2/\bar{n}_a) + (\bar{n}_a - 1)\right\}\hat{\rho}\right], \qquad (15.3)$$

where $\hat{\rho}$ is an estimator of ρ which we discuss below at (15.4). The variance estimate (15.3) is given in Donald and Donner (1987); Rao and Scott (1992) give a slightly different estimator. For large K, an approximate 95% confidence interval for P is

$$p - 1.96\,\widehat{\text{se}}(p) < P < p + 1.96\,\widehat{\text{se}}(p),$$

where $\widehat{\text{se}}(p) = \sqrt{\widehat{\text{Var}}(p)}$. By assuming a specific distribution for Y_{i+}, such as the beta-binomial distribution, one could provide an exact confidence interval for P, but in this chapter we focus on nonparametric methods that are valid in large samples for any distribution.

Note that the average cluster size, the variability of cluster sizes, and the intraclass correlation all affect the variance of p. Researchers may not have control over the cluster size, as in the family study, but in other studies the n_i's can often be designed by the investigator. In longitudinal studies, for example, n_i is the number of time points of observation and repeated measurement, while in periodontal studies, n_i is the number of measurements sites in the oral cavity. If $n_i = n$ for all i, then s^2 is zero, and the variance of p reduces to $(PQ/N)\{1 + (n-1)\rho\}$. When ρ is positive, the naive variance estimate pq/N underestimates the true variance. When ρ is negative, pq/N overestimates the true variance. Note that because the VIF depends on the product of the correlation and cluster size (minus 1), even if the correlation is small, a large cluster size can result in a marked variance inflation. For example, with $\rho = 0.05$ and $n = 100$, the VIF is 5.95, meaning that p has almost six times the variance given by the naive estimate. Variation in cluster sizes further inflates the variance. For example, if half the clusters have $n_i = 50$ and the other half have $n_i = 150$, resulting in the same average $\bar{n}_a = 100$ but with $s^2 = 2500$, the VIF increases to $1 + \{(2500/100) + 100 - 1\}0.05 = 7.2$. Thus variation in cluster sizes modestly increases the VIF, while the average size of the cluster can have a large effect on the VIF when ρ is nonnegligible.

In practice, the intraclass correlation ρ is unknown and needs to be estimated. Using the relationship

$$E\left\{(Y_{ij} - P)(Y_{ik} - P)\right\}/PQ = \rho,$$

a natural estimator for ρ is

$$\hat{\rho} = \frac{2 \sum\limits_{i=1}^{K} \sum\limits_{j>k} (Y_{ij}-p)(Y_{ik}-p)}{\sum\limits_{i=1}^{K} n_i(n_i-1)pq}.\tag{15.4}$$

Because data are often presented only in terms of Y_{i+}, a computationally more convenient expression for the numerator of (15.4) is given by

$$2 \sum_{i=1}^{K} \sum_{j>k} (Y_{ij}-p)(Y_{ik}-p)$$

$$= \sum_{i=1}^{K} \left\{ Y_{i+}(Y_{i+}-1) - 2p(n_i-1)Y_{i+} + n_i(n_i-1)p^2 \right\}.$$

To illustrate, Table 15.1 presents a subset of the data from a toxicologic experiment originally reported by Weil (1970) and analyzed by Williams (1975) and Rao and Scott (1992). The table gives the number Y_{i+} of pups

Table 15.1. *Number of pups surviving 21 lactation days among pups alive 4 days after birth for 16 litters of pregnant rats given a chemically treated diet*

	Number of Pups	
Litter No. $(=i)$	Survived 21 Days $(=Y_{i+})$	Alive after 4 Days $(=n_i)$
1	12	12
2	11	11
3	10	10
4	9	9
5	10	11
6	9	10
7	9	10
8	8	9
9	8	9
10	4	5
11	7	9
12	4	7
13	5	10
14	3	6
15	3	10
16	0	7

surviving 21 lactation days among the number n_i of pups alive 4 days after birth from $K = 16$ pregnant rats whose diet was chemically treated. The estimated proportion of all pups in a similar situation who would survive 21 lactation days is $p = \Sigma_i Y_{i+}/\Sigma_i n_i = 112/145 = 0.7724$. To calculate the standard error of p, we first estimate the correlation to be $\hat{\rho} = 0.3205$ using (15.4). With $N = 145$, $\bar{n}_a = 9.0625$, and $s^2 = 3.4336$, the variance inflation factor from (15.2) is $\text{VIF} = 3.705$, and (15.3) yields

$$\widehat{\text{Var}}(p) = \frac{(0.7724)(0.2276)}{145} \times 3.705 = 0.004493$$

with estimated standard error $\widehat{\text{se}}(p) = 0.004493^{1/2} = 0.0670$. A 95% confidence interval for P is then

$$p \pm 1.96\,\widehat{\text{se}}(p) = (0.641, 0.904).$$

15.2. INFERENCE FOR TWO PROPORTIONS

Next consider a 2×2 table with data correlated due to cluster sampling. We now have a binary exposure variable, X_{ij}, in addition to the binary outcome Y_{ij} for the jth member in the ith cluster. There are two cases to consider. In one case, exposure does not vary among the members (subunits) in the same cluster (independent unit); in the other case, exposure does vary. When X_{ij} does not vary within a cluster, we can denote exposure as X_i with a single subscript, and we can continue to aggregate the binary outcomes to single cluster counts Y_{i+}, using X_i to keep track of which clusters are exposed and which are unexposed. When X_{ij} does vary within a cluster, it is no longer appropriate to aggregate the data to single cluster counts. Instead, the data should be aggregated separately by exposure group, thus: $Y_{i1+} = \Sigma_{j=1}^{n_i} X_{ij} Y_{ij}$ and $Y_{i2+} = \Sigma_{j=1}^{n_i}(1 - X_{ij})Y_{ij}$. In either case, the two group proportions can be estimated as if the data were independent, but the standard errors cannot—they have different forms depending on whether or not exposure varies within clusters.

When exposure does not vary within clusters, we may use the layout of Table 15.2 to represent the data. The cell counts can be expressed in terms of X_i and Y_{ij} as follows.

$$a = \sum_{i=1}^{K} \sum_{j=1}^{n_i} X_i Y_{ij} = \sum_{i=1}^{K} X_i Y_{i+},$$

$$b = \sum_{i=1}^{K} \sum_{j=1}^{n_i} X_i (1 - Y_{ij}),$$

Table 15.2. *Data layout from a two-sample study when exposures do not vary within clusters*

		Outcome (Y)		
		1	0	Total
Exposure (X)	1	a	b	$a + b = \Sigma_i X_i n_i = N_1$
	0	c	d	$c + d = \Sigma_i (1 - X_i) n_i = N_2$
	Total	$a + c = \Sigma_i Y_{i+}$	$b + d = \Sigma_i (n_i - Y_{i+})$	N

$$c = \sum_{i=1}^{K} \sum_{j=1}^{n_i} (1 - X_i) Y_{ij} = \sum_{i=1}^{K} (1 - X_i) Y_{i+},$$

$$d = \sum_{i=1}^{K} \sum_{j=1}^{n_i} (1 - X_i)(1 - Y_{ij}).$$

Now let $P_1 = P(Y = 1 | X = 1)$ and $P_2 = P(Y = 1 | X = 0)$. In testing $P_1 = P_2$, a natural test statistic is

$$z = \frac{p_1 - p_2}{\sqrt{\text{Var}(p_1 - p_2)}},$$

where $p_1 = a/(a + b)$ and $p_2 = c/(c + d)$. Here z is distributed approximately as a standard normal variable in large samples. In the case we are considering, a and c are statistically independent—see Problem 15.3. The variance of $p_1 - p_2$ then needs only a simple adjustment as in the single sample case, namely,

$$\text{Var}(p_1 - p_2) = \frac{P_1 Q_1 f_1}{a + b} + \frac{P_2 Q_2 f_2}{c + d}, \tag{15.5}$$

where f_1 and f_2 are the variance inflation factors defined for the groups of clusters with $X_i = 1$ and $X_i = 0$, respectively. Specifically, after obtaining $\hat{\rho}_1$ from (15.4) using only those clusters with $X_i = 1$, we calculate

$$\bar{n}_1 = \frac{\sum_{i=1}^{K} X_i n_i}{\sum_{i=1}^{K} X_i},$$

$$s_1^2 = \frac{\sum_{i=1}^{K} X_i (n_i - \bar{n}_i)^2}{\sum_{i=1}^{K} X_i},$$

Table 15.3. *Number of pups surviving 21 lactation days among pups alive 4 days after birth for 16 litters of pregnant rats given a control diet*

	Number of Pups	
Litter No. $(= i)$	Survived 21 Days $(= Y_{i+})$	Alive after 4 Days $(= n_i)$
1	13	13
2	12	12
3	9	9
4	9	9
5	8	8
6	8	8
7	12	13
8	11	12
9	9	10
10	9	10
11	8	9
12	11	13
13	4	5
14	5	7
15	7	10
16	7	10

and

$$f_1 = 1 + \left\{ \left(s_1^2 / \bar{n}_1 \right) + \left(\bar{n}_1 - 1 \right) \right\} \rho_1;$$

$\hat{\rho}_2$, $\bar{n}_2$, s_2^2, and f_2 are obtained similarly, using only those clusters with $X_i = 0$, and replacing X_i by $1 - X_i$ in the above expressions.

To illustrate the first case, consider the data presented in Table 15.1 together with the data shown in Table 15.3 from another 16 pregnant rats who were fed a control diet. Letting $X_{ij} = 0$ for the control group and $X_{ij} = 1$ for the chemically treated group, it is clear that X_{ij} does not vary among the pups in the same litter, such that, $X_{i1} = X_{i2} = \cdots = X_{in_i} = X_i$.

The data are summarized in the following 2×2 layout:

		Outcome		
		Survived	Died	Total
Exposure	Treated diet	112	33	145
	Control diet	142	16	158
	Total	254	49	303

For the control group with $N_2 = 158$, we obtain $p_2 = 142/158 = 0.8987$, $\hat{\rho}_2 = 0.01657$, $\bar{n}_2 = 9.875$, $s_2^2 = 4.984$, $f_2 = 1.155$, $\widehat{\text{Var}}(p_2) = 0.0006656$, and $\text{se}(p_2) = 0.0258$. To test H_0: $P_1 = P_2$, the z-score is $z = (0.8987 - 0.7724)/(0.004493 + 0.0006656)^{1/2} = 1.758$, and we do not reject H_0 at the $\alpha = 0.05$ level.

When exposure does vary within a cluster, we need to retain the double subscript notation for X_{ij}, and separate out Y_{i1+} and Y_{i2+} for exposed and unexposed subunits, respectively. We also let k_i be the number of subunits in the ith cluster with $X_{ij} = 1$. In this case $a = \sum_{i=1}^{K} Y_{i1+}$ and $c = \sum_{i=1}^{K} Y_{i2+}$ are not statistically independent, because some subunits in a cluster may contribute to a and others in the same cluster to c. The variance of $p_1 - p_2$ must now include the covariance between p_1 and p_2, as follows:

$$\text{Var}(p_1 - p_2) = \frac{P_1 Q_1 f_1}{a+b} + \frac{P_2 Q_2 f_2}{c+d} - 2\frac{\text{Cov}(a, c | \{X_{ij}\})}{(a+b)(c+d)}. \quad (15.6)$$

where f_1 and f_2 denote the variance inflation factors calculated from the two sets of K subclusters, one with cluster sizes $k_1, \ldots, k_K$ and the other with cluster sizes $n_1 - k_1, \ldots, n_K - k_K$, and where $\text{Cov}(a, c | \{X_{ij}\})$ denotes the conditional covariance of a and c given the set of exposures $\{X_{ij}\}$. Deriving this covariance involves careful counting of pairs (Y_{ij}, Y_{ik}) such that Y_{ij} belongs to group 1 and Y_{ik} belongs to group 2:

$$\text{Cov}(a, c | \{X_{ij}\}) = \text{Cov}\left(\sum_{i=1}^{K} \sum_{j=1}^{n_i} X_{ij} Y_{ij}, \sum_{i=1}^{K} \sum_{k=1}^{n_i} (1 - X_{ik}) Y_{ik} \,\Big|\, \{X_{ij}\}\right)$$

$$= \sum_{i=1}^{K} \text{Cov}\left(\sum_{j=1}^{n_i} X_{ij} Y_{ij}, \sum_{k=1}^{n_i} (1 - X_{ik}) Y_{ik} \,\Big|\, \{X_{ij}\}\right)$$

$$= \sum_{i=1}^{K} \sum_{j \neq k} X_{ij} (1 - X_{ik}) \text{Cov}\left(Y_{ij}, Y_{ik} | X_{ij} = 1, \; X_{ik} = 0\right)$$

$$= \rho_{12} \sqrt{P_1 Q_1 P_2 Q_2} \sum_{i=1}^{K} k_i (n_i - k_i), \quad (15.7)$$

where ρ_{12} denotes the conditional correlation between two binary responses within the same cluster, one with $X_{ij} = 1$, the other with $X_{ik} = 0$: $\rho_{12} = \text{Cov}(Y_{ij}, Y_{ik} | X_{ij} = 1, X_{ik} = 0)/\sqrt{P_1 Q_1 P_2 Q_2}$. This correlation can be estimated in the same manner as in the single-proportion case. A consistent estimate of

p_{12} is given by

$$
\hat{\rho}_{12} = \frac{\displaystyle\sum_{i=1}^{K}\sum_{j \neq k} X_{ij}(1 - X_{ik})(Y_{ij} - p_1)(Y_{ik} - p_2)}{\displaystyle\sum_{i=1}^{K} k_i(n_i - k_i)\sqrt{p_1 q_1 p_2 q_2}}
$$

$$
= \frac{\displaystyle\sum_{i=1}^{K}\{Y_{i1+} - k_i p_1\}\{Y_{i2+} - (n_i - k_i)p_2\}}{\displaystyle\sum_{i=1}^{K} k_i(n_i - k_i)\sqrt{p_1 q_1 p_2 q_2}}. \tag{15.8}
$$

15.3. DESIGN CONSIDERATIONS

Consider an experiment comparing a treatment with a control where the two groups are assembled in clusters. Just as standard errors depend on whether or not exposure varies within clusters, so do power and sample size calculations. Suppose that the experimenter has a choice of allocating treatments within clusters or between clusters. Allocating treatments randomly within clusters will result in exposure varying within clusters, whereas allocating them randomly to entire clusters will result in exposure not varying within clusters. Variance formulas (15.5) and (15.6) suggest that allocating within clusters gives a smaller standard error for the difference estimator. Indeed, the clusters serve as a natural blocking factor.

When exposure does not vary within clusters, the sample size formula (4.14) given in Chapter 4 can be modified to give the required sample size per group (without use of continuity correction and with equal total group sizes, $N_1 = N_2 = N'$). Assuming equal cluster sizes, $n_i = \bar{n}$ for all i, the modified formula is (see Donner, Birkett, and Buck, 1981)

$$
N' = \frac{\left(z_{\alpha/2}\sqrt{2\,\overline{PQ}\bar{f}} + z_\beta\sqrt{f_1 P_1 Q_1 + f_2 P_2 Q_2}\right)^2}{(P_1 - P_2)^2}, \tag{15.9}
$$

where $\bar{P} = (P_1 + P_2)/2 = 1 - \bar{Q}$ and where $\bar{f} = (f_1 + f_2)/2 = 1 + \rho(\bar{n} - 1)$ is the variance inflation factor calculated under the null hypothesis. A sample version of $\bar{f}$ would be used to estimate the variance, $2\,\overline{PQ}\bar{f}$, of $p_1 - p_2$ under the null hypothesis. When exposure varies within clusters, we assume there will be the same number of clusters, $K = 2N'/\bar{n}$, with $k_i = \bar{n}/2$ exposed and $n_i - k_i = \bar{n}/2$ unexposed in each cluster, so that the total sample size remains N' per group. Then $\bar{f}$ may be replaced by $\bar{f} - \bar{n}\rho/2$, and $P_1 Q_1 f_1 + P_2 Q_2 f_2$ may be replaced by $P_1 Q_1 f_1 + P_2 Q_2 f_2 - \bar{n}\rho_{12}\sqrt{P_1 Q_1 P_2 Q_2}$, using f_1, f_2, and ρ_{12} as defined in the previous section.

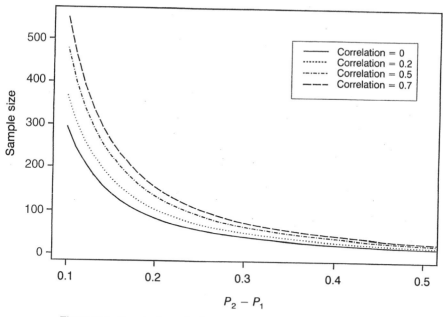

Figure 15.1. Required sample size versus difference in rates ($P_1 = 0.2$).

To calculate power and sample size, we need information on correlation, average cluster size, and the variance of cluster sizes. A naive power calculation ignoring the cluster effect will overstate the actual power and understate actual required sample sizes. When the intraclass correlations are positive, for fixed total sample size N and total number of clusters K, maximum power is achieved when the cluster sizes are equal. If cluster sizes can be designed, then for fixed total sample size, smaller-size clusters yield greater power (but require more clusters) than larger-size clusters. When $\rho = 0$, power is equivalent to sampling $N = Kn$ independent units, while if $\rho = 1$, power is equivalent to sampling only K independent units. When $0 < \rho < 1$, power corresponds to sample sizes between K and Kn. Figure 15.1 illustrates the effect of ρ on sample size. The figure plots the sample size N' per group required to achieve 80% power as a function of $P_2 - P_1$ for $\rho = 0$, 0.2, 0.5, and 0.7, when $\alpha = 0.05$ (two-tailed), $P_1 = 0.2$, $\bar{n} = 5$, and $s^2 = 0$.

15.4. 2 × 2 × 2 TABLES

15.4.1. Hypothesis Testing

A pair of 2×2 tables with correlated data raises several problems according to the dependence structure and the hypotheses to be tested. Sometimes cell counts in different tables are correlated, sometimes cell counts from different

Table 15.4. *Notation for a two-group, two-wave panel study with binary outcomes*

		Observed Frequencies						
		Time 1				Time 2		
		Outcome $(= Y_1)$				Outcome $(= Y_2)$		
		1	0	Total		1	0	Total
Exposure $(= X)$	1	a_1	b_1	n_1	1	a_2	b_2	n_1
	0	c_1	d_1	n_2	0	c_2	d_2	n_2

		Observed Proportions						
		Time 1				Time 2		
		Outcome $(= Y_1)$				Outcome $(= Y_2)$		
		1	0	Total		1	0	Total
Exposure $(= X)$	1	p_{11}	q_{11}	1	1	p_{12}	q_{12}	1
	0	p_{21}	q_{21}	1	0	p_{22}	q_{22}	1

rows within a table are correlated, and sometimes the cells themselves are clustered counts. Different dependence structures lead to different test statistics, and we consider each of these situations in this section.

Dependent Tables

Consider a two-group comparison in which each individual in each group provides a binary outcome at each of two points in time. Let p_{ij} denote the observed proportion of positive responses in group i at time j for $i = 1, 2$ and $j = 1, 2$, with corresponding unknown population proportions $\underline{P} = (P_{11}, P_{12}, P_{21}, P_{22})'$. The observed frequencies and proportions may be summarized in a pair of 2×2 tables as in Table 15.4 These fourfold tables differ from those shown in Chapter 10 because of the correlation between the cell counts in different tables.

Several questions may now be posed, depending on the study objectives. The first question is whether or not, at each time point, the two groups have the same response proportions, that is, $P_{11} = P_{21}$ and $P_{12} = P_{22}$. We write this null hypothesis as

$$H_{01}: \begin{pmatrix} P_{11} - P_{21} \\ P_{12} - P_{22} \end{pmatrix} = 0.$$

It can be shown that

$$\begin{pmatrix} P_{11} - P_{21} \\ P_{12} - P_{22} \end{pmatrix}$$

is distributed asymptotically as a bivariate normal random variable with mean

$$\begin{pmatrix} P_{11} - P_{21} \\ P_{12} - P_{22} \end{pmatrix}$$

and variance-covariance matrix

$$\Sigma_1 = \begin{pmatrix} \dfrac{P_{11}Q_{11}}{n_1} + \dfrac{P_{21}Q_{21}}{n_2} & \mathrm{Cov}(p_{11}, p_{12}) + \mathrm{Cov}(p_{21}, p_{22}) \\ \mathrm{Cov}(p_{11}, p_{12}) + \mathrm{Cov}(p_{21}, p_{22}) & \dfrac{P_{12}Q_{12}}{n_1} + \dfrac{P_{22}Q_{22}}{n_2} \end{pmatrix}.$$

$$(15.10)$$

The variance-covariance matrix may be estimated by substituting p_{ij} for P_{ij}, and the covariance terms may be estimated by

$$\widehat{\mathrm{Cov}}(p_{11}, p_{12}) = \frac{\hat{\rho}_1}{n_1} \sqrt{p_{11} q_{11} p_{12} q_{12}}$$

$$(15.11)$$

$$\widehat{\mathrm{Cov}}(p_{21}, p_{22}) = \frac{\hat{\rho}_2}{n_1} \sqrt{p_{21} q_{21} p_{22} q_{22}},$$

where

$$\hat{\rho}_i = \frac{\sum_{h=1}^{n_i}(Y_{hi1} - p_{i1})(Y_{hi2} - p_{i2})}{n_i\sqrt{p_{i1} q_{i1} p_{i2} q_{i2}}} = \frac{\sum_{h=1}^{n_i} Y_{hi1} Y_{hi2} - n_i p_{i1} p_{i2}}{n_i\sqrt{p_{i1} q_{i1} p_{i2} q_{i2}}}, \quad (15.12)$$

and where we have indexed all n_i binary observations in group i at time j as Y_{hij} ($h = 1, \ldots, n_i$). Under hypothesis H_{01}, instead of using separate estimates p_{ij} in (15.10) and (15.11), the pooled proportions $p_{+j} = 1 - q_{+j}$ may be used, where $p_{+1} = (a_1 + c_1)/(n_1 + n_2)$ and $p_{+2} = (a_2 + c_2)/(n_1 + n_2)$.

Note that $\sum_h Y_{hi1} Y_{hi2}$ (hence $\hat{\rho}_i$), which is not available from the marginal tables in Table 15.4, must be calculated from the joint outcome frequencies. There is no reason that $\hat{\rho}_1$ must equal $\hat{\rho}_2$ under H_{01}, even when the observed proportions are equal across groups at each time point, that is, $p_{11} = p_{21}$ and $p_{12} = p_{22}$. This can be seen by cross-classifying Y_{hi1} and Y_{hi2} in a 2×2 table; different values of $\sum_h Y_{hi1} Y_{hi2}$ in the $(1,1)$ cell are consistent with the observed margins a_1 and a_2 in group 1 (or c_1 and c_2 in group 2). The separate estimates in (15.12) should therefore be used if there is evidence of different strengths of correlation in the two groups between time 1 and 2 measurements. A stronger form of the null hypothesis (see H_{05} below) posits a common distribution for (Y_1, Y_2) in each group, in which case the intraclass correlations are the same and may be estimated by pooling the data:

$$\hat{\rho} = \frac{\sum_{h=1}^{n_1+n_2}(Y_{h1}-P_{+1})(Y_{h2}-P_{+2})}{(n_1+n_2)\sqrt{P_{+1}q_{+1}P_{+2}q_{+2}}} = \frac{\sum_{h=1}^{n_1+n_2}Y_{h1}Y_{h2}-(n_1+n_2)P_{+1}P_{+2}}{(n_1+n_2)\sqrt{P_{+1}q_{+1}P_{+2}q_{+2}}}.$$

$$(15.13)$$

After settling on an estimated version of Σ_1, say $\hat{\Sigma}_1$, hypothesis H_{01} may be tested by the statistic

$$T_1 = (p_{11}-p_{21}, p_{12}-p_{22})\hat{\Sigma}_1^{-1}\begin{pmatrix} p_{11}-p_{21} \\ p_{12}-p_{22} \end{pmatrix}, \qquad (15.14)$$

which has an asymptotic chi squared distribution with 2 df as n_1 and n_2 become large.

The second question is whether or not, in each group, the probability of a positive response remains constant over time, that is, $P_{11} = P_{12}$ and $P_{21} = P_{22}$. The null hypothesis is

$$H_{02}: \begin{pmatrix} P_{11}-P_{12} \\ P_{21}-P_{22} \end{pmatrix} = 0.$$

In this case, $p_{11}-p_{12}$ and $p_{21}-p_{22}$, which involve different groups of subjects, are statistically independent and are each asymptotically normal. The pair

$$\begin{pmatrix} p_{11}-p_{12} \\ p_{21}-p_{22} \end{pmatrix}$$

is asymptotically bivariate normal with mean

$$\begin{pmatrix} P_{11}-P_{12} \\ P_{21}-P_{22} \end{pmatrix}$$

and variance-covariance matrix Σ_2, where Σ_2 is a diagonal matrix with diagonal elements

$$\{(P_{11}Q_{11}+P_{12}Q_{12})/n_1\} - 2\text{Cov}(p_{11},p_{12})$$

and (15.15)

$$\{(P_{21}Q_{21}+P_{22}Q_{22})/n_2\} - 2\text{Cov}(p_{21},p_{22}).$$

Σ_2 is estimated by $\hat{\Sigma}_2$, substituting p_{ij} for P_{ij} and using (15.11) and (15.12).

H_{02} may be tested by the statistic

$$T_2 = (p_{11} - p_{12}, p_{21} - p_{22}) \hat{\Sigma}_2^{-1} \begin{pmatrix} p_{11} - p_{12} \\ p_{21} - p_{22} \end{pmatrix}$$

$$= \frac{(p_{11} - p_{12})^2}{\{(p_{11}q_{11} + p_{12}q_{12})/n_1\} - 2\widehat{\mathrm{Cov}}(p_{11}, p_{12})}$$

$$+ \frac{(p_{21} - p_{22})^2}{\{(p_{21}q_{21} + p_{22}q_{22})/n_2\} - 2\widehat{\mathrm{Cov}}(p_{21}, p_{22})}, \qquad (15.16)$$

which has an asymptotic chi squared distribution with 2 df.

The third question is whether or not the changes from time 1 to time 2 are the same for the two groups, such that, $P_{12} - P_{11} = P_{22} - P_{21}$, which is equivalent to asking whether or not the group differences are the same at each time point, such that, $P_{21} - P_{11} = P_{22} - P_{12}$. This null hypothesis can be expressed as

$$H_{03}: (P_{12} - P_{11}) - (P_{22} - P_{21}) = (P_{21} - P_{11}) - (P_{22} - P_{12}) = 0.$$

The difference $(p_{12} - p_{11}) - (p_{22} - p_{21})$ is asymptotically normal with mean $(P_{12} - P_{11}) - (P_{22} - P_{21})$ and variance

$$\Sigma_3 = (-1, 1) \Sigma_2 \begin{pmatrix} -1 \\ 1 \end{pmatrix} = \frac{P_{11}Q_{11} + P_{12}Q_{12}}{n_1} - 2\mathrm{Cov}(p_{11}, p_{12})$$

$$+ \frac{P_{21}Q_{21} + P_{22}Q_{22}}{n_2} - 2\mathrm{Cov}(p_{21}, p_{22}). \quad (15.17)$$

Hypothesis H_{03} may be tested by the statistic

$$T_3 = \{(p_{12} - p_{11}) - (p_{22} - p_{21})\}^2 / \hat{\Sigma}_3, \qquad (15.18)$$

where

$$\hat{\Sigma}_3 = (-1, 1) \hat{\Sigma}_2 \begin{pmatrix} -1 \\ 1 \end{pmatrix}.$$

T_3 is asymptotically chi squared with 1 df.

The first hypothesis is equivalent to the assertion that, at each time point, there is an *odds ratio* of 1 comparing response probabilities for group 1 versus group 2, and the second hypothesis is equivalent to the assertion that, for each group, there is an odds ratio of 1 comparing response probabilities for time 1 versus time 2. The third hypothesis, however, is not equivalent to the assertion that the odds ratios for the two tables are the same; that

Table 15.5. *Observed and expected cell frequencies for two multinomial distributions with a 2×2 response design*

		Observed Frequencies			
Exposure	$(Y_1, Y_2) =$ (1,1)	(1,0)	(0,1)	(0,0)	Total
1	$n_{11}(1)$	$n_{10}(1)$	$n_{01}(1)$	$n_{00}(1)$	n_1
0	$n_{11}(2)$	$n_{10}(2)$	$n_{01}(2)$	$n_{00}(2)$	n_2
Total	n_{11}	n_{10}	n_{01}	n_{00}	$n_1 + n_2$

		Expected Frequencies			
Exposure	$(Y_1, Y_2) =$ (1,1)	(1,0)	(0,1)	(0,0)	Total
1	$n_1 \pi_{11}(1)$	$n_1 \pi_{10}(1)$	$n_1 \pi_{01}(1)$	$n_1 \pi_{00}(1)$	n_1
0	$n_2 \pi_{11}(2)$	$n_2 \pi_{10}(2)$	$n_2 \pi_{01}(2)$	$n_2 \pi_{00}(2)$	n_2

hypothesis is

$$H_{04}: \frac{P_{11}/Q_{11}}{P_{21}/Q_{21}} = \frac{P_{12}/Q_{12}}{P_{22}/Q_{22}}.$$

Both H_{03} and H_{04} specify no interaction between group and time, but H_{03} is on an additive scale, while H_{04} is on a multiplicative scale, and these need not hold simultaneously. Test statistics for H_{04} will be discussed in Section 15.5 in the context of generalized estimating equations.

Note that hypotheses H_{01} through H_{04} concern the *marginal* proportions of positive outcome at each time point; they do not address *subject-specific* changes. There are four possible joint events for binary outcomes observed at two time points: (1,1), (1,0), (0,1), and (0,0). These constitute a multinomial response, and we can ask whether or not the underlying multinomial probabilities are the same for the two groups. Casting the raw data into a 2×4 table, the observed and expected cell frequencies may be denoted as in Table 15.5.

As mentioned above, Table 15.5 contains information not available from the marginal frequencies in Table 15.4. Formally,

$$\pi_{jk}(i) = P(Y_1 = j, Y_2 = k | X = 2 - i),$$

with $\displaystyle\sum_{j=0}^{1} \sum_{k=0}^{1} \pi_{jk}(i) = 1$ for $i = 1$ and 2.

The equality of the joint distribution of (Y_1, Y_2) between the two groups is hypothesis H_5:

$$H_5: \begin{pmatrix} \pi_{11}(1) \\ \pi_{10}(1) \\ \pi_{01}(1) \\ \pi_{00}(1) \end{pmatrix} = \begin{pmatrix} \pi_{11}(2) \\ \pi_{10}(2) \\ \pi_{01}(2) \\ \pi_{00}(2) \end{pmatrix} = \begin{pmatrix} \pi_{11} \\ \pi_{10} \\ \pi_{01} \\ \pi_{00} \end{pmatrix}.$$

Expression (9.38), which is equivalent to (9.3), gives the appropriate statistic for testing the equality of two multinomial probability vectors. We denote that statistic by T_5:

$$T_5 = \sum_{j=0}^{1} \sum_{k=0}^{1} \frac{\{\hat{\pi}_{jk}(1) - \hat{\pi}_{jk}(2)\}^2}{\hat{\pi}_{jk}(1/n_1 + 1/n_2)}, \tag{15.19}$$

where $\hat{\pi}_{jk}(i)$ are the sample proportions $n_{jk}(i)/n_i$ corresponding to $\pi_{jk}(i)$, and $\hat{\pi}_{jk}$ is obtained from the marginal proportions $\hat{\pi}_{jk} = n_{jk}/(n_1 + n_2)$. As in Section 9.4, T_5 is asymptotically chi squared with 3 df.

The methods of Chapter 11 for polytomous logistic regression may also be applied. Indeed, the double-dichotomy response design was illustrated by the breathlessness and wheeze example of Section 11.4.1. Specifically, we can write

$$\ln \frac{P\{(Y_1, Y_2) = (j, k) | X = x\}}{P\{(Y_1, Y_2) = (0, 0) | X = x\}}$$

$$= \varphi^{(1)}(x) \cdot t^{(1)}(j, k) + \varphi^{(2)}(x) \cdot t^{(2)}(j, k) + \varphi^{(12)}(x) \cdot t^{(12)}(j, k),$$

where $t^{(1)}(j, k) = 1$ if and only if $j = 1$, $t^{(2)}(j, k) = 1$ if and only if $k = 1$, and $t^{(12)}(j, k) = t^{(1)}(j, k)t^{(2)}(j, k)$, and where

$$\varphi^{(1)}(x) = \beta_0^{(1)} + \beta_1^{(1)}x,$$

$$\varphi^{(2)}(x) = \beta_0^{(2)} + \beta_1^{(2)}x,$$

and

$$\varphi^{(12)}(x) = \beta_0^{(12)} + \beta_1^{(12)}x,$$

Hypothesis H_5 is equivalent to H_5: $\beta_1^{(1)} = \beta_1^{(2)} = \beta_1^{(12)} = 0$. Other hypotheses about specific parameters may be tested as well.

We use data from the Northern Manhattan Stroke Study (NOMASS) to illustrate analyses of $2 \times 2 \times 2$ tables with correlated outcomes. As discussed

Table 15.6. *Functional status by stroke mechanism at time of stroke (time 1) and two years later (time 2) from NOMASS*

Stroke Mechanism $(=X)$	Time 1 Functional Status $(=Y_1)$			Time 2 Functional Status $(=Y_2)$		
	Normal	Impaired	Total	Normal	Impaired	Total
IATH	5	20	25	17	8	25
Other	26	205	231	106	125	231
Total	31	225	256	123	133	256

in Section 14.4 and in Sacco et al. (1998) and Paik, Sacco, and Lin (2000), NOMASS was designed to identify determinants of stroke and stroke outcomes in an urban population of white, black, and Hispanic residents of northern Manhattan. One of the research questions is whether or not the stroke mechanism (X) of intracranial atherosclerosis (IATH) versus other stroke mechanisms affects functional status (Y) at the time of stroke (time 1) and two years later (time 2). The data analyzed here (Table 15.6) are from a subset of patients whose functional outcomes are observed at both time points. A larger data set with other covariate information is analyzed in Section 15.5.

To test H_{01}, that the IATH group and non-IATH group have the same functional status (at each time point), we compute $p_{11} = 0.2$, $p_{12} = 0.68$, $p_{21} = 0.1126$, $p_{22} = 0.4589$. From (15.12), we compute $\hat{\rho}_1 = 0.3440$ and $\hat{\rho}_2 = 0.1943$, using $\Sigma_h Y_{h11} Y_{h12} = 5$ and $\Sigma_h Y_{h21} Y_{h22} = 19$ (see Table 15.7 below). If separate estimates for all terms in (15.10)–(15.12) are used to estimate Σ_1 in (15.10), we find

$$\hat{\Sigma}_1 = \begin{pmatrix} 0.006832 & 0.002692 \\ 0.002692 & 0.009779 \end{pmatrix}.$$

Then

$$T_1 = (0.2 - 0.1126, 0.68 - 0.4589)$$

$$\times \begin{pmatrix} 0.006832 & 0.002692 \\ 0.002692 & 0.009779 \end{pmatrix}^{-1} \begin{pmatrix} 0.2 - 0.1126 \\ 0.68 - 0.4589 \end{pmatrix} = 5.116.$$

Under the null hypothesis, however, the pooled proportion $p_{+1} = 31/256 = 0.1211$ can be used instead of P_{11} and P_{21} in (15.10) and instead of p_{11} and p_{21} in (15.11); and $p_{+2} = 123/256 = 0.4805$ can be used instead of P_{12} and

P_{22} in (15.10) and instead of p_{12} and p_{22} in (15.11). Then

$$\hat{\Sigma}_1 = \begin{pmatrix} 0.004718 & 0.002373 \\ 0.002373 & 0.011065 \end{pmatrix}$$

and $T_1 = 4.7994$. If one were to treat $\hat{\rho}_1$ and $\hat{\rho}_2$ as equal and use (15.13) to estimate the common value ρ, the estimate is $\hat{\rho} = 0.2182$,

$$\hat{\Sigma}_1 = \begin{pmatrix} 0.004718 & 0.001577 \\ 0.001577 & 0.011065 \end{pmatrix},$$

and $T_1 = 5.115$, very close to the value with all terms estimated separately. In none of these instances do we reject H_{01} at the 0.05 level for chi squared on 2 df.

Next, we test H_{02}, that the rates of functional impairment at the two time points are the same (for the IATH and non-IATH groups). Now

$$\hat{\Sigma}_2 = \begin{pmatrix} 0.01185 & 0 \\ 0 & 0.00121 \end{pmatrix}$$

and

$$T_2 = (0.2 - 0.68, 0.1126 - 0.4589)$$

$$\times \begin{pmatrix} 0.01185 & 0 \\ 0 & 0.00121 \end{pmatrix}^{-1} \begin{pmatrix} 0.2 - 0.68 \\ 0.1126 - 0.4589 \end{pmatrix} = 118.6,$$

which is highly significant as a chi squared variate on 2 df.

To test the interaction hypothesis H_{03}, we calculate

$$\hat{\Sigma}_3 = (-1, 1) \begin{pmatrix} 0.01185 & 0 \\ 0 & 0.00121 \end{pmatrix} \begin{pmatrix} -1 \\ 1 \end{pmatrix} = 0.01306,$$

and $T_3 = 1.369$. We do not reject H_{03}, that there is no interaction between time and group membership.

Table 15.7. *Joint response frequencies at times 1 and 2 by stroke mechanism for the NOMASS data*

Stoke Mechanism	$(Y_1, Y_2) =$	(1, 1)	(1, 0)	(0, 1)	(0, 0)	Total
IATH		5	0	12	8	25
Other		19	7	87	118	231
Total		24	7	99	126	256

Table 15.8. *Notation for overdispersed response data (collapsing over time) by exposure in two strata*

		Observed Frequencies							
		Stratum 1					Stratum 2		
		Outcome					Outcome		
		1	0	Total			1	0	Total
Exposure	1	a_1	b_1	n_{11}		1	a_2	b_2	n_{12}
	0	c_1	d_1	n_{21}		0	c_2	d_2	n_{22}

		Observed Proportions							
		Stratum 1					Stratum 2		
		Outcome					Outcome		
		1	0	Total			1	0	Total
Exposure	1	p_{11}	q_{11}	1		1	p_{12}	q_{12}	1
	0	p_{21}	q_{21}	1		0	p_{22}	q_{22}	1

To test H_{05}, that the response profile is the same for the two groups, we require the joint frequencies in Table 15.7. The test statistic T_5 is

$$T_5 = \frac{\left(\frac{8}{25}\right) - \left(\frac{118}{231}\right)^2}{\frac{119}{256}\left(\frac{1}{25} + \frac{1}{231}\right)} + \frac{\left(\frac{12}{25} - \frac{87}{231}\right)^2}{\frac{99}{256}\left(\frac{1}{25} + \frac{1}{231}\right)} + \cdots + \frac{\left(\frac{5}{25} - \frac{19}{231}\right)^2}{\frac{24}{256}\left(\frac{1}{25} + \frac{1}{231}\right)} = 6.386.$$

Since T_5 is smaller than the critical value for chi squared on 3 df at the 0.05 level (7.81 from Table A.2), we do not reject H_5 ($p > 0.10$).

Overdispersed Cell Counts with Independent Rows and Tables

Suppose we wish to study the relation between functional impairment and stroke mechanism irrespective of time point, but stratifying the data by age at the time of stroke in two intervals. In each age group one subject contributes two data points, functional status at time one and time two. The data may be arranged as in Table 15.8. Unlike Table 15.4, the two fourfold tables in Table 15.8 contain different subjects, so the cell counts in different tables are independent. Moreover, the stroke type does not change over time and the two rows in each table contain different subjects, so the rows in each table are independent. However, the cell counts in a given row are *not* distributed as binomial random variables given the row margin, because the cells represent sums of correlated binary variables. The variances of the cell counts given the row margins have the form (15.1).

The observed proportions are $p_{11} = a_1/n_{11}$, $p_{11} = a_2/n_{12}$, $p_{11} = c_1/n_{21}$, and $p_{22} = c_2/n_{22}$, with underlying expected values $P_{ij} = E(p_{ij})$. Note that the row margins for each table are allowed to differ, i.e., $n_{11} \neq n_{12}$ and $n_{21} \neq n_{22}$. When cell counts are overdispersed, but rows and tables are statistically independent, the hypotheses H_{01}, H_{02}, and H_{03} are similar to those presented above, but the variance-covariance matrices Σ_1, Σ_2, and Σ_3 are different. We denote the variance inflation factor defined in (15.2) for the ith row of the jth table by f_{ij}, such that

$$\text{Var}(p_{ij}) = \frac{P_{ij}Q_{ij}f_{ij}}{n_{ij}}.$$

Due to the independence between tables, $\text{Cov}(p_{11}, p_{12}) = \text{Cov}(p_{21}, p_{22}) = 0$, and the covariance term in Σ_1 disappears. Then, estimating the separate variance inflation factors $\hat{f}_{ij}$ as in (15.3) and (15.4), we obtain

$$T_1 = \frac{(p_{11} - p_{21})^2}{(\hat{f}_{11} p_{11} q_{11}/n_{11}) + (\hat{f}_{21} p_{21} q_{21}/n_{21})}$$

$$+ \frac{(p_{12} - p_{22})^2}{(\hat{f}_{12} p_{12} q_{12}/n_{12}) + (\hat{f}_{22} p_{22} q_{22}/n_{22})}, \qquad (15.20)$$

which is asymptotically chi squared with 2 df;

$$T_2 = \frac{(p_{11} - p_{12})^2}{(\hat{f}_{11} p_{11} q_{11}/n_{11}) + (\hat{f}_{12} p_{12} q_{12}/n_{12})}$$

$$+ \frac{(p_{21} - p_{22})^2}{(\hat{f}_{21} p_{21} q_{21}/n_{21}) + (\hat{f}_{22} p_{22} q_{22}/n_{22})} \qquad (15.21)$$

with 2 df; and

$$T_3 = \frac{\{(p_{11} - p_{12}) - (p_{21} - p_{22})\}^2}{(\hat{f}_{11} p_{11} q_{11}/n_{11}) + (\hat{f}_{12} p_{12} q_{12}/n_{12}) + (\hat{f}_{21} p_{21} q_{21}/n_{21}) + (\hat{f}_{22} p_{22} q_{22}/n_{22})}$$

$$(15.22)$$

with 1 df.

Table 15.9 presents the NOMASS data from Table 15.6 stratified by age. Note that in either table, a subject contributes two counts.

H_{01} specifies that for each age group, the proportions who exhibit normal functional status are the same with or without IATH. Because $n_i = n = 2$ for all subjects, we have $f_{11} = f_{12} = f_{21} = f_{22} = 1 + \hat{\rho} = 1.2182$. Then $T_1 = 5.5965$, which is not significant at the 0.05 level. For hypothesis H_{02}, we obtain $T_2 = 26.6189$, and conclude that functional status depends on age. For H_{03},

Table 15.9. *Functional status and stroke mechanism from NOMASS data,
collapsed over time and stratified by age at stroke > 70 years and ≤ 70 years*

| Stroke Mechanism | Age > 70 | | | Age ≤ 70 | | |
| | Functional Status | | | Functional Status | | |
	Normal	Impaired	Total	Normal	Impaired	Total
IATH	17	9	26	5	19	24
Other	78	120	198	54	210	264
Total	95	129	224	59	229	288

we fail to reject the hypothesis with $T_3 = 3.0948$, indicating no significant interaction between stroke mechanism and age group.

15.4.2. Inference for the Mantel-Haenszel Odds Ratio with Clustered Data

When several fourfold tables are statistically independent, we can estimate an assumed common odds ratio and test whether it equals one using the methods of Chapter 10. As mentioned at (10.53), the Mantel-Haenszel odds ratio $\hat{\omega}_{MH}$ at (10.52) satisfies the estimating equation

$$\sum_{j=1}^{g} \frac{a_j d_j - b_j c_j \omega}{N_j} = 0, \qquad (15.23)$$

where $N_j = a_j + b_j + c_j + d_j$, and g is the number of independent strata. The Mantel-Haenszel odds ratio does not require iterative computation. It is a consistent estimator for a fixed number of tables with large sample sizes per stratum or for a large number of strata with small sample sizes.

When the data in different tables are correlated, some adjustments are needed. One approach is to use the method of generalized estimating equations discussed in Section 15.5. An alternative approach is to use an adjusted Mantel-Haenszel odds ratio or test statistic. Fortunately, (10.52) is consistent even when data are correlated. This is true essentially because the estimating equation (15.23) is unbiased, that is, the left-hand side has zero expectation. The use of unbiased estimating equations is discussed further in Section 15.5. The only problem is that the variance of the logarithm of the Mantel-Haenszel odds ratio given at (10.58) is not correct for correlated data. Similarly, the numerator of the Mantel-Haenszel chi squared statistic can be used as is, but the variance term in the denominator needs to reflect the correlation between tables. Donald and Donner (1987) show that when exposure does not vary within the cluster, one may simply divide the Mantel-Haenszel chi squared statistic shown in (10.62) by the variance inflation factor f; the adjusted statistic then has a chi squared distribution with 1 df.

Alternative variance estimators have been proposed for the Mantel-Haenszel odds ratio. Donald and Donner (1987) consider the case of covariates that are constant within clusters, and suggest using the correction factor in Hauck's variance formula. Denoting the correction factor for the ith row and the jth table by f_{ij}, let

$$v_j^* = \frac{f_{1j}}{n_{1j}P_{1j}Q_{1j}} + \frac{f_{2j}}{n_{2j}P_{2j}Q_{2j}}. \tag{15.24}$$

Then with $g = 2$,

$$\mathrm{Var}(\hat{\omega}_{\mathrm{MH}}) = \frac{\omega^2 \Sigma_{j=1}^g w_j v_j^*}{\left(\Sigma_{j=1}^g w_j\right)^2}, \tag{15.25}$$

where $w_j = P_{2j}Q_{2j}/(n_{1j}^{-1} + n_{2j}^{-1})$. Liang (1985) proposed an empirical variance estimator which is useful when the number of strata is large:

$$\widehat{\mathrm{Var}}(\hat{\omega}_{\mathrm{MH}}) = \frac{\sum_{j=1}^g \left(\dfrac{a_j d_j}{N_j} - \hat{\omega}_{\mathrm{MH}} \dfrac{b_j c_j}{N_j} \right)^2}{\left(\sum_{j=1}^g \dfrac{b_j c_j}{N_j} \right)^2}. \tag{15.26}$$

Zhang and Boos (1997) proposed two modified statistics using another unbiased empirical variance estimator. An extension of the variance formula given in Robins, Breslow, and Greenland (1986) and Phillips and Holland (1987) is not straightforward and is not yet available. Rao and Scott (1992) and Donner and Hauck (1988) proposed modified Mantel-Haenszel odds ratios using new weights which include corrections for correlation.

The above-mentioned adjustments are limited to the case in which exposure is constant within clusters and when tables and table rows are independent. Begg (1999) proposed an adjustment for the Mantel-Haenszel chi squared statistic, and Begg and Panageas (1999) proposed an adjustment for the variance of the Mantel-Haenszel odds ratio, which are applicable when exposure is constant within clusters or varies across subunits within clusters, or when tables are dependent as in Table 15.4.

An alternative way to obtain a consistent variance estimate is to use the jackknife technique: delete independent units one at a time and estimate the variance from the sum of squared differences of the delete-one estimates from the full estimate. The same technique is applied at (15.40) below for GEE estimates.

Using the data in Table 15.9, were we to ignore the fact that the cell counts are clustered, we would obtain $\hat{\omega}_{\mathrm{MH}} = 1.9044$, and $\widehat{\mathrm{se}}(\hat{\omega}_{\mathrm{MH}}) = 0.6596$.

The Mantel-Haenszel chi squared statistic without continuity correction is 3.9722, which would be significant at the 0.05 level. Taking the clustering into account, $\hat{\omega}_{MH}$ remains the same, but the standard error using (15.25) is 0.7279, and the variance-inflation-adjusted Mantel-Haenszel chi squared statistic is 3.2607. This fails to reach significance at the 0.05 level, and we do not reject the hypothesis of no association.

15.5.* EXTENSIONS OF LOGISTIC REGRESSION FOR CORRELATED OUTCOMES

In this section we consider certain extensions of the logistic regression model to accommodate correlation among binary outcomes. These modifications vary depending on the study aims and analytic assumptions. The discussion is intended for the more advanced reader. The main focus is on generalized estimating equations in Section 15.5.1 and random effects models in Section 15.5.2. Other techniques are touched on briefly, such as summarization by individual or time in Section 15.5.3, Markov models in Section 15.5.4, and multivariate binary distributions in Section 15.5.5.

As before, let Y_{ij} be a binary outcome for the jth subunit of the ith independent unit, where $i = 1, \ldots, K$ and $j = 1, \ldots, n_i$. Let $Y_i = (Y_{i1}, Y_{i2}, \ldots, Y_{in_i})'$ denote the ith independent vector of binary responses, and let X_{ij} be a vector of covariates of length p, which includes the intercept constant. We collect the n_i vectors into the $p \times n_i$ matrix $X_i = [X_{i1}| \cdots |X_{in_i}]$.

15.5.1. Generalized Estimating Equations

Suppose the marginal probability of a positive outcome is of primary interest. "Marginal" is used in the sense that the probability is not conditional on the outcomes at previous time points, although it is conditional on X—the probabilities throughout this section are all conditional on X. We denote the marginal probability by $P_{ij} = P_{ij}(X_{ij}) = P(Y_{ij} = 1|X_{ij})$, and assume that the logit of P_{ij} is linear in X, i.e.,

$$\ln \frac{P(Y_{ij} = 1|X_{ij})}{P(Y_{ij} = 0|X_{ij})} = \ln \frac{P(X_{ij})}{1 - P(X_{ij})} = \beta' X_{ij}. \tag{15.27}$$

Estimating Equations
An equation which yields an estimator as a solution is called an *estimating equation*, and the function equated to zero is called an *estimating function*. The quasiscore function introduced in Section 12.3 is an example of an estimating function, as is the left-hand side of (15.23). Suppose we fit the logistic regression model (15.27) as if all the Y_{ij}'s were independent. Because the specified likelihood function is generally not the correct likelihood

function when the Y_{ij}'s are correlated, the equation solved to obtain the estimate is not the correct score equation, but rather an estimating equation. Although the solution of the estimating equation is not the maximum likelihood estimate, it turns out nevertheless to be *consistent*, i.e., the estimator converges to the true parameter value in probability as K becomes large, primarily because the estimating function, like the correct score function, has zero expectation. We say that an estimating equation is *unbiased* if the corresponding estimating function has zero expectation for any true value of the parameters. A well-known estimating equation for continuous data is the set of normal equations whose solution gives ordinary least-squares estimates, which are consistent estimators even when the error terms are not normal, due mainly to unbiasedness of the normal equations. While the parameter estimates from an unbiased estimating equation are consistent, the standard errors computed as if all Y_{ij}'s were independent are incorrect, and so are the associated p-values and confidence intervals; so, much of the effort in this subject is devoted to proper evaluation of the standard errors of the estimates.

Liang and Zeger (1986) and Zeger and Liang (1986) proposed the method of generalized estimating equations (GEEs) as an extension of generalized linear models (McCullagh and Nelder, 1989) for correlated outcomes. The key idea of GEEs in such applications is to use an unbiased estimating equation. GEE models for correlated binary outcomes are described next.

GEEs for Multivariate Binary Data

Let $E(Y_i) = P_i$, where $P_i = (P_{i1}, \ldots, P_{in_i})'$. Since Y_{ij} is binary, $\mathrm{Var}(Y_{ij}) = P_{ij}(1 - P_{ij})$. Next, assume the variance-covariance matrix of Y_i is

$$V_i = V_i\left(\alpha, \beta | X_{i1}, \ldots, X_{in_i}\right) = A_i(P_i)^{1/2} R_i(\alpha) A_i(P_i)^{1/2}, \quad (15.28)$$

where A_i is an $n_i \times n_i$ diagonal matrix with jth diagonal element $P_{ij}(1 - P_{ij})$ and $R_i(\alpha)$ is a correlation matrix that may depend upon an additional parameter α. When $\alpha = 0$, we take $R_i(0)$ as the identity matrix. If α is known, an estimate of β, say $\hat{\beta}$, can be obtained by solving the estimating equation

$$U(\beta, \alpha) = \sum_{i=1}^{K} \frac{\partial P_i'}{\partial \beta} V_i^{-1}(Y_i - P_i) = 0. \quad (15.29)$$

In the present case of a binary outcome with logistic link function, if $\alpha = 0$, $\partial P_i' / \partial \beta = X_i A_i$ and the estimating function $U(\beta, \alpha)$ is equal to the score function $\sum_i X_i(Y_i - P_i) = \sum_i \sum_j X_{ij}(Y_{ij} - P_{ij})$ from logistic regression (see Section 11.4.3). If the Y_{ij}'s were indeed independent, $U(\beta, 0)$ would be the correct score function, that is, the derivative of the log likelihood given by the product of Bernoulli distributions. The main distinction between a score function and an estimating function is that the score function derives from the likelihood function while an estimating function, constructed *ab initio*, is not necessarily derived from a target function to be maximized. Both have zero expectation.

Such unbiased estimating equations are key to proving the consistency and asymptotic normality of $\hat{\beta}$. To see why heuristically, first note that $U(\hat{\beta}, \alpha) = 0$ so, by a Taylor expansion about the true value β^* of β,

$$0 = U(\hat{\beta}, \alpha) = U(\beta^*, \alpha) + \frac{\partial U(\beta'', \alpha)}{\partial \beta'}(\hat{\beta} - \beta^*),$$

where the matrix $\partial U / \partial \beta'$ is evaluated at β'' satisfying $|\beta'' - \hat{\beta}| < |\beta^* - \hat{\beta}|$. This leads to

$$\hat{\beta} - \beta^* = \left(-\frac{\partial U(\beta'', \alpha)}{\partial \beta'}\right)^{-1} U(\beta^*, \alpha).$$

Since $U(\beta^*, \alpha)$ is a sum of random vectors with mean zero and finite variance, it is of order $\sqrt{K}$ in probability, while $-(\partial U / \partial \beta')(\beta'', \alpha)$ is a sum of positive terms, and is thus of order K. Therefore $\hat{\beta}$ converges in probability to β^* as K becomes large, that is, $\hat{\beta}$ is consistent.

Now let $W_0(\beta, \alpha) = E\{(-\partial U / \partial \beta')(\beta, \alpha)\}$. We use W rather than I to distinguish the expected value of $-\partial U / \partial \beta'$ from the Fisher information matrix $I(\beta)$, which, under independence, equals $I(\beta) = W_0(\beta, 0) = \sum_i X_i V_i X_i' = \sum_i \sum_j P_{ij} Q_{ij} X_{ij} X_{ij}'$. Then we have

$$W_0(\beta, \alpha) = \sum_{i=1}^{K} \frac{\partial P_i'}{\partial \beta} V_i^{-1} \frac{\partial P_i}{\partial \beta'}. \tag{15.30}$$

It can be shown that $-(\partial U / \partial \beta')(\beta'', \alpha)$ converges to $W_0(\beta^*, \alpha)$, from which it follows that $\hat{\beta} - \beta^*$ has the same asymptotic distribution as $W_0(\beta^*, \alpha)^{-1} U(\beta^*, \alpha)$, which we denote by

$$\hat{\beta} - \beta^* \approx W_0(\beta^*, \alpha)^{-1} U(\beta^*, \alpha). \tag{15.31}$$

The central limit theorem implies that $U(\beta^*, \alpha)$ is asymptotically multivariate normal, and (15.31) shows that $\hat{\beta} - \beta^*$ is also asymptotically multivariate normal. A similar argument was used for the quasilikelihood method in Section 12.3.

Liang and Zeger (1986) called $R_i(\alpha)$ a "working correlation" matrix to reflect the fact that $R_i(\alpha)$ does not actually have to be the true correlation matrix of Y_i. With that in mind, the true variance of $U(\beta^*, \alpha)$, call it

$W_1(\beta^*, \alpha)$, is

$$W_1(\beta^*, \alpha) = \text{Var}\left\{ \sum_{i=1}^{K} \frac{\partial P_i'}{\partial \beta} V_i^{-1}(Y_i - P_i) \right\}$$

$$= E\left\{ \sum_{i=1}^{K} \frac{\partial P_i'}{\partial \beta} V_i^{-1}(Y_i - P_i)(Y_i - P_i)'V_i^{-1} \frac{\partial P_i}{\partial \beta'} \right\}.$$

If $R_i(\alpha)$ is correctly specified, $E(Y_i - P_i)(Y_i - P_i)' = V_i$, and the right-hand side becomes

$$E\left\{ \sum_{i=1}^{K} \frac{\partial P_i'}{\partial \beta} V_i^{-1}(Y_i - P_i)(Y_i - P_i)'V_i^{-1} \frac{\partial P_i}{\partial \beta'} \right\} = \sum_{i=1}^{K} \frac{\partial P_i'}{\partial \beta} V_i^{-1} \frac{\partial P_i}{\partial \beta'},$$

resulting in $W_1 = W_0$. Even when $R_i(\alpha)$ is misspecified, however, the variance of $U(\beta^*, \alpha)$ can be consistently estimated by

$$\hat{W}_1 = \sum_{i=1}^{K} \frac{\partial P_i'}{\partial \beta} V_i^{-1}(Y_i - P_i)(Y_i - P_i)'V_i^{-1} \frac{\partial P_i}{\partial \beta'}, \qquad (15.32)$$

evaluated at α and $\beta = \hat{\beta}$. Using equation (15.31), we see that the variance of $\hat{\beta}$ is of the so-called *sandwich* form:

$$W_0^{-1} W_1 W_0^{-1}, \qquad (15.33)$$

which can be consistently estimated by $\hat{W}_0^{-1} \hat{W}_1 \hat{W}_0^{-1}$. This sandwich estimate enables us to draw correct inferences even when the correlation structure is misspecified. Misspecification of the correlation structure does not affect the consistency of $\hat{\beta}$ and its variance estimate, but it reduces statistical efficiency, resulting in larger standard errors and wider confidence intervals than would obtain with the correct specification. See below under "Efficiency."

Estimation of α

Since the consistency of $\hat{\beta}$ is unaffected by misspecification of R, we could specify R as the identity matrix, in which case solving $U(\beta, 0) = 0$ is equivalent to fitting an ordinary logistic regression. When $R(\alpha)$ is chosen as some other function of an unknown parameter α, we need to estimate α. Note that α is assumed common to all i. The correlation matrix may be different for different units, but should be completely determined by α. Liang and Zeger (1986) give several examples of correlation structures. A simple example is the intraclass correlation matrix,

$$
R_i(\alpha) = \begin{pmatrix}
1 & \alpha & \alpha & \cdots & \alpha \\
\alpha & 1 & \alpha & \cdots & \alpha \\
\alpha & \alpha & 1 & \cdots & \alpha \\
\vdots & \vdots & \vdots & \ddots & \vdots \\
\alpha & \alpha & \alpha & \cdots & 1
\end{pmatrix}
$$

In this case, an estimate of α is given by

$$
\hat{\alpha} = \frac{2 \displaystyle\sum_{i=1}^{K} \sum_{j>k} \frac{Y_{ij} - \hat{P}_{ij}}{\sqrt{\hat{P}_{ij}(1 - \hat{P}_{ij})}} \frac{Y_{ik} - \hat{P}_{ik}}{\sqrt{\hat{P}_{ik}(1 - \hat{P}_{ik})}}}{\displaystyle\sum_{i=1}^{K} n_i(n_i - 1)}. \tag{15.34}
$$

Another example is an autoregressive process of order 1 (AR-1), where the (j, k)th element of $R_i(\alpha)$ is $\alpha^{|j-k|}$:

$$
R_i(\alpha) = \begin{pmatrix}
1 & \alpha & \alpha^2 & \cdots & \alpha^{n_i-1} \\
\alpha & 1 & \alpha & \cdots & \alpha^{n_i-2} \\
\alpha^2 & \alpha & 1 & \cdots & \alpha^{n_i-3} \\
\vdots & \vdots & \vdots & \ddots & \vdots \\
\alpha^{n_i-1} & \alpha^{n_i-2} & \alpha^{n_i-3} & \cdots & 1
\end{pmatrix}.
$$

In this case, α can be estimated as a coefficient in a regression model where $(Y_{ij} - \hat{P}_{ij})/\sqrt{\hat{P}_{ij}(1 - \hat{P}_{ij})}$ is the dependent variable and $(Y_{i,j-1} - \hat{P}_{i,j-1})/\sqrt{\hat{P}_{i,j-1}(1 - \hat{P}_{i,j-1})}$ is the independent variable with intercept constrained to be zero.

Muñoz et al. (1992) proposed a flexible family of correlation structures in which the (j, k)th element of $R_i(\alpha)$ is $\alpha^{|j-k|^\delta}$. With the additional parameter δ, this family can express various types of correlation structure including AR-1 ($\delta = 1$) and intraclass correlation ($\delta = 0$).

When the number of subunits is the same for all units ($n_i = n$ for all i), if we assume that $R_i(\alpha) = R$ is constant, we can estimate all $n(n - 1)/2$ unknown parameters without specifying any particular structure as follows:

$$
\hat{R} = K^{-1} \sum_{i=1}^{K} \hat{A}_i^{-1/2} (Y_i - \hat{P}_i)(Y_i - \hat{P}_i)' \hat{A}_i^{-1/2}. \tag{15.35}
$$

We see that the estimation of α depends on β, and the estimation of β in turn depends on α. Each step can be iterated in alternating fashion until both parameters converge. For the asymptotic properties of $\hat{\beta}$ to hold, Liang and Zeger (1986) required the estimate of α to be $\sqrt{K}$-consistent. Under this assumption, the statistical uncertainty introduced by replacing α by $\hat{\alpha}$ is of a small order of magnitude that does not affect the asymptotic distribution of $\hat{\beta}$.

Inference

In likelihood-based inference, we can draw inferences from any of three types of test statistic: the Wald test, score test, or likelihood ratio test. The Wald test is based on the asymptotic normality of maximum likelihood estimators. The score test is based on the asymptotic normality of the score function evaluated at the null-hypothesis value of the parameters of interest, with restricted maximum likelihood estimates (mle's) used for nuisance parameters. The likelihood ratio test is based on the asymptotic chi squared distribution of twice the difference of the log likelihood functions evaluated at corresponding mle's for two nested models. Since the GEE estimator is not derived from a likelihood function, these three test statistics do not exist *per se*. However, analogous test statistics can be constructed which are called Wald-type, score-type, or likelihood-ratio-type statistics. Consider a partition of the entire parameter, $\beta = (\beta_1', \beta_2')'$, where β_1 is the parameter of interest of length q, and β_2 is a nuisance parameter of length $p - q$. Suppose we are interested in testing the hypothesis $H_0: \beta_1 = \beta_{10}$.

Wald-Type Statistics

A Wald-type statistic can be formed by

$$T_W = \left(\hat{\beta}_1 - \beta_{10} \right)' \widehat{\mathrm{Var}}\left(\hat{\beta}_1 \right)^{-1} \left(\hat{\beta}_1 - \beta_{10} \right), \qquad (15.36)$$

where $\hat{\beta}_1$ is a $q \times 1$ subvector of the GEE estimate $\hat{\beta}$, and $\widehat{\mathrm{Var}}(\hat{\beta}_1)$ is the corresponding estimated $q \times q$ submatrix of the sandwich variance $W_0^{-1} W_1 W_0^{-1}$ at (15.33). The test statistic is asymptotically chi squared with q df.

To illustrate, consider hypothesis H_{04} given in Section 15.4.1 to test for interaction between group and time. First, we can set up a marginal logistic regression model

$$\ln \frac{P\left(Y_{ij} = 1 | X_i, T_j \right)}{P\left(Y_{ij} = 0 | X_i, T_j \right)} = \gamma_0 + \gamma_1 X_i + \gamma_2 T_j + \gamma_3 X_i T_j,$$

where X_i is the group membership indicator for the ith subject and T_j is an indicator for time point 2. H_{04} is equivalent to the hypothesis that $\gamma_3 = 0$. Here $(\gamma_0, \gamma_1, \gamma_2)$ are nuisance parameters. The Wald-type test statistic is

$T_W = \hat{\gamma}_3^2 / \widehat{\mathrm{Var}}(\hat{\gamma}_3)$, where $\hat{\gamma}_3$ is the GEE estimator and $\widehat{\mathrm{Var}}(\hat{\gamma}_3)$ is the (4,4) element of the sandwich variance estimate.

Score-Type Statistics

Lefkopoulou, Moore, and Ryan (1989) examined score-type statistics for GEE inferences under the independent working correlation structure, $R = I$. These statistics can be constructed in the same way for general $R(\alpha)$ structures. One partitions the estimating function $U(\beta, \alpha) = (U_1(\beta_1, \beta_2, \alpha)',$ $U_2(\beta_1, \beta_2, \alpha)')'$ where $U_1(\beta_1, \beta_2, \alpha)$ is a q-variate subvector of the estimating function $U(\beta, \alpha)$ corresponding to β_1. The score-type statistic is then

$$T_S = U_1\big(\beta_{10}, \hat{\beta}_2(\beta_{10}), \alpha\big)' \widehat{\mathrm{Var}}\big\{U_1\big(\beta_{10}, \hat{\beta}_2(\beta_{10}), \alpha\big)\big\}^{-1}$$
$$\times U_1\big(\beta_{10}, \hat{\beta}_2(\beta_{10}), \alpha\big), \tag{15.37}$$

where $\hat{\beta}_2(\beta_{10})$ is the solution of $U(\beta_{10}, \beta_2, \alpha) = 0$, i.e., the GEE estimate of β_2 under the restriction $\beta_1 = \beta_{10}$. Consider a similar partition for the matrices W_0 and W_1:

$$W_0 = E \begin{pmatrix} -\dfrac{\partial U_1}{\partial \beta_1'} & -\dfrac{\partial U_1}{\partial \beta_2'} \\[2mm] -\dfrac{\partial U_2}{\partial \beta_1'} & -\dfrac{\partial U_2}{\partial \beta_2'} \end{pmatrix} = \begin{pmatrix} D_{11} & D_{12} \\ D_{21} & D_{22} \end{pmatrix}, \quad \text{say,}$$

and

$$W_1 = \begin{pmatrix} M_{11} & M_{12} \\ M_{21} & M_{22} \end{pmatrix},$$

where by symmetry $D_{21} = D_{12}$ and $M_{21} = M_{12}$. To obtain the variance of $U_1(\beta_{10}, \hat{\beta}_2(\beta_{10}), \alpha)$, we consider the following Taylor approximation:

$$U_1\big(\beta_{10}, \hat{\beta}_2(\beta_{10}), \alpha\big) \approx U_1\big(\beta_{10}, \beta_2, \alpha\big) + \frac{\partial U_1(\beta_{10}, \beta_2, \alpha)}{\partial \beta_2}\big\{\hat{\beta}_2(\beta_{10}) - \beta_2\big\}$$
$$\approx U_1\big(\beta_{10}, \beta_2, \alpha\big) - D_{12}D_{22}^{-1}U_2\big(\beta_{10}, \beta_2, \alpha\big). \tag{15.38}$$

The second approximate equality holds because $\hat{\beta}_2(\beta_{10}) - \beta_2 \approx$ $D_{22}^{-1}U_2(\beta_{10}, \beta_2, \alpha)$, just as was derived at (15.31) for the entire parameter vector. Then from (15.38),

$$\mathrm{Var}\big\{U\big(\beta_{10}, \hat{\beta}_2(\beta_{10}), \alpha\big)\big\} = M_{11} + D_{12}D_{22}^{-1}M_{22}D_{22}^{-1}D_{21} - 2D_{12}D_{22}^{-1}M_{21}.$$
$$\tag{15.39}$$

Expression (15.38) is analogous to the profile score function in the theory of maximum likelihood. It can be thought of as analogous to a residual from the projection of $U_1(\beta_{10}, \beta_2, \alpha)$ onto the space spanned by $U_2(\beta_{10}, \beta_2, \alpha)$. When $R = I$, the right-hand side of (15.38) is uncorrelated with $U_2(\beta_{10}, \beta_2, \alpha)$, but not otherwise.

The test statistic T_S has an asymptotic chi squared distribution with q df. Replacing α by $\hat{\alpha}$, the estimate of α under the null, does not affect the asymptotic distribution of the test statistic. One drawback is that the computation of the score statistic requires a specialized program.

Likelihood-Ratio-Type Statistics
When the Y_{ij}'s are independent, the log-likelihood function is

$$L(\beta|Y) = \sum_{i=1}^{K} \left[\sum_{j=1}^{n_i} Y_{ij} \ln \frac{P_{ij}}{1 - P_{ij}} - (1 - Y_{ij}) \ln(1 - P_{ij}) \right],$$

and the log-likelihood ratio statistic for testing $\beta_1 = \beta_{10}$ in the presence of the nuisance parameter β_2 is

$$T_L = 2\left[L(\hat{\beta}_1, \hat{\beta}_2) - L\{\beta_{10}, \hat{\beta}_2(\beta_{10})\} \right],$$

where $\hat{\beta}_2(\beta_{10})$ is the maximizer of L under the restriction $\beta_1 = \beta_{10}$.

In GEEs, one does not start with an explicit likelihood function. Instead, Rotnitzky and Jewell (1990) consider the distribution of T_L when the Y_{ij}'s are correlated. They show that T_L can be expressed as a weighted sum of independent chi squared variables with 1 df. Suppose we write

$$T_L \approx \sum_{j=1}^{q} d_j \chi_j^2,$$

where $\chi_1^2, \ldots, \chi_q^2$ are q independent chi squared random variables with 1 df. The weights $d_1 \geq d_2 \geq \cdots \geq d_q$ are eigenvalues of $D_{11.2}^{-1} V_1$, where

$$D_{11.2} = D_{11} - D_{12} D_{22}^{-1} D_{21},$$

$$V_1 = M_{11} + D_{12} D_{22}^{-1} M_{22} D_{22}^{-1} D_{21} - 2 D_{12} D_{22}^{-1} M_{21},$$

and all submatrices of D and M in $D_{11.2}$ and V_1 are evaluated at $\alpha = 0$. When there are no nuisance parameters, $D_{11.2} = W_0$ and $V_1 = W_1$.

Rotnitzky and Jewell (1990) also derive the distributions of the naive Wald and score tests formed as if all observations were independent. Those statistics are asymptotically equivalent to T_L.

Computation

GEE estimates under the independent working correlation structure can be obtained using any software that fits logistic regression models. The coefficient standard errors reported by the software are the square roots of the diagonal elements of $\hat{W}_0^{-1}$, so to compute the correct values we need to calculate $\hat{W}_1$ as well. Some programs have a routine to fit GEE and report the sandwich variance. SAS® (PROC GENMOD), Stata® (XTGEE), and SUDAAN® (PROC MULTILOG) are among the commercially available programs that have these features.

The sandwich variance estimate can also be estimated by the *jackknife* method. Let $\hat{\beta}_{-i}$ be the GEE estimate obtained after deleting the ith independent unit or cluster. The jackknife variance

$$V_J = \sum_{i=1}^{K} \left(\hat{\beta}_{-i} - \hat{\beta} \right)\left(\hat{\beta}_{-i} - \hat{\beta} \right)' \tag{15.40}$$

consistently estimates the sandwich variance $W_0^{-1}W_1W_0^{-1}$. Use of the jackknife variance to estimate the sandwich variance is discussed in Paik (1988), Ziegler (1997), and Lipsitz, Dear, and Zhao (1994).

Efficiency

When the correlation structure is correctly specified, the variance of $\hat{\beta}$ is the inverse of W_0^*, where the asterisk indicates that the correlation matrix R is correctly specified. Otherwise the variance of $\hat{\beta}$ is $W_0^{-1}W_1W_0^{-1}$. By applying the maximization lemma of quadratic forms (see Problem 15.8), we find that the asymptotic relative efficiency (ARE) of a linear combination of $\hat{\beta}$ lies between the largest and smallest eigenvalues of $W_0^{-1}W_1W_0^{-1}W_0^*$. When the dimension of β is 1, the ARE of the estimator with misspecified correlation structure is exactly $W_0^{-1}W_1W_0^{-1}W_0^*$. Rotnitzky and Jewell (1990) provide the upper and lower bounds for efficiency under special correlation structures. The efficiency of GEE estimators in the case of misspecified $R(\alpha)$ is examined analytically by Mancl and Leroux (1996) and by simulation in Paik (1988) and Park (1993).

Extensions of GEEs

Extensions of GEEs have been studied by several authors. Prentice (1988) considers modeling not only the mean as a function of the covariates as in the original GEE method, but also correlation as a function of the covariates. The estimating equation for the correlation is stacked with the original GEEs for β to form a joint estimating equation. Paik (1992) considers joint modeling of mean and scale parameters. Liang, Zeger, and Qaqish (1992) modeled the mean together with the odds ratio between repeated binary outcomes instead of the correlation.

Caution in Using GEEs

Because the asymptotic properties of GEE estimators and test statistics depend on large K and fixed n_i, studies with large n_i or small K are not suited to GEE analysis. Even when K is large with fixed n_i, difficulties may arise. Most of these are related to specification of the working correlation structure. For some working correlation structures, such as m-dependence, there is a range of α that yields a non-positive-definite correlation matrix. Users should make sure the estimated correlation matrix is positive definite. A more fundamental problem is the potential ambiguity of the estimated working correlation coefficient. The difficulty is that when α is not a true correlation, but merely a working correlation, it is sometimes unclear what $\hat{\alpha}$ is estimating. As previously noted, one of the assumptions used to derive consistency and asymptotic normality of $\hat{\beta}$ is that the estimate of α is $\sqrt{K}$-consistent. Crowder (1995) examines this issue and cautions that in some cases misspecification of $R(\alpha)$ may lead to a breakdown of the asymptotic properties of $\hat{\beta}$.

For these reasons, it is good practice to fit the independent-working-correlation model and examine the empirical correlations before fitting more complicated working correlation structures. Noticeable differences in results should stimulate further checking.

Another important issue is missing data. GEE naturally handles varying numbers of subunits per independent unit, so when varying numbers occur due to dropout in a longitudinal study, there is no obstacle to fitting a GEE model. However, the results of the analysis are valid only when such dropout occurs completely at random. (See Chapter 16 for a full discussion of missing-data methods and terminology.) If the probability of dropout or other kinds of missingness depends on the observed data (missing at random but not completely at random), or on the unobserved value of Y_{ij} (*nonignorably* missing), GEE estimates are not consistent. To address this problem, Robins, Rotnitzky, and Zhao (1995) propose a weighted form of GEE in which each observation is weighted by the reciprocal of an estimate of the probability of observation. Paik (1997) proposes an imputed form of GEE in which missing outcomes are replaced with estimates of their conditional expectation given the observed data. Fitzmaurice, Molenberghs, and Lipsitz (1995) examine the bias in GEE estimates when the missingness mechanism is nonignorable. Xie and Paik (1997a, 1997b) propose an imputation approach when covariates are missing. Ziegler, Kastner, and Blettner (1998) give an extensive annotated bibliography on GEEs.

Example 15.5.1. NOMASS Functional Outcome Data. We return to the Northern Manhattan Stroke Study (NOMASS) to illustrate the use of GEE methods. The research goal considered here is to estimate the effect of the stroke mechanism and associated syndromes on functional status at baseline (prior to the stroke) and two years later, adjusting for other known stroke risk factors.

Table 15.10. *GEE estimates and standard errors for a logistic regression model of functional outcomes from NOMASS data*

	Independent Working Correlation			Intraclass Working Correlation		
	Estimate	SE	p-Value	Estimate	SE	p-Value
Intercept	−5.9866	1.0904	< 0.0001	−6.0456	1.0794	< 0.0001
IATH	0.8801	0.5421	0.1045	0.8553	0.5496	0.1196
LHS	1.0818	0.4128	0.0088	1.0770	0.4153	0.0095
Time	2.9040	0.6819	< 0.0001	2.9107	0.6930	< 0.0001
IATH × time	0.1621	0.6346	0.7984	0.2117	0.6291	0.7364
LHS × time	0.3619	0.5106	0.4784	0.3603	0.5091	0.4792
Age	0.0475	0.0114	< 0.0001	0.0480	0.0113	< 0.0001
Female	−0.5846	0.2399	0.0148	−0.5910	0.2412	0.0143
Education	−0.4383	0.2815	0.1195	−0.4333	0.2825	0.1250
Race	0.7592	0.5969	0.2034	0.7857	0.6026	0.1922
Race × time	−0.9137	0.6921	0.1868	−0.9193	0.7025	0.1907

Two hundred ninety-four patients who survived for two years after stroke were included in the analysis. Functional status is dichotomized as *impaired* ($Y = 1$) if the Barthel Activities of Daily Living (ADL) scale is less than 95, indicating any type of dependence in daily living. These outcomes were observed two years after stroke for 256 of the 294 patients. At baseline (before stroke), 35 of 294 were impaired; two years after stroke, 127 of 256 were impaired. Covariates of interest include (i) age (continuous), (ii) sex (female versus male), (iii) race (nonwhite versus white), (iv) education (at least high school versus less than high school), (v) large hemisphere syndromes (LHS) (present versus absent), and (vi) intracranial atherosclerosis (IATH) (present versus absent). For each binary covariate the second category in parentheses is designated as the reference group. LHS includes such stroke syndromes as unconsciousness, major paralysis, and aphasia. IATH is one of several mechanisms by which stroke occurs.

The results of two GEE models are shown in Table 15.10. Computations were carried out using SAS® (code given in Table 15.11). The left panel in Table 15.10 uses an independent working correlation structure. The results indicate that patients are still more likely to be functionally impaired two years after stroke than before the stroke. The risk of impairment increases with age and is higher for men. IATH and LHS increase the odds of functional impairment at baseline by factors of $e^{0.88} = 2.4$ and $e^{1.08} = 2.9$, respectively, adjusting for other factors. The effects of IATH and LHS were a little larger at time 2, but not significantly so.

The right-hand panel of Table 15.10, which uses an intraclass correlation structure, reveals coefficient estimates and standard errors only slightly different from those using the independent working correlation structure. This implies that there was little improvement in efficiency, ostensibly be-

Table 15.11. *SAS® code for the GEE analysis of Table 15.10*

```
/* independence correlation model */
title 'Model 1.1 -- GEE independence correlation model';
proc genmod data=stroke3;
class subj;
model y=iath large time iath*time large*time age sex edu
race race*time / dist=binomial link=logit type3;
repeated subject=subj / corr=ind corrw;
run;
/* intraclass correlation model */
title 'Model 1.2 -- GEE intraclass correlation model';
proc genmod data=stroke3;
class subj;
model y=iath large time iath*time large*time age sex edu
race race*time / dist=binomial link=logit;
repeated subject=subj / corr=exch corrw;
run;
```

cause the correlation between the two measurements was weak (intraclass correlation = 0.0965). Also note that, because there are only two time points under consideration, the AR-1 structure or any other correlation structure would be identical to the intraclass correlation structure and would yield identical results.

Example 15.5.2. Cognitive Function among Stroke Patients. The next example exhibits a somewhat larger influence of the working correlation structure on the coefficient standard errors. Tatemichi et al. (1992) studied cognitive function among 241 elderly stroke patients in a longitudinal design with six time points: 7–10 days after the stroke, again at 3 months, and then yearly for 4 years. The outcome of interest at each time point was whether or not the subject had normal cognitive function, defined operationally as a score of 24 or higher on the 30-item Mini Mental State Examination (MMSE). The numbers of patients observed by time point were 241 (at 7–10 days), 237 (at 3 months), 183 (at year 1), 158 (at year 2), 98 (at year 3), and 35 (at year 4). As mentioned above, variable length of follow up is handled naturally by GEEs, but the validity of the results holds only when the dropout data are missing completely at random (MCAR). Here we use standard GEE under MCAR. Paik (1997) analyzes these data using an extended GEE method without this assumption, which almost certainly does not hold.

Let $Y_{it} = 1$ if the ith individual's MMSE score is above 24 at time t; otherwise $Y_{it} = 0$. We assume that if a patient is alive at time t, then

$$\text{logit}\{E(Y_{it})\} = \beta_0 + \sum_{k=1}^{5} \beta_k I(t = k + 1) + \beta_6 \, \text{Age}_i + \beta_7 \, \text{Edu}_i + \beta_8 \, \text{Sev}_i,$$

Table 15.12. *Coefficient estimates and their standard errors under various working correlation structures for cognitive function data*

Parameter	Independent Working Corr.			Intraclass Working Corr.		AR1 Working Corr.	
	Est.	Naive SE	SE	Est.	SE	Est	SE
Intercept	3.8034	0.6716	1.0901	3.1323	1.0538	3.4221	1.0483
Time2	0.4512	0.2134	0.1477	0.4465	0.1451	0.4428	0.1454
Time3	0.5737	0.2309	0.1823	0.6062	0.1714	0.6064	0.1714
Time4	0.5401	0.2395	0.1960	0.5374	0.1830	0.4977	0.1820
Time5	0.1583	0.2723	0.2297	0.1021	0.1962	0.1476	0.2099
Time6	0.0951	0.4049	0.3652	0.2427	0.2765	0.2826	0.3002
Age	−0.0706	0.0095	0.0155	−0.0619	0.0149	−0.0655	0.0148
Sev	−1.2442	0.1677	0.2782	−1.2502	0.2692	−1.2437	0.2675
Edu	0.1747	0.0192	0.0298	0.1792	0.0290	0.1754	0.0296

where Age_i denotes age of the ith patient at the time of entry, Edu_i denotes years of education, and Sev_i is a binary stroke severity indicator (1 = severe, 0 = not severe). The proportions of patients with normal cognitive function were observed to be 0.52, 0.61, 0.65, 0.66, 0.61, and 0.63 at 7–10 days, 3 months, and 1, 2, 3, and 4 years, respectively. Table 15.12 shows the coefficient estimates and their standard errors under independent, intraclass, and AR-1 working correlation structures.

The columns labeled "SE" report the sandwich estimator standard errors; the column labelled "Naive SE" reports the standard errors obtained by incorrectly assuming the repeated outcomes are independent when fitting the logistic regression model. We see that the standard errors for time-constant variables such as age, stroke severity, and education are understated. This is an extension to logistic regression of the variance inflation phenomenon we studied earlier. On the other hand, the standard errors are overstated for the time-varying variables, Time2 to Time6. As suggested by expression (15.6), when the covariates vary within a cluster, the variance of the estimate decreases on correctly taking the correlation into account. Also notice that under the assumption of the intraclass or AR-1 correlation structures, the standard errors of the estimates are slightly smaller than those under the independent correlation structure. This reflects how the estimation of β becomes more efficient as the working correlation approaches the true correlation structure.

When an intraclass correlation structure is assumed, the estimated correlation is $\hat{\alpha} = 0.5022$. With AR-1 structure, we obtain $\hat{\alpha} = 0.5549$ from the regression of lagged standardized residuals, with estimated working correlation matrix

1.0000	0.5549	0.3079	0.1708	0.0948	0.0526
0.5549	1.0000	0.5549	0.3079	0.1708	0.0948
0.3079	0.5549	1.0000	0.5549	0.3079	0.1708
0.1708	0.3079	0.5549	1.0000	0.5549	0.3079
0.0948	0.1708	0.3079	0.5549	1.0000	0.5549
0.0526	0.0948	0.1708	0.3079	0.5549	1.0000

If no correlation structure is assumed, the estimated empirical correlation matrix is

1.0000	0.5462	0.4024	0.4482	0.5177	0.5609
0.5462	1.0000	0.5419	0.4349	0.4742	0.4833
0.4024	0.5419	1.0000	0.5435	0.5502	0.5350
0.4482	0.4349	0.5435	1.0000	0.5524	0.7015
0.5177	0.4742	0.5502	0.5524	1.0000	0.8188
0.5609	0.4833	0.5350	0.7015	0.8188	1.0000

One should not rely heavily on this estimate, as there are too few measurements at later time points to estimate the correlations stably. Nevertheless, the empirical correlation matrix clearly suggests that the intraclass correlation structure describes the data better than the AR-1 structure.

Cognitive function improves after the initial damage of stroke, then appears to decline after 2 years, a phenomenon not seen in the unadjusted proportions. Older patients and those with more severe stroke had more cognitive impairment. Those with more years of education were more likely to have normal cognitive function.

15.5.2. Random Effects Models

Suppose that in any given cluster i there is a unit-specific factor, call it b_i, shared by each subunit, and that, conditional on the factor, the measurements Y_{ij} for $j = 1, \ldots, n_i$ are *conditionally independent*; that is, for any $j \neq k$,

$$P\left(Y_{ij} = 1 \mid Y_{ik} = 1, b_i\right) = P\left(Y_{ij} = 1 \mid Y_{ik} = 0, b_i\right) = P\left(Y_{ij} = 1 \mid b_i\right)$$

Even though the Y_{ij}'s are conditionally independent, variability in b_i from cluster to cluster induces an observable *marginal correlation*, such that $P(Y_{ij} = 1 \mid Y_{ik} = 1) \neq P(Y_{ij} = 1 \mid Y_{ik} = 0)$. The shared factor is called a *random effect*, and statistical models with such features are called *random effects models*. Consider, for example, a family study where the outcomes are binary indicators of some condition, such as malnutrition or obesity, for each family member. Suppose some families have a propensity to have the condition while others do not, and that, conditional on the propensity, each member does or does not have the condition as an independent event. Probabilistically, the situation is equivalent to the toss of a coin to determine outcomes for family members, but every family has its own coin with a different probability of heads. Under these circumstances, if a sample of families is selected and the binary outcomes from two members of each family cross-classified, the resulting fourfold table would show a marginal correlation between outcomes due to the shared propensity factor.

The random effects models considered in this section can be viewed as extensions of those in Section 9.6 to a regression setting. Given b_i, the response outcomes are assumed to be conditionally independent with

$$P(Y_{ij} = 1 | X_{ij}, b_i) = \frac{\exp(\beta_0 + \beta_1 X_{ij} + b_i)}{1 + \exp(\beta_0 + \beta_1 X_{ij} + b_i)}. \qquad (15.41)$$

The marginal covariance between Y_{ij} and Y_{ik} is positive because the conditional probabilities of Y_{ij} and Y_{ik} in (15.41) vary in the same way through their dependence on b_i; that is, they co-vary. Specifically,

$$
\begin{aligned}
&\text{Cov}(Y_{ij}, Y_{ik} | X_{ij}, X_{ik}) \\
&\quad = E\{\text{Cov}(Y_{ij}, Y_{ik} | X_{ij}, X_{ik}, b_i) | X_{ij}, X_{ik}\} \\
&\qquad + \text{Cov}\{E(Y_{ij} | X_{ij}, b_i), E(Y_{ik} | X_{ik}, b_i) | X_{ij}, X_{ik}\} \\
&\quad = 0 + \text{Cov}\{P(Y_{ij} = 1 | X_{ij}, b_i), P(Y_{ik} = 1 | X_{ik}, b_i) | X_{ij}, X_{ik}\} > 0. \quad (15.42)
\end{aligned}
$$

The reader is asked to show (Problem 15.5) that the last term in (15.42) is positive. Model (15.41) is also called a *subject-specific* model (Stiratelli, Laird, and Ware, 1984; Zeger, Liang, and Albert, 1988). Note that the interpretation of the parameter β_1 is different from that of the corresponding nonintercept terms β_1 of the coefficient β in the marginal model (15.27). The odds ratio parameter in (15.41) for a binary exposure X_{ij},

$$\exp(\beta_1) = \frac{P(Y_{ij} = 1 | X_{ij} = 1, b_i) / P(Y_{ij} = 0 | X_{ij} = 1, b_i)}{P(Y_{ij} = 1 | X_{ij} = 0, b_i) / P(Y_{ij} = 0 | X_{ij} = 0, b_i)},$$

applies within each cluster i, whereas $\exp(\beta_1)$ in (15.27) refers to the odds ratio constructed from the marginal probabilities in the population. In a family study, for example, with X_{ij} a smoking indicator and no other covariates, β_1 might represent the log odds ratio on lung disease for a smoking member compared to a nonsmoking member in the same family. In the marginal model, β_1 would be the log odds ratio on lung disease for smokers compared to nonsmokers in the population. Because conditioning on the family-specific factor b_i allows more control for confounding factors at the family level, β_1 from the random effects model is of direct interest in etiologic research.

There are two ways to draw inferences from a random effects model. One is to assume a distribution for b_i, obtain the marginal likelihood, and maximize it. The other is to find a sufficient statistic for b_i, condition on it, and maximize the conditional likelihood, which depends on β but not on b_i.

Marginal Likelihood
Let b_i be independent and identically distributed as $F(b_i)$. In parametric models, $F(b_i)$ is a known distribution with unknown parameters. The marginal probability becomes

$$P\left(Y_{ij} = 1 | X_{ij}\right) = \int P\left(Y_{ij} = 1 | X_{ij}, b_i\right) dF(b_i). \qquad (15.43)$$

Although the logistic regression model (15.41) is linear in X_{ij} and b_i, the marginal probability (15.43) generally is not of logit form. Suppose, for example, that b_i is distributed as a normal deviate with mean 0 and unknown variance σ^2. The marginal likelihood for cluster i is then

$$\int_{-\infty}^{\infty} \left\{ \prod_{j=1}^{n_i} P\left(Y_{ij} = 1 | X_{ij}, b_i\right)^{Y_{ij}} P\left(Y_{ij} = 0 | X_{ij}, b_i\right)^{1-Y_{ij}} \right\}$$
$$\times \frac{1}{\sqrt{2\pi\sigma^2}} \exp\left(-\frac{b_i^2}{2\sigma^2}\right) db_i,$$

and the full likelihood $L_M(\beta, \sigma^2)$ is a product of such factors for each independent unit i. This likelihood does not have a closed form, and maximizing L_M over (β, σ^2) involves numerical integration. Another drawback of this approach is that the random effect b_i is not directly observable, and distributional assumptions such as normality are difficult to verify and are often gratuitous. Nonparametric models which do not require specification of the parametric form of F are studied by Davidian and Gallant (1993).

Conditional Likelihood
When interest centers on the regression coefficient β_1 for X, but not on β_0 or on b_i, the conditional likelihood method eliminates the nuisance parameters altogether. First, the contribution of cluster i to the full likelihood given

b_i is

$$\prod_{j=1}^{n_i} P(Y_{ij} = 1|X_{ij}, b_i)^{Y_{ij}} P(Y_{ij} = 0|X_{ij}, b_i)^{1-Y_{ij}}$$

$$= \exp\left(\sum_{j=1}^{n_i} Y_{ij} \ln \frac{P(Y_{ij} = 1|X_{ij}, b_i)}{P(Y_{ij} = 0|X_{ij}, b_i)} + \ln P(Y_{ij} = 0|X_{ij}, b_i) \right)$$

$$= \exp\left(\sum_{j=1}^{n_i} Y_{ij}(\beta_0 + \beta_1 X_{ij} + b_i) - \ln\{1 + \exp(\beta_0 + \beta_1 X_{ij} + b_i)\} \right)$$

$$= \exp\left[(\beta_0 + b_i) \sum_{j=1}^{n_i} Y_{ij} + \beta_1 \sum_{j=1}^{n_i} X_{ij} Y_{ij} \right.$$

$$\left. - \sum_{j=1}^{n_i} \ln\{1 + \exp(\beta_0 + \beta_1 X_{ij} + b_i)\} \right]. \qquad (15.44)$$

Although $\sum_{j=1}^{n_i} Y_{ij}$ carries information about $\beta_0 + b_i$, it carries little information about β_1. Conditioning on $y_{i+} = \sum_{j=1}^{n_i} Y_{ij}$, the contribution to the conditional likelihood becomes

$$\frac{\prod_{j=1}^{n_i} P(Y_{ij} = 1|X_{ij}, b_i)^{Y_{ij}} P(Y_{ij} = 0|X_{ij}, b_i)^{1-Y_{ij}}}{\sum_{Y_i} \prod_{j=1}^{n_i} P(Y_{ij} = 1|X_{ij}, b_i)^{Y_{ij}} P(Y_{ij} = 0|X_{ij}, b_i)^{1-Y_{ij}}}, \qquad (15.45)$$

where the summation in the denominator is over all possible binary vectors $Y_i = (Y_{i1}, \ldots, Y_{in_i})$ that satisfy $Y_{i1} + \cdots + Y_{in_i} = y_{i+}$. Equation (15.45) simplifies dramatically with (15.44)—the resulting conditional likelihood function is

$$L_C(\beta_1) = \prod_{i=1}^{K} \frac{\exp\left(\beta_1 \sum_{j=1}^{n_i} X_{ij} Y_{ij} \right)}{\sum_{Y_i} \exp\left(\beta_1 \sum_{j=1}^{n_i} X_{ij} Y_{ij} \right)}. \qquad (15.46)$$

Conditional likelihood was used in Chapter 14 to analyze matched sample studies. In a longitudinal study with observations at times $t_{i1}, \ldots, t_{in_i}$, each subject provides a matched sample of outcomes $Y_{i1}, \ldots, Y_{in_i}$ with corresponding covariates $X_{i1}, \ldots, X_{in_i}$. Different outcomes associated with different levels of the covariates allow estimation of β_1. This method is especially effective in studying factors influencing change in structural growth models.

Table 15.13. *Maximum marginal likelihood estimates and standard errors from random effects model (15.41) for functional outcomes from NOMASS data*

Parameter	Estimate	Standard Error	p-Value
Intercept	−6.9007	1.3528	< 0.0001
IATH	0.9510	0.6326	0.1338
LHS	1.2806	0.5010	0.0111
Time	3.3849	0.8170	< 0.0001
IATH × time	0.3278	0.8236	0.6909
LHS × time	0.4061	0.6575	0.5373
Age	0.0545	0.0132	< 0.0001
Female	−0.6785	0.2928	0.0212
Education	−0.5183	0.3172	0.1034
Race	0.8479	0.6677	0.2051
Race × time	−1.0449	0.7757	0.1790
σ^2	1.0555	0.8132	0.1953

See Levin (1986) for an application to spontaneous abortion, whose risk increases with maternal age. Estimation of the parameters of a subject-specific growth curve model for the increase in risk is considered in the presence of substantial woman-to-woman heterogeneity in the risk of miscarriage (the random effect).

Note that β_0 and b_i are eliminated by conditioning, so this approach cannot be used for drawing inferences about them. A potential disadvantage of the conditional approach is that if $Y_{ij} = 1$ for all j, or $Y_{ij} = 0$ for all j, or if X_{ij} is constant within units, those units do not contribute to the likelihood, i.e., all data in those units are uninformative. If many units are uninformative, there is a loss of efficiency compared to the parametric marginal likelihood approach.

Table 15.13 shows the results of fitting the random effects model (15.41) to the NOMASS functional outcome data using maximum marginal likelihood, assuming one normally distributed random intercept and X_{ij} as in Table 15.10. SAS® code is given in Table 15.14.

As noted above, the interpretation of coefficients in the random effects model is quite different from that in the marginal model (15.27). For example, the coefficient of LHS is the change in log odds on functional impairment when a subject has LHS compared to when the same subject does not have LHS, one of which situations is counterfactual. Note also that each coefficient in Table 15.13 is larger than the corresponding coefficient in Table 15.10, albeit with larger standard errors. This is typical of subject-specific models compared to marginal models—for a subject-specific effect to persist when probabilities are averaged over many random units, it would typically need to be larger than the effect based on population averages. The estimate of σ^2, 1.05, indicates that 68% of all units have b_i ranging from

Table 15.14. *SAS*® *code for the random effects model using maximum marginal likelihood*

```
title 'Model 2 -- random effects model';
proc nlmixed data=stroke3;
/* define the parameters and their starting values */
parms b0=-4 biath=0.7 blarge=1 btime=2.5 biat=-0.1 blargt=0
bage=0 bsex=-0.5 bedu=-0.3 brace=0.1 bracet=-0.3 s2a=2;
/* define the linear predictor component */
xlinear=(b0+a)+biath*(iath)+blarge*(large)+btime*(time)
+biat*(iath*time)+ biargt*(large*time)+bage*(age)
+ bsex*(sex)+bedu*(edu)+ brace*(race)+bracet*(race*time);
expx=exp(xlinear);
p=expx=exp(xlinear);
model y ~ binary(p);
random a ~ normal (0,s2a) subject=subj;
run;
```

$-\sqrt{1.05}$ to $\sqrt{1.05}$. This means, for example, that the probabilities of functional impairment at time 2 for subjects who have the same risk factor profile as the reference group range between

$$\left(\frac{e^{-6.90+3.38-\sqrt{1.05}}}{1+e^{-6.90+3.38-\sqrt{1.05}}}, \frac{e^{-6.90+3.38+\sqrt{1.05}}}{1+e^{-6.90+3.38+\sqrt{1.05}}} \right) = (0.01, 0.08).$$

The conditional likelihood method does not estimate coefficients for the covariates that are constant in time, which are essentially matching factors. These include IATH, LHS, Age (at stroke), Female, Education, and Race. The time-dependent covariates, $X_3 =$ time, $X_4 =$ IATH $\times$ time, $X_5 =$ LHS $\times$ time, and $X_{11} =$ Race $\times$ time, can be estimated by conditional maximum likelihood. The model essentially becomes a regression model for the log odds ratio on impairment at time 2 versus time 1, as a function of IATH, LHS, and Race, as follows (we omit the data-analytic results for brevity):

$$\ln \frac{P(Y_{i2} = 1 | \text{IATH, LHS, Race}) / P(Y_{i2} = 0 | \text{IATH, LHS, Race})}{P(Y_{i1} = 1 | \text{IATH, LHS, Race}) / P(Y_{i1} = 0 | \text{IATH, LHS, Race})}$$

$$= \beta_4 + \beta_5 \text{ IATH} + \beta_6 \text{ LHS} + \beta_{11} \text{ Race}.$$

15.5.3. Summarizing by Individual or by Time

An analytic strategy to finesse the problem of high dimensionality of repeated measurements is to summarize the data in some way down to one or two dimensions. One way is to *summarize by individual.* In longitudinal studies, one can summarize the time course of measurements for each individual by an average, or by a slope and intercept. In periodontal research, an average can be taken at each site in the mouth. A strength of such a tactic, insofar as it can address the scientific questions of interest, is that the summary measures are independent. Of course, if scientific interest resides in responses at the subunit level, then this type of analysis is inappropriate. As for the random effects model, analyses summarizing by individual typically assume conditional independence of measurements within the same individual.

Alternatively, one can *summarize by time*. In this case subject data are independent at each time point, so an assumption of conditional independence given time is automatically satisfied. The summary measures for each time point are correlated, however, and must be taken into account when combining the summary measures.

Summarizing by Individual

Korn and Whittemore (1979) summarize repeated measurements by estimating individual regression coefficients for each subject. Their model, called a *random regression* model, is useful when the number of subunits is large, such as in diary studies (see, e.g., Neugebauer et al., 1994). Here we consider the simplest case of a single-sample study with a linear logistic regression model with random coefficients. Let X_{ij} denote the time of observation at the jth measurement for the ith subject. The model can be described in two stages. At the first stage, given individual regression coefficients (β_{0i}, β_{1i}), it is assumed that

$$P\left(Y_{ij} = 1 | X_{ij}, \beta_{0i}, \beta_{1i}\right) = \frac{\exp\left(\beta_{0i} + \beta_{1i}X_{ij}\right)}{1 + \exp\left(\beta_{0i} + \beta_{1i}X_{ij}\right)} \qquad (15.47)$$

with conditional independence of the Y_{ij}'s given the X_{ij}'s and the (β_{0i}, β_{1i})'s. At the second stage, the unobservable (β_{0i}, β_{1i})'s are assumed to arise from a bivariate normal distribution with mean (α_0, α_1) and dispersion matrix D, an unknown 2×2 symmetric matrix. Let $(\hat{\beta}_{0i}, \hat{\beta}_{1i})$ be the maximum likelihood estimates of the logistic regression coefficients for the ith subject. By the asymptotic normality of mles when the number of measurements per individual is large, it is reasonable to treat $(\hat{\beta}_{0i}, \hat{\beta}_{1i})$ given (β_{0i}, β_{1i}) as a bivariate normal random variable with mean (β_{0i}, β_{1i}) and variance-covariance matrix $I_i^{-1}(\beta_{0i}, \beta_{1i})$, the inverse information matrix. Korn and Whittemore (1979) treat the $I_i^{-1}(\beta_{0i}, \beta_{1i})$ terms as known and fixed at their values at the mles for each individual.

Under these assumptions, the marginal distribution of $(\hat{\beta}_{0i}, \hat{\beta}_{1i})$ is approximately bivariate normal with mean (α_0, α_1) and variance $I_i^{-1} + D$. The marginal likelihood of normal densities can be maximized to estimate the unknown parameters (α_0, α_1) and D. The maximum likelihood estimate of (α_0, α_1) turns out to be a weighted average of the individual $(\hat{\beta}_{0i}, \hat{\beta}_{1i})$'s (see Problem 15.6).

Dawson and Lagakos (1993) also summarize by individual, but take account of missing data. The summary measures are stratified by the various patterns of missing data and then combined. These authors use this technique for a two-group comparison. Their method is valid as long as the missingness probabilities are the same for the two groups.

Summarizing by Time

Several authors consider obtaining summary statistics by time and combining the time-specific statistics (Moulton and Zeger, 1989; Wei and Stram, 1988; Wei and Johnson, 1985). These methods are useful when the number of time points is limited. The essence of the method is as follows. Let n be the maximum of n_i over i. At the jth time point ($j = 1, \ldots, n$), we assume that

$$P(Y_{ij} = 1 | X_{ij}, \beta_{0j}, \beta_{1j}) = \frac{\exp(\beta_{0j} + \beta_{1j}X_{ij})}{1 + \exp(\beta_{0j} + \beta_{1j}X_{ij})}. \quad (15.48)$$

One obtains the estimate ($\hat{\beta}_{0j}, \hat{\beta}_{1j}$) by fitting model (15.48) using all available data at time j. Inference can be based on the multivariate normality of the stacked coefficient estimators, $\hat{\beta} = (\hat{\beta}_{01}, \hat{\beta}_{11}, \hat{\beta}_{02}, \hat{\beta}_{12}, \ldots, \hat{\beta}_{0n}, \hat{\beta}_{1n})'$. Actually, this model fits into the GEE framework if the interaction terms include time and all covariates in the model.

Wei and Johnson (1985) also consider the two-sample problem. They propose using U statistics for each time point and combining these dependent test statistics as a weighted average. Based on the multivariate normality of the stacked time-specific U statistics, the distribution of the combined statistic can be obtained. The authors show that the optimal weight is the inverse of the covariance matrix of the stacked time-specific U statistics.

15.5.4. Models Conditioning on Previous Outcomes

In some cases the conditional probability of a positive outcome given the previous outcomes is of primary interest. This probability can be modeled directly as follows:

$$P(Y_{ij} = 1 | X_{ij}, Y_{i,j-1}, Y_{i,j-2}, \ldots, Y_{i1})$$

$$= \frac{\exp(\beta_0 + \beta_1 X_{ij} + \beta_2 Y_{i,j-1} + \cdots + \beta_j Y_{i1})}{1 + \exp(\beta_0 + \beta_1 X_{ij} + \beta_2 Y_{i,j-1} + \cdots + \beta_j Y_{i1})}. \quad (15.49)$$

While the association among repeated measurements is treated as a nuisance in the models presented in Sections 15.5.1 through 15.5.3, coefficients $\beta_2, \ldots, \beta_j$ in (15.49) give direct measures of association between repeated measurements. Inferences concerning β can be drawn conveniently by maximizing the following likelihood function:

$$L = \prod_{i=1}^{g} \prod_{j=1}^{n_i} P\left(Y_{ij} = 1 \mid X_{ij}, Y_{i,j-1}, Y_{i,j-2}, \ldots, Y_{i1}\right)^{Y_{ij}}$$

$$\times P\left(Y_{ij} = 0 \mid X_{ij}, Y_{i,j-1}, Y_{i,j-2}, \ldots, Y_{i1}\right)^{1-Y_{ij}}. \tag{15.50}$$

A peculiarity of this model is that the marginal distributions of the Y_{ij} have different forms depending on j. For example, for $j = 1$, the marginal probability is of logit form, but for $j = 2$, it is not. Also note that (15.49) implies a certain joint distribution for Y_i.

In a one-step Markov model (see, e.g., Diggle, Liang, and Zeger, 1996), the probability of a positive outcome is assumed to depend only on the immediately preceding outcome. That is, Y_{ij} is conditionally independent of $Y_{i,j-2}, \ldots, Y_{i1}$ given $Y_{i,j-1}$. As a result, we have

$$P\left(Y_{ij} = 1 \mid X_{ij}, Y_{i,j-1}, Y_{i,j-2}, \ldots, Y_{i1}\right) = P\left(Y_{ij} = 1 \mid X_{ij}, Y_{i,j-1}\right).$$

In this case, the likelihood (15.50) reduces to

$$L_V = \prod_{i=1}^{K} \prod_{j=1}^{n_i} P\left(Y_{ij} = 1 \mid X_{ij}, Y_{i,j-1}\right)^{Y_{ij}} P\left(Y_{ij} = 0 \mid X_{ij}, Y_{i,j-1}\right)^{1-Y_{ij}}. \tag{15.51}$$

Suppose one is interested in the conditional probability given the immediately preceding outcome only, but is not willing to assume that Y_{ij} is independent of $(Y_{i,j-2}, Y_{i,j-3}, \ldots, Y_{i1})$ conditional on $Y_{i,j-1}$ as in the Markov model. In this case L_V is not a likelihood function, but inferences can still be drawn correctly by maximizing L_V. This approach can be justified using the theory of estimating equations. Let

$$\mu_{ij} = P\left(Y_{ij} = 1 \mid X_{ij}, Y_{i,j-1}\right) = \frac{\exp\left(\beta_0 + \beta_1 X_{ij} + \beta_2 Y_{i,j-1}\right)}{1 + \exp\left(\beta_0 + \beta_1 X_{ij} + \beta_2 Y_{i,j-1}\right)}$$

and $\mu_i = (\mu_{i1}, \mu_{i2}, \ldots, \mu_{in_i})'$. Then the maximizer of L_V is a solution of

$$\sum_{i=1}^{K} \frac{\partial \mu_i'}{\partial \beta} V_i^{-1}(Y_i - \mu_i) = 0, \tag{15.52}$$

where V_i is a diagonal matrix with elements $\mu_{ij}(1 - \mu_{ij})$. Equation (15.52) is an unbiased estimating equation as long as μ_{ij} is correctly specified. Using arguments similar to those used to justify GEEs, $\hat{\beta}$ can be shown to be asymptotically normal with mean equal to the true value of β and with variance given by

$$
\left(\sum_{i=1}^{K} \frac{\partial \mu_i'}{\partial \beta} V_i^{-1} \frac{\partial \mu_i}{\partial \beta'} \right)^{-1} \left\{ \sum_{i=1}^{K} \frac{\partial \mu_i'}{\partial \beta} V_i^{-1} (Y_i - \mu_i)(Y_i - \mu_i)' V_i^{-1} \frac{\partial \mu_i}{\partial \beta'} \right\}
$$

$$
\times \left(\sum_{i=1}^{K} \frac{\partial \mu_i'}{\partial \beta} V_i^{-1} \frac{\partial \mu_i}{\partial \beta'} \right)^{-1}. \quad (15.53)
$$

As for GEEs, a more efficient estimator can be obtained when the variance is modeled as $V_i = A_i^{1/2} R_i(\alpha) A_i^{1/2}$.

15.5.5. Multivariate Binary Distributions

Multivariate binary data can be analyzed with a likelihood approach given a multivariate joint distribution for the outcomes. When $n_i = n$ for all i, the methods of Chapter 11 for polytomous logistic regression with a $2 \times \cdots \times 2$ response variable is most useful when interest centers on the logit parameters rather than the marginal probabilities of individual outcomes. In other cases, the challenge is to find a rich and flexible class of multivariate binary distributions that captures the features of interest. Several authors have proposed multivariate distributions for binary data (Bahadur, 1961; Fitzmaurice, Laird, and Lipsitz, 1994). Among them, Prentice and Zhao (1991) study a multivariate binary distribution of quadratic exponential form:

$$
f(Y_i | \theta_i, \lambda_i) = \Delta_i^{-1} \exp\{Y_i \theta_i + w_i \lambda_i - C_i(Y_i)\}, \quad (15.54)
$$

where $\theta_i = (\theta_{i1}, \ldots, \theta_{in_i})'$, $w_i = (Y_{i1}Y_{i2}, Y_{i1}Y_{i3}, Y_{i2}Y_{i3}, \ldots)'$, $\lambda_i = (\lambda_{i12}, \lambda_{i13}, \lambda_{i23}, \ldots)'$, $\Delta_i = \Delta_i(\theta_i, \lambda_i)$ is a normalizing constant, and $C_i(Y_i)$ is an arbitrary function of Y_i. One of the attractive features of the quadratic exponential form is that both conditional and marginal distributions of any subset of the components of Y_i belong to the same family of distributions (see Problem 15.7). The dimensions of θ_i, λ_i, and w_i are determined by Y_i. It is not hard to verify that the expected values of Y_i and w_i have the following form (Problem 15.8):

$$
E(Y_i) = \frac{\partial \ln \Delta_i}{\partial \theta_i} \quad \text{and} \quad E(w_i) = \frac{\partial \ln \Delta_i}{\partial \lambda_i}. \quad (15.55)
$$

To proceed, we model the mean of Y_i, $P_i = E(Y_i)$, and the mean of w_i, say $\eta_i = E(w_i)$. For example,

$$
P_{ij} = \frac{\exp(\beta_{0j} + \beta_1 X_{ij})}{1 + \exp(\beta_0 + \beta_1 X_{ij})}, \quad (15.56)
$$

and

$$\eta_{ijk} = \mathrm{Cov}(Y_{ij}, Y_{ik}) + P_{ij}P_{ik} = \alpha_{jk}\sqrt{\mathrm{Var}(Y_{ij})\,\mathrm{Var}(Y_{ik})} + P_{ij}P_{ik}. \quad (15.57)$$

Let $\eta_i = (\eta_{i12}, \eta_{i13}, \eta_{i23}, \dots)'$, and let α be the vector of length $n(n-1)/2$, $\alpha = (\alpha_{12}, \alpha_{13}, \alpha_{23}, \dots, \alpha_{n-1,\,n})$. Note that P is linked to the regression parameter β, and η is linked to the correlation parameter α. In this quadratic exponential family, the likelihood equation for β has the same form as a GEE when R is correctly specified.

The likelihood equation becomes

$$\frac{\partial \ln \prod_{i=1}^{K} f(Y_i|X_i)}{\partial(\beta', \alpha')'} = \sum_{i=1}^{K} \begin{pmatrix} \dfrac{\partial P_i}{\partial \beta'} & 0 \\[2ex] \dfrac{\partial \eta_i}{\partial \beta'} & \dfrac{\partial \eta_i}{\partial \alpha'} \end{pmatrix}$$

$$\times \begin{pmatrix} \mathrm{Var}(Y_i) & \mathrm{Cov}(Y_i, w_i) \\ \mathrm{Cov}(w_i, Y_i) & \mathrm{Var}(w_i) \end{pmatrix}^{-1} \begin{pmatrix} Y_i - P_i \\ w_i - \eta_i \end{pmatrix} = 0. \quad (15.58)$$

Computation of $(\hat{\beta}, \hat{\alpha})$ starts from an initial value $(\beta^{(0)}, \alpha^{(0)})$, and updates are made by Newton-Raphson iteration:

$$\begin{pmatrix} \beta^{(\nu+1)} \\ \alpha^{(\nu+1)} \end{pmatrix} = \begin{pmatrix} \beta^{(\nu)} \\ \alpha^{(\nu)} \end{pmatrix} + \left\{ -\frac{\partial^2 \ln f(Y_i|X_i)}{\partial(\beta', \alpha')'\partial(\beta', \alpha')} \right\}^{-1}\Bigg|_{\substack{\beta=\beta^{(\nu)} \\ \alpha=\alpha^{(\nu)}}}$$

$$\times \left\{ \frac{\partial \ln f(Y_i|X_i)}{\partial(\beta', \alpha')'} \right\}\Bigg|_{\substack{\beta=\beta^{(\nu)} \\ \alpha=\alpha^{(\nu)}}}$$

It is clear that solving (15.58) requires evaluation of $\mathrm{Cov}(Y_i, w_i)$ and $\mathrm{Var}(w_i)$, which involve the third and fourth moments of Y. This evaluation is carried out by direct computation, for example,

$$\mathrm{Var}(w_i) = \sum (w_i - \eta_i)(w_i - \eta_i)' f(y_i | \theta_i, \lambda_i), \quad (15.59)$$

where the summation is over all possible realizations y_i of Y_i. To compute (15.59), we need to know θ_i and λ_i. The updating formula for θ_i and λ_i given initial values $(\beta^{(0)}, \alpha^{(0)})$ and $(\theta^{(0)}, \lambda^{(0)})$ is

$$\left(\theta_i^{(\nu+1)\prime}, \lambda_i^{(\nu+1)\prime} \right)' = \left(\theta_i^{(\nu)\prime}, \lambda_i^{(\nu)\prime} \right)' + \left\{ E \begin{pmatrix} Y_i - P_i^{(\nu)} \\ w_i - \eta_i^{(\nu)} \end{pmatrix} \begin{pmatrix} Y_i - P_i^{(\nu)} \\ w_i - \eta_i^{(\nu)} \end{pmatrix}' \right\}^{-1} E \begin{pmatrix} Y_i - P_i^{(\nu)} \\ w_i - \eta_i^{(\nu)} \end{pmatrix},$$

where the expectations are calculated directly as in (15.59) using $f(y_i | \theta_i^{(\nu)}, \lambda_i^{(\nu)})$.

PROBLEMS

15.1. Verify the variance formula (15.1).

15.2. Verify formula (15.2) for the variance inflation factor.

15.3. Verify algebraically that the cell counts a and c in Table 15.2 are independent when exposure does not vary within clusters. [*Hint.* Show

$$\mathrm{Cov}(a, c) = \mathrm{Cov}\left\{ \sum_{i=1}^{K} Y_{i+} X_i, \ \sum_{i=1}^{K} Y_{i+} (1 - X_i) \right\} = \sum_{i=1}^{K} \mathrm{Var}(Y_{i+}) \, X_i (1 - X_i).]$$

15.4. Show that

$$\mathrm{Var}\left(\sum_{j=1}^{n_i} Y_{ij} \right) = \mathrm{Var}\left\{ \sum_{j=1}^{n_i} Y_{ij} X_{ij} + \sum_{j=1}^{n_i} Y_{ij} (1 - X_{ij}) \right\}$$

$$= k_i P_1 Q_1 \{ 1 + (k_i - 1) \rho_1 \} + (n_i - k_i) P_2 Q_2 \{ 1 + (n_i - k_i - 1) \rho_2 \}$$

$$+ 2 k_i (n_i - k_i) \rho_{12} \sqrt{P_1 Q_1 P_2 Q_2} \, .$$

15.5. Let $f(u)$ and $g(u)$ be two functions that are either both strictly increasing or both strictly decreasing. Let U be any nondegenerate random variable such that $Ef(U)$ and $Eg(U)$ are finite.

(a) Show that $\mathrm{Cov}\{f(U), g(U)\} > 0$. [*Hint.* Express $\mathrm{Cov}\{f(U), g(U)\}$ as

$$\mathrm{Cov}\{f(U), g(U)\} = Ef(U)\{g(U) - Eg(U)\}$$

$$= E[\{f(U) - f(u^*)\}\{g(U) - Eg(U)\}]$$

for any fixed number u^*. Suppose f and g are both strictly increasing. Then there is a value u^* such that $g(u) > Eg(U)$ for all $u > u^*$ and $g(u) < Eg(U)$ for all $u < u^*$. Conclude that the factors $f(U) - f(u^*)$ and $g(U) - Eg(U)$ always have the same sign, and therefore the expected value of their product is positive.]

(b) Let $f(b_i)$ be (15.41) with $X = X_{ij}$, let $g(b_i)$ be (15.41) with $X = X_{ik}$, and let $U = b_i$. Conclude that $\mathrm{Cov}\{P(Y_{ij} = 1 | X_{ij}, b_i), \ P(Y_{ik} = 1 | X_{ik}, b_i) | X_{ij}, X_{ik}\} > 0$ and therefore that $\mathrm{Cov}(Y_{ij}, Y_{ik} | X_{ij}, X_{ik}) > 0$ even though $\mathrm{Cov}(Y_{ij}, Y_{ik} | X_{ij}, X_{ik}, b_i) = 0$.

15.6. (Korn and Whittemore, 1979.) In Section 15.5.3, the log marginal likelihood for α and D can be written

$$\sum_{i=1}^{n} -\tfrac{1}{2}|W_i + D| - \sum_{i=1}^{n} \tfrac{1}{2}\left(\hat{\beta}_{0i} - \alpha_0, \hat{\beta}_{1i} - \alpha_1\right)(W_i + D)^{-1}$$
$$\times \left(\hat{\beta}_{0i} - \alpha_0, \hat{\beta}_{0i} - \alpha_1\right)'.$$

Verify that when D is known, the maximum likelihood estimate of (α_0, α_1) can be written as

$$(\hat{\alpha}_0, \hat{\alpha}_1)' = \left\{ \sum_{i=1}^{n} (W_i + D) \right\}^{-1} \sum_{i=1}^{n} (W_i + D)^{-1}\left(\hat{\beta}_{0i}, \hat{\beta}_{1i}\right)'.$$

15.7. Binary distribution (15.54) in the bivariate case can be written

$$f(Y_1, Y_2 | \theta, \lambda) = \Delta^{-1} \exp\{Y_1\theta_1 + Y_2\theta_2 + Y_1 Y_2 \lambda - C(Y_1, Y_2)\},$$

where $\Delta = \Delta(\theta, \lambda)$ is a normalizing constant and $C(Y_1, Y_2)$ is an arbitrary function. Verify that both the marginal distribution of Y_1 and the conditional distribution of Y_2 given Y_1 belong to the same family.

15.8. Using the fact that $E(\partial f(Y_i)/\partial\theta_i) = 0$ and that $E(\partial f(Y_i)/\partial\lambda_i) = 0$, derive the following relationships:

$$E(Y_i) = \frac{\partial \ln \Delta_i}{\partial\theta_i} \quad \text{and} \quad E(w_i) = \frac{\partial \ln \Delta_i}{\partial\lambda_i}.$$

15.9. (ARE of GEE estimators.) The maximization lemma for quadratic forms states that if B is a $p \times p$ positive definite matrix with eigenvalues $\lambda_1 \geq \lambda_2 \geq \cdots \geq \lambda_p > 0$ and associated normalized eigenvectors $e_1, e_2, \ldots, e_p$, then

$$\max_{x \neq 0} \frac{x'Bx}{x'x} = \lambda_1 \quad \text{when } x = e_1$$

and

$$\min_{x \neq 0} \frac{x'Bx}{x'x} = \lambda_p \quad \text{when } x = e_p$$

Consider a linear combination of the GEE regression coefficients, $c'\beta$. When R is correctly specified, the variance of $\hat{\beta}$ is $c'W_0^{*-1}c$, where W_0^* denotes W_0 with correct specification of R. When $R = I$, the variance of $\hat{\beta}$ is $c'W_0^{-1}W_1W_0^{-1}c$. Use the maximization lemma to derive maximum and minimum values of the asymptotic relative efficiency (ARE) of the GEE estimator with and without correct specification of R.

REFERENCES

Bahadur, R. R. (1961). A representation of the joint distribution of responses to n dichotomous items. Pp. 158–168 in H. Solomon (Ed.), *Studies in item analysis and prediction*. Stanford Mathematical Studies in the Social Sciences VI. Stanford: Stanford University Press.

Begg, M. D. (1999). Analyzing k 2×2 tables under cluster sampling. *Biometrics*, **55**, 302–307.

Begg, M. D. and Panageas, K. S. (1999). Interval estimation of the common odds ratio from k 2×2 tables under cluster sampling. *Statist. in Med.*, **18**, 1087–1100.

Crowder, M. (1995). On the use of a working correlation matrix in using generalized linear models for repeated measures. *Biometrika*, **82**, 407–410.

Davidian, M. and Gallant, R. (1993). The nonlinear mixed effects model with a smooth random effects density. *Biometrika*, **80**, 475–488.

Dawson, J. D. and Lagakos, S. W. (1993). Size and power of two sample tests of repeated measures data. *Biometrics*, **49**, 1022–1032.

Diggle, P. J., Liang, K.-Y., and Zeger, S. L. (1996). *Analysis of longitudinal data*. Clarendon Press.

Donald, A. and Donner, A. (1987). Adjustments to the Mantel-Haenszel chi-square statistic and odds ratio variance estimator when the data are clustered. *Statist. in Med.*, **6**, 491–499.

Donner, A., Birkett, N., and Buck, C. (1981). Randomization by cluster. Sample size requirements and analysis. *Am. J. Epidemiol.*, **114**, 906–914.

Donner, A. and Hauck, W. (1988). Estimation of a common odds ratio in case control studies of familial aggregation. *Biometrics*, **44**, 369–378.

Fitzmaurice, G. M., Laird, N. M., and Lipsitz, S. R. (1994). Analysing incomplete longitudinal binary responses: A likelihood-based approach. *Biometrics*, **50**, 601–612.

Fitzmaurice, G. M., Molenberghs, G., and Lipsitz, S. R. (1995). Regression models for longitudinal binary responses with informative drop-outs. *J. R. Statist. Soc., Ser. B*, **57**, 691–704.

Korn, E. L. and Whittemore, A. S. (1979). Methods for analyzing panel studies of acute health effects of air pollution. *Biometrics*, **35**, 795–802.

Lachin, J. M. and Wei, L. J. (1988). Estimators and tests in the analysis of multiple nonindependent 2×2 tables with partially missing observations. *Biometrics*, **44**, 513–528.

Lefkopoulou, M., Moore, D., and Ryan, L. (1989). The analysis of multiple correlated binary outcomes: Application to rodent teratology experiments. *J. Am. Statist. Assoc.*, **84**, 810–815.

Levin, B. (1986). Empirical Bayes estimation in heterogeneous matched binary samples with systematic aging effects. Pp. 179–194 in J. Van Ryzin (Ed.), *Adaptive statistical procedures and related topics*, Inst. of Math. Statist. Lecture Notes—Monograph Series, Vol. 8.

Liang, K.-Y. (1985). Odds ratio inference with dependent data. *Biometrika*, **72**, 678–682.

Liang, K.-Y. and Zeger, S. L. (1986). Longitudinal data analysis using generalized linear models. *Biometrika*, **73**, 13–22.

Liang, K.-Y., Zeger, S. L., and Qaqish, B. (1992). Multivariate regression analyses for categorical data. *J. R. Statist. Soc., Ser. B*, **54**, 3–40.

Lipsitz, S. R., Dear, K. B. G., and Zhao, L. (1994). Jackknife estimators of variance for parameter estimates from estimating equations with applications to clustered survival data. *Biometrics*, **50**, 842–846.

Mancl, L. A. and Leroux, B. G. (1996). Efficiency of regression estimates for clustered data. *Biometrics*, **52**, 500–511.

McCullagh, P. and Nelder, J. A. (1989). *Generalized linear models*, 2nd ed. London: Chapman and Hall.

Moulton, L. H. and Zeger, S. L. (1989). Analyzing repeated measures on generalized linear models via bootstrap. *Biometrics*, **45**, 381–394.

Muñoz, A., Carey, V., Schouten, J. P., Segal, M., and Rosner, B. (1992). A parametric family of correlation structures for the analysis of longitudinal data. *Biometrics*, **48**, 733–742.

Neugebauer, R., Paik, M., Hauser, W. A., Nadel, E., Leppik, I., and Susser M. (1994). Stressful life events and seizure frequency in patients with epilepsy. *Epilepsia*, **35**, 336–343.

Paik, M. C. (1988). Repeated measurement analysis for nonnormal data in small samples. *Comm. Statist.*, **B17**, 1155–1171.

Paik, M. C. (1992). Parametric variance function estimation for nonnormal repeated measurement data. *Biometrics*, **48**, 19–30.

Paik, M. C. (1997). The generalized estimating equation approach when data are not missing completely at random. *J. Am. Statist. Assoc.*, **92**, 1320–1329.

Paik, M. C., Sacco, R. L., and Lin, I.-F. (2000). Bivariate binary data analysis with missing outcomes. *Biometrics*, **56**, 1145–1156.

Park, T. (1993). A comparison of the generalized estimating equation approach with the maximum likelihood approach for repeated measurements. *Statist. in Med.*, **12**, 1723–1732.

Phillips, A. and Holland, P. W. (1987). Estimators of the variance of the Mantel-Haenszel log-odds-ratio estimate. *Biometrics*, **43**, 425–431.

Prentice, R. L. (1988). Correlated binary regression with covariates specific to each binary observation. *Biometrics*, **43**, 1033–1048.

Prentice, R. L. and Zhao, L. P. (1991). Estimating equations for parameters in means and covariances of multivariate discrete and continuous responses. *Biometrics*, **47**, 825–39.

Rao, J. N. K. and Scott, A. J. (1992). A simple method for the analysis of clustered binary data. *Biometrics*, **48**, 577–585.

Robins, J., Breslow, N., and Greenland, S. (1986). Estimators of the Mantel-Haenszel variance consistent in both sparse data and large-strata limiting models. *Biometrics*, **42**, 311–323.

Robins, J. M., Rotnitzky, A., and Zhao, L. P. (1995). Analysis of semiparametric regression models for repeated outcomes in the presence of missing data. *J. Am. Statist. Assoc.*, **90**, 106–121.

Rotnitzky, A. and Jewell, N. P. (1990). Hypothesis testing of regression parameters in semiparametric generalized linear models for cluster correlated data. *Biometrika*, **77**, 485–497.

Sacco, R. L., Boden-Albala, B., Gan, R., Chen, X., Kargman, D. E., Shea, S., Paik, M. C., and Hauser, W. A. (1998). Stroke incidence among white, black, and hispanic residents of the same community: The Northern Manhattan Stroke Study. *Am. J. Epidemiol.*, **147**, 259–268.

Stiratelli, R., Laird, N., and Ware, J. H. (1984). Random-effects models for serial observations with binary response. *Biometrics*, **40**, 961–971.

Tatemichi, T. K., Paik, M., Bagiella, E., Desmond, D. W., Pirro, M., and Hanzawa, L. K., (1992). Dementia after stroke is a predictor of long-term survival. *Stroke*, **25**, 1915–1919.

Wei, L. J. and Johnson, W. E. (1985). Combining dependent tests with incomplete repeated measurements. *Biometrika*, **72**, 359–364.

Wei, L. J. and Stram, D. O. (1988). Analyzing repeated measurements with possibly missing observations by modeling marginal distributions. *Statist. in Med.*, **7**, 139–148.

Weil, C. S. (1970). Selection of valid number of sampling units and a consideration of their combination in toxicological studies involving reproductions, teratogenesis or carcinogenesis. *Food and Cosmetics Toxicology* **8**, 177–182.

Williams, D. A. (1975). The analysis of binary responses from toxicological experiments involving reproduction and teratogenicity. *Biometrics*, **31**, 949–952.

Xie, F. and Paik, M. C. (1997a). Generalized estimating equation model for binary outcomes with missing covariates. *Biometrics*, **53**, 1458–1466.

Xie, F. and Paik, M. C. (1997b). Multiple imputation methods for the missing covariates in generalized estimating equation. *Biometrics*, **53**, 1538–1546.

Zeger, S. L. and Liang, K.-Y. (1986). Longitudinal data analysis for discrete and continuous outcomes. *Biometrics*, **42**, 121–130.

Zeger, S. L., Liang, K.-Y., and Albert, P. S. (1988). Models for longitudinal data: A generalized estimating equation approach. *Biometrics*, **44**, 1049–1060.

Zeger, S. L. and Qaqish, B. (1988). Markov regression models for time series: A quasilikelihood approach. *Biometrics*, **44**, 1019–1031.

Zhang, J. and Boos, D. D. (1977). Mantel-Haenszel test statistics for correlated binary data. *Biometrics*, **53**, 1185–1198.

Zhao, L. P., Prentice, R. L., and Self, S. G. (1992). Multivariate mean parameter estimation by using a partly exponential model. *J. R. Statist. Soc.*, *Ser. B*, **54**, 805–811.

Ziegler, A., Kastner, C., and Blettner, M. (1998). The generalized estimating equations: An annotated bibliography. *Biometrical Journal*, **40**, 115–139.

CHAPTER 16

Missing Data

Unlike the data used in most textbook illustrations, data collected in the real world are often incomplete. Study participants refuse to continue in follow up, for example, or decline to answer questions they consider embarrassing. Laboratory samples become contaminated, or assays yield uninterpretable results. Investigators, fieldworkers, or technicians make errors. Data are lost. Sometimes even in the design of a study, one will knowingly create missing data. Such is the case of the two-stage design discussed in the next chapter, where for reasons of cost or other practical reasons, only a subsample of the entire sample can be studied in appropriate detail or with the most reliable instruments; the details or reliable measurements are then missing for the rest.

In this chapter we consider methods appropriate for drawing inferences in the presence of missing data. Section 16.1 identifies three types of nonresponse or "missingness mechanisms." Section 16.2 discusses inference for data missing at random in a 2×2 table with a monotone missingness pattern. Section 16.3 discusses methods for analyzing several 2×2 tables, Section 16.4 does the same for logistic regression models when covariate data are missing at random, and Section 16.5 considers missing outcomes in logistic regression. Section 16.6 presents methods appropriate for nonignorably missing data, and Section 16.7 discusses the case of nonmonotone missingness.

16.1. THREE TYPES OF NONRESPONSE MECHANISM

Consider a simple 2×2 table where S indicates smoking status (smoker versus nonsmoker) and H indicates blood pressure status (hypertensive versus normotensive). We are interested in three parameters: $D_{S|H}$, the

Statistical Methods for Rates and Proportions, Third Edition
By Joseph L. Fleiss, Bruce Levin, and Myunghee Cho Paik
ISBN 0-471-52629-0   Copyright © 2003 John Wiley & Sons, Inc.

difference in smoking rates between hypertensive and normotensive subjects; $D_{H|S}$, the difference in hypertension rates between smokers and nonsmokers; and ω, the odds ratio:

$$D_{S|H} = P(S = 1 | H = 1) - P(S = 1 | H = 0),$$

$$D_{H|S} = P(H = 1 | S = 1) - P(H = 1 | S = 0),$$

and

$$\omega = \frac{P(S = 1 | H = 1)/P(S = 0 | H = 1)}{P(S = 1 | H = 0)/P(S = 0 | H = 0)}$$

$$= \frac{P(H = 1 | S = 1)/P(H = 0 | S = 1)}{P(H = 1 | S = 0)/P(H = 0 | S = 0)}.$$

For a sample of 200 subjects, suppose that smoking status is known for all 200 but that blood pressure has been measured for only 100, with the results shown in Table 16.1 The first four rows represent completely observed records. The last two rows represent incompletely observed records. We can divide these data between two tables, as in Table 16.2(a) and 16.2(b).

Table 16.1. *Smoking and hypertension (hypothetical data)*

S	H	Frequencies
1	1	30
1	0	20
0	1	10
0	0	40
1	?	80
0	?	20
		200

Table 16.2. *Tables with complete and incomplete data*

		(a) Complete Table					(b) Incomplete Table		
			H					H	
		1	0	Total			1	0	Total
S	1	30	20	50		S 1	?	?	80
	0	10	40	50		0	?	?	20
	Total	40	60	100		Total	?	?	100

If we restrict the analysis to the completely observed records in Table 16.2(a), the estimates of $D_{S|H}$, $D_{H|S}$, and ω based on the sample proportions are

$$d_{S|H} = \frac{30}{40} - \frac{20}{60} = 0.42,$$

$$d_{H|S} = \frac{30}{50} - \frac{10}{50} = 0.40,$$

and

$$o = \frac{30/10}{20/40} = 6.$$

Under what conditions do these estimates accurately reflect the parameters of interest? To answer this question, we need first to understand the relation between the variables and the mechanism causing the data to be missing. There are three types of nonresponse mechanism (Rubin, 1976). For the time being, we continue to assume S is completely observed.

(a) *Missing Completely at Random* (MCAR). The missingness of H depends on neither S nor H. If the subjects with complete data constitute a truly random sample (i.e., are a random subsample of our random sample), we do not expect marked differences between Table 16.2(a) and a table with complete observations for all 200 subjects. Smoking rates for hypertensive and normotensive subjects would be similar in each table, as would hypertension rates for smokers and nonsmokers. Analysis of the observed data thus yields unbiased estimates of the parameters $D_{S|H}$, $D_{H|S}$, and ω (and their standard errors). In general, whatever the mechanism is that causes the data to be missing, the estimates remain unbiased provided that the mechanism is independent of S and H.

(b) *Missing at Random* (MAR). The missingness of H depends on S but not H. Suppose, for example, that compared to smokers, nonsmokers are more likely to complete the study protocol (i.e., come to the investigator's office for sphygmomanometry) because they are more health-conscious. As explained in the next section, Table 16.2(a) would then provide an accurate estimate of hypertension rates given smoking status, $P(H|S)$, but an inaccurate estimate of smoking rates given hypertension status, $P(S|H)$. Thus the hypertension rate difference $D_{H|S}$, and the odds ratio ω [because it can be expressed in terms of $P(H|S)$], can be consistently estimated from the observed data. Section 16.2.1 describes a consistent method to estimate the smoking rate difference $D_{S|H}$.

(c) *Nonignorable* (NI) *Missingness*. The missingness of H depends on H even after conditioning on S. If, for example, hypertensive subjects who

Table 16.3. *Observation indicator and data*

R_H	S	H	Frequencies
1	1	1	30
1	1	0	20
1	0	1	10
1	0	0	40
0	1	?	80
0	0	?	20
			200

smoke are more (or less) likely to have missing data than nonhypertensive subjects who smoke, then both the hypertension rate given smoking status and the smoking rate given hypertension status differ between the tables with complete and incomplete data. None of the three parameters can be consistently estimated from the completely observed data. Inferences require assumptions about the relationships between S, H, and the reasons that data are missing, assumptions which are difficult to verify. These are discussed further in Section 16.6. No analysis with NI missingness is complete without sensitivity analyses.

It is evident that some types of missingness are more damaging than others. To help clarify the discussion, we define an *observation indicator*. Let R_H take the value 1 if H is observed, 0 if H is missing. The data in Table 16.1 can then be presented as in Table 16.3. Note that the variable R_H is completely observed. Even when H is missing, R_H is known (if H is missing, $R_H = 0$). The observation indicator is sometimes called a *missingness indicator*, even though a 1 indicates the opposite. Similarly, when we talk of response mechanisms or models for $P(R_H|S, H)$, we are also apt to think of these as *nonresponse mechanisms*.

The *missingness probability* is defined as $P(R_H = 0|S, H)$. For the three response mechanisms, the missingness probabilities satisfy

$$\text{MCAR:} \quad P(R_H = 0|S, H) = P(R_H = 0),$$

$$\text{MAR:} \quad P(R_H = 0|S, H) = P(R_H = 0|S), \qquad (16.1)$$

$$\text{NI:} \quad P(R_H = 0|S, H) \neq P(R_H = 0|S).$$

Sometimes we can use these probabilities to rule out certain types of nonresponse mechanisms. For example, from Table 16.3, we can construct Table 16.4. The sample estimates of the missingness probabilities are

$$p(R_H = 1|S = 1) = 50/130 \quad \text{and} \quad p(R_H = 1|S = 0) = 50/70.$$

Table 16.4. *Observed smoking data and observation indicator R_H*

		R_H 1	R_H 0	Total
S	1	50	80	130
	0	50	20	70
	Total	100	100	200

Table 16.5. *Nonmonotonically missing data*

S	H	Frequencies
1	1	30
1	0	20
0	1	10
0	0	40
1	?	40
0	?	20
?	1	20
?	0	20
		200

Because the two proportions differ significantly, the data suggest that the nonresponse mechanism is not MCAR. Distinguishing between MAR and NI requires a test statistic to determine whether or not R_H is independent of H given S. Again, the test statistic must rely on unverifiable model assumptions which we discuss in Section 16.6.

We now consider cases in which both S and H are incompletely observed. Suppose we have the situation in Table 16.5. As before, we divide these data between two tables (Table 16.6).

Table 16.6(b) has unknown column totals as well as unknown row totals, whereas Table 16.2(b) has unknown column totals only. We therefore define

Table 16.6. *Tables with complete and incomplete data for nonmonotonically missing data*

		(a) Complete Table H 1	H 0	Total			(b) Incomplete Table H 1	H 0	Total
S	1	30	20	50	S	1	?	?	?
	0	10	40	50		0	?	?	?
	Total	40	60	100		Total	?	?	100

Table 16.7. *Observation indicators for nonmonotonically missing data*

R_S	R_H	S	H	Frequencies
1	1	1	1	30
1	1	1	0	20
1	1	0	1	10
1	1	0	0	40
1	0	1	?	40
1	0	0	?	20
0	1	?	1	20
0	1	?	1	20
				200

a second observation indicator, R_S, taking the value 1 if S is observed, 0 if S is missing. An array of observation indicators (R_S, R_H) is called a *missingness pattern*. If all patterns in the array are nondecreasing [(1, 1) or (0, 1)] or nonincreasing [(1, 1) or (1, 0)], the missingness pattern is said to be *monotone*. Thus, the data in Table 16.3 have a monotone missingness pattern, because there are only two patterns: (1, 1) and (1, 0), both of which are nonincreasing. In Table 16.7, on the other hand, there are three patterns: (1, 1), (1, 0), and (0, 1); the missingness pattern is *nonmonotone*.

As we will see, missingness patterns play an important role in deciding which method we select to handle missing data.

16.2. DATA MISSING AT RANDOM IN A 2 × 2 TABLE

In this section, we discuss the missing-data problem and its solutions in the simple setting of a 2 × 2 table. When data are MCAR, as mentioned above, statistical inferences drawn from the completely observed records are valid, that is, estimates are consistent and tests have their nominal error rates. Reliance on the completely observed records is called *complete record* (CR) *analysis*. CR analysis is identical to the analyses covered earlier in this book, so here we focus on methods for data that are MAR, making comparisons of these methods with CR analysis along the way. We consider first the analysis of a monotonic missingness pattern, postponing discussion of the nonmonotone case to Section 16.7.

16.2.1. Point Estimation

For the data in Table 16.1, smoking status is completely observed, but hypertension status is incompletely observed. We assume that the missingness of H depends on S but not on H. Under the assumed MAR mechanism we have [by Problem 16.1(a)]

$$P(H|S, R_H = 1) = P(H|S, R_H = 0) = P(H|S). \qquad (16.2)$$

Because we can estimate $P(H|S, R_H = 1)$ consistently from the completely observed data, by (16.2) we also estimate $P(H|S)$ consistently by CR analysis and, consequently, $D_{H|S}$ and ω as well. However, we cannot estimate $P(S|H)$ consistently by CR analysis, because [by Problem 16.1(b)]

$$P(S|H, R_H = 1) \neq P(S|H),$$

so the rate of smoking given hypertension among completely observed records is different than what it would be if there were no missing data. To estimate $P(S|H)$ there are two ways to proceed: by imputation or by weighting.

Imputation
A natural way to handle missing data is to use our best estimate of the value we would have observed had we been able. This approach, known as *imputation*, does not always give valid point estimates, although in the case of a 2×2 table, it does. The standard error, on the other hand, is not estimated consistently, because an imputed value lacks the variability of actual data. How to estimate standard errors correctly is discussed in Section 16.2.2.

If all of the data were observed, we would work from a display like Table 16.8. Because some H's are missing, we partition the table as shown in Table 16.9. The subscripts o and m denote, respectively, observed and missing cell counts. Denote the observed data $(a_o, b_o, c_o, d_o, m_1, m_2)$ by O. If all data were observed, we would estimate $P(S = 1|H = 1)$ by the sample proportion $p_{S|H} = a/(a + c)$. When a and c are partially missing, the best estimates of a and c are their conditional expectations given the observed data, $E(a|O)$ and $E(c|O)$. The conditional expectation of a given the observed data is

$$E(a|O) = E(a \mid a_o, b_o, c_o, d_o, m_1, m_2) = a_o + E(a_m|O)$$

Table 16.8. *Summary table when no data are missing*

		H		
		1	0	Total
S	1	a	b	$a + b$
	0	c	d	$c + d$
	Total	$a + c$	$b + d$	n

Table 16.9. *Tables with complete and incomplete data*

		(a) Complete Table				(b) Incomplete Table		
		H					H		
		1	0	Total			1	0	Total
S	1	a_o	b_o	$a_o + b_o$	S	1	a_m	b_m	m_1
	0	c_o	d_o	$c_o + d_o$		0	c_m	d_m	m_2
	Total	$a_o + c_o$	$b_o + d_o$	n_o		Total	$a_m + c_m$	$b_m + d_m$	n_m

and that for c is

$$E(c|O) = E(c | a_o, b_o, c_o, d_o, m_1, m_2) = c_o + E(c_m|O).$$

Once estimates of the conditional mean of the cell counts, say $\hat{E}(a_m|O)$ and $\hat{E}(c_m|O)$ are obtained, $P(S = 1|H = 1)$ is estimated by

$$\hat{P}(S = 1|H = 1) = \frac{a_o + \hat{E}(a_m|O)}{a_o + \hat{E}(a_m|O) + c_o + \hat{E}(c_m|O)}. \qquad (16.3)$$

$P(S = 1|H = 0)$ is estimated similarly, using the observed frequencies b_o and d_o and the estimated conditional means $\hat{E}(b_m|O)$ and $\hat{E}(d_m|O)$, and from these we estimate $D_{S|H}$ by subtraction. These imputation estimates are consistent if the conditional expectation estimates are consistent.

There are two apparent ways to estimate the conditional expectation of the missing cell counts. Applying the observed sample cell proportion a_o/n_o to the missing data total, we can estimate $E(a_m|O)$ by $n_m a_o/n_o$. This estimate is valid if

$$P(S, H|R_H = 1) = P(S, H|R_H = 0) = P(S, H),$$

which holds only if data are MCAR [Problem 16.1(c)]. If that were the case, then a_o/n_o would give a consistent estimate of the cell probability $P(S = 1, H = 1)$, c_o/n_o would give a consistent estimate of the cell probability $P(S = 0, H = 1)$, and similarly for the other cells, as well as the row and column conditional probabilities. Consequently, this method of estimating the conditional cell expectations would allow us to obtain consistent estimates for all three parameters $D_{H|S}$, $D_{S|H}$, and ω.

Alternatively, applying the row proportions as observed in the complete data to the row totals of missing data, we can estimate $E(a_m|O)$ by $\hat{a}_m = m_1 \hat{P}(H = 1|S = 1) = m_1 a_o/(a_o + b_o)$ and $E(c_m|O)$ by $\hat{c}_m = m_2 \hat{P}(H = 1|S = 0) = m_2 c_o/(c_o + d_o)$. These estimates are valid under the less restrictive MAR condition (16.2) which we are assuming. We reiterate that only the row probabilities $P(H|S)$ are estimated consistently from the complete data; neither the column probabilities $P(S|H)$ nor the individual cell probabilities are. For example, a_o/n_o is not a consistent estimate for $P(S = 1, H = 1)$, and c_o/n_o is not a consistent estimate for $P(S = 0, H = 1)$. But $a_o/(a_o + b_o)$ is a consistent estimate of $P(H = 1|S = 1)$, and $c_o/(c_o + d_o)$ is a consistent estimate of $P(H = 1|S = 0)$, so it is clear that we can use these in $\hat{a}_m$ to estimate $E(a_m|O)$ and in $\hat{c}_m$ to estimate $E(c_m|O)$ in order to obtain a consistent method of imputation under MAR.

Therefore we estimate $P(S = 1|H = 1)$ using (16.3) by

$$\hat{P}(S = 1|H = 1) = \frac{a_o + \hat{a}_m}{a_o + \hat{a}_m + c_o + \hat{c}_m}. \tag{16.4}$$

With $\hat{b}_m = m_1 \hat{P}(H = 0|S = 1) = m_1 b_o/(a_o + b_o)$ and $\hat{d}_m = m_2 \hat{P}(H = 0|S = 0)$
$= m_2 d_o/(c_o + d_o)$, we also have

$$\hat{P}(S = 1|H = 0) = \frac{b_o + \hat{b}_m}{b_o + \hat{b}_m + d_o + \hat{d}_m},$$

so that we have the following consistent imputation estimates for $D_{S|H}$, $D_{H|S}$, and ω:

$$\hat{D}_{S|H} = \frac{a_o + \hat{a}_m}{a_o + \hat{a}_m + c_o + \hat{c}_m} - \frac{b_o + \hat{b}_m}{b_o + \hat{b}_m + d_o + \hat{d}_m},$$

$$\hat{D}_{H|S} = \frac{a_o + \hat{a}_m}{a_o + \hat{a}_m + b_o + \hat{b}_m} - \frac{c_o + \hat{c}_m}{c_o + \hat{c}_m + d_o + \hat{d}_m},$$

and

$$\hat{\omega} = \frac{(a_o + \hat{a}_m)(d_o + \hat{d}_m)}{(b_o + \hat{b}_m)(c_o + \hat{c}_m)}.$$

Let us compare the CR and imputation estimates a little more closely. First consider the imputation scheme conditioning on the total margin, which is valid only under MCAR. With $\hat{P}(S = 1, H = 1) = a_o/n_o$, we have

$$a_o + \hat{E}(a_m|O) = a_o + \frac{n_m a_o}{n_o} = a_o\left(1 + \frac{n_m}{n_o}\right).$$

Replacing the other missing cell counts with their expectations produces similar expressions with the same factor $1 + n_m/n_o$, so that substitution in (16.3) reduces to the CR estimate $a_o/(a_o + c_o)$ for $P(S = 1|H = 1)$. Similarly, the imputation estimates for $D_{S|H}$, $P(H = 1|S = 1)$, $D_{H|S}$, and ω are identical with the corresponding CR estimates.

Now consider the imputation scheme conditioning on the row margins, which is valid under MAR. The CR estimate of $P(H = 1|S = 1)$ is, say, $\tilde{P}(H = 1|S = 1) = a_o/(a_o + b_o)$, while the imputation estimate is $\hat{P}(H = 1|S = 1) = (a_o + \hat{a}_m)/(a_o + \hat{a}_m + b_o + \hat{b}_m)$. These too are identical, because

$$a_o + \hat{a}_m = a_o\left(1 + \frac{m_1}{a_o + b_o}\right)$$

and

$$b_o + \hat{b}_m = b_o\left(1 + \frac{m_1}{a_o + b_o}\right),$$

and the common factor in parentheses cancels out. Similarly, the imputation estimates for $D_{H|S}$ and ω are identical to the CR estimates $\{a_o/(a_o + b_o)\} - \{c_o/(c_o + d_o)\}$ and $o = a_o d_o/b_o c_o$, respectively. However, a similar cancellation does not occur for the two estimates of $P(S = 1|H)$, because, for example, from (16.4),

$$\hat{P}(S = 1|H = 1) = \frac{a_o\{1 + m_1/(a_o + b_o)\}}{a_o\{1 + m_1/(a_o + b_o)\} + c_o\{1 + m_2/(c_o + d_o)\}} \neq \frac{a_o}{a_o + c_o}.$$

To summarize, for the case we are considering of the 2×2 table under MAR, we find some but not all of the CR and imputation estimates to be equal. In other applications, however, even when complete record analysis is valid, CR and imputation estimates are seldom algebraically identical.

Example 16.2.1. Consider again the data in Tables 16.1 and 16.2. Since the imputation estimates of $D_{H|S}$ and ω are identical to the CR estimates, we focus on the estimation of $D_{S|H}$. The estimated expected cell counts under MAR are $\hat{a}_m = 80 \times 30/50 = 48$, $\hat{b}_m = 80 \times 20/50 = 32$, $\hat{c}_m = 20 \times 10/50 = 4$, and $\hat{d}_m = 20 \times 40/50 = 16$. The observed and estimated cell counts are shown in Table 16.10.

Table 16.10. *Observed complete and estimated expected incomplete cell frequencies for the data of Table 16.2*

		(a) Complete Table					(b) Estimated Expected Table		
		H					*H*		
		1	0	Total			1	0	Total
S	1	30	20	50	*S*	1	48	32	80
	0	10	40	50		0	4	16	20
	Total	40	60	100		Total	52	48	100

Table 16.11. *Combined observed complete and estimated expected missing cell frequencies from Table 16.10*

		\multicolumn{2}{H}		
		1	0	Total
S	1	78	52	130
	0	14	56	70
	Total	92	108	200

When the two tables are combined, we have Table 16.11. The estimates for $P(S = 1|H = 1)$ and $P(S = 1|H = 0)$ are thus

$$\hat{P}(S = 1|H = 1) = 78/92 = 39/46 = 0.8478$$

and

$$\hat{P}(S = 1|H = 0) = 52/108 = 13/27 = 0.4815,$$

giving $\hat{D}_{S|H} = 0.8478 - 0.4815 = 0.3663$, about 5 percentage points lower than the CR estimate of $0.75 - 0.3333 = 0.4167$. Note that the imputation estimate of the odds ratio is $(78 \times 56)/(52 \times 14) = 6$, numerically identical to the complete-record estimate, $(30 \times 40)/(20 \times 10)$.

Weighting
Another way to handle missing data is to compensate for the missingness by weighting the observed data. We begin by noting that, whereas we cannot consistently estimate $P(S|H)$ using completely observed records only, we can consistently estimate $P(S|H, R_H = 1)$ and $P(R_H = 1|S)$ under MAR. Bayes theorem gives us a connection between $P(S|H, R_H = 1)$ and $P(S|H)$:

$$\frac{P(S = 1|H, R_H = 1)}{P(S = 0|H, R_H = 1)} = \frac{P(S = 1|H)}{P(S = 0|H)} \cdot \frac{P(R_H = 1|S = 1, H)}{P(R_H = 1|S = 0, H)}, \quad (16.5)$$

and MAR gives us another relation: $P(R_H = 1|S, H) = P(R_H = 1|S)$. Substituting this last in (16.5) and rearranging terms, we have

$$\frac{P(S = 1|H)}{P(S = 0|H)} = \frac{P(S = 1|H, R_H = 1)/P(R_H = 1|S = 1)}{P(S = 0|H, R_H = 1)/P(R_H = 1|S = 0)}.$$

The quantities appearing on the right-hand side can be consistently estimated under MAR. This formula suggests an old survey sampling trick (Horvitz and Thompson, 1952): to weight observed quantities inversely by their probability of observation, thereby compensating for the missing data.

To estimate $P(S = 1 | H = 1)$ in our numerical example, we first calculate

$$\frac{\hat{P}(S = 1 | H = 1, R_H = 1)}{\hat{P}(R_H = 1 | S = 1)} = \frac{30/40}{50/130} = \frac{39}{20}$$

and

$$\frac{\hat{P}(S = 1 | H = 1, R_H = 1)}{\hat{P}(R_H = 1 | S = 0)} = \frac{10/40}{50/70} = \frac{7}{20}.$$

Therefore the estimate of $P(S = 1 | H = 1)/P(S = 0 | H = 1)$ is $\frac{39}{7}$, so the estimate of $P(S = 1 | H = 1)$ is $39/(39 + 7) = \frac{39}{46}$. Similarly,

$$\frac{\hat{P}(S = 1 | H = 0, R_H = 1)}{\hat{P}(R_H = 1 | S = 1)} = \frac{20/60}{50/130} = \frac{13}{15}$$

and

$$\frac{\hat{P}(S = 0 | H = 0, R_H = 1)}{\hat{P}(R_H = 1 | S = 1)} = \frac{40/60}{50/70} = \frac{14}{15}.$$

The estimate of $P(S = 1 | H = 0)$ is then $13/(13 + 14) = \frac{13}{27}$.

Note that these estimates are numerically identical to the imputation estimates. This is no coincidence. Going back to the imputation method, the conditional expectation of the cell count in the upper left-hand corner of the full-data Table 16.8 is $E(a | O) = a_o\{1 + m_1/(a_o + b_o)\} = a_o\{(a_o + b_o)/(m_1 + a_o + b_o)\}^{-1}$, and $(a_o + b_o)/(m_1 + a_o + b_o)$ estimates $P(R_H = 1 | S = 1)$. Thus the imputation and weighting estimates yield identical results in 2×2 tables. In general, however, the two approaches do not yield equivalent estimates (Little, 1986), and they have different asymptotic properties as well.

Two Paradigms

Imputation and weighting represent two distinct paradigms for handling missing data, each one tackling the problem from a different angle: imputation *fills in* missing data, whereas weighting *blows up* observed data. Imputation fills in the best guess for the missing data, makes a "completed" data set, and analyzes it. Weighting blows up each observed datum by the inverse of the probability of observing it, essentially replicating the observed data to stand in for the missing data. For example, if only one record is observed out of ten sampled with the other nine records missing, weighting the observed record by a factor of 10 (the reciprocal probability of observation) replicates the observed record nine times to stand in for the missing records. The weighting factor depends on how underrepresented each observed record is among all records with the same characteristics.

16.2.2. Variance Estimation

We cannot estimate the variance of the imputation estimate (16.4) by

$$\frac{(a_o + \hat{a}_m)(c_o + \hat{c}_m)}{(a_o + \hat{a}_m + c_o + \hat{c}_m)^3},$$

as we would if the imputed data had actually been observed. Calculating the variance of an imputation estimate is generally challenging. Problem 16.2 derives an empirical variance estimate by a general method used for estimating equations. Other methods include the jackknife and multiple imputation, which we discuss in subsequent sections. Here we present a relatively simple formula for the estimated variance of $\hat{D}_{S|H}$ using the delta method.

To keep the notation concise, let $\pi_1 = P(S = 1 | H = 1)$ and $\pi_2 = P(S = 1 | H = 0)$ denote the conditional probabilities we are interested in estimating; let $p_1 = a_o/(a_o + b_o)$ and $p_2 = c_o/(c_o + d_o)$; and let $q_1 = b_o/(a_o + b_o) = 1 - p_1$ and $q_2 = d_o/(c_o + d_o) = 1 - p_2$. We provide an estimate of the variance of $\hat{D}_{S|H}$ conditional on the total number $n_1 = a_o + b_o + m_1$ of smokers ($S = 1$) and $n_2 = c_o + d_o + m_2$ of nonsmokers ($S = 0$). Conditioning on n_1 and n_2 renders the random variables p_1 and p_2 conditionally independent. Now let $f_1 = n_1/(n_1 + n_2)$ and $f_2 = n_2/(n_1 + n_2)$, and let

$$\bar{p} = \frac{n_1 p_1 + n_2 p_2}{n_1 + n_2} = f_1 p_1 + f_2 p_2 \quad \text{and} \quad \bar{q} = \frac{n_1 q_1 + n_2 q_2}{n_1 + n_2} = f_1 q_1 + f_2 q_2.$$

With this notation we can write the imputation estimates (16.4) for π_1 and $1 - \pi_1$ as

$$\hat{\pi}_1 = \frac{n_1 p_1}{n_1 p_1 + n_2 p_2} = \frac{f_1 p_1}{\bar{p}} \quad \text{and} \quad 1 - \hat{\pi}_1 = \frac{n_2 p_2}{n_1 p_1 + n_2 p_2} = \frac{f_2 p_2}{\bar{p}},$$

the imputation estimates for π_2 and $1 - \pi_2$ as

$$\hat{\pi}_2 = \frac{n_1 q_1}{n_1 q_1 + n_2 q_2} = \frac{f_1 q_1}{\bar{q}} \quad \text{and} \quad 1 - \hat{\pi}_2 = \frac{n_2 q_2}{n_1 q_1 + n_2 q_2} = \frac{f_2 q_2}{\bar{q}},$$

and the imputation estimate for $D_{S|H}$ as

$$\hat{D}_{S|H} = \hat{\pi}_1 - \hat{\pi}_2 = \frac{f_1 p_1}{\bar{p}} - \frac{f_1 q_1}{\bar{q}}$$

[see Problem 16.3(a)]. In Problem 16.3(b) and (c), the reader is asked to use the delta method to derive the large sample variances of the estimates $\hat{\pi}_1$

and $\hat{\pi}_2$, and their covariance. Specifically, these are estimated by

$$\widehat{\text{Var}}(\hat{\pi}_1) = \{\hat{\pi}_1(1 - \hat{\pi}_1)\}^2 \left(\frac{q_1/p_1}{n_1 - m_1} + \frac{q_2/p_2}{n_2 - m_2} \right),$$

$$\widehat{\text{Var}}(\hat{\pi}_2) = \{\hat{\pi}_2(1 - \hat{\pi}_2)\}^2 \left(\frac{p_1/q_1}{n_1 - m_1} + \frac{p_2/q_2}{n_2 - m_2} \right),$$

and

$$\widehat{\text{Cov}}(\hat{\pi}_1, \hat{\pi}_2) = -\{\hat{\pi}_1(1 - \hat{\pi}_1)\hat{\pi}_2(1 - \hat{\pi}_2)\}^2 \left(\frac{p_1/q_1}{n_1 - m_1} + \frac{p_2/q_2}{n_2 - m_2} \right),$$

Putting these together in Problem 16.3(d), we have the variance estimate for $\hat{D}_{S|H}$:

$$\widehat{\text{Var}}(\hat{\pi}_1 - \hat{\pi}_2) = \{\hat{\pi}_1(1 - \hat{\pi}_1)\}^2 \left(\frac{q_1/p_1}{n_1 - m_1} + \frac{q_2/p_2}{n_2 - m_2} \right)$$

$$+ \{\hat{\pi}_2(1 - \hat{\pi}_2)\}^2 \left(\frac{p_1/q_1}{n_1 - m_1} + \frac{p_2/q_2}{n_2 - m_2} \right)$$

$$+ 2\{\hat{\pi}_1(1 - \hat{\pi}_1)\hat{\pi}_2(1 - \hat{\pi}_2)\} \left(\frac{1}{n_1 - m_1} + \frac{1}{n_2 - m_2} \right)$$

$$= \frac{1}{n_1 - m_1} \left\{ \hat{\pi}_1(1 - \hat{\pi}_1)\sqrt{\frac{q_1}{p_1}} + \hat{\pi}_2(1 - \hat{\pi}_2)\sqrt{\frac{p_1}{q_1}} \right\}^2$$

$$+ \frac{1}{n_2 - m_2} \left\{ \hat{\pi}_1(1 - \hat{\pi}_1)\sqrt{\frac{q_2}{p_2}} + \hat{\pi}_2(1 - \hat{\pi}_2)\sqrt{\frac{p_2}{q_2}} \right\}^2.$$

$$(16.6)$$

In our numerical example, $p_1 = 0.6$, $q_1 = 0.4$, $p_2 = 0.2$, $q_2 = 0.8$, $n_1 = 130$, $n_2 = 70$, $f_1 = 130/200 = 0.65$, $f_2 = 70/200 = 0.35$, $\bar{p} = (0.65)(0.6) + (0.35)(0.2) = 0.46$, $\bar{q} = (0.65)(0.4) + (0.35)(0.8) = 0.54$, $\hat{\pi}_1 = (0.65)(0.6)/0.46 = \frac{39}{46}$, $\hat{\pi}_2 = (0.65)(0.4)/0.54 = \frac{13}{27}$. Then $\widehat{\text{Var}}(\hat{\pi}_1) = 0.001554$, $\widehat{\text{Var}}(\hat{\pi}_2) = 0.002182$, $\widehat{\text{Cov}}(\hat{\pi}_1, \hat{\pi}_2) = -0.001288$, and $\widehat{\text{Var}}(\hat{\pi}_1 - \hat{\pi}_2) = 0.006312$.

Note how expression (16.6) increases as m_1 and m_2 increase, reflecting the additional uncertainty in $\hat{\pi}_1 - \hat{\pi}_2$ as the missingness increases. Note also that the estimated variance of $\hat{\pi}_1 - \hat{\pi}_2$, 0.006312, is about 70% larger than the estimated variance would be if the imputed data had actually been observed:

$$\frac{(a_o + \hat{a}_m)(c_o + \hat{c}_m)}{(a_o + \hat{a}_m + c_o + \hat{c}_m)^3} + \frac{(b_o + \hat{b}_m)(d_o + \hat{d}_m)}{(b_o + \hat{b}_m + d_o + \hat{d}_m)^3} = \frac{\hat{\pi}_1(1 - \hat{\pi}_1)}{(n_1 + n_2)\bar{p}} + \frac{\hat{\pi}_2(1 - \hat{\pi}_2)}{(n_1 + n_2)\bar{q}}$$

$$= \frac{(78)(14)}{92^3} + \frac{(52)(56)}{108^3}$$

$$= 0.003714.$$

16.3. DATA MISSING AT RANDOM IN SEVERAL 2 × 2 TABLES

Let C be a stratification variable with K levels. We assume there is a common odds ratio ω between S and H across the levels of C and our goal is to estimate ω. As discussed in Chapters 10 and 11, there are two widely used estimators of the common odds ratio, the maximum likelihood estimator and the Mantel-Haenszel estimator. Here we focus on the Mantel-Haenszel odds ratio; the next section covers maximum likelihood estimation in logistic regression models with incomplete data, which we can apply to the K 2×2 tables.

16.3.1. Complete Record, Weighting, and Imputation Methods for the Mantel-Haenszel Estimator, and Variance Estimation by the Jackknife

When either the exposure or outcome variable is MAR, the Mantel-Haenszel odds ratio based on complete records is consistent. When the stratifying variable is MAR, the complete record estimator is not consistent and one must turn to imputation or weighting methods.

Missing Exposure or Outcome
Suppose H is partially missing, but S and C are completely observed. Let R_H be the observation indicator for H. Table 16.12 replicates Table 16.9 for each table $i = 1, \ldots, K$.

When there are no missing data, the Mantel-Haenszel odds ratio

$$\hat{\omega}_{MH} = \frac{\sum_{i=1}^{K} a_i d_i / n_i}{\sum_{i=1}^{K} b_i c_i / n_i}$$

is the solution of the unbiased estimating equation

$$\sum_{i=1}^{K} \frac{a_i d_i - \omega b_i c_i}{n_i} = 0$$

Table 16.12. *Notation for complete and incomplete portions of several 2 × 2 tables*

		(a) Complete Table					(b) Incomplete Table		
		H					H		
		1	0	Total			1	0	Total
S	1	a_{oi}	b_{oi}	$a_{oi} + b_{oi}$	S	1	a_{mi}	b_{mi}	m_{1i}
	0	c_{oi}	d_{oi}	$c_{oi} + d_{oi}$		0	c_{mi}	d_{mi}	m_{2i}
	Total	$a_{oi} + c_{oi}$	$b_{oi} + d_{oi}$	n_{oi}		Total	$a_{mi} + c_{mi}$	$b_{mi} + d_{mi}$	n_{mi}

(see Section 15.5.1 for the basic theory of estimating equations). Using complete records only, the analogous estimating equation

$$\sum_{i=1}^{K} \frac{a_{oi}d_{oi} - \omega b_{oi}c_{oi}}{n_{oi}} = 0 \qquad (16.7)$$

is unbiased if the left-hand side has zero expectation. We demonstrate this as follows. In each table, the rows are conditionally independent given $n_{1i} = a_{oi} + b_{oi} + m_{1i}$ and $n_{2i} = c_{oi} + d_{oi} + m_{2i}$. Conditioning further on the observed sums $a_{oi} + b_{oi} = n_{1i} - m_{1i}$ and $c_{oi} + d_{oi} = n_{2i} - m_{2i}$, we have

$$E\left(\frac{a_{oi}d_{oi} - \omega b_{oi}c_{oi}}{n_{oi}} \middle| n_{i1}, n_{i2}, a_{oi} + b_{oi}, c_{oi} + d_{oi} \right)$$

$$= \frac{(n_{1i} - m_{1i})(n_{2i} - m_{2i})}{n_{oi}} (P_{1i}Q_{2i} - \omega Q_{1i}P_{2i}),$$

where $P_{1i} = P(H = 1 | S = 1, C = i, R_H = 1) = 1 - Q_{1i}$ and $P_{2i} = P(H = 1 | S = 0, C = i, R_H = 1) = 1 - Q_{2i}$. Under MAR, $P_{1i} = P(H = 1 | S = 1, C = i)$ and $P_{2i} = P(H = 1 | S = 0, C = i)$, so the factor $P_{1i}Q_{2i} - \omega Q_{1i}P_{2i}$ equals zero by definition of ω. Thus, unconditionally, each term in the sum of (16.7) has zero expectation.

It follows that the complete-record Mantel-Haenszel odds ratio is consistent when H is MAR. A symmetric argument can be applied when the roles of H and S are reversed.

Alternatively, we can obtain a Mantel-Haenszel-type estimate by imputation. For each table $i = 1, \ldots, K$, let the observed data be denoted by $O_i = (a_{oi}, b_{oi}, c_{oi}, d_{oi}, m_{1i}, m_{2i})$ with $n_i = a_{oi} + b_{oi} + c_{oi} + d_{oi} + m_{1i} + m_{2i} = n_{1i} + n_{2i} = n_{oi} + n_{mi}$. When data are missing, we wish to use the unbiased estimating equation

$$\sum_{i=1}^{K} \frac{\begin{aligned}[\{a_{oi} + E(a_{mi}|O_i)\}\{d_{oi} + E(d_{mi}|O_i)\} \\ - \omega\{b_{oi} + E(b_{mi}|O_i)\}\{c_{oi} + E(c_{mi}|O_i)\}]\end{aligned}}{n_i} = 0,$$

whose solution is

$$\hat{\omega} = \frac{\sum_{i=1}^{K} \dfrac{\{a_{oi} + E(a_{mi}|O_i)\}\{d_{oi} + E(d_{mi}|O_i)\}}{n_i}}{\sum_{i=1}^{K} \dfrac{\{b_{oi} + E(b_{mi}|O_i)\}\{c_{oi} + E(c_{mi}|O_i)\}}{n_i}}, \qquad (16.8)$$

so we need to estimate the expected values of the missing cell counts. As in the case of a single fourfold table, there are two estimators for these counts. For the upper left-hand cell, the estimators are (i) $\hat{a}_{mi}^{(1)} = n_{mi} a_{oi}/n_{oi}$ and (ii) $\hat{a}_{mi}^{(2)} = m_{1i} a_{oi}/(a_{oi} + b_{oi})$. Estimator (i) is consistent if

$$P(S, H|C, R_H = 1) = P(S, H|C, R_H = 0) = P(S, H|C),$$

which holds if the missingness is independent of both S and H given C, or, equivalently, if

$$P(R_H|C, S, H) = P(R_H|C),$$

i.e., if the missingness is MCAR, in which case the individual cell probabilities $P(S, H|C)$ are estimated consistently using the completely observed records. The estimated conditional expectation of the total cell count a_i becomes

$$\hat{E}(a_i|O_i) = a_{oi} + \hat{a}_{mi}^{(1)} = a_{oi}(1 + n_{mi}/n_{oi}) = a_{oi}n_i/n_{oi},$$

and, on estimating the other conditional expectations similarly, equation (16.8) reduces to

$$\hat{\omega}^{(1)} = \frac{\displaystyle\sum_{i=1}^{K} \frac{\{a_{oi} + \hat{a}_{mi}^{(1)}\}\{d_{oi} + \hat{d}_{mi}^{(1)}\}}{n_i}}{\displaystyle\sum_{i=1}^{K} \frac{\{b_{oi} + \hat{b}_{mi}^{(1)}\}\{c_{oi} + \hat{c}_{mi}^{(1)}\}}{n_i}} = \frac{\displaystyle\sum_{i=1}^{K} \frac{a_{oi}d_{oi}}{n_i^{\#}}}{\displaystyle\sum_{i=1}^{K} \frac{b_{oi}c_{oi}}{n_i^{\#}}}, \tag{16.9}$$

where $n_i^{\#} = n_{oi}^2/n_i$.

Estimator (ii) is consistent if

$$P(H|S, C, R_H = 1) = P(H|S, C, R_H = 0) = P(H|S, C),$$

which holds if the missingness is independent of H given S and C, or, equivalently, if

$$P(R_H|S, C, H) = P(R_H|S, C),$$

that is, H is MAR, in which case only the row probabilities $P(H|S, C)$ can be estimated consistently from the complete records. The estimated conditional expectation of the total cell count a_i is

$$\hat{E}(a_i|O_i) = a_{oi} + \hat{a}_{mi}^{(2)} = a_{oi}\left(1 + \frac{m_{1i}}{a_{oi} + b_{oi}}\right) = a_{oi}\frac{n_{1i}}{n_{1i} - m_{1i}},$$

and estimating the other conditional expectations similarly, we obtain

$$
\hat{\omega}^{(2)} = \frac{\sum_{i=1}^{K} \dfrac{\{a_{oi} + \hat{a}_{mi}^{(2)}\}\{d_{oi} + \hat{d}_{mi}^{(2)}\}}{n_i}}{\sum_{i=1}^{K} \dfrac{\{b_{oi} + \hat{b}_{mi}^{(2)}\}\{c_{oi} + \hat{c}_{mi}^{(2)}\}}{n_i}} = \frac{\sum_{i=1}^{K} \dfrac{a_{oi} d_{oi}}{n_i^*}}{\sum_{i=1}^{K} \dfrac{b_{oi} c_{oi}}{n_i^*}}, \tag{16.10}
$$

where $n_i^* = n_i(n_{1i} - m_{1i})(n_{2i} - m_{2i})/(n_{1i} n_{2i})$.

An unbiased estimating equation can also be constructed using the method of weighting by the inverse probability of missingness. The equation is

$$
\sum_{i=1}^{K} \Biggl\{ \frac{\dfrac{a_{oi}}{P(R_H = 1 \mid S = 1, H = 1, C = i)} \cdot \dfrac{d_{oi}}{P(R_H = 1 \mid S = 0, H = 0, C = i)}}{n_i}
$$

$$
- \omega \frac{\dfrac{b_{oi}}{P(R_H = 1 \mid S = 1, H = 0, C = i)} \cdot \dfrac{c_{oi}}{P(R_H = 1 \mid S = 0, H = 1, C = i)}}{n_i} \Biggr\}.
$$

$$\tag{16.11}$$

Under MCAR, $P(R_H = 1 \mid S, H, C) = P(R_H = 1 \mid C)$, so the solution to (16.11) is

$$
\hat{\omega}(P^{(1)}) = \frac{\sum_{i=1}^{K} \dfrac{a_{oi} d_{oi}/n_i}{\{P(R_H = 1 \mid C = i)\}^2}}{\sum_{i=1}^{K} \dfrac{b_{oi} c_{oi}/n_i}{\{P(R_H = 1 \mid C = i)\}^2}},
$$

where $P^{(1)}$ is the vector of probabilities $P(R_H = 1 \mid C = i)$ for $i = 1, \ldots, K$. Estimating the vector of $P(R_H = 1 \mid C = i)$ by $\hat{P}^{(1)} = n_{oi}/n_i$ and replacing $P^{(1)}$ by $\hat{P}^{(1)}$ in $\hat{\omega}(P^{(1)})$, we conclude that the weighting estimator of the odds ratio $\hat{\omega}(\hat{P}^{(1)})$ is identical to the imputation estimate (16.9).

Under MAR, $P(R_H = 1 \mid S, H, C) = P(R_H = 1 \mid S, C)$, so the solution to (16.11) is

$$
\hat{\omega}(P^{(2)}) = \frac{\sum_{i=1}^{K} \dfrac{a_{oi} d_{oi}/n_i}{P(R_H = 1 \mid S = 1, C = i) P(R_H = 1 \mid S = 0, C = i)}}{\sum_{i=1}^{K} \dfrac{b_{oi} c_{oi}/n_i}{P(R_H = 1 \mid S = 1, C = i) P(R_H = 1 \mid S = 0, C = i)}},
$$

where $P^{(2)}$ is the vector of probabilities $P(R_H = 1 \mid S = j, C = i)$ for $j = 0, 1$ and $i = 1, \ldots, K$. Estimating the vector of $P(R_H = 1 \mid S = j, C = i)$ by $\hat{P}^{(2)} = \{(n_{ji} - m_{ji})/n_{ji}\}$ and replacing $P^{(2)}$ by $\hat{P}^{(2)}$ in $\hat{\omega}(P^{(2)})$, we conclude that the weighting estimator of the odds ratio $\hat{\omega}(\hat{P}^{(2)})$ is identical to the imputation estimate (16.10).

We note that the use of n_i in (16.11) is in accord with the idea of blowing up the observed data that characterizes the weighting method. One could also use n_{oi} instead, and doing so simplifies calculation of the variance of the estimated log odds ratio, which we next consider. In that case, $n_i^{\#}$ in (16.9) is replaced by $n_{oi}^{\#} = n_{oi}^3/n_i^2$, and n_i^* in (16.10) is replaced by $n_{oi}^* = n_{oi}(n_{1i} - m_{1i})(n_{2i} - m_{2i})/(n_{1i}n_{2i})$.

Variance Estimation
With P denoting $P^{(1)}$ under MCAR or $P^{(2)}$ under MAR, and $\hat{P}$ denoting $\hat{P}^{(1)}$ or $\hat{P}^{(2)}$, $\hat{\omega}(\hat{P})$ is given approximately by

$$\hat{\omega}(\hat{P}) \approx \hat{\omega}(P) + (\hat{P} - P)' \frac{\partial \hat{\omega}(P)}{\partial P}. \tag{16.12}$$

It can be shown that when n_{oi} is used in estimating equation (16.11) instead of n_i, $E\{\partial \hat{\omega}(P)/\partial P\}$ is approximately zero, and that there are only negligible contributions to the total variance of the estimate due to the variance of the second term and the covariance between the first and second terms in (16.12). Then the variance of $\ln \hat{\omega}(\hat{P})$ is estimated by formula (10.58) for the standard Mantel-Haenszel odds ratio after replacing R_i, S_i, P_i, and Q_i by R_i^*, S_i^*, P_i^*, and Q_i^*, respectively, where $R_i^* = a_{oi}d_{oi}/n_{oi}^*$, $S_i^* = b_{oi}c_{oi}/n_{oi}^*$, $P_i^* = (a_{oi} + d_{oi})/n_{oi}^*$, and $Q_i^* = (b_{oi} + c_{oi})/n_{oi}^*$.

The variance of the imputation estimate [equal to the weighting estimate using (16.11) with n_i] cannot be obtained in the same way, because the corresponding derivatives in (16.12) do not have zero expectation. The method of Problem 16.2 can be used, but is complicated. Instead, we indicate how to use the *jackknife* technique to estimate $\mathrm{Var}(\ln \hat{\omega}^{(1)})$ or $\mathrm{Var}(\ln \hat{\omega}^{(2)})$. The jackknife deletes one independent record at a time, each time recalculating the quantities of interest, called *delete-one* statistics. The jackknife variance estimate is then the sum of squared differences between the delete-one statistics and the overall estimate.

When all records are completely observed in a 2×2 table, the asymptotic variance of the sample log odds ratio $\ln(ad/bc)$ is estimated by $(1/a) + (1/b) + (1/c) + (1/d)$. If a record from the upper left-hand cell is deleted, then the log odds ratio becomes $\ln\{(a - 1)d/(bc)\}$ and the contribution to the jackknife variance estimate is

$$\left(\ln \frac{(a - 1)d}{bc} - \ln \frac{ad}{bc} \right)^2 = \left\{ \ln\left(1 - \frac{1}{a}\right) \right\}^2.$$

Repeating the argument for deletion of records from other cells, the jackknife variance estimate is expressible in closed form as

$$a\left\{\ln\left(1-\frac{1}{a}\right)\right\}^2 + b\left\{\ln\left(1-\frac{1}{b}\right)\right\}^2 + c\left\{\ln\left(1-\frac{1}{c}\right)\right\}^2 + d\left\{\ln\left(1-\frac{1}{d}\right)\right\}^2.$$

Note that when cell counts are large, $\ln\{1-(1/a)\} \approx 1/a$, and the jackknife estimate approaches the asymptotic variance $(1/a)+(1/b)+(1/c)+(1/d)$.

The jackknife variance estimate for the imputation log Mantel-Haenszel odds ratio $\ln\hat{\omega}^{(1)}$ or $\ln\hat{\omega}^{(2)}$ is calculated in similar fashion, each time deleting one of the $n_1 + \cdots + n_K$ records and recalculating the delete-one log odds ratios from (16.9) or (16.10). The equivalence of the variance estimate to a known asymptotic variance formula has yet to be verified. However, simulation studies by the authors have shown that the jackknife estimate provides nominal error rates and coverage probabilities under a variety of conditions.

Missing Stratifying Variable

Now suppose that S and H are completely observed but that C is missing for some records, so that the tables into which to cross-classify S and H are unknown. The margins m_{1i} and m_{2i} in Table 16.12(b) are now individually unknown, although we know each cell of the pooled missing data as in Table 16.13(b). The observed data vectors are now $O_i = (a_{oi}, b_{oi}, c_{oi}, d_{oi}, a_{m+}, b_{m+}, c_{m+}, d_{m+})$ for $i = 1, \ldots, K$.

C is missing at random if the observation indicator R_C is conditionally independent of C given S and H, so that the missingness of C may depend on S or H or both, but not on the missing value of C. If the missingness depends on both S and H, the complete record Mantel-Haenszel odds ratio is not consistent for any table, because $E(a_{oi}d_{oi} - \omega b_{oi}c_{oi}) \neq 0$. If the missingness does not depend on both S and H, for example, if R_C is independent of (C, S) given H, or if R_C is independent of (C, H) given S, then the complete record Mantel-Haenszel odds ratio is consistent. However, statistical efficiency is lost, as illustrated below.

The following imputation estimator corrects the bias when the complete record odds ratio is biased, and improves efficiency when the complete record odds ratio is unbiased. The imputation Mantel-Haenszel odds ratio

Table 16.13. *Pooled data obtained by summing Tables 16.12 for $i = 1, \ldots, K$*

		(a) Complete Table					(b) Incomplete Table		
		H					H		
		1	0	Total			1	0	Total
S	1	a_{o+}	b_{o+}	$a_{o+}+b_{o+}$	S	1	a_{m+}	b_{m+}	m_{1+}
	0	c_{o+}	d_{o+}	$c_{o+}+d_{o+}$		0	c_{m+}	d_{m+}	m_{2+}
	Total	$a_{o+}+c_{o+}$	$b_{o+}+d_{o+}$	n_{o+}		Total	$a_{m+}+c_{m+}$	$b_{m+}+d_{m+}$	n_{m+}

has the same form as (16.8), but the conditional expectations are different. We estimate these by

$$\hat{E}(a_{mi}|O_i) = a_{m+}\frac{a_{oi}}{a_{o+}},$$

$$\hat{E}(b_{mi}|O_i) = b_{m+}\frac{b_{oi}}{b_{o+}},$$

$$\hat{E}(c_{mi}|O_i) = c_{m+}\frac{c_{oi}}{c_{o+}},$$

$$\hat{E}(d_{mi}|O_i) = d_{m+}\frac{d_{oi}}{d_{o+}}.$$

The resulting estimator is

$$\hat{\omega} = \frac{\displaystyle\sum_{i=1}^{K} a_{oi}d_{oi}/n_{1i}^*}{\displaystyle\sum_{i=1}^{K} b_{oi}c_{oi}/n_{2i}^*},$$

where

$$n_{1i}^* = \hat{n}_i \frac{a_{o+}}{a_{mi}+a_{o+}} \cdot \frac{d_{o+}}{d_{m+}+d_{o+}},$$

$$n_{2i}^* = \hat{n}_i \frac{b_{o+}}{b_{mi}+b_{o+}} \cdot \frac{c_{o+}}{c_{m+}+c_{o+}},$$

and

$$\hat{n}_i = n_{oi} + \hat{E}(a_{mi}|O_i) + \hat{E}(b_{mi}|O_i) + \hat{E}(c_{mi}|O_i) + \hat{E}(d_{mi}|O_i).$$

Note that $n_{1i}^*/\hat{n}_i$ and $n_{2i}^*/\hat{n}_i$ are estimators of $P(R_C = 1|S = 1, H = 1) \cdot P(R_C = 1|S = 0, H = 0)$ and $P(R_C = 1|S = 1, H = 0) \cdot P(R_C = 1|S = 0, H = 1)$ respectively, so that the weighting estimate has the same form as the imputation estimate. If n_{oi} is used instead of n_i for the weighting estimate, we replace n_{1i}^* and n_{2i}^* with

$$n_{o1i}^* = n_{oi} \frac{a_{o+}}{a_{m+}+a_{o+}} \cdot \frac{d_{o+}}{d_{m+}+d_{o+}}$$

and

$$n_{o2i}^* = n_{oi} \frac{b_{o+}}{b_{m+}+b_{o+}} \cdot \frac{c_{o+}}{c_{m+}+c_{o+}},$$

respectively.

Table 16.14. *Hypothetical data for two 2 × 2 tables*

R_H	S	H	C	Frequencies
1	1	1	1	12
1	1	1	0	18
1	1	0	1	25
1	1	0	0	19
1	0	1	1	8
1	0	1	0	11
1	0	0	1	13
1	0	0	0	17
0	1	?	1	29
0	1	?	0	25
0	0	?	1	10
0	0	?	0	13
				200

Explicit variance formulas are even more elaborate than those in the missing-exposure case, because the terms across the stratifying variables are correlated. Further research is needed to confirm whether or not the jackknife technique is consistent in this case.

Example 16.3.1. To illustrate the imputation Mantel-Haenszel odds ratio $\hat{\omega}^{(2)}$ and weighting counterpart, consider Table 16.14, in which H is partially missing and S and C are completely observed. Table 16.15 shows the data in the layout of Table 16.12.

The complete-record Mantel-Haenszel odds ratio from Table 16.15(a) is 1.110, with log odds ratio 0.1045 and variance 0.1428 from (10.58), yielding a 95% confidence interval for ω of (0.529, 2.328). The jackknife variance estimate of the complete record log odds ratio is 0.1503, with corresponding 95% confidence interval (0.519, 2.373) for ω.

For the weighting odds ratio using n_{oi}, we have $n_{o1}^* = 22.026$, $n_{o2}^* = 26.49$, and $\hat{\omega}(\hat{P}^{(2)}) = 1.098$ with logarithm 0.0935. The modified version of the asymptotic variance (10.58) is 0.1429, yielding a 95% confidence interval for ω of (0.523, 2.303), while the jackknife variance estimate is 0.1535, with corresponding 95% confidence interval (0.509, 2.366) for ω.

For the imputation odds ratio, we have $n_1^* = 36.84$, $n_2^* = 41.98$, and $\hat{\omega}^{(2)} = 1.107$. The jackknife variance estimate is 0.1520 yielding a 95% confidence interval for ω of (0.516, 2.377).

To illustrate the case of a missing stratifying variable, we present the results of a small simulation experiment (200 replications) in which the stratifying variable C is MAR. Two missingness conditions are illustrated: (i) R_C depends on both S and H, but not C: logit $\{P(R_C = 1|S, H, C)\} = -1 + 2S + 2SH$; and (ii) R_C is independent of C and H given S: logit $\{P(R_C = 1|S, H, C)\} = -1 + 2S$. The underlying mechanism generating S

Table 16.15. *Complete and incomplete portions of Table 16.14*

$C = 1$

		(a) Complete Table					(b) Incomplete Table		
		H					*H*		
		1	0	Total			1	0	Total
S	1	12	25	37	*S*	1	?	?	29
	0	8	13	21		0	?	?	10
	Total	20	38	58		Total	?	?	39

$C = 0$

		(a) Complete Table					(b) Incomplete Table		
		H					*H*		
		1	0	Total			1	0	Total
S	1	18	19	37	*S*	1	?	?	25
	0	11	17	28		0	?	?	13
	Total	29	36	65		Total	?	?	38

given H and C is logit $\{P(S = 1 | H, C)\} = -1 + H + C$, so that the true log odds ratio between S and H is 1. Here C has two levels, and the conditional distribution of C given H is $P(C = 1 | H) = 0.2 + 0.6H$, with $P(H = 1) = 0.5$.

Table 16.16 gives results for four estimates: (a) full data (for comparison—missing data precludes use of the full data estimate in practice), (b) complete record, (c) imputation, and (d) weighting. The table also shows the simulation mean squared error for each estimate. The results show that the imputation and weighting estimates correct the bias incurred by complete record analysis under condition (i), and improve efficiency under condition (ii).

Table 16.16. *Simulation results for four estimators of the log odds ratio between S and H with a missing stratifying variable C under two different MAR missingness conditions*

Method	(i) R_C Depends on Both S and H		(ii) R_C is Independent of H Given S	
	Mean Point Estimate	Mean Squared Error	Mean Point Estimate	Mean Squared Error
(a) Full data	1.0026	0.0441	1.0026	0.0441
(b) Complete record	1.2905	0.1966	1.0260	0.1145
(c) Imputation	0.9936	0.0639	0.9975	0.0647
(d) Weighting	1.0108	0.0691	1.0112	0.0669

16.3.2. Multiple Imputation

Single imputation as presented in the preceding sections produces consistent point estimates under appropriate MCAR or MAR assumptions. Naive application of standard error formulas for complete data, however, does not produce accurate estimates of the true uncertainty. To obtain valid standard errors requires special methods like the jackknife or those presented in Section 16.2.2 or Problem 16.2. The multiple imputation technique of Rubin (1976) also provides valid standard errors. Rubin (1987) provides formulas for these, together with estimates of the amount of information lost due to missingness.

The key idea of multiple imputation is to generate each missing value repeatedly while mimicking the actual variation that might have been observed in the data had they not been missing. Repeating the imputations in this way allows one to gauge how sensitive the results are to imputation, and thereby to provide valid standard errors. For each of, say, m^* repeated imputations, after the data sets have been *completed* by pooling the observed and imputed data, ordinary point estimates and standard errors are prepared. The multiple imputation point estimate is then the average of the m^* ordinary point estimates, and the multiple imputation standard error is given by formula (16.16) below. We note that the term "multiple" derives from imputing data repeatedly, not from the possible use of a multiple regression model to generate the imputed values. "Repeated imputation" is an apt description of the procedure.

For 2×2 tables it would appear plausible to generate the missing cell a_m as a binomial random variable with index m_1 and parameter $p_1 = a_o / (a_o + b_o)$. This imputation underestimates the true uncertainty, however, because it ignores the fact that p_1 is itself an estimate, not the true probability $P_1 = P(H = 1 | S = 1)$. This defect is corrected as follows.

Rubin originally proposed multiple imputation in the context of a fully Bayesian analysis, and suggested imputing the missing data by first sampling parameter values from their posterior distribution given the observed data, and then generating the missing data randomly from distributions governed by the sampled parameters. For 2×2 tables, this involves sampling a value P_1^* from the posterior distribution of P_1 and then generating a binomial random variable a_m^* with index m_1 and parameter P_1^*. The value c_m^* is imputed similarly by sampling P_2^* from the posterior distribution of $P_2 = P(H = 1 | S = 0)$ and generating c_m^* as $\text{Bin}(m_2, P_2^*)$. Setting $b_m^* = m_1 - a_m^*$ and $d_m^* = m_2 - c_m^*$ completes one imputation of the missing data. The completed table with cells $a_o + a_m^*$, $b_o + b_m^*$, etc. is used to estimate the log odds ratio, say, together with its standard error. The entire process is then repeated m^* times. The additional variation introduced by using randomly generated P_1^* and P_2^* corrects for the fact that p_j is an estimate of P_j.

For example, suppose that *a priori* (before observation of the data), P_1 has a beta distribution with parameters α_0 and β_0 (see Section 9.6.4 for a definition of the beta distribution). Then *a posteriori* (after observation of a_o

and b_o), P_1 has a beta distribution with parameters $\alpha_1 = a_o + \alpha_0$ and $\beta_1 = b_o + \beta_0$. Because the conditional distribution of the imputed value of the missing cell, a_m^*, is $\text{Bin}(m_1, P_1^*)$ given $P_1 = P_1^*$, the marginal distribution of a_m^* is beta-binomial, with mean $Ea_m^* = m_1 \alpha_1 / (\alpha_1 + \beta_1) = m_1 \pi_1$, say, with $\pi_1 = \alpha_1 / (\alpha_1 + \beta_1)$, and variance given by

$$\text{Var}(a_m^*) = m_1 \pi_1 (1 - \pi_1)\{1 + (m_1 - 1) D^2\} \qquad (16.13)$$

where

$$D^2 = \frac{\text{Var}(P_1^*)}{\pi_1(1 - \pi_1)} = \frac{1}{\alpha_1 + \beta_1 + 1}$$

$$= \frac{1}{a_o + b_o + \alpha_0 + \beta_0 + 1} = \frac{1}{n_1 - m_1 + \alpha_0 + \beta_0 + 1}. \qquad (16.14)$$

D^2 represents additional variation due to uncertainty in P_1. When the observed sample size $a_o + b_o = n_1 - m_1$ is large compared to α_0 and β_0, π_1 approaches p_1, so we are essentially sampling a_m^* with mean $m_1 p_1$ as if a_m^* were binomial, but with a variance inflation factor $1 + (m_1 - 1)D^2$ approaching $1 + (m_1 - 1)/(n_1 - m_1) = (n_1 - 1)/(n_1 - m_1)$. If the number of missing records m_1 is a small fraction of n_1, the imputation distribution is essentially binomial; if m_1 is a nonzero fraction of n_1, the imputations have greater-than-binomial variance.

Rubin and Schenker (1986) proposed a simple alternative technique called the *approximate Bayesian bootstrap*. This method generates P_1^* as the sample proportion from a bootstrap sample drawn from the observed set of a_o ones and b_o zeros. A *bootstrap sample* is generally drawn *with* replacement after each draw of a record from the observed set of data. Generating parameters by bootstrap sampling, and using these to govern the distributions for imputing missing data, also appropriately reflects uncertainty in the unknown parameters.

For 2 × 2 tables, the bootstrap generates P_1^* as a scaled binomial random variable with mean p_1 and variance $p_1 q_1 / (n_1 - m_1)$. Thus the imputed missing cell a_m^* has mean $m_1 p_1$ and variance

$$\text{Var}(a_m^*) = m_1 p_1 (1 - p_1)\{1 + (m_1 - 1) D^2\} \qquad \text{with} \quad D^2 = 1/(n_1 - m_1).$$

In a Bayesian framework, this corresponds to use of an improper beta prior (negative $\alpha_0 + \beta_0 = -1$), but the variance inflation factor is slightly larger than with a proper prior with positive α_0 and β_0. The inflation factor is approximately the same as with a proper prior if $n_1 - m_1$ is large compared to α_0 and β_0. We note that use of a value of D^2 larger than (16.14) is not unreasonable if the MAR assumption itself is questionable, for in that case there is uncertainty attaching to the use of the estimate p_1 to generate a_m^* in the first place, even if the observed sample size is large.

We illustrate the multiple imputation procedure for estimation of the log Mantel-Haenszel odds ratio in several 2×2 tables. Let $\ln \hat{\omega}_{MH}^{(k)}$ denote the standard Mantel-Haenszel log odds ratio from the kth completed data set ($k = 1, \ldots, m^*$), and let s_k^2 denote its nominal estimated variance from (10.58). The multiple imputation point estimate of $\lambda = \ln \omega$ is then the simple average

$$\hat{\lambda} = \frac{1}{m^*} \sum_{k=1}^{m^*} \ln \hat{\omega}_{MH}^{(k)}. \tag{16.15}$$

When m^* is large, (16.15) will be close to the imputation estimates presented earlier.

The multiple imputation variance of the point estimate is obtained by combining within- and between-imputation components of variance:

$$\widehat{\text{Var}}(\hat{\lambda}) = \left\{ \frac{1}{m^*} \sum_{k=1}^{m^*} s_k^2 \right\} + \left(1 - \frac{1}{m^*} \right) \left\{ \frac{1}{m^* - 1} \sum_{k=1}^{m^*} \left(\ln \hat{\omega}_{MH}^{(k)} - \hat{\lambda} \right)^2 \right\}. \tag{16.16}$$

The first term estimates the expected value of $\text{Var}(\ln \hat{\omega}_{MH}^{(k)})$ over the imputation distribution for the missing data. The factor in braces in the second term estimates how variable the completed data point estimates are due to the imputation of the missing data. The leading factor is a correction for bias when m^* is small.

The simplicity of Rubin's variance formula (16.16) is the reward earned only after careful and often laborious imputation of the missing data. A problem arises, however, with the use of (16.16) for the particular application to the Mantel-Haenszel estimate of the odds ratio which we discuss at the end of the section.

For imputing the missing data of Table 16.15, we use the approximate Bayesian bootstrap. The first step is to draw m^* bootstrap samples to generate P_{ji}^* for each table ($i = 1$ and 2 for $C = 1$ and 0, respectively) and each row ($j = 1$ and 2 for $S = 1$ and 0, respectively). For each repetition $k = 1, \ldots, m^*$ this may be accomplished by generating four binomial random variables $B_{ji}^{(k)}$, with indices 37, 21, 37, and 28, as per the observed margins $n_{ji} - m_{ji}$, and with parameters $p_{11} = \frac{12}{37}$, $p_{21} = \frac{8}{21}$, $p_{12} = \frac{18}{37}$, and $p_{22} = \frac{11}{28}$, respectively, and then dividing by the corresponding observed margins. Once the binomial parameters $P_{ji}^{*(k)}$ are generated for each k, an independent binomial random variable is generated for each of a_{m1}, c_{m1}, a_{m2}, and c_{m2}, with sample sizes $m_{11} = 29$, $m_{21} = 10$, $m_{12} = 25$, and $m_{22} = 13$, respectively. These are used to complete the data sets, and the Mantel-Haenszel log odds ratios $\ln \hat{\omega}_{MH}^{(k)}$ and variance estimates s_k^2 are calculated.

Using $m^* = 25$, the mean log odds ratio in one calculation was 0.08294, which is the multiple imputation point estimate $\hat{\lambda}$ in (16.15). This corresponds to an odds ratio estimate of $\exp(0.08294) = 1.086$, slightly less than the single imputation and weighting estimates from the previous section. The mean of the 25 variance estimates s_k^2 was 0.09180, which is the first term of (16.16). The sample variance of the 25 log odds ratios was 0.02876, and multiplying by the leading factor $1 - 1/m^* = 0.96$ provides the second term, 0.02761. Summing, the multiple imputation variance estimate is 0.1194, and taking the square root yields the multiple imputation standard error 0.3456. A 95% confidence interval for ω is given by $\exp(0.08294 \pm 1.96 \times 0.3456) = (0.552, 2.139)$.

The multiple imputation variance estimate is about 20% smaller than the jackknife estimates obtained in the previous section (0.12 versus 0.15). Comparing the excess of the jackknife variance over the mean complete data variance [i.e., the first term of (16.16)], $0.15 - 0.092 = 0.058$, with the excess of the multiple imputation variance over the mean complete data variance, $0.12 - 0.092 = 0.028$, shows that the jackknife corresponds roughly to the use of a beta prior in the multiple imputation procedure with variance inflation factor about twice as large as that of the approximate Bayesian bootstrap.

Robins and Wang (2000) study the consistency of the multiple imputation variance formula (16.16) when the ordinary point estimates are solutions of an estimating equation and derive a general variance formula which differs from (16.16). The difference vanishes when the estimating equation is a score function (so that the ordinary point estimates are maximum likelihood estimates). In general, however, the difference is nonzero because the negative derivative of an estimating function is not its variance (whereas the negative derivative of a score function is its variance). The difference is often positive, in which case the variance given by (16.16) is conservative, but positivity is not guaranteed in all cases. Our example of the Mantel-Haenszel log odds ratio, which is not a maximum likelihood estimate, illustrates this point. It would appear prudent, then, to avoid using (16.16) for the Mantel-Haenszel log odds ratio. The single imputation method of Section 16.3.1 with the jackknife variance estimate is preferred.

16.4.* LOGISTIC REGRESSION WHEN COVARIATES ARE MISSING AT RANDOM

Another way to estimate the common odds ratio underlying several 2×2 tables is to use logistic regression, which can also handle more general situations (Chapter 11). In this section, we consider the problem of missing data when there are two explanatory factors, one of which has missing data. Extension to the case of many covariates, only one of which has missing values, is straightforward. If more than one covariate has missing values, extensions become complicated, requiring multivariate regression models (Section 15.5).

Let Y_i be a binary response indicating whether or not the ith subject has an event. Let X_i be a binary covariate with missing values. Let Z_i be a vector of completely observed covariates. With $P(X_i, Z_i)$ denoting $P(Y_i = 1 | X_i, Z_i)$, we assume that

$$\ln \frac{P(X_i, Z_i)}{1 - P(X_i, Z_i)} = \beta_0 + \beta_X X_i + \beta_Z Z_i, \tag{16.17}$$

where $\beta = (\beta_0, \beta_X, \beta_Z)'$ contains the unknown parameters of interest. Let R_i be the observation indicator for X_i. If no data are missing, the likelihood function is

$$L = L(\beta | \{X_i\}, \{Y_i\}, \{Z_i\}) = \prod_{i=1}^{n} P(X_i, Z_i)^{Y_i} \{1 - P(X_i, Z_i)\}^{1-Y_i}.$$

The maximum likelihood estimate is obtained by solving

$$\frac{\partial}{\partial \beta} \ln L = \sum_{i=1}^{n} \begin{pmatrix} 1 \\ X_i \\ Z_i \end{pmatrix} \{Y_i - P(X_i, Z_i)\} = 0.$$

We denote the contribution of the ith unit to the score function by u_i:

$$u_i = \begin{pmatrix} 1 \\ X_i \\ Z_i \end{pmatrix} \{Y_i - P(X_i, Z_i)\}.$$

When values of X_i are missing, the corresponding equation using complete records only is

$$U_C = \sum_{i=1}^{n} R_i \begin{pmatrix} 1 \\ X_i \\ Z_i \end{pmatrix} \{Y_i - P(X_i, Z_i)\} = \sum_{i=1}^{n} R_i u_i = 0, \tag{16.18}$$

The solution to equation (16.18) is consistent only if the data are MCAR. If R_i depends on Y_i (MAR) or on X_i given Z_i (NI), the solution for β is not consistent, because $E(U_C) \neq 0$ under either of these conditions.

In this section, we focus on the following MAR case:

$$P(R | Y, X, Z) = P(R | Y, Z).$$

Under this condition,

$$P(X | Y, Z, R = 0) = P(X | Y, Z, R = 1) = P(X | Y, Z). \tag{16.19}$$

For an estimator to be consistent, its estimating function must have expectation zero (Section 15.5). Since U_C has nonzero expectation, we need to adjust the estimating function. There are four approaches to adjustment: (1) likeli-hood analysis (Murphy and Van der Vaart, 2001); (2) imputation, which adds $E(u_i|Y_i, Z_i)$ to U_C if the ith record is incomplete (Pepe and Fleming, 1991; Reilley and Pepe, 1995); (3) weighting, which weights the completely ob-served data by the reciprocal of the probability of observation (Zhao and Lipsitz, 1992); and (4) modeling $P(Y|X, Z, R = 1)$ from the observed data (Wang, 1999). The first two approaches require additional assumptions for either $P(X|Z)$ or $P(X|Y, Z)$. The last two approaches require an additional model assumption for $P(R|X, Y, Z)$. All four approaches have unbiased estimating equations.

Before discussing each approach, we consider the implications of making assumptions about $P(X|Z)$ or $P(X|Y, Z)$. Both the likelihood and the imputation approaches replace missing u_i with an estimate of the conditional mean of u_i given the observed data, $E(u_i|Y_i, Z_i)$. An attractive feature of specifying $P(X|Y, Z)$ is that we can directly estimate $E(u_i|Y_i, Z_i)$. Suppose that $P(X = 1|Y, Z)$ has a linear logistic form, say,

$$\ln \frac{P(X = 1|Y, Z)}{1 - P(X = 1|Y, Z)} = \delta_0 + \delta_Y Y + \delta_Z Z. \tag{16.20}$$

Because equation (16.19) holds under MAR, we obtain a consistent estimate of $\delta = (\delta_0, \delta_Y, \delta_Z)'$ by fitting a logistic regression model with X as the outcome and Y and Z as covariates, using completely observed records only. Substitution of the maximum likelihood estimate of δ in (16.20) produces estimated probabilities $\hat{P}(X_i|Y_i, Z_i)$, and these are used to estimate $E(u_i|Y_i, Z_i)$ for given β:

$$\hat{E}(u_i|Y_i, Z_i) = \hat{P}(X_i = 1|Y_i, Z_i) \begin{pmatrix} 1 \\ 1 \\ Z_i \end{pmatrix} \{Y_i - P(1, Z_i)\}$$

$$+ \hat{P}(X_i = 0|Y_i, Z_i) \begin{pmatrix} 1 \\ 0 \\ Z_i \end{pmatrix} \{Y_i - P(0, Z_i)\}. \tag{16.21}$$

Suppose, alternatively, that $P(X|Z)$ has a prespecified form, such as

$$\ln \frac{P(X = 1|Z)}{1 - P(X = 1|Z)} = \gamma_0 + \gamma_Z Z. \tag{16.22}$$

Then we need an extra step to compute $E(u_i|Y_i, Z_i)$, to wit,

$$E(X_i|Y_i, Z_i) = P(X_i = 1|Y_i, Z_i)$$

$$= \frac{P(Y_i|X_i = 1, Z_i)P(X_i = 1|Z_i)}{\sum_{x=0}^{1} P(Y_i|X_i = x|Z_i)P(X_i = x|Z_i)}. \tag{16.23}$$

A drawback to modeling $P(X|Y, Z)$ is that both $P(Y|X, Z)$ and $P(X|Y, Z)$ specify a relationship between Y and X, generating a potential conflict between the two assumptions (16.17) and (16.20). See Section 14.1. When both linear logistic models are correctly specified, we have $\delta_Y = \beta_X$, by invariance of the odds ratio, but careful analysis requires attention to the goodness of fit of both models.

Likelihood analysis with specification of $P(X|Z)$ instead of $P(X|Y, Z)$ produces a simpler score function and information matrix (discussed below). For this reason, we present the likelihood approach with a model based on $P(X|Z)$. Imputation analysis with specification of $P(X|Y, Z)$ instead of $P(X|Z)$ is simpler because we can use complete records to model $P(X|Y, Z)$, whereas the estimate of γ in (16.22) obtained from complete records is not consistent, because $P(X|Z, R = 0) \neq P(X|Z, R = 1)$. For this reason we present the imputation approach with a model for $P(X|Y, Z)$.

For both $P(X|Z)$ and $P(X|Y, Z)$, we consider the case in which the functional form is known up to a fixed number of unknown parameters. Pepe and Fleming (1991) discuss imputation which requires no parametric assumptions about $P(X|Y, Z)$ when Z is categorical and data are MCAR. Paik (2000) and Murphy and Van der Vaart (2001) consider a likelihood approach under MAR conditions which requires no parametric assumptions about $P(X|Z)$. Here we present a parametric model for $P(X|Z)$ which allows Z to be a continuous or categorical variable.

16.4.1. Likelihood Approach

The likelihood approach involves specifying the joint distribution $P(R, Y, X|Z)$. There are two ways of partitioning the joint distribution: $P(R|Y, X, Z) \cdot P(Y, X|Z)$ (the *selection model*) and $P(Y, X|Z, R) \cdot P(R|Z)$ (the *pattern mixture model*). The parameters of interest in $P(Y, X|Z)$ can be directly estimated in the selection model. The pattern mixture model estimates $P(Y, X|Z, R)$, which must be averaged using $P(R|Z)$ as weights to draw inferences about $P(Y, X|Z)$. Sometimes a pattern mixture model best addresses the question of interest (e.g., Little 1994; Fitzmaurice, Laird, and Shneyer, 2001). Here, however, we focus on the selection model approach.

Likelihood Function and Score Equations
When data are missing, each record's contribution to the likelihood function differs depending on whether or not X_i is observed. If (Y_i, X_i, Z_i) are all observed, the contribution to the likelihood function, conditional on Z_i, is

$$P(R_i = 1, Y_i, X_i|Z_i) = P(R_i = 1|Y_i, X_i, Z_i) \cdot P(Y_i, X_i|Z_i)$$
$$= P(R_i = 1|Y_i, X_i, Z_i) \cdot P(Y_i|X_i, Z_i) \cdot P(X_i|Z_i),$$

which we write as

$$L_{i1} = P(R_i = 1|Y_i, X_i, Z_i)P(X_i|Z_i)$$
$$\times \{P(Y_i = 1|X_i, Z_i)\}^{Y_i}\{1 - P(Y_i = 1|X_i, Z_i)\}^{1-Y_i}.$$

If only (Y_i, Z_i) are observed, the contribution to the likelihood function is

$$P(R_i = 0, Y_i | Z_i) = P(R_i = 0, Y_i, X_i = 1 | Z_i) + P(R_i = 0, Y_i, X_i = 0 | Z_i)$$

$$= P(R_i = 0 | Y_i, X_i = 1, Z_i) \cdot P(Y_i | X_i = 1, Z_i) \cdot P(X_i = 1 | Z_i)$$

$$+ P(R_i = 0 | Y_i, X_i = 0, Z_i) \cdot P(Y_i | X_i = 0, Z_i) \cdot P(X_i = 0 | Z_i),$$

which we write as

$$L_{i2} = \sum_{x=0}^{1} P(R_i = 0 | Y_i, X_i = x, Z_i) P(X_i = x | Z_i)$$

$$\times \{P(Y_i = 1 | X_i = x, Z_i)\}^{Y_i} \{1 - P(Y_i = 1 | X_i = x, Z_i)\}^{1-Y_i}.$$

Combining the contributions from all records, the likelihood function is

$$L = \prod_{i=1}^{n} L_{i1}^{R_i} L_{i2}^{1-R_i}. \tag{16.24}$$

The likelihood function thus comprises three elements: $P(R_i | Y_i, X_i, Z_i)$, $P(Y_i | X_i, Z_i)$, and $P(X_i | Z_i)$. For $P(Y_i | X_i, Z_i)$ and $P(X_i | Z_i)$, we use the models of equation (16.17) and equation (16.22). For the missingness probability, $P(R_i | Y_i, X_i, Z_i)$, we do not need a model specification under MAR: $P(R_i | Y_i, X_i, Z_i)$ equals $P(R_i | Y_i, Z_i)$, which factors out of the summation over x in L_{i2}. Assuming $P(R_i | Y_i, Z_i)$ is parametrically independent of β and γ, the factors involving $P(R_i | Y_i, Z_i)$ do not affect the maximization of the likelihood function over β and γ.

The score equation for β derived from (16.24) has the following form (Problem 16.4):

$$U_\beta = \frac{\partial \ln L}{\partial \beta} = \sum_{i=1}^{n} R_i u_i + (1 - R_i) E(u_i | Y_i, Z_i, R_i = 0)$$

$$= \sum_{i=1}^{n} R_i \begin{pmatrix} Y_i - P(X_i, Z_i) \\ X_i \{Y_i - P(X_i, Z_i)\} \\ Z_i \{Y_i - P(X_i, Z_i)\} \end{pmatrix}$$

$$+ (1 - R_i) \begin{pmatrix} Y_i - E\{P(X_i, Z_i) | Y_i, Z_i, R_i = 0\} \\ E[X_i \{Y_i - P(X_i, Z_i)\} | Y_i, Z_i, R_i = 0] \\ Z_i [Y_i - E\{P(X_i, Z_i) | Y_i, Z_i, R_i = 0\}] \end{pmatrix} = 0. \tag{16.25}$$

The score equation for γ is

$$U_\gamma = \frac{\partial \ln L}{\partial \gamma}$$

$$= \sum_{i=1}^{n} R_i \begin{pmatrix} X_i - \mu_i \\ Z_i(X_i - \mu_i) \end{pmatrix} + (1 - R_i) \begin{pmatrix} E(X_i|Y_i, Z_i, R_i = 0) - \mu_i \\ Z_i\{E(X_i|Y_i, Z_i, R_i = 0) - \mu_i\} \end{pmatrix} = 0,$$

$$(16.26)$$

where $\mu_i = E(X_i|Z_i)$. Note that under MAR mechanisms, equation (16.19) holds and $E(X|Y, Z, R = 0) = E(X|Y, Z)$, so the condition $R = 0$ in the score equations can be dropped. Thus we write

$$U_\beta = \frac{\partial \ln L}{\partial \beta} = \sum_{i=1}^{n} R_i u_i + (1 - R_i) E(u_i|Y_i, Z_i)$$

$$= \sum_{i=1}^{n} R_i \begin{pmatrix} Y_i - P(X_i, Z_i) \\ X_i\{Y_i - P(X_i, Z_i)\} \\ Z_i\{Y_i - P(X_i, Z_i)\} \end{pmatrix}$$

$$+ (1 - R_i) \begin{pmatrix} Y_i - E\{P(X_i, Z_i)|Y_i, Z_i\} \\ E[X_i\{Y_i - P(X_i, Z_i)\}|Y_i, Z_i] \\ Z_i[Y_i - E\{P(X_i, Z_i)|Y_i, Z_i\}] \end{pmatrix} = 0 \qquad (16.27)$$

and

$$U_\gamma = \frac{\partial \ln L}{\partial \gamma} = \sum_{i=1}^{n} R_i \begin{pmatrix} X_i - \mu_i \\ Z_i(X_i - \mu_i) \end{pmatrix}$$

$$+ (1 - R_i) \begin{pmatrix} E(X_i|Y_i, Z_i) - \mu_i \\ Z_i\{E(X_i|Y_i, Z_i) - \mu_i\} \end{pmatrix} = 0, \qquad (16.28)$$

We then solve equations (16.27) and (16.28) simultaneously to obtain $(\hat\beta, \hat\gamma)$, the mle of β and γ. These equations differ from the full-data score equations for β and γ, because we replace statistics involving missing X_i with their conditional expectations given the observed data. Computation of $\hat\beta$ and $\hat\gamma$ may be organized in one of three ways, which we present in order of decreasing complexity.

Single Joint Newton-Raphson Iteration for $\hat\beta$ and $\hat\gamma$
This is the standard Newton-Raphson method. The conditional expectations required in (16.27) and (16.28) are viewed as functions of β and γ. From

(16.23),

$$E\left(X_i|Y_i=1,Z_i\right) = P\left(X_i=1|Y_i=1,Z_i\right)$$

$$= \frac{P(Y_i=1|X_i=1,Z_i)P(X_i=1|Z_i)}{\sum_{x=0}^{1}P(Y_i=1|X_i=x,Z_i)P(X_i=x|Z_i)}$$

$$= \frac{\dfrac{\exp(\beta_0+\beta_X+\beta_ZZ_i)}{1+\exp(\beta_0+\beta_X+\beta_ZZ_i)} \cdot \dfrac{\exp(\gamma_0+\gamma_ZZ_i)}{1+\exp(\gamma_0+\gamma_ZZ_i)}}{\dfrac{\exp(\beta_0+\beta_X+\beta_ZZ_i)}{1+\exp(\beta_0+\beta_X+\beta_ZZ_i)} \cdot \dfrac{\exp(\gamma_0+\gamma_ZZ_i)}{1+\exp(\gamma_0+\gamma_ZZ_i)} + \dfrac{\exp(\beta_0+\beta_ZZ_i)}{1+\exp(\beta_0+\beta_ZZ_i)} \cdot \dfrac{1}{1+\exp(\gamma_0+\gamma_ZZ_i)}}$$

$$= \frac{\dfrac{\exp(\beta_X+\gamma_0+\gamma_ZZ_i)}{1+\exp(\beta_0+\beta_X+\beta_ZZ_i)}}{\dfrac{\exp(\beta_X+\gamma_0+\gamma_ZZ_i)}{1+\exp(\beta_0+\beta_X+\beta_ZZ_i)} + \dfrac{1}{1+\exp(\beta_0+\beta_ZZ_i)}} \tag{16.29}$$

and

$$E\left(X_i|Y_i=0,Z_i\right) = P\left(X_i=1|Y_i=0,Z_i\right)$$

$$= \frac{P(Y_i=0|X_i=1,Z_i)P(X_i=1|Z_i)}{\sum_{x=0}^{1}P(Y_i=0|X_i=x,Z_i)P(X_i=x|Z_i)}$$

$$= \frac{\dfrac{1}{1+\exp(\beta_0+\beta_X+\beta_ZZ_i)} \cdot \dfrac{\exp(\gamma_0+\gamma_ZZ_i)}{1+\exp(\gamma_0+\gamma_ZZ_i)}}{\dfrac{1}{1+\exp(\beta_0+\beta_X+\beta_ZZ_i)} \cdot \dfrac{\exp(\gamma_0+\gamma_ZZ_i)}{1+\exp(\gamma_0+\gamma_ZZ_i)} + \dfrac{1}{1+\exp(\beta_0+\beta_ZZ_i)} \cdot \dfrac{1}{1+\exp(\gamma_0+\gamma_ZZ_i)}}$$

$$= \frac{\dfrac{\exp(\gamma_0+\gamma_ZZ_i)}{1+\exp(\beta_0+\beta_X+\beta_ZZ_i)}}{\dfrac{\exp(\gamma_0+\gamma_ZZ_i)}{1+\exp(\beta_0+\beta_X+\beta_ZZ_i)} + \dfrac{1}{1+\exp(\beta_0+\beta_ZZ_i)}}. \tag{16.30}$$

Also,

$$E\{P(X_i,Z_i)|Y_i=1,Z_i\} = \sum_{x=0}^{1} P\left(X_i=x|Y_i=1,Z_i\right)P(x,Z_i)$$

$$= \frac{\dfrac{\exp(\beta_X+\gamma_0+\gamma_ZZ_i)}{1+\exp(\beta_0+\beta_X+\beta_ZZ_i)} \cdot \dfrac{\exp(\beta_0+\beta_X+\beta_ZZ_i)}{1+\exp(\beta_0+\beta_X+\beta_ZZ_i)} + \dfrac{1}{1+\exp(\beta_0+\beta_ZZ_i)} \cdot \dfrac{\exp(\beta_0+\beta_ZZ_i)}{1+\exp(\beta_0+\beta_ZZ_i)}}{\dfrac{\exp(\beta_X+\gamma_0+\gamma_ZZ_i)}{1+\exp(\beta_0+\beta_X+\beta_ZZ_i)} + \dfrac{1}{1+\exp(\beta_0+\beta_ZZ_i)}}$$

$$\tag{16.31}$$

and

$$E\{P(X_i, Z_i) \mid Y_i = 0, Z_i\} = \sum_{x=0}^{1} P(X_i = x \mid Y_i = 0, Z_i) P(x, Z_i)$$

$$= \frac{\dfrac{\exp(\gamma_0 + \gamma_Z Z_i)}{1 + \exp(\beta_0 + \beta_X + \beta_Z Z_i)} \cdot \dfrac{\exp(\beta_0 + \beta_X + \beta_Z Z_i)}{1 + \exp(\beta_0 + \beta_X + \beta_Z Z_i)} + \dfrac{1}{1 + \exp(\beta_0 + \beta_Z Z_i)} \cdot \dfrac{\exp(\beta_0 + \beta_Z Z_i)}{1 + \exp(\beta_0 + \beta_Z Z_i)}}{\dfrac{\exp(\gamma_0 + \gamma_Z Z_i)}{1 + \exp(\beta_0 + \beta_X + \beta_Z Z_i)} + \dfrac{1}{1 + \exp(\beta_0 + \beta_Z Z_i)}}.$$

$$(16.32)$$

The expressions for $E[X_i\{Y_i - P(X_i, Z_i)\} \mid Y_i, Z_i]$ are similar, but only the first term of the sum in the numerator of (16.31) or (16.32) appears. The above expressions are substituted into (16.27) and (16.28) to arrive at the explicit set of equations involving β and γ,

$$\begin{pmatrix} U_\beta(\beta, \gamma) \\ U_\gamma(\beta, \gamma) \end{pmatrix} = 0,$$

to solve by the Newton-Raphson method.

The equations are complicated. Moreover, the Newton-Raphson algorithm requires differentiating U_β and U_γ to obtain the observed information matrix,

$$I(\beta, \gamma) = \begin{bmatrix} -\dfrac{\partial U_\beta(\beta, \gamma)}{\partial \beta'} & -\dfrac{\partial U_\beta(\beta, \gamma)}{\partial \gamma'} \\ -\dfrac{\partial U_\gamma(\beta, \gamma)}{\partial \beta'} & -\dfrac{\partial U_\gamma(\beta, \gamma)}{\partial \gamma'} \end{bmatrix}. \qquad (16.33)$$

Given an initial value, say $(\hat{\beta}^{(0)}, \hat{\gamma}^{(0)})'$, the approximations to the mle are updated by

$$\begin{pmatrix} \hat{\beta}^{(\nu+1)} \\ \hat{\gamma}^{(\nu+1)} \end{pmatrix} = \begin{pmatrix} \hat{\beta}^{(\nu)} \\ \hat{\gamma}^{(\nu)} \end{pmatrix} + I(\hat{\beta}^{(\nu)}, \hat{\gamma}^{(\nu)})^{-1} \begin{pmatrix} U_\beta(\hat{\beta}^{(\nu)}, \hat{\gamma}^{(\nu)}) \\ U_\gamma(\hat{\beta}^{(\nu)}, \hat{\gamma}^{(\nu)}) \end{pmatrix}$$

until the iterates converge.

An advantage of carrying out the differentiations is that $I(\hat{\beta}, \hat{\gamma})^{-1}$ is a consistent estimate of the asymptotic variance-covariance matrix of the mle $(\hat{\beta}, \hat{\gamma})$ which is produced as a by-product of the calculation.

Iterative Separate Estimation of $\hat{\beta}$ and $\hat{\gamma}$—the **EM** *Algorithm*

The following modification of the joint estimation procedure simplifies the calculations to a certain extent. Given approximations $(\hat{\beta}^{(\nu)}, \hat{\gamma}^{(\nu)})'$ for $\nu = 0, 1, 2, \ldots$, the conditional expectations $E(X_i|Y_i, Z_i)$ are calculated from (16.23) as before, but are then treated as numerical constants, say $c_i^{(\nu)} = c_i^{(\nu)}(\hat{\beta}^{(\nu)}, \hat{\gamma}^{(\nu)}) = E(X_i|Y_i, Z_i)$, in the expressions for $E\{P(X_i, Z_i)|Y_i, Z_i\}$ and $E[X_i\{Y_i - P(X_i, Z_i)\}|Y_i, Z_i]$ in (16.27), rather than as functions of β and γ. For example,

$$E\{P(X_i, Z_i)|Y_i, Z_i\} = P(1, Z_i)c_i^{(\nu)} + P(0, Z_i)\left(1 - c_i^{(\nu)}\right)$$

$$= \frac{\exp(\beta_0 + \beta_X + \beta_Z Z_i)}{1 + \exp(\beta_0 + \beta_X + \beta_Z Z_i)} c_i^{(\nu)}$$

$$+ \frac{\exp(\beta_0 + \beta_Z Z_i)}{1 + \exp(\beta_0 + \beta_Z Z_i)}\left(1 - c_i^{(\nu)}\right).$$

The left-hand side of equation (16.27) is then a relatively simple function of β alone:

$$U_\beta^{(\nu)}(\beta) = \sum_{i=1}^n R_i \begin{pmatrix} Y_i - P(X_i, Z_i) \\ X_i\{Y_i - P(X_i, Z_i)\} \\ Z_i\{Y_i - P(X_i, Z_i)\} \end{pmatrix}$$

$$+ (1 - R_i) \begin{pmatrix} Y_i - \{P(1, Z_i)c_i^{(\nu)} + P(0, Z_i)(1 - c_i^{(\nu)})\} \\ \{Y_i - P(1, Z_i)\}c_i^{(\nu)} \\ Z_i[Y_i - \{P(1, Z_i)c_i^{(\nu)} + P(0, Z_i)(1 - c_i^{(\nu)})\}] \end{pmatrix}$$

$$(16.34)$$

and the equation $U_\beta^{(\nu)}(\beta) = 0$ is solved by a Newton-Raphson algorithm for $\hat{\beta}^{(\nu+1)}$. The derivative of $U_\beta^{(\nu)}(\beta)$ with respect to β, evaluated at $\hat{\beta}^{(\nu)}$, is still required, but is also relatively simple—see Problem 16.5. In similar fashion, $E(X_i|Y_i, Z_i) = c_i^{(\nu)}$ is treated as if it were observed data in (16.28). The left-hand side of (16.28) is viewed as the function

$$U_\gamma^{(\nu)}(\gamma) = \sum_{i=1}^n R_i \begin{pmatrix} X_i - \mu_i \\ Z_i(X_i - \mu_i) \end{pmatrix} + (1 - R_i) \begin{pmatrix} c_i^{(\nu)} - \mu_i \\ Z_i\{c_i^{(\nu)} - \mu_i\} \end{pmatrix}, \quad (16.35)$$

which depends only on γ through μ_i. The equation $U_\gamma^{(\nu)}(\gamma) = 0$ is solved separately for $\hat{\gamma}^{(\nu+1)}$. The derivative of $U_\gamma^{(\nu)}(\gamma)$ with respect to γ, evaluated at $\hat{\gamma}^{(\nu)}$, is given in Problem 16.5. Once $\hat{\beta}^{(\nu+1)}$ and $\hat{\gamma}^{(\nu+1)}$ are in hand, the conditional expectations $E(X_i|Y_i, Z_i)$ are updated to $c_i^{(\nu+1)}$ and the entire process is repeated until it converges.

This procedure is an EM (expectation-maximization) algorithm (Dempster, Laird, and Rubin, 1977). The E-step evaluates the conditional expectations of the missing data given the observed data at current estimates of the parameters; the M-step maximizes the likelihood function as if the conditional expectations were observed data. Dempster, Laird, and Rubin (1977) prove that, on iterating these two steps, the likelihood of the observed data increases with each iteration and the algorithm becomes stationary at the maximum likelihood estimate.

A disadvantage to this method is that it does not produce standard errors for $(\hat{\beta}, \hat{\gamma})$ directly; these must be calculated separately, either from $I(\hat{\beta}, \hat{\gamma})^{-1}$ at (16.33) as in the joint method (thus negating the simplification provided by the EM algorithm), or by some other method such as the jackknife.

The E-M Algorithm Using the Expanded-Dataset Method

The estimating function $U_{\beta}^{(\nu)}(\beta)$ in the preceding method, while simpler than $U_{\beta}(\beta, \gamma)$ in the joint method, is not a regular logistic regression score function, so special programming is still required to solve $U_{\beta}^{(\nu)}(\beta) = 0$. There is a clever way, however, to use any software package which provides for *case weighting* to solve the equations $U_{\beta}^{(\nu)}(\beta) = 0$ and $U_{\gamma}^{(\nu)}(\gamma) = 0$ simply. The procedure constructs an *expanded dataset* by replacing each record with missing X_i by two records, one with $X_i = 1$ and the other with $X_i = 0$. The duplicated records are then weighted by $P(X_i = 1 | Y_i, Z_i, R_i = 0)$ and $P(X_i = 0 | Y_i, Z_i, R_i = 0)$, respectively. The necessary steps for computation are as follows:

(i) Prepare an expanded dataset by duplicating each record with missing X_i, one with $X_i = 1$ and the other with $X_i = 0$. The expanded dataset has n' records, where $n' = \sum_{i=1}^{n} R_i + 2\sum_{i=1}^{n}(1 - R_i)$. The duplicated records keep Y_i and Z_i fixed as observed.

(ii) Given initial values of β and γ, create *case weights* w_i for $i = 1, \ldots, n'$. For observed records, $w_i = 1$. For the duplicated record with $X_i = 1$, $w_i = P(X_i = 1 | Y_i, Z_i, R_i = 0)$, and for the duplicated record with $X_i = 0$, $w_i = P(X_i = 0 | Y_i, Z_i, R_i = 0)$. Under MAR, these are obtained from (16.23).

(iii) Fit two separate, weighted logistic regression models, one for Y given X and Z, the other for X given Z, using the expanded dataset of size n' with case weights w_i, to obtain updated estimates of β and γ.

(iv) Using the new estimates of β and γ, update the case weights w_i in step (ii) and the estimates of β and γ in step (iii). Repeat until convergence.

Lipsitz and Ibrahim (1996) use this technique in a survival analysis context. As mentioned above, a separate calculation is required to obtain standard errors. We describe the use of the jackknife for this purpose below.

We pause here to ask: What happens if we choose to specify a model for $P(X|Y,Z)$ as in (16.20) with parameter δ instead of specifying a model for $P(X|Z)$ as in (16.22) with parameter γ? To write down the likelihood function in terms of L_{i1} and L_{i2}, we must deduce the form of $P(X|Z)$ given the specified $P(X|Y,Z)$ from Bayes theorem (Problem 16.6):

$$P(X=1|Z)$$

$$= \frac{P(Y|X=0,Z)P(X=1|Y,Z)}{P(Y|X=0,Z)P(X=1|Y,Z) + P(Y|X=1,Z)P(X=0|Y,Z)}.$$

$$(16.36)$$

Equation (16.36) shows that $P(X|Z)$ is a function of both β and δ, unlike $P(X|Z)$ in (16.22), which depends on γ but not β. It follows that the score function for β has a more complicated form than (16.27) and the observed information matrix is more complicated than $I(\beta,\gamma)$ in (16.33).

16.4.2. Imputation

Observe that the score function U_β in (16.25) has zero expectation (Problem 16.7), a critical property of an estimating function. Observe further that certain slight modifications of U_β do not change its unbiasedness. First, if we replace u_i with any other unbiased estimating function, for example, the quasiscore function of Wedderburn (1974), the resulting estimating function remains unbiased. Even if u_i is not a score function, it is unbiased as long as it depends on Y_i only through $Y_i - P(X_i, Z_i)$. Second, if the conditional mean $E(u_i|Y_i, Z_i)$ is estimated consistently using a method other than maximum likelihood estimation of $\hat{\gamma}$ by solving (16.28) followed by calculation of (16.23), the unbiasedness of the estimating function is unaffected and the estimate of β as the solution of equation (16.27) is consistent. The imputation method described below is obtained via a modification of the second kind. We call the methods incorporating such modifications *imputation methods*. Estimators of β obtained by imputation methods have different asymptotic properties than maximum likelihood estimates.

As mentioned at the beginning of this section, $P(X|Y,Z)$ can be consistently estimated using only complete records, but $P(X|Z)$ cannot. Suppose model (16.22) for $P(X|Z)$ is correct. If we fit the model using only the complete records and then compute the conditional mean using equation (16.23), we obtain an inconsistent estimate of γ, thus an inconsistent estimate of $E(X|Y,Z)$, and, consequently, an inconsistent estimate of β. On the other hand, suppose (16.20) for $P(X|Y,Z)$ is correct. When we fit that model using complete records and compute the conditional expectation of X given (Y,Z) directly from the model, we obtain consistent estimates for δ and $E(X|Y,Z)$, and thus β, because X is conditionally independent of R given (Y,Z). These considerations motivate the following imputation method for estimating β.

First, using complete records, solve the following estimating equation for δ, calling the solution $\tilde{\delta}$:

$$U_\delta(\delta) = \sum_{i=1}^{n} R_i \begin{pmatrix} 1 \\ Y_i \\ Z_i \end{pmatrix} \left\{ X_i - \frac{\exp(\delta_0 + \delta_Y Y_i + \delta_Z Z_i)}{1 + \exp(\delta_0 + \delta_Y Y_i + \delta_Z Z_i)} \right\} = 0. \quad (16.37)$$

Using $\tilde{\delta}$, estimates of the conditional expectations $E(X_i|Y_i, Z_i)$, $E\{P(X_i, Z_i)|Y_i, Z_i\}$, and $E\{X_i P(X_i, Z_i)|Y_i, Z_i\}$ are easily computed. For example,

$$\tilde{E}\{P(X_i, Z_i)|Y_i, Z_i\} = P(1, Z_i)\tilde{c}_i + P(0, Z_i)(1 - \tilde{c}_i),$$

where

$$\tilde{c}_i = \tilde{E}(X_i|Y_i, Z_i) = \frac{\exp(\tilde{\delta}_0 + \tilde{\delta}_Y Y_i + \tilde{\delta}_Z Z_i)}{1 + \exp(\tilde{\delta}_0 + \tilde{\delta}_Y Y_i + \tilde{\delta}_Z Z_i)}. \quad (16.38)$$

The estimated expectations are inserted in (16.27), analogous to (16.34):

$$\tilde{U}_\beta(\beta) = U_\beta(\beta, \tilde{\delta}) = \sum_{i=1}^{n} R_i \begin{pmatrix} Y_i - P(X_i, Z_i) \\ X_i\{Y_i - P(X_i, Z_i)\} \\ Z_i\{Y_i - P(X_i, Z_i)\} \end{pmatrix}$$

$$+ (1 - R_i) \begin{pmatrix} Y_i - \{P(1, Z_i)\tilde{c}_i + P(0, Z_i)(1 - \tilde{c}_i)\} \\ \{Y_i - P(1, Z_i)\}\tilde{c}_i \\ Z_i[Y_i - \{P(1, Z_i)\tilde{c}_i + P(0, Z_i)(1 - \tilde{c}_i)\}] \end{pmatrix}. \quad (16.39)$$

While the separate-solution method in the likelihood approach repeatedly solves (16.27) and (16.28), updating the conditional expectations after each solution, the imputation method has just two steps: First, solve (16.37) to estimate $\tilde{\delta}$ and obtain $\tilde{c}_i$; second, solve $\tilde{U}_\beta(\beta) = 0$ once for the solution $\tilde{\beta}$.

Note that whereas the likelihood approach estimates γ from all available data, the imputation estimate of δ derives from complete records only. By viewing the imputation estimator $(\tilde{\beta}, \tilde{\delta})$ as the solution of the joint estimating equation,

$$U_J(\beta, \delta) = \begin{pmatrix} U_\beta(\beta, \delta) \\ U_\delta(\delta) \end{pmatrix} = \sum_{i=1}^{n} U_{Ji} = 0, \quad (16.40)$$

we can derive its asymptotic properties: imputation estimates are consistent and asymptotically normally distributed; specifically,

$$\begin{pmatrix} \tilde{\beta} - \beta \\ \tilde{\delta} - \delta \end{pmatrix} \sim N\left(0, \Gamma^{-1} \operatorname{Var}(U_J)\Gamma^{-1}\right),$$

where

$$\Gamma = \Gamma(\beta, \delta) = E \begin{pmatrix} -\dfrac{\partial U_\beta(\beta, \delta)}{\partial \beta'} & 0 \\[2ex] -\dfrac{\partial U_\beta(\beta, \delta)}{\partial \delta'} & -\dfrac{\partial U_\delta(\delta)}{\partial \delta'} \end{pmatrix}.$$

The asymptotic variance of the imputation estimator has the sandwich form typical for estimators derived from estimating equations (Section 15.5): the "meat" $\operatorname{Var}(U_J)$ sandwiched between the "bread" Γ^{-1}. Problem 16.8 provides the derivatives required for Γ. To estimate the variance-covariance matrix of $(\tilde{\beta}, \tilde{\delta})$, $\operatorname{Var}(U_J)$ may be estimated by the empirical variance evaluated at $(\tilde{\beta}, \tilde{\delta})$, $\sum_i U_{Ji} U'_{Ji}$, and substituted in the sandwich formula with Γ^{-1} evaluated at $(\tilde{\beta}, \tilde{\delta})$. This approach requires evaluation of Γ. Alternatively, the variance-covariance matrix of $(\tilde{\beta}, \tilde{\delta})$ may be estimated directly by the jackknife (see below).

Imputation estimates can be computed using standard software by the expanded-dataset method. The first step, preparing the expanded dataset, is identical to the likelihood case.

(i) Prepare an expanded dataset by duplicating each record with missing X_i, one with $X_i = 1$ and the other with $X_i = 0$. The expanded dataset has n' records, where $n' = \sum_{i=1}^n R_i + 2\sum_{i=1}^n (1 - R_i)$ The duplicated records keep Y_i and Z_i fixed as observed.

(ii) Create case weights w_i for $i = 1, \ldots, n'$. For observed records, $w_i = 1$. For the duplicated record with $X_i = 1$, $w_i = P(X_i = 1 | Y_i, Z_i, R_i = 0)$, and for the duplicated record with $X_i = 0$, $w_i = P(X_i = 0 | Y_i, Z_i, R_i = 0)$. Under MAR, these are obtained from the fitted logistic regression model (16.20). Calculate $\tilde{\delta}$ by solution of (16.37) using complete records only, and $\tilde{c}_i$ from (16.38). Then set $w_i = \tilde{c}_i$ for duplicated records with $X_i = 1$, or set $w_i = 1 - \tilde{c}_i$ for duplicated records with $X_i = 0$.

(iii) Fit model (16.17) using weighted logistic regression with the expanded dataset of size n' and case weights w_i to obtain the final estimate $\tilde{\beta}$.

Although the above algorithm has an "expectation" step and a "maximization" step, it is not an EM algorithm, because we did not maximize a likelihood function.

Standard-Error Calculation with the Jackknife

Standard errors are easily calculated using the jackknife technique for both the maximum likelihood estimator and the imputation estimator. Let T denote $(\hat{\beta}, \hat{\gamma})'$ or $(\tilde{\beta}, \tilde{\delta})'$. The jackknife variance estimate is $\sum_{i=1}^{n} (T_{-i} - T)(T_{-i} - T)'$, where T_{-i} denotes the estimate obtained by deleting the ith record. When $R_i = 0$, duplicated records are deleted pairwise to calculate T_{-i}.

Lipsitz, Dear, and Zhao (1994) justify the jackknife variance estimate for Cox models for correlated survival data. A similar justification applies here.

16.4.3. Weighting

In weighting methods, each observed record is weighted by the inverse of its probability of observation. The theoretical estimating equation is

$$W_{\beta} = \sum_{i=1}^{n} \frac{R_i}{\pi_i} u_i = \sum_{i=1}^{n} \frac{R_i}{\pi_i} \begin{pmatrix} Y_i - P(X_i, Z_i) \\ X_i\{Y_i - P(X_i, Z_i)\} \\ Z_i\{Y_i - P(X_i, Z_i)\} \end{pmatrix} = 0, \qquad (16.41)$$

where

$$\pi_i = P(R_i = 1 | X_i, Y_i, Z_i).$$

Due to the weighting procedure, $E(W_{\beta}) = 0$. Because π is unknown (unless data are missing by design), we need to replace π by an estimate, $\hat{\pi}$. Recall that, under MAR, $P(R = 1 | X, Y, Z) = P(R = 1 | Y, Z)$; since (R, Y, Z) are completely observed, we can estimate $P(R = 1 | Y, Z)$ from all records. With the following parametric model for $P(R = 1 | Y, Z)$,

$$\ln \frac{\pi}{1 - \pi} = \alpha_0 + \alpha_Y Y + \alpha_Z Z, \qquad (16.42)$$

the estimating equation for α is

$$U_{\alpha} = \sum_{i=1}^{n} \left\{ R_i - \frac{\exp(\alpha_0 + \alpha_Y Y_i + \alpha_Z Z_i)}{1 + \exp(\alpha_0 + \alpha_Y Y_i + \alpha_Z Z_i)} \right\} \begin{pmatrix} 1 \\ Y_i \\ Z_i \end{pmatrix} = 0. \quad (16.43)$$

The analysis is conducted in two steps: First, fit model (16.42) using the observation indicator R as an outcome. Second, using complete records, fit a weighted logistic regression model for Y_i with the inverse of the predicted values, $\hat{\pi}^{-1}$, as the case-weights. Since the estimator is the solution of

$$\begin{pmatrix} W_{\beta} \\ U_{\alpha} \end{pmatrix} = 0,$$

the asymptotic variance is obtained as a sandwich-type estimator in the same manner as the variance of the imputation estimator (Zhao, Lipsitz, and Lew, 1996). Alternatively, the variance can be estimated by the jackknife technique or by the method of Robins, Rotnitzky, and Zhao (1994).

Robins, Rotnitzky, and Zhao (1994) modify (16.43) by subtracting a correction term so that the estimating function is orthogonal to the score function of the nuisance parameters, α. Although this estimator is asymptotically efficient, calculating the correction term is not trivial. For the particular case of one missing covariate, the modified estimating equation has the form

$$\sum_{i=1}^{n} \frac{R_i}{\pi_i} u_i - \left(\frac{R_i}{\pi_i} - 1 \right) E(u_i | Y_i, Z_i). \tag{16.44}$$

This estimating equation is also examined by Lipsitz, Ibrahim, and Zhao (1999) for nonparametric estimation of $E(u_i | Y_i, Z_i)$. Interestingly, the estimating equation (16.44) guarantees consistency when the model specification of either the nonresponse mechanism or the conditional expectation is correct.

16.4.4. Models Conditioning on the Observation Indicator

As discussed above, complete record analysis gives inconsistent estimates of $P(Y|X, Z)$ under MAR conditions. Wang (1999) suggested modeling $P(Y|X, Z, R = 1)$, which can be estimated consistently using complete records. If we assume a model for the probability of observation $P(R|X, Z, Y)$, then $P(Y|X, Z, R = 1)$ can be expressed in terms of the models for $P(Y|X, Z)$ and $P(R|X, Z, Y)$:

$$\ln \frac{P(Y=1|X, Z, R=1)}{P(Y=0|X, Z, R=1)} = \ln \frac{P(Y=1|X, Z)}{P(Y=0|X, Z)} + \ln \frac{P(R=1|X, Z, Y=1)}{P(R=1|X, Z, Y=0)}.$$

Under MAR conditions, $P(R|X, Y, Z) = P(R|Y, Z)$, so

$$\ln \frac{P(Y=1|X, Z, R=1)}{P(Y=0|X, Z, R=1)} = \beta_0 + \beta_X X + \beta_Z Z + \ln \frac{P(R=1|Y=1, Z)}{P(R=1|Y=0, Z)}.$$

Assuming (16.42),

$$\ln \frac{P(R=1|Y=1, Z)}{P(R=1|Y=0, Z)} = \alpha_0 + \alpha_Y + \alpha_Z Z + \ln \frac{1 + \exp(\alpha_0 + \alpha_Z Z)}{1 + \exp(\alpha_0 + \alpha_Y + \alpha_Z Z)}.$$

An estimating equation for β is

$$Q_\beta = \sum_{i=1}^{n} R_i\{Y_i - P(Y_i = 1|X_i, Z_i, R_i = 1)\}\begin{pmatrix} 1 \\ X_i \\ Z_i \end{pmatrix} = 0.$$

For α, we use equation (16.43).

To compute the estimate of β and α using standard software, we first estimate α, say $\hat{\alpha}$, from (16.43), then compute $\ln\{P(R = 1|Y = 1, Z)/P(R = 1|Y = 0, Z)\}$ evaluated at $\hat{\alpha}$, say $g(Z, \hat{\alpha})$, and declare it as an *offset*. The estimate from the logistic regression model with Y as outcome, (X, Z) as covariates and $g(Z, \hat{\alpha})$ as offset is the solution of the joint estimating equation

$$\begin{pmatrix} Q_\beta \\ U_\alpha \end{pmatrix} = 0.$$

As in the case of imputation or weighting estimators, the asymptotic variance has the sandwich form. The jackknife also consistently estimates the variance.

Liang and Qin (2000) propose a pseudolikelihood approach which eliminates the offset term and therefore the need to specify a missingness model such as (16.42).

16.4.5. Comparisons

Of the four methods for handling missing data, the likelihood approach is most efficient but requires the most restrictive assumptions. Weighting and models that condition on the observation indicator require specification of the nonresponse mechanism; the consistency of the estimate therefore depends on correct specification of the mechanism. The imputation approach requires specification of an imputation model for the missing data; the consistency of the estimate therefore depends on the correct specification of the model. In general, imputation methods, unlike likelihood methods, do not require specification of a full joint distribution. They require specification only of: (i) the imputation model, i.e., the conditional expectation of the missing data given the observed data; and (ii) the main analysis model for the outcome of interest. These two specifications are usually less restrictive than specifying a full joint distribution for X, Y, and R given Z. Even if we assume a parametric model for the joint distribution, we may choose an imputation method for computational simplicity. The resulting estimators are not as efficient as maximum likelihood estimates, but can be useful in practice when computation is substantially easier and the loss of the efficiency is small. Table 16.17 provides an example.

Between imputation and weighting, imputation tends to yield more efficient estimates. Intuitively, if we have a strong predictor of missing data,

Table 16.17. *Estimates and standard errors of β using three different methods under MAR*

Method	Estimate	β_0	β_X	β_Z
Likelihood	parameter	0.3666	0.1057	0.3529
	se	0.2704	0.3934	0.3072
Imputation	parameter	0.3666	0.1056	0.3529
	se	0.2704	0.3934	0.3072
Weighting	parameter	0.3881	0.1014	0.3095
	se	0.2929	0.3947	0.3835

imputation capitalizes on this information (Paik, 1997). The weighting approach, on the other hand, cannot benefit from such information. Wang (1999) shows that in some situations estimates from a conditional model are more efficient than those from a weighting approach. Under MCAR, the conditional model approach of Wang (1999) reduces to a valid complete-record analysis. Weighting estimates are sometimes less efficient than the complete-record estimate under MCAR. Reilly and Pepe (1998) and Kuk, Mak, and Li (2001) discuss the advantages and disadvantages of different estimation methods.

16.4.6. Example

We use the hypothetical data presented in Tables 16.14 and 16.15 to illustrate the results of the likelihood, imputation, and weighting methods. We reinterpret S as a binary outcome Y, H as a covariate X with some values missing, and C as a completely observed binary covariate Z. Table 16.17 shows that the maximum likelihood estimates and the imputation estimates are almost identical. The maximum likelihood estimate of the log odds ratio ($\hat{\beta}_X = 0.1057$) and its standard error (0.3934) are very close to the logarithm of the imputation Mantel-Haenszel odds ratio ($0.1016 = \ln 1.107 = \ln \hat{\omega}^{(2)}$) and its standard error ($0.3918 = \sqrt{0.1520}$) in Section 16.3.

The standard errors of $\hat{\beta}_X$ are similar for all three methods, but the standard error of $\hat{\beta}_Z$ from the weighting method is about 25% larger than those of the maximum likelihood and imputation estimates. This inflation makes intuitive sense because records not used in the weighting method carry information about the effect of Z on Y. Table 16.18 contains the parameter estimates and standard errors for the imputation and weighting models. The table shows that the standard errors of coefficients in the imputation models for the likelihood method (γ_0 and γ_Z) are smaller than the standard errors for the corresponding coefficients in the imputation method (δ_0 and δ_Z), but this fact is not manifest in the standard errors of $\hat{\beta}$. As for the estimate of α in the weighting model, the Wald tests for H_0: $\alpha_Y = 0$ and H_0: $\alpha_Z = 0$ are not significant, suggesting that the nonresponse mechanism is MCAR rather than MAR. However, studies are usually not designed to detect nonzero components of α, so failure to reject H_0 may be due to lack of power.

Table 16.18. *Estimates and standard errors of parameters of the imputation and weighting models (16.22), (16.20), and (16.42) under MAR*

Method	Estimate	γ_0	γ_Z
Likelihood	parameter	-0.2128	-0.4245
	se	0.2546	0.3804

Method	Estimate	δ_0	δ_Y	δ_Z
Imputation	parameter	-0.2765	0.1056	-0.4331
	se	0.3392	0.3934	0.3851

Method	Estimate	α_0	α_Y	α_Z
Weighting	parameter	0.8032	-0.4323	-0.1077
	se	0.2910	0.3168	0.2977

Readers may find SAS® code to compute the estimates in Tables 16.17 and 16.18 at http://www.wiley.com/statistics.

16.5.* LOGISTIC REGRESSION WHEN OUTCOMES ARE MISSING AT RANDOM

Now we turn to the case in which the outcome variable Y is MAR and the covariates X and Z are completely observed. Denoting the observation indicator of Y by R, we assume the missingness depends on (X, Z) but not on Y, such that, $P(R|X, Y, Z) = P(R|X, Z)$, in which case $P(Y|X, Z, R = 1) = P(Y|X, Z, R = 0) = P(Y|X, Z)$. This equality implies that complete record analysis is valid. We encountered this situation in the analysis of the 2×2 table of Section 16.2.1, where the missingness of hypertension status (Y in the present context) was assumed to depend only on smoking (now X). The probability of hypertension given smoking status was consistently estimated using only completely observed records.

Under the present assumptions, both the likelihood and the imputation estimating functions reduce to complete-record analysis. We write the score equation for β explicitly:

$$\frac{\partial \ln L}{\partial \beta} = \sum_{i=1}^n R_i u_i + (1 - R_i) E(u_i | X_i, Z_i, R_i = 0)$$

$$= \sum_{i=1}^n R_i \{Y_i - P(X_i, Z_i)\} \begin{pmatrix} 1 \\ X_i \\ Z_i \end{pmatrix}$$

$$+ (1 - R_i)\{E(Y|X_i, Z_i) - P(X_i, Z_i)\} \begin{pmatrix} 1 \\ X_i \\ Z_i \end{pmatrix}.$$

Since $E(Y_i|X_i, Z_i) = P(X_i, Z_i)$, the contribution from the incomplete records is zero, and the score equation reduces to

$$\frac{\partial \ln L}{\partial \beta} = \sum_{i=1}^{n} R_i \begin{pmatrix} Y_i - P(X_i, Z_i) \\ X_i\{Y_i - P(X_i, Z_i)\} \\ Z_i\{Y_i - P(X_i, Z_i)\} \end{pmatrix} = 0.$$

Weighting analysis requires a weighted logistic regression, where the case weights are the inverse probabilities of observation, which depend on the covariates. The weighted logistic regression estimates are less efficient than the unweighted logistic regression estimates from the complete-record analysis.

16.6.* NONIGNORABLE MISSINGNESS

When missingness in a covariate is nonignorable (NI), the observation indicator depends on the unobserved value of X. The methods described under MAR are no longer valid, because the probability of observing X, $P(R|X, Y, Z)$, cannot be factored out as an isolated term in the likelihood function. We must therefore model $P(R|X, Y, Z)$ explicitly.

Work attempting to estimate the parameters of interest together with the probability of response first appeared in the econometrics literature (e.g., Nelson, 1977). Baker and Laird (1988) discussed NI missing categorical data within a likelihood framework; Wu and Bailey (1988) and Wu and Carroll (1988) considered the continuous case. More recently, Lipsitz, Ibrahim, Chen, and Peterson (1999) studied a likelihood-based method for handling NI missing covariates in logistic regression models.

16.6.1. Inference under Nonignorable Missingness

To understand the characteristics of valid inference under nonignorable missingness, it is helpful to examine the likelihood and score functions. The likelihood function is of the form shown in (16.24), but the response mechanism $P(R|Y, X, Z)$ is nonignorable. The score function is of the form given in (16.25), but the conditional expectations are different. Under MAR, $E(u_i|Y_i, Z_i, R_i = 0) = E(u_i|Y_i, Z_i, R_i = 1) = E(u_i|Y_i, Z_i)$. Under NI, this relationship is no longer true. Using Bayes' theorem,

$$E(X_i|Y_i, Z_i, R_i = 0) = P(X_i = 1|Y_i, Z_i, R_i = 0)$$

$$= \frac{P(X_i = 1|Y_i, Z_i)\{1 - \pi_i(1)\}}{P(X_i = 1|Y_i, Z_i)\{1 - \pi_i(1)\} + P(X_i = 0|Y_i, Z_i)\{1 - \pi_i(0)\}}, \quad (16.45)$$

where $\pi_i(x) = P(R_i = 1|X_i = x, Y_i, Z_i)$ for $x = 0$ or 1, so that $E(X_i|Y_i, Z_i, R_i = 0)$ is a function of π_i as well as $E(X_i|Y_i, Z_i)$. We consider the case in which $P(X_i|Z_i)$ is given by (16.45), $P(X_i|Y_i, Z_i)$ is given by (16.23), and π has a known functional form up to some unknown parameters. Suppose π_i has a linear logistic form:

$$\ln \frac{\pi_i}{1 - \pi_i} = \alpha_0 + \alpha_X X_i + \alpha_Y Y_i + \alpha_Z Z_i. \tag{16.46}$$

A score equation for α is

$$\sum_{i=1}^{n} R_i (R_i - \pi_i) \begin{pmatrix} 1 \\ X_i \\ Y_i \\ Z_i \end{pmatrix} + (1 - R_i) E \left\{ (R_i - \pi_i) \begin{pmatrix} 1 \\ X_i \\ Y_i \\ Z_i \end{pmatrix} \Big| Y_i, Z_i, R_i = 0 \right\} = 0. \tag{16.47}$$

The maximum likelihood estimates of (β, γ, α) can be obtained solving equations (16.25), (16.26), and (16.47) simultaneously. Parameter estimation under NI missingness thus requires (i) solving a third estimating equation (16.47) and (ii) including the probabilities of response from (16.46) in the computation of conditional expectation—(16.23) for $P(X_i|Y_i, Z_i)$ first, then $P(X_i|Y_i, Z_i)$ and π_i in (16.45) to produce $E(X_i|Y_i, Z_i, R_i = 0)$.

The computation of the estimate and its standard error can be carried out using standard software as follows:

(i) Prepare an expanded dataset by duplicating each record with missing X_i, one with $X_i = 1$ and the other with $X_i = 0$. The expanded dataset has n' records, where $n' = \sum_{i=1}^{n} R_i + 2\sum_{i=1}^{n}(1 - R)$. The duplicated records keep Y_i and Z_i fixed as observed.

(ii) Given initial values of (β, γ, α), create case weights w_i for $i = 1, \dots, n'$. For observed records, $w_i = 1$. For the duplicated record with $X_i = 1$, $w_i = P(X_i = 1|Y_i, Z_i, R_i = 0)$, and for the duplicated record with $X_i = 0$, $w_i = P(X_i = 0|Y_i, Z_i, R_i = 0)$. Under NI, these are obtained from (16.45) with $P(X_i = 1|Y_i, Z_i)$ as given in (16.23).

(iii) Fit three separate, weighted logistic regression models, one for Y given X and Z, the next for X given Z, and the last for R given X, Y, and Z, using the expanded dataset of size n' with case weights w_i to obtain updated estimates of (β, γ, α).

(iv) Using the new estimates of (β, γ, α), update the case-weights w_i in step (ii) and the estimates of (β, γ, α) in step (iii). Repeat until convergence.

The standard error can be computed using the jackknife (Section 16.4.2). Using the data given in Tables 16.14 and 16.15, we fit the above described

Table 16.19. *Maximum likelihood estimates and standard errors of β under NI*

Estimate	β_0	β_X	β_Z
parameter	0.3666	0.1056	0.3529
se	0.2704	0.3934	0.3072

Table 16.20. *Estimates and standard errors of parameters of the imputation model (16.22) and probability-of-response model (16.46) under NI*

Estimate	γ_0	γ_Z
parameter	-0.2131	-0.4241
se	0.2539	0.3788

Estimate	α_0	α_X	α_Y	α_Z
parameter	0.8032	-0.0001	-0.4323	-0.1077
se	0.2911	0.0006	0.3167	0.2978

model. The estimates and standard errors in Tables 16.19 and 16.20 are very close to those obtained under MAR (Tables 16.17 and 16.18). We also see that the estimate of α_X is nearly zero, suggesting that the nonresponse mechanism is MAR rather than NI. The SAS code to compute the maximum likelihood estimates under NI is provided in http://www.wiley.com/statistics.

16.6.2. Sensitivity Analysis

The maximum likelihood estimation of β under conditions of nonignorable missingness sometimes suffers from technical difficulties such as nonidentifiability (different sets of parameter values give identical likelihood) or nonconvergence. Even if we surmount these difficulties, maximum likelihood estimation is valid only when all models are correctly specified, a circumstance difficult to verify. In addition to the routine model-checking effort one should conduct even without missing data, it is advisable to conduct sensitivity analyses (Little and Rubin, 1999). A sensitivity analysis treats the relation between the observation indicator and the missing variable as known and, given that relation, estimates the parameters of interest. When there is a nonidentifiability problem, stipulating the dependence between the observation indicator and the missing variable makes the rest of the parameters identifiable (Rotnitzky, Robins, and Scharfstein, 1998; Scharfstein, Rotnitzky, and Robins, 1998). Even when all parameters are identifiable, sensitivity analysis provides information about how much estimates of the parameters of interest change as the severity of nonignorability increases.

For example, consider the case of a 2×2 table. A saturated model for the probability of observation is

$$\ln \frac{\pi}{1 - \pi} = \alpha_0 + \alpha_X X + \alpha_Y Y + \alpha_{XY} XY.$$

Under this model, the parameters become unidentifiable. We can set α_{XY} at certain values and observe the resultant changes in the odds ratio between X and Y. Note that the dependence of π on missing data X characterizes the severity of nonignorable missingness. MAR corresponds to $\alpha_X = \alpha_{XY} = 0$, so the magnitude of α_X and α_{XY} measures the deviation from MAR, that is, the severity of nonignorability. We can assess the sensitivity of our inferences by assigning α_{XY} a range of plausible values and calculating maximum likelihood estimates of the log odds ratio and $(\alpha_0, \alpha_X, \alpha_Y)$. Most software packages handle this computation if $\alpha_{XY} XY$ is declared as an "offset."

We can conduct a similar sensitivity analysis in a less formal way through a simple extreme-case scenario. For example, if the missing variable is binary, we know that it is either 1 or 0. Thus, one extreme case is when all missing X's are 1 or all are 0. However, the maximum impact on the sample log odds ratio, $\ln o$, does not occur when all missing X's have the maximum (or minimum) value (i.e., $\alpha_X \to \pm\infty$). Rather, the log odds ratio is maximized (or minimized) when all missing X's with $Y = 1$ are 1 (or 0), and all missing X's with $Y = 0$ are 0 (or 1) (i.e., $\alpha_{XY} \to \pm\infty$).

Consider the smoking and hypertension data in Table 16.2. The odds ratio estimate is maximized when all the data in the incomplete table are in the diagonal cells, as shown in Table 16.21. In this scenario, $\alpha_{XY} = -\infty$. The odds ratio estimate is $o = \{(30 + 80) \times (40 + 20)\}/\{(20 + 0) \times (10 + 0)\} = 33$. Conversely, the odds ratio estimate is minimized when all the data are in the off-diagonal cells, as in Table 16.22. In this scenario, $\alpha_{XY} = -\infty$. The odds ratio estimate is $o = \{(30 + 0) \times (40 + 0)\}/\{(20 + 80) \times (10 + 20)\} = 0.25$.

At one extreme, the odds ratio is 33; at the other, it is 0.25. Less extreme odds ratio estimates can be obtained changing one cell count at a time. The second most extreme cases would be the two incomplete tables shown in Table 16.23.

Table 16.21. One extreme-case scenario for the missing data of Table 16.2

		(a) Complete Table					(b) Incomplete Table		
		\multicolumn{3}{c} H				H		
		1	0	Total			1	0	Total
S	1	30	20	50	S	1	80	0	80
	0	10	40	50		0	0	20	20
	Total	40	60	100		Total	80	20	100

Table 16.22. *Another extreme-case scenario for the missing data of Table 16.2*

		(a) Complete Table						(b) Incomplete Table		
			H						H	
		1	0	Total				1	0	Total
S	1	30	20	50		S	1	0	80	80
	0	10	40	50			0	20	0	20
	Total	40	60	100			Total	80	20	100

Table 16.23. *Two near-extreme-case scenarios for the missing data of Table 16.2*

		(a) Incomplete Table 1						(b) Incomplete Table 2		
			H						H	
		1	0	Total				1	0	Total
S	1	79	1	80		S	1	80	0	80
	0	0	20	20			0	1	19	20
	Total	79	21	100			Total	81	19	100

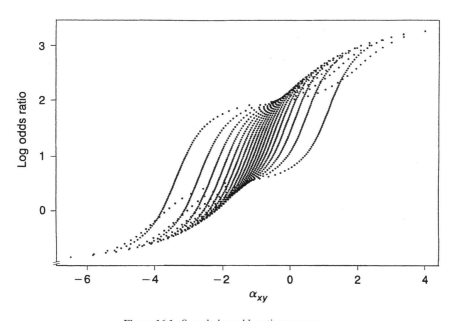

Figure 16.1. Sample log odds ratio versus α_{XY}.

We can continue changing the cell counts in the incomplete table, maintaining fixed row margins. Each such table corresponds to a certain value of α_{XY}. A plot of the resultant log odds ratios versus α_{XY} is informative. Figure 16.1 shows all possible pairs $(\alpha_{XY}, \ln o)$ generated by changing cell counts in the incomplete table. The two horizontal lines represent the logs of the extreme values computed for the data in Tables 16.21 and 16.22 (maximum = $\ln 33 = 3.4965$, minimum = $\ln 0.25 = -1.3863$). Recall that $\alpha_X = \alpha_{XY} = 0$ corresponds to MAR.

16.7.* NONMONOTONE MISSINGNESS

So far, we have considered monotonically missing data only. Now we turn to the situation in which covariate Z is completely observed, but X and Y are partially observed. There are four possible patterns of missingness (Table 16.24): (i) (X, Y, Z) are all observed; (ii) X is missing and (Y, Z) are observed; (iii) Y is missing and (X, Z) are observed; and (iv) X and Y are missing and Z is observed. Let R_X and R_Y be the observation indicators for X and Y, respectively.

Consider the (non)response mechanism

$$P(R_X | X, Y, Z) = P(R_X | Y, Z). \qquad (16.48)$$

Although this mechanism looks the same as the mechanism assumed under MAR in the case of a missing covariate, the nonresponse mechanism here is nonignorable: the missingness of X may depend on an unobserved value of Y.

Under (16.48), complete-record analysis is not valid, because generally

$$P(Y | X, Z, R_X = 1, R_Y = 1) \neq P(Y | X, Z).$$

If

$$P(R_Y | X, Y, Z) = P(R_Y | Z) \qquad (16.49a)$$

and

$$P(R_X | X, Y, Z, R_Y) = P(R_X | Z, R_Y), \qquad (16.49b)$$

Table 16.24. *Nonmonotonically missing data (hypothetical)*

Pattern	Y	X	Z	R_X	R_Y
(i)	o	o	o	1	1
(ii)	o	?	o	1	0
(iii)	?	o	o	0	1
(iv)	?	?	o	0	0

the nonresponse mechanism is MCAR, and it follows that

$$P(Y|X, Z, R_X = 1, R_Y = 1) = P(Y|X, Z)$$

(Problem 16.9). In this case, complete-record analysis is valid.

A more elaborate set of assumptions is required for non-monotonically missing data to be MAR, which we specify below to illustrate the likelihood and imputation methods of analysis. The weighting method can be applied as in the monotone case by weighting the completely observed records [pattern (i)] by $1/P(R_X = 1, \ R_Y = 1 | X \ Y, Z)$ (Rotnitzky and Robins, 1997; Robins, 1997).

Likelihood Approach

For the moment, we do not assume (16.48). The likelihood function requires specification of the joint distribution of $P(R_X, R_Y, X, Y|Z)$. We partition the joint distribution as for selection models:

$$P(R_X, R_Y, X, Y|Z) = P(R_X, R_Y|X, Y, Z)P(Y|X, Z)P(X|Z).$$

The full likelihood function for the nonmonotonically missing data in Table 16.24 is

$$L = \prod_{i=1}^{n} L_{i1}^{R_{X_i} R_{Y_i}} L_{i2}^{(1-R_{X_i})R_{Y_i}} L_{i3}^{R_{X_i}(1-R_{Y_i})} L_{i4}^{(1-R_{X_i})(1-R_{Y_i})},$$

where

$$L_{i1} = P(Y_i|X_i, Z_i)^{Y_i} \{1 - P(Y_i|X_i, Z_i)\}^{1-Y_i}$$
$$\times P(X_i|Z_i)P(R_{X_i} = 1, R_{Y_i} = 1|X_i, Y_i, Z_i),$$

$$L_{i2} = \sum_{x=0}^{1} P(Y_i|x, Z_i)^{Y_i} \{1 - P(Y_i|x, Z_i)\}^{1-Y_i}$$
$$\times P(x|Z_i)P(R_{X_i} = 0, R_{Y_i} = 1|x, Y_i, Z_i),$$

$$L_{i3} = \sum_{y=0}^{1} P(y|X_i, Z_i)^{y} \{1 - P(y|X_i, Z_i)\}^{1-y} P(X_i|Z_i)$$
$$\times P(R_{X_i} = 1, R_{Y_i} = 0|X_i, y, Z_i),$$

$$L_{i4} = \sum_{x=0}^{1} \sum_{y=0}^{1} P(y|x, Z_i)^{y} \{1 - P(y|x, Z_i)\}^{1-y}$$
$$\times P(x|Z_i)P(R_{X_i} = 0, R_{Y_i} = 0|x, y, Z_i).$$

L_{i1}, L_{i2}, L_{i3}, and L_{i4} represent the contributions to the likelihood function of patterns (i) through (iv), respectively. The resulting score function for β is

$$\frac{\partial \ln L}{\partial \beta} = \sum_{i=1}^{n} \Big\{ R_{X_i} R_{Y_i} u_i + (1 - R_{X_i}) R_{Y_i} E(u_i | Y_i, Z_i, R_{X_i} = 0, R_{Y_i} = 1)$$

$$+ R_{X_i}(1 - R_{Y_i}) E(u_i | X_i, Z_i, R_{X_i} = 1, R_{Y_i} = 0)$$

$$+ (1 - R_{X_i})(1 - R_{Y_i}) E(u_i | Z_i, R_{X_i} = 0, R_{Y_i} = 0) \Big\} = 0. \quad (16.50)$$

This score function differs from the full data score function only in that missing statistics have been replaced by their conditional expectations. If X is missing and Y is observed [pattern (ii)], u_i is replaced with $E(u_i | Y_i, Z_i, R_{X_i} = 0, R_{Y_i} = 1)$; if Y is missing and X is observed [pattern (iii)], u_i is replaced with $E(u_i | X_i, Z_i, R_{X_i} = 1, R_{Y_i} = 0)$; if both X and Y are missing [pattern (iv)], u_i is replaced with $E(u_i | Z_i, R_{X_i} = 0, R_{Y_i} = 0)$. Then the problem is reduced to finding $P(X | Y, Z, R_X = 0, R_Y = 1)$, $P(Y | X, Z, R_X = 1, R_Y = 0)$, and $P(X, Y | Z, R_X = 0, R_Y = 0)$. These probabilities can be expressed as

$$P(X = x | Y, Z, R_X = 0, R_Y = 1)$$

$$= \frac{P(R_X = 0, R_Y = 1 | X = x, Y, Z) P(Y | X = x, Z) P(X = x | Z)}{\sum_{i=0}^{1} P(R_X = 0, R_Y = 1 | X = i, Y, Z) P(Y | X = i, Z) P(X = i | Z)},$$

$$P(Y = y | X, Z, R_X = 1, R_Y = 0)$$

$$= \frac{P(R_X = 1, R_Y = 0 | X, Y = y, Z) P(Y = y | X, Z) P(X | Z)}{\sum_{j=0}^{1} P(R_X = 1, R_Y = 0 | X, Y = j, Z) P(Y = j | X, Z) P(X | Z)},$$

and

$$P(X = x, Y = y | Z, R_X = 0, R_Y = 0)$$

$$= \frac{P(R_X = 0, R_Y = 0 | X = x, Y = y, Z) P(Y = y | X = x, Z) P(X = x | Z)}{\sum_{i=0}^{1} \sum_{j=0}^{1} P(R_X = 0, R_Y = 0 | X = i, Y = j, Z) P(Y = j | X = i, Z) P(X = i | Z)}.$$

In addition to assuming the models for $P(Y | X, Z)$ and $P(X | Z)$ as in (16.17) and (16.22), we need to model the probabilities of response for X and Y. Further partitioning of the joint distribution of R_X and R_Y is possible:

$$P(R_X, R_Y | X, Y, Z) = P(R_X | X, Y, Z, R_Y) P(R_Y | X, Y, Z)$$

$$= P(R_Y | X, Y, Z, R_X) P(R_X | X, Y, Z).$$

Which partition is preferable is determined by the nature of the study. If Y is observed first, for example, and the observation of X depends on whether Y is observed or not, the first partition is the natural choice. We proceed with the first partitioning. Let π_X denote the conditional probability of observing X given R_Y and (X, Y, Z):

$$\pi_X = P(R_X = 1 | X, Y, Z, R_Y)$$

and π_Y the probability of observing Y given X, Y, Z:

$$\pi_Y = P(R_Y = 1 | X, Y, Z).$$

As in previous cases, we assume that the functional forms of π_X and π_Y are known up to some unknown parameters.

We now specialize the development by assuming

$$\ln \frac{\pi_X}{1 - \pi_X} = \alpha_0 + \alpha_Y Y + \alpha_Z Z + \alpha_{R_Y} R_Y \tag{16.51}$$

and

$$\ln \frac{\pi_Y}{1 - \pi_Y} = \eta_0 + \eta_X X + \eta_Z Z. \tag{16.52}$$

Note that π_X does not depend on X (given Y, Z, and R_Y) and π_Y does not depend on Y (given X and Z, ignoring R_X). This does not imply that (16.48) is true, however, because $P(R_X | X, Y, Z)$ is a weighted average of $P(R_X | X, Y, Z, R_Y)$ for $R_Y = 1$ or 0, with weights $\pi_Y = P(R_Y | X, Y, Z)$. While the averaged items are assumed independent of X in (16.51), the weights π_Y from (16.52) still may depend on X. The missingness is still nonmonotonically nonignorable because π_X depends on Y and π_Y depends on X. Looking ahead to the discussion of MAR, however, the assumptions embodied in (16.51) and (16.52) are natural to make.

To compute conditional expectations for the score function for β, we fit three more models to estimate γ, α, and η. Assuming (16.22), the score function for γ is

$$\frac{\partial \ln L}{\partial \gamma} = \sum_{i=1}^{n} \left\{ R_X \begin{pmatrix} X_i - \mu_i \\ Z_i(X_i - \mu_i) \end{pmatrix} \right.$$

$$+ (1 - R_{X_i}) R_{Y_i} \begin{pmatrix} E(X_i | Y_i, Z_i, R_{X_i} = 0, R_{Y_i} = 1) - \mu_i \\ Z_i \{ E(X_i | Y_i, Z_i, R_{X_i} = 0, R_{Y_i} = 1) - \mu_i \} \end{pmatrix}$$

$$\left. + (1 - R_{X_i})(1 - R_{X_i}) \begin{pmatrix} E(X_i | Z_i, R_{X_i} = 0, R_{Y_i} = 0) - \mu_i \\ Z_i \{ E(X_i | Z_i, R_{X_i} = 0, R_{Y_i} = 0) - \mu_i \} \end{pmatrix} \right\}$$

$$= 0. \tag{16.53}$$

For α, we have

$$
\frac{\partial \ln L}{\partial \alpha} = \sum_{i=1}^{n} \left\{ R_{Y_i} \begin{pmatrix} 1 \\ Y_i \\ Z_i \\ R_{Y_i} \end{pmatrix} (R_{X_i} - \pi_{X_i}) \right.
$$

$$
+ R_{X_i}(1 - R_{Y_i}) \begin{pmatrix} R_{X_i} - E(\pi_{X_i}|X_i, Z_i, R_{X_i} = 1, R_{Y_i} = 0) \\ E\{Y_i(R_{X_i} - \pi_{X_i})|X_i, Z_i, R_{X_i} = 1, R_{Y_i} = 0\} \\ Z_i\{R_{X_i} - E(\pi_{X_i}|X_i, Z_i, R_{X_i} = 1, R_{Y_i} = 0)\} \\ R_{Y_i}\{R_{X_i} - E(\pi_{X_i}|X_i, Z_i, R_{X_i} = 1, R_{Y_i} = 0)\} \end{pmatrix}
$$

$$
\left. + (1 - R_{X_i})(1 - R_{Y_i}) \begin{pmatrix} R_{X_i} - E(\pi_{X_i}|Z_i, R_{X_i} = 0, R_{Y_i} = 0) \\ E\{Y_i(R_{X_i} - \pi_{X_i})|Z_i, R_{X_i} = 0, R_{Y_i} = 0\} \\ Z_i\{R_{X_i} - E(\pi_{X_i}|Z_i, R_{X_i} = 0, R_{Y_i} = 0)\} \\ R_{Y_i}\{R_{X_i} - E(\pi_{X_i}|Z_i, R_{X_i} = 0, R_{Y_i} = 0)\} \end{pmatrix} \right\}
$$

$$
= \sum_{i=1}^{n} \left\{ R_{Y_i} \begin{pmatrix} 1 \\ Y_i \\ Z_i \\ 1 \end{pmatrix} (R_{X_i} - \pi_{X_i}) \right.
$$

$$
+ R_{X_i}(1 - R_{Y_i}) \begin{pmatrix} 1 - E(\pi_{X_i}|X_i, Z_i, R_{X_i} = 1, R_{Y_i} = 0) \\ E\{Y_i(1 - \pi_{X_i})|X_i, Z_i, R_{X_i} = 1, R_{Y_i} = 0\} \\ Z_i\{1 - E(\pi_{X_i}|X_i, Z_i, R_{X_i} = 1, R_{Y_i} = 0)\} \\ 0 \end{pmatrix}
$$

$$
\left. + (1 - R_{X_i})(1 - R_{Y_i}) \begin{pmatrix} -E(\pi_{X_i}|Z_i, R_{X_i} = 0, R_{Y_i} = 0) \\ E\{Y_i(-\pi_{X_i})|Z_i, R_{X_i} = 0, R_{Y_i} = 0\} \\ -Z_i E(\pi_{X_i}|Z_i, R_{X_i} = 0, R_{Y_i} = 0) \\ 0 \end{pmatrix} \right\} = 0. \quad (16.54)
$$

Similarly for η,

$$
\frac{\partial \ln L}{\partial \eta} = \sum_{i=1}^{n} \left\{ R_{X_i} \begin{pmatrix} 1 \\ X_i \\ Z_i \end{pmatrix} (R_{Y_i} - \pi_{Y_i}) \right.
$$

$$
+ (1 - R_{X_i}) R_{Y_i} \begin{pmatrix} R_{Y_i} - E\left(\pi_{Y_i} | Y_i, Z_i, R_{X_i} = 0, R_{Y_i} = 1\right) \\ E\{X_i(R_{Y_i} - \pi_{Y_i}) | Y_i Z_i, R_{X_i} = 0, R_{Y_i} = 1\} \\ Z_i\{R_{Y_i} - E\left(\pi_{Y_i} | Y_i, Z_i, R_{X_i} = 0, R_{Y_i} = 1\right)\} \end{pmatrix}
$$

$$
\left. + (1 - R_{X_i})(1 - R_{Y_i}) \begin{pmatrix} R_{Y_i} - E\left(\pi_{Y_i} | Z_i, R_{X_i} = 0, R_{Y_i} = 0\right) \\ E\{X_i(R_{Y_i} - \pi_{Y_i}) | Z_i, R_{X_i} = 0, R_{Y_i} = 0\} \\ Z_i\{R_{Y_i} - E\left(\pi_{Y_i} | Z_i, R_{X_i} = 0, R_{Y_i} = 0\right)\} \end{pmatrix} \right\}
$$

$$
= \sum_{i=1}^{n} \left\{ R_{X_i} \begin{pmatrix} 1 \\ X_i \\ Z_i \end{pmatrix} (R_{Y_i} - \pi_{Y_i}) \right.
$$

$$
+ (1 - R_{X_i}) R_{Y_i} \begin{pmatrix} 1 - E\left(\pi_{Y_i} | Y_i, Z_i, R_{X_i} = 0, R_{Y_i} = 1\right) \\ E\{X_i(1 - \pi_{Y_i}) | Y_i Z_i, R_{X_i} = 0, R_{Y_i} = 1\} \\ Z_i\{1 - E\left(\pi_{Y_i} | Y_i, Z_i, R_{X_i} = 0, R_{Y_i} = 1\right)\} \end{pmatrix}
$$

$$
\left. + (1 - R_{X_i})(1 - R_{Y_i}) \begin{pmatrix} -E\left(\pi_{Y_i} | Z_i, R_{X_i} = 0, R_{Y_i} = 0\right) \\ -E\{X_i\pi_{Y_i} | Z_i, R_{X_i} = 0, R_{Y_i} = 0\} \\ -Z_i E\left(\pi_{Y_i} | Z_i, R_{X_i} = 0, R_{Y_i} = 0\right) \end{pmatrix} \right\} = 0.
$$

$$
(16.55)
$$

By solving equations (16.50), (16.53), (16.54), and (16.55) simultaneously, we obtain maximum likelihood estimates of β, γ, α, and η. Solving the four equations simultaneously may seem overwhelming, but it can be accomplished with widely available software. We describe the details below.

Computation

The first step is to create an expanded dataset. We duplicate records with pattern (ii), one with $X = 1$ and the other with $X = 0$; the case weights attached to the duplicated records are $P(X = 1|Y, Z, R_Y = 1, R_X = 0)$ and $P(X = 0|Y, Z, R_Y = 1, R_X = 0)$, respectively. We duplicate records with pattern (iii), one with $Y = 1$ and the other with $Y = 0$; the weights attached to the duplicated records are $P(Y = 1|X, Z, R_Y = 0, R_X = 1)$ and $P(Y = 0|X, Z, R_Y = 0, R_X = 1)$, respectively. We *quadruplicate* records with pattern (iv): $(Y = 1, X = 1)$; $(Y = 1, X = 0)$; $(Y = 0, X = 1)$; and $(Y = 0, X = 0)$. The weights attached to the quadruplicated records are $P(Y = 1, X = 1|Z, R_X = 0, R_Y = 0)$, $P(Y = 1, X = 0|Z, R_X = 0, R_Y = 0)$, $P(Y = 0, X = 1|Z, R_X = 0, R_Y = 0)$, and $P(Y = 0, X = 0|Z, R_X = 0, R_Y = 0)$, respectively.

Given initial values of β, γ, α, and η, we compute the case weights. The weight for observed records is 1. The weight for the duplicated records from pattern (ii) is

$$
\begin{aligned}
w &= P(X|Y, Z, R_X = 0, R_Y = 1; \alpha, \beta, \gamma, \eta) \\[2mm]
&= \frac{P(R_X = 0|Y, Z, R_Y = 1; \alpha)P(R_Y = 1|X, Z; \eta)P(Y|X, Z; \beta)P(X|Z; \gamma)}{\displaystyle\sum_{x=0}^{1} P(R_X = 0|Y, Z, R_Y = 1; \alpha)P(R_Y = 1|X = x, Z; \eta)} \\
&\hspace{5cm} \cdot P(Y|X = x, Z; \beta)P(X = x|Z; \gamma) \\[2mm]
&= \frac{P(R_Y = 1|X, Z; \eta)P(Y|X, Z; \beta)P(X|Z; \gamma)}{\displaystyle\sum_{x=0}^{1} P(R_Y = 1|X = x, Z; \eta)P(Y|X = x, Z; \beta)P(X = x|Z; \gamma)}.
\end{aligned}
$$

The weights associated with the duplicated and quadruplicated records from patterns (iii) and (iv), $P(Y|X, Z, R_X = 1, R_Y = 0)$ and $P(Y, X|Z, R_X = 0, R_Y = 0)$, respectively, are computed similarly. Once the weights are computed, weighted logistic models for X, Y, R_X, and R_Y are fitted using the expanded dataset with the computed weights. Using the new estimates of α, β, γ, and η, the weights are updated and the procedure is repeated until convergence. Standard errors can be computed by the jackknife technique.

We note that solution of the likelihood equations without assumptions (16.51) and (16.52) proceeds as above with some additional equations: in (16.54),

$$
\begin{aligned}
\sum_{i=1}^{n} &\Big[R_{X_i} R_{Y_i} X_i (R_{X_i} - \pi_{X_i}) \\
&+ (1 - R_{X_i}) R_{Y_i} E\{X_i (R_{X_i} - \pi_{X_i})|Y_i, Z_i, R_{X_i} = 0, R_{Y_i} = 1\} \\
&+ R_{X_i}(1 - R_{Y_i}) E\{X_i (R_{X_i} - \pi_{X_i})|X_i, Z_i, R_{X_i} = 1, R_{Y_i} = 0\} \\
&+ (1 - R_{X_i})(1 - R_{Y_i}) E\{X_i (R_{X_i} - \pi_{X_i})|Z_i, R_{X_i} = 0, R_{Y_i} = 0\} \Big] = 0,
\end{aligned}
$$

and in (16.55),

$$\sum_{i=1}^{n} \left[R_{X_i} R_{Y_i} Y_i (R_{Y_i} - \pi_{Y_i}) \right.$$

$$+ R_{X_i}(1 - R_{Y_i}) E\{Y_i(R_{Y_i} - \pi_{Y_i}) | X_i, Z_i, R_{X_i} = 1, R_{Y_i} = 0\}$$

$$+ (1 - R_{X_i}) R_{Y_i} E\{Y_i(R_{Y_i} - \pi_{Y_i}) | Y_i, Z_i, R_{X_i} = 0, R_{Y_i} = 1\}$$

$$\left. + (1 - R_{X_i})(1 - R_{Y_i}) E\{Y_i(R_{Y_i} - \pi_{Y_i}) | Z_i, R_{X_i} = 0, R_{Y_i} = 0\} \right] = 0,$$

Beware of non-identifiability. As noted in Section 16.3, the missingness pattern can be confounded with the nonresponse mechanism (Mark and Gail, 1994). As in Section 16.6, sensitivity analysis is required. Model-checking methods with missing data need further research.

MAR under Nonmonotone Missingness

For the nonmonotonically missing data shown in Table 16.24 to be MAR, more restrictive missingness assumptions than (16.48) are needed. The following set of conditions, for example, satisfy (16.48) and yield a MAR mechanism when missingness is nonmonotone (Problem 16.10):

$$P(R_Y | X, Y, Z) = P(R_Y | Z),$$

$$P(R_X | X, Y, Z, R_Y = 1) = P(R_X | Y, Z, R_Y = 1), \qquad (16.56)$$

$$P(R_X | X, Y, Z, R_Y = 0) = P(R_X | Z, R_Y = 0).$$

Another example of MAR can be found under the nonmonotone missingness pattern of Problem 16.11. Robins and Gill (1997) discuss MAR processes that result in nonmonotonic missingness.

Under assumption (16.56), R_Y depends on neither X nor Y, given Z. If Y is observed ($R_Y = 1$), R_X may depend on Y and Z, but not on X. However, if Y is not observed ($R_Y = 0$), R_X depends on neither X nor the unobserved Y, given Z. Assumption (16.56) specializes (16.51) with $\alpha_Y = 0$ and (16.52) with $\eta_X = 0$. The conditional expectations simplify to

$$P(X | Y, Z, R_X = 0, R_Y = 1)$$

$$= \frac{P(R_X = 0 | Y, Z, R_Y = 1) P(R_Y = 1 | Z) P(Y | X, Z) P(X | Z)}{\sum_{x=0}^{1} P(R_X = 0 | Y, Z, R_Y = 1) P(R_Y = 1 | Z) P(Y | X = x, Z) P(X = x | Z)}$$

$$= \frac{P(Y | X, Z) P(X | Z)}{\sum_{x=0}^{1} P(Y | X = x, Z) P(X = x | Z)},$$

$$P(Y|X, Z, R_X = 1, R_Y = 0)$$

$$= \frac{P(R_X = 1|Z, R_Y = 0)P(R_Y = 0|Z)P(Y|X, Z)P(X|Z)}{\sum\limits_{y=0}^{1} P(R_X = 1|Z, R_Y = 0)P(R_Y = 0|Z)P(Y = y|X, Z)P(X|Z)}$$

$$= \frac{P(Y|X, Z)P(X|Z)}{\sum\limits_{y=0}^{1} P(Y = y|X, Z)P(X|Z)},$$

and

$$P(X, Y|Z, R_X = 0, R_Y = 0)$$

$$= \frac{P(R_X = 0|Z, R_Y = 0)P(R_Y = 0|Z)P(Y|X, Z)P(X|Z)}{\sum\limits_{x=0}^{1}\sum\limits_{y=0}^{1} P(R_X = 0| Z, R_Y = 0)}$$
$$\cdot P(R_Y = 0|Z)P(Y = y|X = x, Z)P(X = x|Z)$$

$$= \frac{P(Y|X, Z)P(X|Z)}{\sum\limits_{x=0}^{1}\sum\limits_{y=0}^{1} P(Y = y|X = x, Z)P(X = x|Z)}. \tag{16.57}$$

These relationships show that the conditional expectations of the missing statistics given the observed data do not involve the nonresponse mechanisms. That is, we do not need to estimate α or η. We can solve just two equations, (16.50) and (16.53), simultaneously to obtain a consistent estimate of β. This is similar to the case of monotone missing data under MAR—when only covariate X is missing and Y is observed, we need assumptions about $P(Y|X, Z)$ and $P(X|Z)$ (or $P(X|Y, Z)$), but not about the probability of nonresponse.

The MAR missingness mechanism shown in (16.56) also simplifies the score function for β shown in equation (16.50). The contributions from patterns (iii) and (iv) become zero: since $E(Y|X, Z, R_X = 1, R_Y = 0) = E(Y|X, Z)$, we have $E(u_i|X_i, Z_i, R_{X_i} = 1, R_{Y_i} = 0) = 0$. Also, the relationship $E(X, Y|Z, R_X = 0, R_Y = 0) = E(X, Y|Z)$ leads to $E(Y|Z, R_X = 0, R_Y = 0) = E\{P(X, Z)|Z, R_X = 0, R_Y = 0\}$, and $E(u|Z, R_X = 0, R_Y = 0) = 0$. The score equation reduces to

$$\frac{\partial \ln L}{\partial \beta} = \sum_{i=1}^{n} R_{X_i} R_{Y_i} u_i + (1 - R_{X_i})R_{Y_i} E(u_i|Y_i, Z_i, R_{X_i} = 0, R_{Y_i} = 1) = 0.$$

$$\tag{16.58}$$

The patterns with missing Y ($R_Y = 0$ regardless of R_X) do not contribute to the score function of β. This result is similar to the case of missing outcome data where the likelihood approach reduces to complete-record analysis. For the score function of γ, the contribution from pattern (iv) becomes zero:

$$(1 - R_X)(1 - R_Y)\left(\frac{1}{Z}\right)\{E(X|Z, R_X = 0, R_Y = 0) - \mu\} = 0,$$

because $E(X|Z, R_X = 0, R_Y = 0) = E(X|Z) = \mu$. While the score function for β utilizes the data with patterns (i) and (ii), the score function for γ utilizes the data with patterns (i), (ii), and (iii).

To estimate β by imputation, the relationship $P(Y|X, Z, R_Y = 1) = P(Y|X, Z)$ proved in Problem 16.10 shows that analysis using patterns (i) and (ii) only ($R_Y = 1$ regardless of R_X) is valid under (16.56). In these patterns, only X is missing and therefore $E(X|Y, Z, R_X = 0, R_Y = 1)$ suffices for imputation. In fact, because

$$E(X|Y, Z, R_X = 0, R_Y = 1) = E(X|Y, Z, R_X = 1, R_Y = 1) = E(X|Y, Z),$$

the imputation model $E(X|Y, Z, R_X = 0, R_Y = 1)$ can be consistently estimated using complete records only. If we restrict our attention to the data

Table 16.25. Hypothetical data for a pair of 2 × 2 tables with nonmonotonically missing X and Y

R_Y	R_X	Y	X	Z	Frequencies
1	1	1	1	1	8
1	1	1	1	0	14
1	1	1	0	1	22
1	1	1	0	0	14
1	1	0	1	1	7
1	1	0	1	0	9
1	1	0	0	1	11
1	1	0	0	0	14
1	0	1	?	1	29
1	0	1	?	0	22
1	0	0	?	1	10
1	0	0	?	0	10
0	1	?	1	1	5
0	1	?	1	0	6
0	1	?	0	1	5
0	1	?	0	0	8
0	0	?	?	1	3
0	0	?	?	0	3

with patterns (i) and (ii) (Y completely observed and X missing monotonically), the method described for missing covariates can be applied. We model $P(X|Y, Z)$ directly as in (16.20), compute the conditional expectation, then solve (16.58). This approach consists of two separate steps (computing expectation and solving for β), whereas the likelihood approach requires alternating the two steps iteratively. Both approaches yield consistent estimates of β.

Table 16.26. *Parameter estimates and standard errors for the coefficients of (16.17) using three different methods*

Method	Estimate	β_0	β_X	β_Z
Likelihood (NI):	parameter	0.4153	−0.0008	0.3308
(16.22), (16.51), (16.52)	se	0.3047	0.4438	0.3356
Likelihood (MAR):	parameter	0.4101	0.0121	0.3313
(16.22), (16.56)	se	0.3063	0.4430	0.3358
Imputation (MAR):	parameter	0.4157	−0.0004	0.3298
(16.20), (16.56)	se	0.3076	0.4449	0.3377

Table 16.27. *Parameter estimates and standard errors of the imputation and missingness models*

Likelihood (NI)	Estimate	γ_0		γ_Z	
(16.22)	parameter	−0.2229		−0.4252	
	se	0.2577		0.3818	

	Estimate	α_0	α_Y	α_Z	α_{R_Y}
(16.51)	parameter	1.8768	−0.5728	−0.2280	−1.0517
	se	0.5712	0.3426	0.3054	0.5257

	Estimate	η_0	η_X	η_Z	
(16.52)	parameter	1.7165	−0.2811	0.2872	
	se	0.3801	0.4911	0.4247	

Likelihood (MAR)	Estimate	γ_0		γ_Z	
(16.22)	parameter	−0.2157		−0.4256	
	se	0.2553		0.3807	

Imputation (MAR)	Estimate	δ_0	δ_Y	δ_Z	
(16.20)	parameter	−0.1965	−0.0004	−0.5917	
	se	0.3772	0.4449	0.4385	

The likelihood approach is more efficient than the imputation approach, because the data with patterns (i), (ii), and (iii) are used for the mle of the nuisance parameter γ, while only pattern (i) is used for the imputation estimate. However, in practice the loss of efficiency by using the imputation approach is typically small (e.g. Table 16.17), because the estimating equations for β are the same and the only difference arises from the imprecision of the nuisance parameter γ.

Example 16.7.1. Consider the nonmonotonically missing data in Table 16.25.

Results of fitting the models under nonmonotonic NI and MAR are shown in Tables 16.26 and 16.27. SAS® code to fit these models is provided in http://www.wiley.com/statistics. The complete-record Mantel-Haenszel odds ratio is 0.9493 with log odds ratio -0.052. The total number of records in the expanded data set is 313. While the estimates under MAR and NI show little difference in Table 16.26, the maximum likelihood estimates under MAR are only slightly more efficient than the imputation estimates under MAR. Note that $\eta_X = 0$ corresponds to MAR, while nonzero η_X supports nonignorable missingness. The Wald test for H_0: $\eta_X = 0$ from the likelihood NI model gives $z = -0.2811/0.4911 = 0.5724$, and we fail to reject H_0. This might explain why the estimates under MAR and nonignorable missingness are similar.

PROBLEMS

16.1. Starting with the definitions in (16.1), use Bayes' theorem to verify the following relations.

(a) Under the MAR mechanism represented by $P(R_H|S, H) = P(R_H|S)$,

$$P(H|S, R_H = 1) = P(H|S).$$

(b) Under MAR, $P(S = 1|H = 1, R_H = 0) \neq P(S = 1|H = 1, R_H = 1)$.

(c) Under the MCAR mechanism represented by $P(R_H|S, H) = P(R_H)$,

$$P(S, H|R_H = 1) = P(S, H|R_H = 0).$$

16.2. Derive an empirical variance estimate for $\hat{\pi}_1$ as follows. Let $\pi_1 = P(S = 1|H = 1)$, $P_1 = P(H = 1|S = 1, R = 1)$, $P_2 = P(H = 1|S = 0, R = 1)$, and let $M = a_o + m_1 P_1 + c_o + m_2 P_2$. The estimate $(\hat{\pi}_1, p_1, p_2)$

of (π_1, P_1, P_2) is the solution of the following three estimating equations:

$$U\begin{pmatrix} \pi_1 \\ P_1 \\ P_2 \end{pmatrix} = \begin{pmatrix} M\pi_1 - (a_o + m_1 P_1) \\ (a_o + b_o)P_1 - a_0 \\ (c_o + d_o)P_2 - c_0 \end{pmatrix} = 0.$$

Then $\hat{\pi}_1 - \pi_1$ is approximately equivalent to the first element of

$$\left\{ \frac{-\partial U}{\partial(\pi_1, P_1, P_2)} \right\}^{-1} U\begin{pmatrix} \pi_1 \\ P_1 \\ P_2 \end{pmatrix},$$

where

$$\frac{\partial U}{\partial(\pi_1, P_1, P_2)} = \begin{pmatrix} M & -m_1(1-\pi_1) & m_2\pi_1 \\ 0 & a_o + b_o & 0 \\ 0 & 0 & c_o + d_o \end{pmatrix},$$

and

$$\left\{ \frac{\partial U}{\partial(\pi_1, P_1, P_2)} \right\}^{-1} = \begin{pmatrix} \dfrac{1}{M} & \dfrac{m_1(1-\pi_1)}{M(a_o+b_o)} & \dfrac{-m_2\pi_1}{M(c_o+d_o)} \\ 0 & \dfrac{1}{a_o+b_o} & 0 \\ 0 & 0 & \dfrac{1}{c_o+d_o} \end{pmatrix}.$$

The variance of $\hat{\pi}_1$ is the upper left corner element of the matrix

$$\left\{ \frac{-\partial U}{\partial(\pi_1, P_1, P_2)} \right\}^{-1} \widehat{\mathrm{Var}}\left\{ U\begin{pmatrix} \pi_1 \\ P_1 \\ P_2 \end{pmatrix} \right\}\left[\left\{ \frac{-\partial U}{\partial(\pi_1, P_1, P_2)} \right\}^{-1} \right]'.$$

To estimate this matrix we evaluate the elements at $(\hat{\pi}_1, p_1, p_2)$, but the analytic derivation of $\mathrm{Var}\{U(\pi_1, P_1, P_2)\}$ is complicated. Instead we estimate $\mathrm{Var}\{U(\pi_1, P_1, P_2)\}$ empirically, by expressing U as a sum of independent random variables, and taking their sum of squared deviations. To this end, let $X_i = I[H_i = 1]$ be the hypertension indicator and $Y_i = I[S_i = 1]$ be the smoking indicator for the ith record. Let R_i be the observation indicator for H_i. Then $a_o = \Sigma_i X_i Y_i R_i$, $m_1 =$

$\Sigma_i(1 - R_i)Y_i$, and the other cell counts can be expressed similarly in terms of X_i, Y_i, and R_i. Then

$$U\begin{pmatrix}\pi_1 \\ P_1 \\ P_2\end{pmatrix} = \sum_i u_i \begin{pmatrix}\pi_1 \\ P_1 \\ P_2\end{pmatrix},$$

where $u_i(\pi_1, P_1, P_2)$ is given by

$$u_i\begin{pmatrix}\pi_1 \\ P_1 \\ P_2\end{pmatrix} = \begin{pmatrix} \{X_iY_iR_i + (1 - R_i)Y_iP_1 + (1 - X_i)Y_iR_i \\ \quad + (1 - R_i)(1 - Y_i)P_2\}\pi_1 - \{X_iY_iR_i + (1 - R_i)Y_iP_1\} \\ \{X_iY_iR_i + (1 - X_i)Y_iR_i\}P_1 - X_iY_iR_i \\ \{X_i(1 - Y_i)R_i + (1 - X_i)(1 - Y_i)R_i\}P_2 - X_i(1 - Y_i)R_i \end{pmatrix}.$$

The empirical variance estimate of $U(\pi_1 P_1, P_2)$ is then

$$\widehat{\mathrm{Var}}\left\{U\begin{pmatrix}\pi_1 \\ P_1 \\ P_2\end{pmatrix}\right\} = \sum_i u_i \begin{pmatrix}\hat{\pi}_1 \\ p_1 \\ p_2\end{pmatrix} u_i \begin{pmatrix}\hat{\pi}_1 \\ p_1 \\ p_2\end{pmatrix}'.$$

16.3. (a) Using the notation of Section 16.2.2, show that the imputation estimates can be written

$$\frac{a_o + \hat{a}_m}{a_o + \hat{a}_m + c_o + \hat{c}_m} = \frac{f_1 p_1}{\bar{p}}$$

and

$$\frac{b_o + \hat{b}_m}{b_o + \hat{b}_m + d_o + \hat{d}_m} = \frac{f_1 q_1}{\bar{q}}.$$

(b) Consider the joint distribution of (a_o, b_o, m_1) given n_1 to be multinomial with sample size n_1 and probability vector (P_a, P_b, P_m). Let $g(P_a, P_b, P_m) = P_a/(P_a + P_b)$. Use the delta method to show that the variance of $g(a_o, b_o, m_1) = a_o/(a_o + b_o) = p_1$ is given by $P_a P_b/\{n_1(P_a + P_b)^3\}$, which is estimated consistently by

$$\frac{(a_o/n_1)(b_o/n_1)}{n_1\{(a_o + b_o)/n_1\}^3} = \frac{a_o b_o}{(a_o + b_o)^3} = \frac{p_1 q_1}{n_1 - m_1}.$$

Similarly, the variance of p_2 is estimated by $p_2 q_2/(n_2 - m_2)$. By conditional independence of p_1 and p_2 given n_1 and n_2, conclude that the variance-covariance matrix of $(p_1, p_2)'$ is

$$\widehat{\mathrm{Cov}}\begin{pmatrix} p_1 \\ p_2 \end{pmatrix} = \begin{pmatrix} \dfrac{p_1 q_1}{n_1 - m_1} & 0 \\ 0 & \dfrac{p_2 q_2}{n_2 - m_2} \end{pmatrix}.$$

(c) Next, let $h\begin{pmatrix} p_1 \\ p_2 \end{pmatrix} = \begin{pmatrix} \hat{\pi}_1 \\ \hat{\pi}_2 \end{pmatrix} = f_1\begin{pmatrix} p_1/\bar{p} \\ q_1/\bar{q} \end{pmatrix}$. Show that

$$\frac{\partial h\begin{pmatrix} p_1 \\ p_2 \end{pmatrix}}{\partial(p_1, p_2)} = f_1 f_2 \begin{pmatrix} p_2/\bar{p}^2 & -p_1/\bar{p}^2 \\ -q_2/\bar{q}^2 & q_1/\bar{q}^2 \end{pmatrix}.$$

Using the results of part (b), show that

$$\mathrm{Cov}\begin{pmatrix} \hat{\pi}_1 \\ \hat{\pi}_2 \end{pmatrix} = \frac{\partial h\begin{pmatrix} p_1 \\ p_2 \end{pmatrix}}{\partial(p_1, p_2)} \mathrm{Cov}\begin{pmatrix} p_1 \\ p_2 \end{pmatrix} \left\{ \frac{\partial h\begin{pmatrix} p_1 \\ p_2 \end{pmatrix}}{\partial(p_1, p_2)} \right\}'$$

is estimated by the matrix

$$\begin{pmatrix} \{\hat{\pi}_1(1-\hat{\pi}_1)\}^2 \left\{ \dfrac{q_1/p_1}{n_1-m_1} + \dfrac{q_2/p_2}{n_2-m_2} \right\} & -\hat{\pi}_1(1-\hat{\pi}_1)\hat{\pi}_2(1-\hat{\pi}_2) \left\{ \dfrac{1}{n_1-m_1} + \dfrac{1}{n_2-m_2} \right\} \\ -\hat{\pi}_1(1-\hat{\pi}_1)\hat{\pi}_2(1-\hat{\pi}_2) \left\{ \dfrac{1}{n_1-m_1} + \dfrac{1}{n_2-m_2} \right\} & \{\hat{\pi}_2(1-\hat{\pi}_2)\}^2 \left\{ \dfrac{p_1/q_1}{n_1-m_1} + \dfrac{p_2/q_2}{n_2-m_2} \right\} \end{pmatrix}.$$

(d) Conclude that the estimated variance of $\hat{\pi}_1 - \hat{\pi}_2$ is given by

$$\widehat{\mathrm{Var}}(\hat{\pi}_1 - \hat{\pi}_2) = \{\hat{\pi}_1(1-\hat{\pi}_1)\}^2 \left(\frac{q_1/p_1}{n_1-m_1} + \frac{q_2/p_2}{n_2-m_2} \right)$$

$$+ \{\hat{\pi}_2(1-\hat{\pi}_2)\}^2 \left(\frac{p_1/q_1}{n_1-m_1} + \frac{p_2/q_2}{n_2-m_2} \right)$$

$$+ 2\{\hat{\pi}_1(1-\hat{\pi}_1)\hat{\pi}_2(1-\hat{\pi}_2)\} \left(\frac{1}{n_1-m_1} + \frac{1}{n_2-m_2} \right).$$

Demonstrate the equivalence of this expression to

$$\widehat{\mathrm{Var}}(\hat{\pi}_1 - \hat{\pi}_2) = \frac{1}{n_1 - m_1}\left\{\hat{\pi}_1(1-\hat{\pi}_1)\sqrt{\frac{q_1}{p_1}} + \hat{\pi}_2(1-\hat{\pi}_2)\sqrt{\frac{p_1}{q_1}}\right\}^2$$

$$+ \frac{1}{n_2 - m_2}\left\{\hat{\pi}_1(1-\hat{\pi}_1)\sqrt{\frac{q_2}{p_2}} + \hat{\pi}_2(1-\hat{\pi}_2)\sqrt{\frac{p_2}{q_2}}\right\}^2.$$

16.4. From the likelihood given in (16.24), derive the score equation for β,

$$U_\beta = \frac{\partial \ln L}{\partial \beta} = \sum_{i=1}^{n} R_i u_i + (1-R_i)E(u_i|Y_i, Z_i, R_i = 0)$$

$$= \sum_{i=1}^{n} R_i \begin{pmatrix} Y_i - P(X_i, Z_i) \\ X_i\{Y_i - P(X_i, Z_i)\} \\ Z_i\{Y_i - P(X_i, Z_i)\} \end{pmatrix}$$

$$+ (1-R_i)\begin{pmatrix} Y_i - E\{P(X_i, Z_i)|Y_i, Z_i, R_i = 0\} \\ E[X_i\{Y_i - P(X_i, Z_i)\}|Y_i, Z_i, R_i = 0] \\ Z_i[Y_i - E\{P(X_i, Z_i)|Y_i, Z_i, R_i = 0\}] \end{pmatrix} = 0.$$

and the score equation for γ,

$$U_\gamma = \frac{\partial \ln L}{\partial \gamma} = \sum_{i=1}^{n} R_i \begin{pmatrix} X_i - \mu_i \\ Z_i(X_i - \mu_i) \end{pmatrix}$$

$$+ (1-R_i)\begin{pmatrix} E(X_i|Y_i, Z_i, R_i = 0) - \mu_i \\ Z_i\{E(X_i|Y_i, Z_i, R_i = 0) - \mu_i\} \end{pmatrix} = 0.$$

16.5. Show that the negative derivative of $U_\beta^{(\nu)}(\beta)$ is

$$-\frac{\partial U_\beta^{(\nu)}}{\partial \beta'} = \sum_{i=1}^{n} R_i P(X_i, Z_i)\{1 - P(X_i, Z_i)\}\begin{pmatrix} 1 \\ X_i \\ Z_i \end{pmatrix}(1, X_i, Z_i')$$

$$+ (1-R_i)\begin{vmatrix} D_{1i} & D_{2i} & D_{1i}Z_i' \\ D_{2i} & D_{2i} & D_{2i}Z_i' \\ D_{1i}Z_i & D_{2i}Z_i & D_{1i}Z_iZ_i' \end{vmatrix},$$

where

$$D_{1i} = c_i^{(\nu)}P(1, Z_i)\{1 - P(1, Z_i)\} + (1 - c_i^{(\nu)})P(0, Z_i)\{0 - P(1, Z_i)\}$$

and

$$D_{2i} = c_i^{(\nu)}P(1, Z_i)\{1 - P(1, Z_i)\}.$$

Show that the negative derivative of $U_\gamma^{(\nu)}(\gamma)$ is

$$-\frac{\partial U_\gamma^{(\nu)}}{\partial \gamma'} = \sum_{i=1}^n \mu_i(1 - \mu_i)\begin{pmatrix} 1 \\ X_i \\ Z_i \end{pmatrix}(1, X_i, Z_i').$$

16.6. Use Bayes' theorem in the form

$$\frac{P(X=1|Y, Z)}{P(X=0|Y, Z)} = \frac{P(Y|X=1, Z)}{P(Y|X=0, Z)} \cdot \frac{P(X=1|Z)}{P(X=0|Z)}$$

to deduce the relationship between $P(X|Z)$ and $P(X|Y, Z)$ shown in (16.36).

16.7. Show that for U_β in (16.25), $EU_\beta = 0$. [*Hint*. Let $U_{\beta i} = R_i u_i + (1 - R_i)E(u_i|Y_i, Z_i, R_i = 0)$, so that $U_\beta = \Sigma_i U_{\beta i}$. Show that

$$E(U_{\beta i}|Y_i, Z_i, R_i = 1) = E(u_i|Y_i, Z_i, R_i = 1)$$

and

$$E(U_{\beta i}|Y_i, Z_i, R_i = 0) = E(u_i|Y_i, Z_i, R_i = 0).$$

Thus $E(U_{\beta i}|Y_i, Z_i) = E(u_i|Y_i, Z_i)$, whence $EU_{\beta i} = Eu_i$. But $E(u_i|X_i, Z_i) = 0$, whence $Eu_i = E\{E(u_i|X_i, Z_i)\} = 0$.]

16.8. Show that the negative derivative of $U_\beta(\beta, \delta)$ in (16.40) with respect to β is

$$-\frac{\partial U_\beta(\beta, \delta)}{\partial \beta'} = \sum_{i=1}^n R_i P(X_i, Z_i)\{1 - P(X_i, Z_i)\}\begin{pmatrix} 1 \\ X_i \\ Z_i \end{pmatrix}(1, X_i, Z_i')$$

$$+ (1 - R_i)\begin{vmatrix} D_{1i} & D_{2i} & D_{1i}Z_i' \\ D_{2i} & D_{2i} & D_{2i}Z_i' \\ D_{1i}Z_i & D_{2i}Z_i & D_{1i}Z_iZ_i' \end{vmatrix},$$

where

$$D_{1i} = c_i^{(\delta)} P(1, Z_i)\{1 - P(1, Z_i)\} + (1 - c_i^{(\delta)}) P(0, Z_i)\{0 - P(1, Z_i)\}$$
$$D_{2i} = c_i^{(\delta)} P(1, Z_i)\{1 - P(1, Z_i)\}.$$

and

$$c_i^{(\delta)} = P(X_i = 1 | Y_i, Z_i) = \frac{\exp(\delta_0 + \delta_Y Y_i + \delta_Z Z_i)}{1 + \exp(\delta_0 + \delta_Y Y_i + \delta_Z Z_i)}.$$

Show that the negative derivative of $U_\beta(\beta, \delta)$ in (16.40) with respect to δ is the asymmetric matrix

$$-\frac{\partial U_\beta(\beta, \delta)}{\partial \delta'} = \sum_{i=1}^{n} (1 - R_i) \begin{pmatrix} d_{1i} & d_{1i} Y_i & d_{1i} Z_i' \\ d_{2i} & d_{2i} Y_i & d_{2i} Z_i' \\ d_{1i} Z_i & d_{1i} Y_i Z_i & d_{1i} Z_i Z_i' \end{pmatrix},$$

where

$$d_{1i} = \{P(1, Z_i) - P(0, Z_i)\} c_i^{(\delta)} (1 - c_i^{(\delta)})$$

and

$$d_{2i} = \{Y_i - P(1, Z_i)\} c_i^{(\delta)} (1 - c_i^{(\delta)}).$$

Show that the negative derivative of $U_\delta(\delta)$ is

$$-\frac{\partial U_\delta(\delta)}{\partial \delta'} = \sum_{i=1}^{n} R_i c_i^{(\delta)} (1 - c_i^{(\delta)}) \begin{pmatrix} 1 \\ Y_i \\ Z_i \end{pmatrix} (1, Y_i, Z_i').$$

16.9. When both Y and X are partially missing as in Section 16.7, show that under assumptions (16.49), complete-record analysis is valid, namely, that

$$P(Y|X, Z, R_X = 1, R_Y = 1) = P(Y|X, Z).$$

16.10. Using the conditions given in (16.56), verify that

$$P(Y|X, Z, R_Y = 1) = P(Y|X, Z, R_Y = 0) = P(Y|X, Z).$$

Show also that (16.48) is satisfied, hence (16.56) is more restrictive than (16.48).

16.11. Instead of (16.56), assume the following nonmonotone missingness pattern:

$$P(R_X|X, Y, Z) = P(R_X|Z),$$

$$P(R_Y|X, Y, Z, R_X = 1) = P(R_Y|X, Z, R_X = 1),$$

$$P(R_Y|X, Y, Z, R_X = 0) = P(R_Y|X, Z, R_X = 0).$$

Show that MAR holds, that is,

$$P(Y|X, Z, R_Y = 1) = P(Y|X, Z, R_Y = 0) = P(Y|X, Z).$$

Show also that (16.48) is satisfied, hence the nonmonotone missingness pattern of this problem is also more restrictive than (16.48).

REFERENCES

Baker, S. G. and Laird, N. M. (1988). Regression analysis for categorical variables with outcome subject to nonresponse. *J. Am. Statist. Assoc.*, **83**, 62–69.

Dempster, A. P., Laird, N. M., and Rubin, D. M. (1977). Maximum likelihood from incomplete data via the EM algorithm. *J. R. Statist. Soc.*, Ser. B, **39**, 1–38.

Fitzmaurice, G. M., Laird, N. M., and Shneyer, L. (2001). An alternative parameterization of the general linear mixture model for longitudinal data with non-ignorable drop-outs. *Statist. in Med.*, **20**, 1009–1021.

Horvitz, D. G. and Thompson, D. J. (1952). A generalization of sampling without replacement from a finite universe. *J. Am. Statist. Assoc.*, **47**, 663–685.

Ibrahim, J. G. and Lipsitz, S. R. (1996). Parameter estimation from incomplete data in binomial regression when the missing data mechanism is non-ignorable. *Biometrics*, **52**, 1071–1078.

Kuk, A. Y. C., Mak, T. K., and Li, W. K. (2001). Estimation procedures for categorical survey data with non-ignorable nonresponse. *Comm. Statist.*, **A30**, 643–663.

Liang, K. Y. and Qin, J. (2000). Regression analysis under non-standard situations: A pairwise pseudolikelihood approach. *J. R. Statist. Soc.*, Ser. B, **62**, 773–786.

Lipsitz, S. R., Dear, K. B. G., and Zhao, L. (1994). Jackknife estimators of variance for parameter estimates from estimating equations with applications to clustered survival data. *Biometrics*, **50**, 842–846.

Lipsitz, S. R. and Fitzmaurice, G. M. (1996). The score test for independence in R × C contingency tables with missing data. *Biometrics*, **52**, 751–762.

Lipsitz, S. R. and Ibrahim, J. G. (1996). A conditional model for incomplete covariates in parametric regression models. *Biometrika*, **83**, 916–922.

Lipsitz, S. R., Ibrahim, J. G., Chen, M.-H., and Peterson, H. (1999). Non-ignorable missing covariates in generalized linear models. *Statist. in Med.*, **18**, 2435–2448.

Lipsitz, S. R., Ibrahim, J. G., and Zhao, L. P. (1999). A weighted estimating equation for missing covariate data with properties similar to maximum likelihood. *J. Am. Statist. Assoc.*, **94**, 1147–1160.

Little, R. J. A. (1986). Survey nonresponse adjustments for estimates of means. *Int. Statist. Rev.*, **54**, 139–158.

Little, R. J. A. (1994). A class of pattern-mixture models for normal incomplete data. *Biometrika*, **81**, 471–483.

Little, R. and Rubin, D. (1987). *Statistical analysis with missing data*. New York: Wiley.

Little, R. J. and Rubin, D. B. (1999). Comment on "Adjusting for non-ignorable drop-out using semiparametric nonresponse models." *J. Am. Statist. Assoc.*, **94**, 1130–1132.

Mark, S. D. and Gail, M. H. (1994). A comparison of likelihood-based and marginal estimating equation methods for analyzing repeated ordered categorical responses with missing data: Application to an intervention trial of vitamin prophylaxis for oesophageal dysplasia. *Statist. in Med.*, **13**, 479–493.

Murphy, S. A. and Van der Vaart, A. W. (2001). Semiparametric mixtures in case-control studies. *J. Multivariate Anal.*, **79**, 1–32.

Nelson, F. D. (1977). Censored regression models with unobserved, stochastic censoring thresholds. *J. Econometrics*, **6**, 309–328.

Paik, M. C. (1997). The generalized estimating equation approach when data are not missing completely at random. *J. Am. Statist. Assoc.*, **92**, 1320–1329.

Paik M. C. (2000). Methods for missing covariates in logistic regression. *Comm. Statist.*, **B29**, 1–20.

Pepe, M. S. and Fleming, T. R. (1991). A nonparametric method for dealing with mismeasured covariate data. *J. Am. Statist. Assoc.*, **86**, 108–113.

Reilly, M. and Pepe, M. S. (1995). A mean score method for missing and auxiliary covariate data in regression models. *Biometrika*, **82**, 299–314.

Reilly, M. and Pepe, M. S. (1998). The relationship between hot-deck multiple imputation and weighted likelihood. *Statist. in Med.*, **16**, 5–20.

Robins, J. M. (1997). Non-response models for the analysis of non-monotone non-ignorable missing data. *Statist. in Med.*, **16**, 21–37.

Robins, J. M. and Gill, R. D. (1997). Non-response models for the analysis of non-monotone ignorable missing data. *Statist in Med.*, **16**, 39–56.

Robins, J. M. and Ritov, Y. (1997). Toward a curse of dimensionality appropriate (coda) asymptotic theory for semi-parametric models. *Statist. in Med.*, **16**, 285–319.

Robins, J. M., Rotnitzky, A., and Zhao, L. P. (1994). Estimation of regression coefficients when some regressors are not always observed. *J. Am. Statist. Assoc.*, **89**, 846–866.

Robins, J. M. and Wang, N. S. (2000). Inference for imputation estimators. *Biometrika*, **87**, 113–124.

Rotnitzky, A. and Robins, J. M. (1997). Analysis of semi-parametric regression models with non-ignorable non-response. *Statist. in Med.*, **16**, 81–102.

Rotnitzky, A., Robins, J. M., and Scharfstein D. O. (1998). Semiparametric regression for repeated outcomes with non-ignorable nonresponse. *J. Am. Statist. Assoc.*, **93**, 1321–1339.

Rubin, D. B. (1976). Inference and missing data. *Biometrika*, **63**, 581–592.

Rubin, D. B. (1987). *Multiple imputation for survey nonresponse*. New York: Wiley.

Rubin, D. B. and Schenker, N. (1986). Multiple imputation for interval estimation from simple random samples with ignorable nonresponse. *J. Am. Statist. Assoc.*, **81**, 366–374.

Scharfstein D. O., Rotnitzky, A., and Robins, J. M. (1999). Adjusting for non-ignorable drop-out using semiparametric nonresponse models. *J. Am. Statist. Assoc.*, **94**, 1096–1146.

Wang, Y.-G. (1999). Estimating equations with nonignorably missing response data. *Biometrics*, **55**, 984–989.

Wedderburn, R. W. M. (1974). Quasi-likelihood functions, generalized linear models, and the Gauss-Newton method. *Biometrika*, **61**, 439–447.

Wu, M. C. and Carroll, R. J. (1988). Estimation and comparison of changes in the presence of informative right censoring by modeling the censoring process. *Biometrics*, **44**, 175–188.

Wu, M. C. and Bailey, K. (1988). Analyzing changes in the presence of informative right censoring caused by death and withdrawal. *Statist. in Med.*, **7**, 337–346.

Zhao, L. and Lipsitz, S. (1992). Designs and analysis of two-stage studies. *Statist. in Med.*, **11**, 769–782.

Zhao, L. P., Lipsitz, S. R., and Lew, D. (1996). Regression analysis with missing covariate data using estimating equations. *Biometrics*, **52**, 1165–1182.

CHAPTER 17

Misclassification: Effects, Control, and Adjustment

We have so far assumed that every subject has been correctly designated as diseased or nondiseased, and as exposed or unexposed to an antecedent factor. This assumption is assuredly not valid. Such assignments, whether by responses to a questionnaire, or by responses during an interview, or by examination of case records, or by physical or chemical tests, or by any means imaginable, can be wrong. For reasons of mishap—chance misreading, failure to hear a response, and so on—or because of unconscious bias, a subject having the disease may be recorded as not having it, or the reverse. Recording the presence or absence of the antecedent factor is equally vulnerable to error.

In sampling methods I and II, either of the two characteristics studied can be misclassified. In sampling method III, only the response variable can be misclassified.

In this chapter, we consider the effects of misclassification, and give some methods for reducing error and for estimating the extent of error. Section 17.1 presents in detail one example of the effects of misclassification. Section 17.2 describes algebraically how misclassification of one variable affects measures of association. Section 17.3 is devoted to the case where both variables are observed with error. In Section 17.4 we consider statistical means of controlling for error. Algebraic results for probabilistic control are presented in Section 17.5, and some techniques for experimental control of error are discussed in Section 17.6. Section 17.7, a discussion of misclassification in the more general setting of logistic regression models, is mathematically more challenging than the preceding sections.

Statistical Methods for Rates and Proportions, Third Edition
By Joseph L. Fleiss, Bruce Levin, and Myunghee Cho Paik
ISBN 0-471-52629-0   Copyright © 2003 John Wiley & Sons, Inc.

Table 17.1. *Association between G-6-PD deficiency and subtype of schizophrenia in Chicago*

	Diagnosis		
G-6-PD Status	Catatonic	Paranoid	Total
Heavy	15	6	21
Not heavy	57	99	156
Total	72	105	177

17.1. AN EXAMPLE OF THE EFFECTS OF MISCLASSIFICATION

Dern, Glynn, and Brewer (1963) studied the frequency of glucose-6-phosphate dehydrogenase (G-6-PD) deficiency in the erythrocytes of African-American male schizophrenic patients in the Chicago area. G-6-PD deficiency, inherited as a sex-linked error of metabolism, is found in about 10% to 15% of the African-American male population. The deficiency is sometimes referred to as fava bean disease because affected individuals who eat fava beans often suffer hemolysis, a breakdown of red blood cells. Antimalarial agents and other drugs also cause hemolysis in affected individuals.

The data provided by Dern, Glynn, and Brewer are summarized in Table 17.1. For these data, chi squared is 7.95, which indicates an association significant at the 0.01 level.

The proportion of catatonics who are deficient, $p_C = 15/72 = 0.208$, is contrasted with the proportion of paranoids who are deficient, $p_P = 6/105 = 0.057$. The odds ratio is

$$o = \frac{15 \times 99}{6 \times 57} = 4.34; \tag{17.1}$$

that is, the odds that a catatonic is G-6-PD deficient are over four times the odds that a paranoid is deficient.

Fieve et al. (1965) repeated the study at five state hospitals in the New York City area. Results from four of the hospitals are given in Table 17.2.

Table 17.2. *Association between G-6-PD deficiency and subtype of schizophrenia in four New York State hospitals*

	Catatonic		Paranoid		
Hospital	N	% Deficient	N	% Deficient	o
Central Islip	32	15.6	80	12.5	1.30
Pilgrim	78	16.7	76	6.6	2.84
Brooklyn	13	30.8	18	11.1	3.56
Kings Park	55	10.9	96	6.3	1.84

Table 17.3. *Association between G-6-PD deficiency and subtype of schizophrenia at Rockland State Hospital*

Catatonic		Paranoid		
N	% Deficient	N	% Deficient	o
28	7.1	29	24.1	0.24

The four individual odds ratios did not differ significantly; the Mantel-Haenszel summary estimate of the common odds ratio,

$$\hat{\omega}_{MH} = 2.09, \tag{17.2}$$

was significantly different from unity at the 0.05 level (see Chapter 10 for methods of comparing and combining different odds ratios). The findings from these four hospitals support Dern, Glynn, and Brewer's (1963) original finding but indicate a reduced degree of association.

At the fifth hospital, Rockland, the odds ratio was again significantly different from unity (Table 17.3). The problem at Rockland State Hospital, clearly, was that the odds ratio was significantly different from unity in the reverse direction from that found previously.

The investigators quickly checked back with the administration at Rockland and breathed a sigh of relief when they discovered that half the schizophrenic patients had been withheld because they were subjects in other research investigations. The investigators therefore returned to Rockland to study all the resident African-American male catatonics and paranoids. The results from the second survey are in Table 17.4. The odds ratio was again significantly different from unity at the 0.05 level, but even smaller than before.

Thus the evidence of an association between G-6-PD deficiency and subtype of schizophrenia unfortunately points in opposite directions. All we need to complete the confusing picture is evidence of no association. Just such data were provided by a sample of 426 patients at a Veterans Administration hospital in Alabama (Bowman et al., 1965). The data are presented in Table 17.5. For these data, $p_C = 10.4\%$, $p_P = 11.8\%$, $o = 0.87$, and chi squared is 0.07.

Table 17.4. *Association between G-6-PD deficiency and subtype of schizophrenia at Rockland State Hospital—second survey*

Catatonic		Paranoid		
N	% Deficient	N	% Deficient	o
37	2.7	87	16.1	0.14

Table 17.5. *Association between G-6-PD deficiency and subtype of schizophrenia at a VA hospital in Alabama*

| | Diagnosis | | |
G-6-PD Status	Catatonic	Paranoid	Total
Deficient	17	31	48
Nondeficient	146	232	378
Total	163	263	426

Table 17.6. *Evidence for various directions of association between G-6-PD deficiency and subtype of schizophrenia*

Direction of Association	Source	o
Association greater among catatonics	Chicago	4.34
	Four New York hospitals	2.09
Association greater among paranoids	Fifth New York hospital	0.14
No difference	Alabama	0.87

There is therefore evidence in the literature for positive association, negative association, and no association. This conflicting evidence is summarized in Table 17.6.

Attempting to account for this confusion, the New York investigators looked first at the experimental techniques used in the three studies. The techniques were not sufficiently dissimilar to explain the discrepancies; in fact, the technique used at Rockland was identical to that used at the other four hospitals in New York.

Differences in the drugs given the patients might conceivably have produced these discrepant findings. Within each study, therefore, odds ratios were calculated for each major category of drug administered at the time of the study. With only a few exceptions, for too few cases to have much impact, the odds ratios for the specific drug categories within a study were in the same direction as the overall value for the study.

Whatever the influences of differences in techniques of blood testing or medication practices, they paled beside the unreliability of psychiatric diagnosis. A large literature indicates just how unreliable psychiatric diagnoses were (Zubin, 1967; Spitzer and Fleiss, 1974). With respect to schizophrenia, for example, only about 70% of patients given a diagnosis of schizophrenia by one diagnostician received the same diagnosis from a second, and about 10% of patients given a diagnosis other than schizophrenia by one diagnostician received a diagnosis of schizophrenia from a second. The few published data for subtypes of schizophrenia suggest that reliability was less for paranoid and catatonic schizophrenia than for schizophrenia in general.

In each of the three studies cited of G-6-PD deficiency and schizophrenia, the then current hospital diagnoses were accepted uncritically, with no attempt made to verify their accuracy. It is thus likely that the most important source of the discrepancies was the unreliability of psychiatric diagnosis.

Prima facie evidence for diagnostic differences among the five New York hospitals comes from the variability of the proportion of patients diagnosed catatonic among those diagnosed either catatonic or paranoid. The differences among the five hospitals in the kinds of patients they receive are not sufficient to account for the differences in their proportions of catatonics. Problem 17.1 is devoted to these differences.

In the years since these studies were conducted, remarkable improvement has occurred in the reliability of psychiatric diagnosis. Documentation of the shortcomings described above spurred subsequent efforts to improve diagnostic reliability (see e.g., Feighner, et al., 1972; Spitzer, Endicott, and Robins, 1978). Today it is widely agreed that the recognition of substantial diagnostic unreliability played a central role in the break with tradition found in the 3rd edition of the Diagnostic and Statistical Manual of the American Psychiatric Association (1980) and continued in its successors (1987, 1994) (Klerman, 1983; Wilson, 1993). These manuals, in contrast to their predecessors, spell out operational criteria for symptoms and explicit decision rules for diagnosis. We return to this point in Section 17.6.

Our discussion has focused on psychiatry, but psychiatry is not uniquely plagued by inaccurate diagnoses. Unreliability exists in the diagnosis of childhood disorders (Derryberry, 1938; Bakwin 1945); in the diagnosis of emphysema (Fletcher, 1952); in the interpretation of electrocardiograms (Davies, 1958); in the interpretation of X-rays (Yerushalmy, 1947; Cochrane and Garland, 1958); in the certification of X-rays (Yerushalmy, 1947; Cochrane and Garland, 1952); and in the certification of causes of death (Markush, Schaaf, and Seigel, 1967). Reviews of diagnostic unreliability in other branches of physical medicine are given by Garland (1960) and Koran (1975a, 1975b).

It may, in fact, be taken as axiomatic that the determination of the presence or absence of any disease or condition and the determination of the exact form of the condition when present are subject to error. Likewise, the determination of the presence or absence of an antecedent factor is subject to error.

17.2. THE ALGEBRA OF MISCLASSIFICATION

Misclassification can turn a truly strong positive association into one that is less strongly positive or even apparently negative; a truly strong negative association into one that is less strongly negative or even apparently positive; and a nil association into one that is apparently strong. These facts contradict the long-standing but erroneous impression that errors of misclassification tend only to reduce the magnitude of association (Newell, 1962).

Assume for simplicity that the classification of a person as diseased or not is accurate, so that the only source of error is in the determination of whether or not the factor under study was present. Let us consider the comparison of women aged 55–64 newly diagnosed as having lung cancer with similarly aged women newly diagnosed as having breast cancer, with respect to whether they ever smoked.

We assume that the diagnoses are accurate but that the determination of smoking history is subject to error. Two sources of error exist, one residing with the informant and one with the person taking the history. With respect to the informant (e.g., the patient herself or a relative):

1. She may misunderstand the intent or phrasing of the question.
2. She may make an honest mistake in reporting what the patient's smoking status was.
3. She may deliberately misrepresent the patient's smoking status (more likely in claiming the patient never smoked when in fact she did than the reverse).

With respect to the person taking the history:

1. She may misunderstand the informant's answer.
2. She may make an honest coding error.
3. She may apply different standards to recording responses for one type of patient versus another. Suppose, for example, that the history-taker bends over backwards to control for possible bias toward finding an association. She may then record the statement, "I smoked once in a while when I was a kid, but never since" as Never Smoked if made by a lung cancer patient but as Ever Smoked if made by a breast cancer patient.

Horwitz and Lysgaard-Hansen (1975) enumerate several other prevalent sources of error and give prescriptions for their control. Here we study the effects of these errors. The analysis is that of Keys and Kihlberg (1963). Others who have analyzed the effects of misclassification on measures of association and on chi squared tests are Rogot (1961), Mote and Anderson (1965), Assakul and Proctor (1967), Koch (1969), Goldberg (1975), and Copeland et al. (1977).

Consider first the lung cancer patients, who, we assume, are identified without error. Let P_L denote the true proportion of lung cancer patients who ever smoked, so that $1 - P_L$ is the true proportion who never smoked. Denote by E_L the complement of sensitivity and by F_L the complement of specificity for the lung cancer patients; that is, E_L is the probability that a lung cancer patient who actually smoked is recorded as not having smoked, and F_L is the probability that a lung cancer patient who actually never smoked is recorded as having smoked. Whereas one would wish to estimate P_L, the true proportion who ever smoked, one can, from the recorded histories, only estimate

$$p_L = (1 - E_L)P_L + F_L(1 - P_L). \qquad (17.3)$$

The estimated proportion of lung cancer patients who ever smoked, p_L, is a fraction, $1 - E_L$, of those who truly ever smoked plus a fraction, F_L, of those who truly never smoked.

The observable proportion p_L may be less than, equal to, or greater than the true proportion P_L depending on the relative magnitudes of E_L and F_L. In fact,

$$p_L > P_L \quad \text{if} \quad \frac{F_L}{E_L + F_L} > P_L,$$

$$p_L = P_L \quad \text{if} \quad \frac{F_L}{E_L + F_L} = P_L,$$

$$p_L < P_L \quad \text{if} \quad \frac{F_L}{E_L + F_L} < P_L.$$

If E_L and F_L are of approximately the same magnitude, there will be overestimation if P_L is less than 0.5 and underestimation if P_L is greater than 0.5. Thus, even if the error rates are equal, the errors do not necessarily cancel out.

Now let P_B denote the true proportion of breast cancer patients who ever smoked, E_B the complement of their sensitivity, and F_B the complement of their specificity. For the breast cancer patients, therefore, one can estimate only the proportion recorded as ever having smoked, say

$$p_B = (1 - E_B)P_B + F_B(1 - P_B). \qquad (17.4)$$

The algebra of the effects of errors on the odds ratio is complicated (Diamond and Lilienfeld, 1962a, 1962b; Goldberg, 1975; see Copeland et al., 1977, for a graphic study). Suppose, therefore, that the association between smoking and type of cancer is measured simply by the difference between the proportions who smoked. Instead of estimating the true difference, say

$$D = P_L - P_B, \qquad (17.5)$$

we can only estimate $d = p_L - p_B$. This difference between the recorded proportions is easily seen to reduce algebraically to

$$d = D + (F_L - F_B) + P_B(E_B + F_B) - P_L(E_L + F_L), \qquad (17.6)$$

which indicates that an estimate for d is typically biased for D.

The estimated difference d may be less than, equal to, or greater than the true difference D. It may even be of opposite sign, which means that an association that is actually in one direction may be estimated as being in the opposite direction.

This possibility of a reversal of the direction of association cannot arise in the special case in which the two sensitivities are equal,

$$1 - E_L = 1 - E_B = 1 - E, \tag{17.7}$$

say, and in which the two specificities are equal,

$$1 - F_L = 1 - F_B = 1 - F, \tag{17.8}$$

say, and the sum of the two error rates is less than 1.0. By substituting (17.7) and (17.8) into (17.6) and simplifying, we find that the difference between the recorded proportions is

$$d = D\{1 - (E + F)\}. \tag{17.9}$$

The first point to notice about (17.9) is that d, the difference that can be estimated, cannot possibly equal D, the true difference, whenever either error rate is nonzero. The second point to notice is that, provided E plus F is less than 1.0, the observed difference is in the same direction as the true difference, but is numerically smaller—that is, is closer to zero. This situation, considered by Bross in a classic paper (1954), has led to the erroneous anticipation that misclassification *always* deflates the difference between two rates. Equal sensitivities and equal specificities must, however, be considered unusual (see, e.g., Lilienfeld and Graham, 1958; Goldberg, 1975). The third point to notice is that when misclassification rates are large, in the sense that $E + F > 1$, a reversal of the direction of association occurs even with nondifferential misclassification.

With respect to the odds ratio, the effect is, again, unpredictable. In the particular case just considered, where $E_L = E_B$ and the sum of the two rates is less than 1, the odds ratio is underestimated, as was the difference between rates. Specifically, if ω is the true odds ratio and o the odds ratio estimated from misclassified data, then if $\omega > 1$, we expect to find $\omega > o > 1$. That is, the estimated odds ratio is greater than unity, but not by as much as the true value.

Even more care must be taken when interpreting analyses that adjust for confounding factors measured with error. Here even nondifferential measurement error in a covariate can cause an *exaggeration* of an association between an outcome variable and an antecedent factor, for example, producing an effect when none truly exists. Remarkably, this exaggeration can occur even if the outcome variable and antecedent factor are measured without error, and even if the mismeasured covariate is a continuous and unbiased estimate of the true value. We discuss this less well-known but important *underadjustment phenomenon* further in Section 17.7.

17.3. THE ALGEBRA OF MISCLASSIFICATION: BOTH VARIABLES IN ERROR

The previous section was concerned only with errors in one of the two variables under study. A general discussion of the more realistic situation in which both variables are subject to misclassification is given by Keys and Kihlberg (1963). The following analysis and example, dealing with the determination of the odds ratio, are by Barron (1977).

Let A denote the presence and $\overline{A}$ the absence of one of the two variables under study, and B and $\overline{B}$ the presence and absence of the other variable. Let $P(AB)$, $P(A\overline{B})$, and so on denote the various probabilities of joint occurrence if both variables are categorized without error, and let

$$\omega = \frac{P(AB)P(\overline{A}\overline{B})}{P(A\overline{B})P(\overline{A}B)} \tag{17.10}$$

denote the odds ratio accurately associating A and B.

Suppose, however, that both variables are subject to misclassification, with probabilities of correct and incorrect classification given in Table 17.7. It is assumed that the two errors operate independently.

Finally, let $p(AB), p(A\overline{B})$, and so on denote the various probabilities of joint occurrence when the variables are ascertained with error. Explicitly,

$$p(AB) = a_1 b_1 P(AB) + a_1 b_2 P(A\overline{B}) + a_2 b_1 P(\overline{A}B) + a_2 b_2 P(\overline{A}\overline{B}), \tag{17.11}$$

$$p(A\overline{B}) = a_1(1 - b_1)P(AB) + a_1(1 - b_2)P(A\overline{B}) + a_2(1 - b_1)P(\overline{A}B)$$
$$+ a_2(1 - b_2)P(\overline{A}\overline{B}), \tag{17.12}$$

$$p(\overline{A}B) = (1 - a_1)b_1 P(AB) + (1 - a_1)b_2 P(A\overline{B}) + (1 - a_2)b_1 P(\overline{A}B)$$
$$+ (1 - a_2)b_2 P(\overline{A}\overline{B}), \tag{17.13}$$

Table 17.7. *Probabilities of correct and incorrect classification of A and B*

True Status	Classified Status		True Status	Classified Status	
	A	$\overline{A}$		B	$\overline{B}$
A	a_1	$1 - a_1$	B	b_1	$1 - b_1$
$\overline{A}$	a_2	$1 - a_2$	$\overline{B}$	b_2	$1 - b_2$

Table 17.8. *Hypothetical joint probabilities of hypertension and endometrial cancer if both were observed without error*

Hypertension	Endometrial Cancer	
	B	$\bar{B}$
A	0.122	0.060
$\bar{A}$	0.211	0.607

and

$$p(\bar{A}\bar{B}) = (1 - a_1)(1 - b_1)P(AB) + (1 - a_1)(1 - b_2)P(A\bar{B})$$
$$+ (1 - a_2)(1 - b_1)P(\bar{A}B) + (1 - a_2)(1 - b_2)P(\bar{A}\bar{B}). \quad (17.14)$$

The observable odds ratio is then

$$o = \frac{p(AB)p(\bar{A}\bar{B})}{p(A\bar{B})p(\bar{A}B)}, \quad (17.15)$$

which bears no necessary relation to ω in (17.10).

Suppose that, if hypertension (A) and endometrial cancer (B) were observed without error in a hospitalized sample, their probabilities of joint occurrence would be as in Table 17.8. Suppose further that the probability of correctly ascertaining the presence of hypertension is $a_1 = 0.90$, of correctly ascertaining the absence of hypertension is $1 - a_2 = 0.98$, of correctly ascertaining the presence of endometrial cancer is $b_1 = 0.95$, and of correctly ascertaining the absence of endometrial cancer is $1 - b_2 = 0.98$. These rates of correct ascertainment, all empirically determined (see Barron, 1977, for references), are all high.

The observable rates of joint occurrence are, by (17.11)–(17.14),

$$p(AB) = 0.110, \quad (17.16)$$

$$p(A\bar{B}) = 0.070, \quad (17.17)$$

$$p(\bar{A}B) = 0.220, \quad (17.18)$$

$$p(\bar{A}\bar{B}) = 0.600. \quad (17.19)$$

The observable value of the odds ratio is then

$$o = \frac{0.110 \times 0.600}{0.970 \times 0.220} = 4.29, \quad (17.20)$$

over 25% lower than the odds ratio from the accurate data of Table 17.8,

$$\omega = \frac{0.122 \times 0.607}{0.060 \times 0.211} = 5.85. \tag{17.21}$$

17.4. STATISTICAL CONTROL FOR ERROR

Occasionally, an investigator has available two or more ways to determine the status of a patient—one quite expensive but reliable (i.e., subject to little error), the others relatively inexpensive but unreliable. To plan a survey or comparative study on even a moderate scale, the investigator must, to keep the cost of the study as low as possible, employ one of the unreliable devices (Rubin, Rosenbaum, and Cobb, 1956).

If the investigator uses *only* an unreliable device, he or she runs the risk of obtaining the kinds of biased estimates described in the preceding sections. By assessing a subsample with both the unreliable and more reliable devices, however, the investigator can estimate, for a relatively small added cost, the rates of misclassification and thus correct the bias.

Consider, as an example, the determination of the current smoking habits of a sample of subjects. The investigator can rely solely on the subject's report, sacrificing reliability for simplicity. A chemical test for the concentrations of thiocyanates in the subject's urine, saliva, or plasma (Densen et al. 1967), on the other hand, would mean paying for precision.

Suppose that a sample of N newly hospitalized women diagnosed with lung cancer is to be evaluated for smoking habits, and suppose that the investigator chooses to rely on each woman's verbal report on her current smoking practice. For simplicity, each woman is characterized as either a heavy smoker (say, smoking ten or more cigarettes per day, on the average) or not. Let P_L denote the proportion who report heavy smoking.

Self-reported smoking status has the virtue of being inexpensive but the drawback of possibly excessive error. Suppose, therefore, that the investigator decides to estimate the degree of error in the patients' reports by taking a subsample of size n out of the total of N lung cancer patients and, in addition, testing their plasma concentration of thiocyanates. A positive result on the test indicates the patient is a heavy smoker; a negative result indicates she is not a heavy smoker.

The results of this blood test cannot establish the patient's true status, not only because the dichotomy between heavy and nonheavy smoking is imprecise but also because the results of the test are themselves subject to random fluctuations. Nevertheless, because of its greater reproducibility, the blood test may be viewed as a standard against which to compare verbal reports.

Let Table 17.9 represent the cross-classification of reported and tested smoking status for the subsample of n lung cancer patients. The notation is that of Tenenbein (1970, 1971). From these data we estimate as n_{00}/n_0 the

Table 17.9. *Smoking status as determined by report and by the standard blood test*

Report	Standard		Total
	Heavy	Not Heavy	
Heavy	n_{00}	n_{01}	n_0
Not Heavy	n_{10}	n_{11}	n_1

proportion of women, among those who report heavy smoking, who would be assigned to the heavy smoking category by the standard, and as n_{10}/n_1 the proportion of women, among those who do not report heavy smoking, who would be assigned to the heavy smoking category by the standard. Recalling that p_L is the overall proportion of women assigned to the heavy smoking category on the basis of verbal report, it is easily checked that an estimate of the overall proportion who would have been so assigned by the standard is

$$\hat{P}_L = \frac{n_{00}}{n_0} p_L + \frac{n_{10}}{n_1} (1 - p_L). \tag{17.22}$$

Whereas the estimated standard error of p_L is simply $\sqrt{p_L(1 - p_L)/N}$, that of $\hat{P}_L$ is more complicated:

$$\widehat{se}(\hat{P}_L) = \sqrt{\frac{\hat{P}_L(1 - \hat{P}_L)}{N} \left\{ 1 + (1 - K)\frac{N - n}{n} \right\}}, \tag{17.23}$$

where

$$K = \frac{1 - p_L}{p_L} \cdot \frac{\left(\hat{P}_L - n_{10}.n_1\right)^2}{\hat{P}_L(1 - \hat{P}_L)}. \tag{17.24}$$

The estimate (17.22) and standard error (17.23) are derived by Tenenbein (1970, 1971), who also gives criteria for choosing a reasonable value of n.

Deming (1977) presents an interesting application of what is essentially Tenenbein's double-sampling scheme to a problem in survey sampling and gives some further criteria for choosing a value of n. Chiacchierini and Arnold (1977) extend Tenenbein's scheme to the case where both variables are subject to error, and Hochberg (1977) extends it to the case of multidimensional cross-classification tables. Other approaches to the estimation of correction factors are described by Harper (1964), Bryson (1965), and Press (1968).

The following numerical example illustrates the algebra presented above. Suppose that, of a total of 200 female lung cancer patients interviewed, 88 respond that they smoke ten or more cigarettes a day. The observed, but biased, rate of heavy smoking among lung cancer patients is, by self-report,

$$p_L = 0.44. \tag{17.25}$$

Table 17.10. *Smoking status of 50 lung cancer patients determined by report and by chemical test*

	Standard		
Report	Heavy	Not Heavy	Total
Heavy	18	2	20
Not Heavy	6	24	30

Suppose, further, that 50 of the 200 patients are also tested for levels of serum thiocyanates, and that the resulting cross-classification is as given in Table 17.10. Then $n_{00}/n_0 = 18/20 = 0.90$ and $n_{10}/n_1 = 6/30 = 0.20$ are the two correction factors, and substitution into (17.22) yields

$$\hat{P}_L = 0.90 \times 0.44 + 0.20 \times 0.56 = 0.51, \tag{17.26}$$

an improved estimate of the rate of heavy smoking in this group. Note that the rate given in (17.25) is an underestimate by more than 10%.

To determine the standard error of $\hat{P}_L$, the quantity K given by (17.24) must first be calculated. It is

$$K = \frac{0.56}{0.44} \cdot \frac{(0.51 - 0.20)^2}{0.51 \times 0.49} = 0.4894. \tag{17.27}$$

Substitution of this value in (17.23) yields

$$\widehat{se}(\hat{P}_L) = \sqrt{\frac{0.51 \times 0.49}{200}\left(1 + 0.5106 \times \frac{150}{50}\right)} = \sqrt{0.0032} = 0.06 \tag{17.28}$$

as the estimated standard error of $\hat{P}_L$.

If the study is a comparative one, such as comparing the rates of heavy smoking among lung cancer and breast cancer patients, then a subsample of the breast cancer patients would also have to undergo the blood test. Problem 17.3 gives some comparative data for analysis.

17.5. PROBABILISTIC CONTROL FOR ERROR

On occasion, external sources provide information on the magnitude of error. In the example presented in Section 17.3, the rates of correct and incorrect ascertainment of hypertension and endometrial cancer were from sources other than those giving rise to the data on association between these two diseases. The notation here is the same as that used in Section 17.3, and the results are those of Barron (1977).

In practice, one obtains the fallible estimates $p(AB)$, $p(A\bar{B})$, and so on, and may have available from one source or another the values of a_1, a_2, b_1, and b_2 (see Table 17.7). Equations (17.11)–(17.14) may be inverted to yield values for the underlying correct probabilities as follows, where

$$p(A) = p(AB) + p(A\bar{B}) \tag{17.29}$$

and

$$p(B) = p(AB) + p(\bar{A}B). \tag{17.30}$$

The correct probabilities are

$$P(AB) = \frac{p(AB) + a_2 b_2 - a_2 p(B) - b_2 p(A)}{(a_1 - a_2)(b_1 - b_2)}, \tag{17.31}$$

$$P(A\bar{B}) = \frac{-p(AB) - a_2 b_1 + a_2 p(B) + b_1 p(A)}{(a_1 - a_2)(b_1 - b_2)}, \tag{17.32}$$

$$P(\bar{A}B) = \frac{-p(AB) - a_1 b_2 + a_1 p(B) + b_2 p(A)}{(a_1 - a_2)(b_1 - b_2)}, \tag{17.33}$$

$$P(\bar{A}\bar{B}) = \frac{p(AB) + a_1 b_1 - a_1 p(B) - b_1 p(A)}{(a_1 - a_2)(b_1 - b_2)}. \tag{17.34}$$

With $p(AB) = 0.110$, $p(A) = 0.110 + 0.070 = 0.180$, and $p(B) = 0.110 + 0.220 = 0.330$ [see (17.16)–(17.18)] and with $a_1 = 0.9$, $a_2 = 0.02$, $b_1 = 0.95$, and $b_2 = 0.02$, the correct probabilities are

$$P(AB) = 0.122, \tag{17.35}$$

$$P(A\bar{B}) = 0.060, \tag{17.36}$$

$$P(\bar{A}B) = 0.211, \tag{17.37}$$

$$P(\bar{A}\bar{B}) = 0.607, \tag{17.38}$$

that is, identical to the values originally presented in Table 17.8.

When independent estimates of the probabilities of correct ascertainment are available, (17.31)–(17.34) may be applied to obtain the correct probabilities, and desired measures of association may be derived from these rather than from the probabilities based on the erroneous observations. Explicit formulas for standard errors are given by Selen (1986) via a likelihood approach.

17.6. EXPERIMENTAL CONTROL OF ERROR

It is almost always possible to modify a contemplated research design to reduce the probable magnitude of error. Only a few of the large number of techniques and ideas can be presented here. One procedure is modeled on the double-blind feature of a properly designed clinical trial. In a double-blind trial, patients are unaware which of the drugs being compared they take, and investigators evaluate their responses without knowing which treatment they received.

Keeping both patients and evaluators in the dark is obviously desirable for studies in which the presence or absence of a disease and the presence or absence of an antecedent factor are determined at nearly the same time (e.g., patients admitted to an acute treatment ward for whom neither previous records nor the opportunity for followup may exist). Diagnosticians who know whether or not the factor is present may favor one or another of the diagnoses under study. A form of control is to instruct diagnosticians not to ask about the antecedent factor unless it is pathognomonic.

Evaluators seeking to establish the presence or absence of the factor may, if they know the diagnosis, favor recording the factor as present or absent. A form of control is to keep evaluators ignorant of the diagnosis.

Patients may respond differently if they know, or even believe, that they have the disease being studied. A form of control is to keep patients ignorant of the diagnosis until all background information of interest has been collected. An ethical problem must be solved here: just how much can be withheld from patients, and for how long, must be determined ad hoc (see Levin, 1954).

We have so far taken for granted that the person responsible for making the diagnosis is not the person responsible for eliciting information on the background factors. The two roles are not always separable, but results from a study in which the same person assumed both roles are always suspect. An example of the bias which may arise is provided by a study of psychiatric concomitants of systemic lupus erythematosus (SLE).

A number of reports suggested that the frequency (both incidence and prevalence) of psychological disturbance among SLE patients is unusually high. As part of a study of this phenomenon (Ganz et al. 1972), a psychologist interviewed, using a structured interview schedule, samples of SLE and rheumatoid arthritis (RA) patients coming to clinics at four New York City hospitals. RA patients were selected as a control group because there are many similarities between the two diseases but few reports of psychiatric complications in RA.

Sixty-eight SLE and 36 RA patients were interviewed, on the basis of which each patient's psychiatric symptomatology was characterized as severe (e.g., extreme anxiety or depression, and, occasionally, delusional thinking), moderate (e.g., slight degrees of worrying and depression), or none. Every attempt was made to keep the interviewer ignorant of the patients' diagnoses.

Table 17.11. *Psychiatric symptomatology by diagnosis—results from interview*

Symptoms	Systemic Lupus Erythematosus		Rheumatoid Arthritis	
	N	(%)	N	(%)
Severe	24	(35%)	9	(25%)
Moderate	19	(28%)	12	(33%)
None	25	(37%)	15	(42%)
Total	68	(100%)	36	(100%)

Table 17.11 gives the results of the categorization of symptomatology elicited by the interview.

The proportions for the two diagnostic categories are similar. The chi squared statistic, with 2 df, for comparing the two distributions is equal to 1.16, not significant at any meaningful level. Thus, on the basis of a structured interview conducted by an interviewer ignorant of the diagnosis, the conclusion is that the degree of psychiatric symptomatology of SLE patients does not differ essentially from that of RA patients.

As part of the study, the physicians notes on the same day as the interview were also examined. The physician had not been told the results of the interview. The same criteria used to characterize the interview data were applied to the case notes (Table 17.12). The case notes were assessed by a person other than the interviewer.

The proportions for the two diagnostic categories are quite different. For example, nearly a third of the SLE patients, as opposed to only 6% of the RA patients, were characterized on the basis of the case notes as having psychiatric symptoms of some kind. The value of chi squared for the data of Table 17.12 is 8.27, indicating a difference significant at the 0.05 level.

A possible explanation of the difference is that a self-perpetuating myth is in operation. As more and more reports indicate a high frequency of psychological disturbance among SLE patients, more and more clinicians are influenced to observe and record its presence. In itself, this awareness is not a bad thing. But if vigilance recording disturbances for SLE patients comes at the expense of equal care for patients with other disorders, then the scientific value of these observations becomes highly questionable.

Table 17.12. *Psychiatric symptomatology by diagnosis—results from case notes*

Symptoms	Systemic Lupus Erythematosus		Rheumatoid Arthritis	
	N	(%)	N	(%)
Severe	5	(7%)	0	(0%)
Moderate	15	(22%)	2	(6%)
None	48	(71%)	34	(94%)
Total	68	(100%)	36	(100%)

It therefore seems clear that an investigator should rely on a person ignorant of the status of the patient for the collection of background and other information. The desirability of a structured interview or questionnaire —where the questions to be asked and the probes to be made are set forth explicitly, and where the responses are precoded—may be less clear.

Establishing the questions to be asked ensures that each interviewer covers the same ground and that each subject is asked the same questions in the same way, reducing differences in interviewing style and biases due to different kinds of patients being interviewed differently. Precoded responses not only procure the data in a form suitable for data entry and analysis, but also reduce errors inherent in interpreting verbal, sometimes anecdotal reports.

Refinement of standardized interviews, with obligatory questions that elicit information about symptoms, and use of stated algorithms to reach a diagnosis, have been crucial in improving reliability (Spitzer et al., 1967; Wing, et al., 1967; Spitzer et al., 1970; Endicott and Spitzer, 1978; Spitzer et al., 1992; Williams et al., 1992; First et al., 1996; Hasin and Miele, 1997). Interviewers can be trained to high levels of interrater reliability using these instruments (Ventura et al., 1998) and, overall, the evidence suggests that these efforts have substantially improved the reproducibility of psychiatric research over that which prevailed prior to the 1980s (see, e.g., Riskind et al., 1987; Skre et al., 1991. Problems and controversy remain (Clark, Watson, and Reynolds, 1995; Nathan and Langenbucher, 1999). The substantial gains in reliability are not uniform across diagnostic categories. The very high levels of comorbidity found with the existing nomenclature cause some to wonder if the categories themselves require revision. And disputes over the advantages of categorical vs. dimensional classification are still very much alive today.

The need for such procedures in psychiatry and bronchopulmonary medicine is due mainly to the variability among clinicians in the way they elicit information from patients and, having elicited the data, in the way they interpret their findings. Similar factors are present in almost every branch of medicine, and there is no compelling reason why the idea of the structured interview cannot be extended. Its applicability is clear in the interview for history (see, e.g., Medical Research Council, 1966), but rather subtle in the assessment of X-ray negatives, electrocardiogram (EKG) tracings, and the like. An important reason for diagnostic disagreement in heart disease, for example, is that different cardiologists interpret EKGs differently; even the same cardiologist may, on two occasions, interpret the same EKG differently. Surely many of these differences would be reduced if cardiologists were instructed to note, on a precoded form, what the abnormalities were that they thought they detected in each wave of the EKG. The same idea can certainly be applied to the recording of lesions thought to be detected from an X-ray negative.

Having information recorded on such forms, in addition to increasing uniformity, serves yet another purpose. The data, provided they are suitably recorded, can be quantified to provide a more objective gradation of disease severity than that based on clinical judgment. The major difficulty in the use of such forms, assuming that someone has the fortitude and patience to develop, validate, and if necessary revise one, is that clinicians unfamiliar with them might resent having to use them. Considering, however, that such techniques bring medical and epidemiological research closer to the ideal of all scientific endeavor—that all criteria be publicly specified and thus that every study be reproducible—not using them is virtually impossible to justify.

17.7.* MISCLASSIFICATION IN LOGISTIC REGRESSION MODELS

In this section we examine misclassification in the general context of the logistic regression model. As we did for the one- and two-sample problems, we indicate the sources of the bias in studies that measure only the misclassified variables with no validation. It is always good practice to plan a validation subsample, and we present a method that allows correct inferences with such data for a misclassified exposure variable.

In addition to the possible causes of misclassification given in Section 17.2, misclassification in a binary variable can often be viewed as the result of dichotomizing an underlying continuous variable measured with error. For example, let a disease indicator Y be 1 if the underlying continuous severity of illness, say η, is greater than a fixed threshold τ, so that $Y = I[\eta > \tau]$. If the dichotomization is based on $\eta^* = \eta + \varepsilon$ rather than η, where ε is a random error, the resulting binary variable $Y^* = I[\eta^* > \tau]$ will not agree completely with Y, causing misclassification in the disease indicator. Measurement error problems are extensively studied in the context of nonlinear regression models by Carroll, Ruppert, and Stefanski (1995).

Statistical problems arising from surrogate variables are similar to those arising from misclassified variables. In the smoking status example of Section 17.4, the more reliable determination by blood test is invasive and expensive, while the less reliable verbal report is noninvasive and inexpensive. The verbal report may therefore have to serve as a surrogate for the blood test determination, but, in all such cases, one must decide whether to use a surrogate by itself and thereby to risk a biased study, or together with a more reliable determination, at least for a subsample, and thereby increase costs. In the latter case, we knowingly permit a degree of measurement error for pragmatic reasons, but retain an ability to adjust the study results statistically on the basis of the validation subsample. Similar remarks apply to surrogate markers for outcome variables, but here an additional uncertainty obtains, especially in the context of clinical trials, where effective modification of a surrogate marker by a treatment does not necessarily translate into effective modification of a clinical outcome of importance by that treatment.

When inferences are drawn ignoring misclassification error, parameter estimates can be biased and hypothesis tests can lose power, even if they maintain the correct Type I error. This problem has been studied by many authors. Greenland and Robins (1985), examining the bias due to exposure misclassification in the presence of other covariates, note that the bias cannot be dealt with by the usual methods for control of confounding. Greenland (1982) points out that misclassification of an exposure produces more severe bias and power loss in matched case-control studies than in unmatched studies. Lagakos (1988) shows that a test statistic based on a misclassified exposure is valid under the null hypothesis, but the asymptotic relative efficiency is the squared correlation between the exposure variable measured with and without error. Hsieh and Walter (1988) and Reade-Christopher and Kupper (1991) study the effect of misclassification error on association measures such as the relative risk and attributable risk. Prentice (1989) and Hsieh (1991) study the case in which an outcome variable is misclassified. Prentice (1989) presents a condition for a misclassified or surrogate outcome to produce a valid hypothesis test in a randomized clinical trial. Hsieh (1991) investigates the effect of a misclassified outcome on attributable risk. Greenland (1988) provides variance estimators for the bias-corrected estimate of a log odds ratio, when the error rates are estimated from an external source or a subsample from the data at hand. Greenland and Brenner (1993) demonstrate how to correct misclassification in ecologic analysis using error rates estimated from an external source.

Below we consider the case of misclassification of an exposure variable alone, an outcome variable alone, both, or neither, but with mismeasurement of another covariate. Let the binary outcome of interest be denoted by Y, the exposure by X, and the other covariates by Z, all measured without error. The misclassified or mismeasured versions will be denoted with asterisks, Y^*, X^*, and Z^*, respectively.

Misclassification of Exposure

To begin, assume the true model for the variables measured without error, $P(Y = 1|X, Z)$, has the linear logistic form

$$\ln \frac{P(Y = 1|X, Z)}{1 - P(Y = 1|X, Z)} = \beta_0 + \beta_X X + \beta_Z Z.$$

$\beta = (\beta_0, \beta_X, \beta_Z)$ contains the parameter(s) of interest. While X need not be a binary exposure for the general linear logistic regression model, we can illustrate all the important ideas simply with the binary case. If only the misclassified X^* is observed, one cannot directly estimate $P(Y|X, Z)$ but only $P(Y|X^*, Z)$. To proceed, suppose that

$$P(Y|X, X^*, Z) = P(Y|X, Z), \tag{17.39}$$

that is, Y is conditionally independent of X^* given X and Z. In the smoking status example, (17.39) would imply that smoking status by verbal report does not alter the likelihood of lung cancer among those whose smoking status by blood test is fixed at X with other covariates fixed at Z. This assumption may be reasonable in many situations and is frequently used in the mismeasurement literature (see, e.g., Begg and Lagakos, 1992). Let the distribution of X given X^* and Z be denoted by $P(X|X^*, Z)$. Table 17.10 provides an example of an empirical determination of $P(X|X^*, Z)$ when there are no covariates Z. Then we have

$$P(Y|X^*, Z) = \sum_{X=0}^{1} P(Y|X, X^*, Z) P(X|X^*, Z)$$

$$= \sum_{X=0}^{1} P(Y|X, Z) P(X|X^*, Z). \qquad (17.40)$$

Although $P(Y|X, Z)$ is linear in the logit scale, $P(Y|X^*, Z)$ is generally not. For example, if $P(X|X^*, Z)$ is itself linear logistic, with

$$\ln \frac{P(X|X^*, Z)}{1 - P(X|X^*, Z)} = \gamma_0 + \gamma_{X^*} X^* + \gamma_Z Z, \qquad (17.41)$$

then

$$P(Y = 1|X^*, Z)$$

$$= \left\{ \frac{\exp(\beta_0 + \beta_Z Z)}{1 + \exp(\beta_0 + \beta_Z Z)} \right\} \left\{ \frac{1}{1 + \exp(\gamma_0 + \gamma_{X^*} X^* + \gamma_Z Z)} \right\}$$

$$+ \left\{ \frac{\exp(\beta_0 + \beta_X + \beta_Z Z)}{1 + \exp(\beta_0 + \beta_X + \beta_Z Z)} \right\} \left\{ \frac{\exp(\gamma_0 + \gamma_{X^*} X^* + \gamma_Z Z)}{1 + \exp(\gamma_0 + \gamma_{X^*} X^* + \gamma_Z Z)} \right\},$$

which is not of linear logistic form unless $\beta_X = 0$. One can verify that if $\beta_X = 0$, then $P(Y|X^*, Z) = P(Y|X, Z)$, so a test statistic for $\beta_X = 0$ using X^* would be valid. However, in estimating β_X, if we specify $P(Y|X^*, Z)$ incorrectly as linear logistic, say

$$\ln \frac{P(Y = 1|X^*, Z)}{1 - P(Y = 1|X^*, Z)} = \beta_0^* + \beta_X^* X^* + \beta_Z^* Z, \qquad (17.42)$$

then the naive estimate for β_X^* is inconsistent for β_X.

If the correct forms of $P(Y|X^*, Z)$ and $P(X|X^*, Z)$ were known, we could solve for $P(Y|X, Z)$ by inverting equations (17.40) for $X^* = 1$ and $X^* = 0$. Usually $P(Y|X^*, Z)$ is not known and $P(X|X^*, Z)$ must be estimated from jointly observed exposures, so we need a more sophisticated estimation procedure, which we consider below.

Misclassification of Outcome
Next suppose the outcome variable Y alone is misclassified. If we observe (Y^*, X, Z), we can only estimate $P(Y^*|X, Z)$ directly, but not $P(Y|X, Z)$. Analogous to (17.40), we have

$$P(Y^*|X, Z) = \sum_{Y=0}^{1} P(Y^*|Y, X, Z) P(Y|X, Z). \qquad (17.43)$$

Again, if $P(Y|X, Z)$ is linear in the logit scale, then $P(Y^*|X, Z)$ generally is not. For example, if we assume that $P(Y^*|Y, X, Z)$ is linear logistic, say

$$\ln \frac{P(Y^* = 1|Y, X, Z)}{1 - P(Y^* = 1|Y, X, Z)} = \alpha_0 + \alpha_Y Y + \alpha_X X + \alpha_Z Z, \qquad (17.44)$$

then

$P(Y^* = 1|X, Z)$

$$= \left\{ \frac{\exp(\alpha_0 + \alpha_X X + \alpha_Z Z)}{1 + \exp(\alpha_0 + \alpha_X X + \alpha_Z Z)} \right\} \left\{ \frac{1}{1 + \exp(\beta_0 + \beta_X X + \beta_Z Z)} \right\}$$
$$+ \left\{ \frac{\exp(\alpha_0 + \alpha_Y + \alpha_X X + \alpha_Z Z)}{1 + \exp(\alpha_0 + \alpha_Y + \alpha_X X + \alpha_Z Z)} \right\} \left\{ \frac{\exp(\beta_0 + \beta_X X + \beta_Z Z)}{1 + \exp(\beta_0 + \beta_X X + \beta_Z Z)} \right\},$$

which is not of linear logistic form, and a naive analysis using Y^* in place of Y would yield an inconsistent estimate of β_X. Even when $\beta_X = 0$, $P(Y^*|X, Z)$ still depends on X through α_X. Therefore, a test for $\beta_X = 0$ based on Y^* will be biased if $\alpha_X \neq 0$. Prentice (1989) points out that α_X should be zero for a hypothesis test for $\beta_X = 0$ to be valid.

Misclassification of Both Exposure and Outcome
Substituting X^* for X in (17.43) and then using (17.40) for $P(Y|X^*, Z)$ we have

$$P(Y^*|X^*, Z) = \sum_{Y=0}^{1} P(Y^*|Y, X^*, Z) P(Y|X^*, Z)$$
$$= \sum_{Y=0}^{1} P(Y^*|Y, X^*, Z) \sum_{X=0}^{1} P(Y|X, Z) P(X|X^*, Z)$$
$$. = \sum_{X=0}^{1} \sum_{Y=0}^{1} P(X|X^*, Z) P(Y^*|Y, X^*, Z) P(Y|X, Z).$$

$$(17.45)$$

Thus, the estimable probability of Y^* given X^* and Z is a linear combination of the correct conditional probabilities of Y given X and Z, with weights given by products of probabilities of correct and incorrect classification, in one case of X given X^* and in the other case of Y^* given Y and X, each given Z. Equation (17.45) is reminiscent of (17.11)–(17.14) for the joint probabilities $P(X^* = x^*, Y^* = y^*)$, especially if the error rates of observing Y^* given Y do not depend on X^*. In that case, if $\beta_X = 0$ then $P(Y^*|X^*, Z)$ does not depend on X^*, so a test of $\beta_X = 0$ will be valid. However, consistent estimation of β_X in the nonnull case is complicated and will not be given by fitting a linear logistic model for Y^* given X^* and Z.

Mismeasurement of Covariate Z (Underadjustment Bias)

Now suppose X and Y are classified without error, but that the covariate Z has measurement error. Bias in the coefficient β_X (still the parameter of interest) that often results in this situation is called *underadjustment bias*. It is most easily understood in the case of a continuous covariate Z which has a bilinear regression relation with its surrogate Z^*, that is,

$$E(Z^*|X, Z) = a + bX + cZ \quad \text{and} \quad E(Z|X, Z^*) = a' + b'X + c'Z^*. \quad (17.46)$$

For simplicity we have also assumed in (17.46) that the correlations and variance ratios between Z^* and Z are the same for both $X = 1$ and $X = 0$, so that both regressions are additive in X and Z. For example, if Z is normally distributed, and $Z^* = Z + \varepsilon$, where ε is normally distributed with $E(\varepsilon|X, Z) = 0$, then Z and Z^* are bivariate normal and have bilinear regressions. In fact, in this case Z^* is an unbiased estimator of the true value of Z for each exposure value X. We have $a = b = 0$, and the regression of Z^* on Z is the same line for both $X = 1$ and $X = 0$.

Now consider for a moment a linear (rather than linear logistic) model for the outcome Y as a function of X and Z:

$$E(Y|X, Z) = E(Y|X, Z, Z^*) = \beta_0 + \beta_X X + \beta_Z Z. \quad (17.47)$$

This equation states that Y depends only on the true covariate value Z rather than the mismeasured value. Then

$$E(Y|X, Z^*) = E\{E(Y|X, Z, Z^*)|X, Z^*\} = \beta_0 + \beta_X X + \beta_Z E(Z|X, Z^*)$$

$$= (\beta_0 + a'\beta_Z) + (\beta_X + b'\beta_Z)X + c'\beta_Z Z^*. \quad (17.48)$$

Thus the adjusted linear effect of X given Z^* will be seen as the adjusted risk difference

$$P(Y = 1|X = 1, Z^*) - P(Y = 1|X = 0, Z^*) = \beta_X + b'\beta_Z \quad (17.49)$$

rather than β_X. Bias in the estimated coefficient of X will therefore occur unless either (i) $\beta_Z = 0$, such that Z has no true effect on Y, or (ii) $b' = 0$, that is, the regression of Z on Z^* is the same for $X = 1$ and $X = 0$. Note, however, that in the case where Z^* is an unbiased estimator of Z or, more generally, when the regression of Z^* on Z is the same for $X = 1$ and $X = 0$, there will be *unequal regressions* of Z on Z^*, that is, $b' \neq 0$, whenever $E(Z|X = 1) \neq E(Z|X = 0)$. That is because the regression of Z on Z^* has a different slope than the regression of Z^* on Z, so that if the regression line of Z^* on Z is the same for both values of X, but with different mean points, the regression lines of Z on Z^* through their respective mean points will be distinct lines.

   If Z is a true potential confounder, that is, correlated with X and with an independent effect on Y, underadjustment bias will occur. Robbins and Levin (1983) analyze this phenomenon for the linear model under consideration and provide a simple formula for the bias. Specifically, the linear regression coefficient (17.49) can be expressed as a linear combination of the true coefficient β_X and the crude risk difference $P_1 - P_0 = P(Y = 1|X = 1) - P(Y = 1|X = 0) = E(Y|X = 1) - E(Y|X = 0)$, with weights ρ and $1 - \rho^2$, respectively, where ρ is the product-moment correlation between Z and Z^*:

$$P(Y = 1|X = 1, Z^*) - P(Y = 1|X = 0, Z^*) = \rho^2 \beta_X + (1 - \rho^2)\{P_1 - P_0\}.$$
$$(17.50)$$

Even if the true adjusted effect of X on Y given Z is zero ($\beta_X = 0$), there will be an apparent effect of X on Y whenever there is an imperfect surrogate ($\rho \neq 1$) and there are exposure group differences in Z or Z^*, even if Z^* is an unbiased estimator of Z. Nondifferential mismeasurement creates a *bias away from zero* when the mismeasurement is in an adjustment covariate. The bias increases as Z^* becomes a poorer surrogate for Z, that is, as ρ decreases in magnitude.

   Note also that underadjustment bias does not occur if the regressions of Z on Z^* are the same for each level of exposure. They are not under the random mismeasurement model, as explained above. Depending on the context, it is an empirical question whether that model or an alternative mismeasurement model specifying that the regressions of Z on Z^* are the same, best describes the facts. It may be, for example, that for given levels of qualifications for a job (Z^*), average productivity (Z) is the same for men and women (X), that is, $E(Z|Z^*, X)$ is the same for men and women. Even if qualifications are an imperfect surrogate for true productivity, and even if men and women have different average levels of qualifications, use of Z^* instead of Z as an adjustment factor in a regression equation of salary levels against sex will not exhibit underadjustment bias. Therefore caution is always in order when considering mismeasurement models. Finkelstein and Levin (2001) discuss these two mismeasurement models and their implications in the Title VII law of equal employment opportunity and antidiscrimination litigation.

Table 17.13. *Hypothetical joint probabilities of an antecedent exposure (X), disease indicator (Y), and a potential confounder Z, all classified without error*

	Z = 1				Z = 0		
	Disease (= Y)				Disease		
Exposure (= X)	1	0	Total	Exposure	1	0	Total
1	0.05	0.05	0.10	1	0.04	0.16	0.20
0	0.05	0.05	0.10	0	0.12	0.48	0.60
Total	0.10	0.10	0.20	Total	0.16	0.64	0.80

Qualitatively similar relations occur with the logistic regression model for Y. We shall merely illustrate here with a numerical example using a binary covariate Z rather than a continuous one. In this case, a surrogate Z^* of Z with misclassification error cannot be an unbiased estimator of the true Z because, even with nondifferential misclassification, $E(Z^*|X, Z) = a_0 + (a_1 - a_0)Z$, where $a_j = P(Z^* = 1|Z = j)$ for $j = 1$ and 0; unless there is perfect agreement, $a_0 \neq 0$ and $a_1 - a_0 \neq 1$. This does not affect the arguments given above—in our example we will still have equal regressions of Z^* on Z given X.

Suppose we have joint probabilities of an antecedent factor X, disease indicator Y, and covariate Z, as in Table 17.13. These are assumed to hold irrespective of Z^*, given Z. The true odds ratios associating X and Y are then each null: $\omega_1 = 1$ and $\omega_0 = (0.04 \times 0.48)/(0.12 \times 0.16) = 1$ in stratum $Z = 1$ and $Z = 0$, respectively. The linear logistic model specified here is

$$\ln \frac{P(Y = 1|X, Z)}{1 - P(Y = 1|X, Z)} = (-\ln 4) + (\ln 4)Z,$$

corresponding to the linear model

$$P(Y = 1|X, Z) = P(Y = 1|X, Z, Z^*) = 0.2 + 0.3Z.$$

Now suppose the distribution of Z^* given X and Z is

$$P(Z^* = 1|X, Z) = \tfrac{1}{13} + \left(\tfrac{3}{4} - \tfrac{1}{13}\right)Z$$

$$= \begin{cases} \tfrac{3}{4} & \text{(if } Z = 1\text{),} \\ \tfrac{1}{13} & \text{(if } Z = 0\text{).} \end{cases} \qquad (17.51)$$

Table 17.14. *Joint distribution of X, Z, and Z* implied by Table 17.12 and (17.51)*

Z^*	$X = 1$ Z 1	0	Total	Z^*	$X = 0$ Z 1	0	Total
1	0.075	0.015	0.090	1	0.075	0.046	0.121
0	0.025	0.185	0.210	0	0.025	0.554	0.579
Total	0.1	0.2	0.3	Total	0.1	0.6	0.7

This expression gives the same conditional probabilities of correct classification (if $Z = 1$) or misclassification (if $Z = 0$) as are in Table 17.10, such as would be the case, say, if we were regarding smoking status as an adjustment covariate rather than as the antecedent risk factor. Note that (17.51) also gives the same classification probabilities for each level of exposure. The joint distribution of Z^*, Z, and X is given by multiplying $P(Z^* = 1|X, Z)$ in (17.51) by the joint distribution of (X, Z) obtained from the margins of Table 17.13. The resulting joint distribution of Z^*, Z, and X is given in Table 17.14 (see Problem 17.5). Note, however, that now the conditional distribution of Z given X and Z^* does depend on X. The conditional probabilities of Z given X and Z^* derived from Table 17.14 can be summarized as follows:

$$P(Z = 1|X, Z^*) = 0.043 + 0.076X + 0.576Z^* + 0.135XZ^*, \quad (17.52)$$

which is an interactive rather than additive model, because the variance ratios and correlations between Z^* and Z differ at the two levels of X: for example, $\rho_1 = 0.38$ for $X = 1$ and $\rho_0 = 0.52$ for $X = 0$. Finally, taking conditional expectations of $P(Y = 1|X, Z) = P(Y = 1|X, Z, Z^*)$ with respect to the conditional distribution of Z given X and Z^* yields

$P(Y = 1|X, Z^*)$

$\quad = E\{P(Y = 1|X, Z, Z^*)|X, Z^*\} = 0.2 + 0.3P(Z = 1|X, Z^*)$

$\quad = (0.2 + 0.3 \times 0.043) + 0.3 \times 0.076X + 0.3 \times 0.576Z^* + 0.3 \times 0.135XZ^*$

$\quad = 0.2129 + 0.0228X + 0.1728Z^* + 0.0405XZ^*$

$\quad = \begin{cases} 0.4490 \text{ for } X = 1 \quad \text{or} \quad 0.3857 \text{ for } X = 0 \quad \text{when } Z^* = 1, \\ 0.2357 \text{ for } X = 1 \quad \text{or} \quad 0.2129 \text{ for } X = 0 \quad \text{when } Z^* = 0. \end{cases} \quad (17.53)$

The odds ratio in the $Z^* = 1$ stratum is $\omega_1^* = (0.4490/0.5510)/(0.3857/0.6143) = 1.30$, and in the $Z^* = 0$ stratum is $\omega_0^* = (0.2357/0.7643)/(0.2129/0.7871) = 1.14$, creating an association between X and Y where none truly exists. An additive logistic model fit to data with these underlying probabilities would estimate a coefficient for β_X falling between $\ln 1.30$ and $\ln 1.14$. Note how the assumption of the misclassification model (17.51) is subtly different from the assumption that $P(Z = 1|Z^*, X)$ is the same irrespective of X, such as was used earlier in Section 17.4 in the context of Table 17.10.

Adjustment with Double Sampling for Misclassification of Exposure

As suggested above, we need to know the relation between the variables measured with and without error in order to estimate the logistic regression parameters of interest. Double sampling or two-stage designs have been widely used to address this problem. At the first stage, the mismeasured variable (surrogate or misclassified variable) is observed for all subjects; at the second stage, a random subsample with sampling fraction f is selected, and the more reliable variable is measured for the selected subsample. This subsample is often called a validation set, for example, when a gold-standard variable is measured at the second stage. The sample fraction f is typically small. In another variation, the second stage is devoted to sampling a second imperfect variable. If the latter variable is inexpensive to measure, the sampling fraction f may be large or even 100%.

Table 17.10 is an example of the results of a validation sample collected cross-sectionally that provides information on $P(X, X^*|Z)$ and therefore also $P(X|X^*, Z)$. If independent samples of X are observed at both levels of the misclassified exposure X^*, then similar information is available. We shall restrict attention to the case where the binary exposure X is the only variable measured with error, and where the second-stage sample is a validation set in which a standard, reliable measurement is available. Only minor modifications are required for the case of two imperfect exposure measures.

The analytical methods for misclassified variables are similar to those for missing data. Since the surrogate or misclassified variable is observed for all records, but the second-stage variable is observed only for the validation set, the problem can be framed as one of a monotonically missing exposure variable; and because the two-stage design uses either cross-sectional or stratified random sampling at the second stage, the missingness mechanism is known to be either MCAR or MAR, respectively (see Chapter 16 for terminology). However, the size of the validation set is relatively small, so an analysis based only on complete records (i.e., using only the standard measurement), while unbiased, would have too little precision. Here we present a likelihood-based method that utilizes all the data. Given the similarity to the missing-data problem, one could also use an imputation or weighting method as described in Chapter 16. Spiegelman and Casella (1997) use the weighting method for misclassified data.

Let S be the indicator for selection into the subsample: if X is observed, $S = 1$. X^* is observed for all records. Since the selection is made at random, we have $P(S = 1|Y, X, Z) = P(S = 1)$. Combining contributions from the validation and nonvalidation subsamples, the likelihood function is

$$L = \prod_{i=1}^{n} L_{i1}^{S_i} L_{i2}^{1-S_i}, \tag{17.54}$$

where

$$L_{i1} = P(S_i = 1) P(Y_i = 1|X_i, Z_i)^{Y_i} \{1 - P(Y_i = 1|X_i, Z_i)\}^{1-Y_i}$$

and

$$L_{i2} = \sum_{x=0}^{1} P(S_i = 0) P(X_i = x|X_i^*, Z_i) P(Y_i = 1|X_i = x, X_i^*, Z_i)^{Y_i}$$

$$\times \{1 - P(Y_i = 1|X_i = x, X_i^*, Z_i)\}^{1-Y_i}$$

$$= P(S_i = 0) \sum_{x=0}^{1} P(X_i = x|X_i^*, Z_i) P(Y_i = 1|X_i = x, Z_i)^{Y_i}$$

$$\times \{1 - P(Y_i = 1|X_i = x, Z_i)\}^{1-Y_i},$$

and where $P(X_i = x|X_i^*, Z_i)$ follows (17.41). Note that, as constant factors, $P(S_i)$ does not affect maximization of the likelihood function over β and γ.

Let $P_i(\beta, X_i, Z_i) = P(Y_i = 1|X_i, Z_i) = 1/\{1 + \exp - (\beta_0 + \beta_X X_i + \beta_Z Z_i)\}$. The score equation for β derived from the logarithm of (17.54) has the following form:

$$\frac{\partial \ln L}{\partial \beta} = \sum_{i=1}^{n} \left(S_i \begin{bmatrix} Y_i - P_i(\beta, X_i, Z_i) \\ X_i\{Y_i - P_i(\beta, X_i, Z_i)\} \\ Z_i\{Y_i - P_i(\beta, X_i, Z_i)\} \end{bmatrix} \right.$$

$$\left. + (1 - S_i) \begin{bmatrix} Y_i - E\{P_i(\beta, X_i, Z_i)|X_i^*, Y_i, Z_i\} \\ E[X_i\{Y_i - P_i(\beta, X_i, Z_i)\}|X_i^*, Y_i, Z_i] \\ Z_i[Y_i - E\{P_i(\beta, X_i, Z_i)|X_i^*, Y_i, Z_i\}] \end{bmatrix} \right) = 0, \tag{17.55}$$

where the expectations are taken with respect to the conditional distribution of X_i given X_i^*, Y_i, and Z_i, which we evaluate momentarily. Also, let

$\mu_i(\gamma) = \mu_i(\gamma, X_i^*, Z_i) = E(X_i|X_i^*, Z_i)$. The score equation for γ is

$$
\frac{\partial \ln L}{\partial \gamma} = \sum_{i=1}^{n} \left(S_i \begin{bmatrix} X_i - \mu_i(\gamma) \\ X_i^*\{X_i - \mu_i(\gamma)\} \\ Z_i\{X_i - \mu_i(\gamma)\} \end{bmatrix} \right.
$$

$$
\left. + (1 - S_i) \begin{bmatrix} E(X_i|X_i^*, Y_i, Z_i) - \mu_i(\gamma) \\ X_i^*\{E(X_i|X_i^*, Y_i, Z_i) - \mu_i(\gamma)\} \\ Z_i\{E(X_i|X_i^*, Y_i, Z_i) - \mu_i(\gamma)\} \end{bmatrix} \right) = 0. \quad (17.56)
$$

Equations (17.55) and (17.56) differ from equations (16.27) and (16.28) for logistic regression models with missing covariates only in that the conditioning arguments in the expectations include X_i^* in addition to Y_i and Z_i.

The conditional distribution of X_i given X_i^*, Y_i, and Z_i is obtained from Bayes theorem:

$$
P(X_i = 1|X_i^*, Y_i, Z_i)
$$

$$
= \frac{P(Y_i|X_i = 1, Z_i)P(X_i = 1|X_i^*, Z_i)}{P(Y_i|X_i = 1, Z_i)P(X_i = 1|X_i^*, Z_i) + P(Y_i|X_i = 0, Z_i)P(X_i = 0|X_i^*, Z_i)},
$$

which can be evaluated for given values of β and γ from the logistic model for Y_i and (17.41) for $P(X_i|X_i^*, Z_i)$. The conditional expectation of X_i given X_i^*, Y_i, and Z_i is thus

$$
E(X_i|X_i^*, Y_i, Z_i) = P(X_i = 1|X_i^*, Y_i, Z_i), \quad (17.57)
$$

the conditional expectation of $P_i(\beta, X_i, Z_i)$ is

$$
E\{P_i(\beta, X_i, Z_i)|X_i^*, Y_i, Z_i\} = P_i(\beta, 1, Z_i)P(X_i = 1|X_i^*, Y_i, Z_i)
$$

$$
+ P_i(\beta, 0, Z_i)P(X_i = 0|X_i^*, Y_i, Z_i), \quad (17.58)
$$

and the conditional expectation of $X_i P_i(\beta_i, X_i, Z_i)$ is

$$
E\{X_i P_i(\beta, X_i, Z_i)|X_i^*, Y_i, Z_i\} = P_i(\beta, 1, Z_i)P(X_i = 1|X_i^*, Y_i, Z_i). \quad (17.59)
$$

Computation of $\hat{\beta}$ and $\hat{\gamma}$ can be carried out iteratively using a Newton-Raphson algorithm using expressions (17.55)–(17.59). A simpler way is to use the expanded-dataset method described in Section 16.4. When one has missing data, a record with a missing binary value is duplicated, one with the value 1 filled in, the other with the value 0. In the case of mismeasured data, even though the mismeasured value is observed as a 1, say, we add a duplicate record with the value appearing as $X = 0$, and, vice versa, if the value observed is a 0, we add a duplicate record with the value $X = 1$. Given an initial value of β and γ, the conditional expectations $P(X_i = 1 | X_i^*, Y_i, Z_i)$ and $P(X_i = 0 | X_i^*, Y_i, Z_i)$ are evaluated and used as weights for the duplicated records, just as for the missing data procedure. Then with the expanded data set and weights, two regular weighted logistic regression models are fit, one for X and one for Y, which yield new estimates for β and γ. The entire process is iterated until convergence occurs.

The use of double sampling to estimate misclassification errors and to correct for bias in logistic regression coefficients has been studied by many authors. A double sampling scheme for estimating misclassification probabilities was first proposed by Tenenbein (1970, 1971). Palmgren (1987) finds that double sampling is irrelevant for testing equality of two proportions when the probabilities of misclassification are equal in the two populations. Chernoff and Haitovsky (1990) provide optimal designs to compare two proportions. Zelen and Haitovsky (1991) examine the asymptotic relative efficiency of tests based on a misclassified outcome in 2×2, $2 \times 2 \times K$, and paired sample cases. These authors also suggest conditional resampling, in which the sampling probability depends on Y. Chen (1979) and Espeland and Odoroff (1985) propose likelihood methods for utilizing the validation sample to adjust for misclassification error in log-linear models. Correcting bias due to misclassification of the outcome variable in the context of logistic regression is studied by Pepe (1992), Magder and Hughes (1997), and Cheng and Hsueh (1999). For measurement error in exposure, Stefansky (1985) and Armstrong (1985) propose a method applicable to generalized linear models with continuous or categorical covariates. Spiegelman (1994) considers sample size issues, and Elton and Duffy (1983) investigate a likelihood-based method. The case in which both outcome and exposure variables are prone to error is considered by Espeland and Hui (1987). Some authors present methods based on an estimating-equation approach (Liu and Liang, 1991, 1992; Wang, Carroll, and Liang, 1996; Wang and Pepe, 2000). Interesting applications in epidemiology and economics can be found in Lee and Forey (1996), Stewart et al. (1998), and Pfeffermann, Skinner, and Humphreys (1998). Wacholder, Armstrong, and Hartge (1993) examine the case where the validation set is also measured with error. When two imperfect exposure measurements are available, Duffy, Rohan, and Day (1989) and Kosinski and Flanders (1999) propose likelihood-based methods.

PROBLEMS

17.1. The text cited the differences among the five New York state hospitals in the proportions of patients diagnosed catatonic, out of all those diagnosed either catatonic or paranoid.

(a) The frequencies are given below. Calculate the indicated proportions.

Hospital	Catatonic	Paranoid	Total	Proportion Catatonic
Central Islip	32	80	112	$= p_1$
Pilgrim	78	76	154	$= p_2$
Brooklyn	13	18	31	$= p_3$
Kings Park	55	96	151	$= p_4$
Rockland	37	87	124	$= p_5$
Total	215	357	572	$= \bar{p}$

(b) The chi squared statistic for comparing a series of proportions is given by (9.4). Calculate chi squared for the proportions determined in (a).

(c) Refer the value just calculated to Table A.2 with 4 df. At what significance level would the hypothesis of no difference in proportions be rejected? What would you conclude about the standards for the differential diagnosis of catatonic and paranoid schizophrenia in the five hospitals?

17.2. Suppose that the rate of smoking among women aged 55–64 who were newly diagnosed as having lung cancer is $P_L = 0.50$, and suppose that the error rates are $E_L = 0.25$ and $F_l = 0.05$.

(a) What is the value of p_L [see (17.3)], the estimated proportion of such women who ever smoked?

Suppose that the rate of smoking among women aged 55–64 who were newly diagnosed as having breast cancer is $P_B = 0.40$, and suppose that the error rates are $E_B = E_F = 0.10$.

(b) What is the value of p_B [see (17.4)], the estimated proportion of such women who ever smoked?

(c) What is the value of $P_L - P_B$? What is the value of $p_L - p_B$? How do these compare?

(d) What is the odds ratio as a function of P_L and P_B? What is the odds ratio as a function of p_L and p_B? How do these compare?

17.3. We considered, in Section 17.4, a means of correcting for the bias in an observed proportion. We now consider the comparison of two proportions, both of which are subject to error.

(a) The value of p_L, the rate of heavy smoking among lung cancer patients based on verbal report, was 0.44. Suppose that 200 women with cancer of the breast are interviewed, with 60 of them indicating that they are heavy smokers. What is the value of p_B, the rate of heavy smoking among breast cancer patients? What is the value of the odds ratio measuring the degree of association between type of cancer and heavy smoking?

(b) Based on the determination of smoking status by both response to interview and chemical test for 50 lung cancer patients, the rate of heavy smoking was adjusted to $P_L = 0.51$. Suppose that 50 breast cancer patients are likewise given a chemical test in addition to an interview, with the following results:

Chemical Test

Report	Heavy	Not Heavy	Total
Heavy	18	0	18
Not Heavy	2	30	32

What are the values of the two correction factors, n_{00}/n_0 and n_{10}/n_1, which are to be applied to p_B? What value of P_B results from the adjustment

$$P_B = \frac{n_{00}}{n_0} p_B + \frac{n_{10}}{n_1}(1 - p_B)?$$

What is the value of the odds ratio associated with the adjusted rates? Does the association between heavy smoking and type of cancer now appear weaker or stronger than in (a)?

(c) Suppose instead that the cross-classification for the subsample of 50 breast cancer patients yielded the following results:

Chemical Test

Report	Heavy	Not Heavy	Total
Heavy	16	2	18
Not Heavy	7	25	32

What are the values of the correction factors, n_{00}/n_0 and n_{10}/n_1? What is the resulting value of P_B? What is the resulting value of the odds ratio? Does the association appear weaker or stronger than in (a)?

17.4. Suppose that the value of the correction factor n_{00}/n_0 was the same for the two kinds of patients and that the value of the correction factor n_{10}/n_1 was likewise the same. What is a simple expression for $P_L - P_B$ as a function of $p_L - p_B$ and of the difference $n_{00}/n_0 - n_{10}/n_1$?

17.5. Confirm the numerical values in Table 17.14 and expressions (17.52) and (17.53). [*Hint.* Use Bayes' theorem to write

$$P(Z|X, Z^*) = \frac{P(Z^*|Z, X)P(Z|X)}{P(Z^*|X)}$$

$$= \frac{P(Z^*|Z, X) \, P(Z|X)}{P(Z^*|Z = 1, X)P(Z = 1|X) + P(Z^*|Z = 0, X)P(Z = 0|X)} \cdot]$$

REFERENCES

American Psychiatric Association (1980). *DSM-III: Diagnostic and statistical manual of mental disorders*. 3rd ed., Washington, DC: American Psychiatric Press.

American Psychiatric Association (1987). *DSM-III-R: Diagnostic and statistical manual of mental disorders*. 3rd ed., revised. Washington, DC: American Psychiatric Press.

American Psychiatric Association (1994). *DSM-IV: Diagnostic and statistical manual of mental disorders*. 4th ed., Washington, DC: American Psychiatric Press.

Armstrong, B. (1985). Measurement error in the generalised linear model. *Comm. Statist.*, **B14**, 529–544.

Assakul, K. and Proctor, C. H. (1967). Testing independence in two-way contingency tables with data subject to misclassification. *Psychometrika*, **32**, 67–76.

Bakwin, H. (1945). Pseudodoxia pediatrica. *New Engl. J. Med.*, **232**, 691–697.

Barron, B. A. (1977). The effects of misclassification on the estimation of relative risk. *Biometrics*, **33**, 414–418.

Begg, M. D. and Lagakos, S. (1992). Effects of mismodeling on tests of association based on logistic regression models. *Ann. Statist.*, **20**, 1929–1952.

Bowman, J. E., Brewer, G. J., Frischer, H., Carter, L. L., Eisenstein, R. B., and Bayrakci, C. (1965). A re-evaluation of the relationship between glucose-6-phosphate dehydrogenase deficiency and the behavioral manifestations of schizophrenia. *J. Lab. Clin. Med.*, **65**, 222–227.

Bross, I. (1954). Misclassification in 2 × 2 tables. *Biometrics*, **10**, 478–486.

Bryson, M. R. (1965). Errors of classification in a binomial population. *J. Am. Statist. Assoc.*, **60**, 217–224.

Carroll, R. J., Ruppert, D., and Stefanski, L. A. (1995). *Measurement error in nonlinear models*. London: Chapman & Hall.

Chen, T. T. (1979). Log-linear models for categorical data with misclassification and double sampling. *J. Am. Statist. Assoc.*, **74**, 481–488.

Cheng, K. F. and Hsueh, H. M. (1999). Correcting bias due to misclassification in the estimation of logistic regression models. *Statist. Probab. Lett.*, **44**, 229–240.

Chernoff, H. and Haitovsky, Y. (1990). Locally optimal design for comparing two probabilities from binomial data subject to misclassification. *Biometrika*, **77**, 797–805.

Chiacchierini, R. P. and Arnold, J. C. (1977). A two-sample test for independence in 2×2 contingency tables with both margins subject to misclassification. *J. Am. Statist. Assoc.*, **72**, 170–174.

Clark, L. A., Watson, D., and Reynolds, S. (1995). Diagnosis and classification of psychopathology: Challenges to the current system and future directions. *Annual Review of Psychology*, **46**, 121–153.

Cochrane, A. L. and Garland, L. H. (1952). Observer error in interpretation of chest films: International investigation. *Lancet*, **2**, 505–509.

Copeland, K. T., Checkoway, H., McMichael, A. J., and Holbrook, R. H. (1977). Bias due to misclassification in the estimation of relative risk. *Am. J. Epidemiol.*, **105**, 488–495.

Davies, L. G. (1958). Observer variation in reports on electrocardiograms. *Brit. Heart J.*, **20**, 153–161.

Deming, W. E. (1977). An essay on screening, or on two-phase sampling, applied to surveys of a community. *Int. Statist. Rev.*, **45**, 29–37.

Densen, P. M., Davidow, B., Bass, H. E., and Jones, E. W. (1967). A chemical test for smoking exposure. *Arch. Environ. Health*, **14**, 865–874.

Dern, R. J., Glynn, M. F., and Brewer, G. J. (1963). Studies on the correlation of the genetically determined trait G-6-PD deficiency with behavioral manifestations in schizophrenia. *J. Lab. Clin. Med.*, **62**, 319–329.

Derryberry, M. (1938). Reliability of medical judgments on malnutrition. *Public Health Rep.*, **53**, 263–268.

Diamond, E. L. and Lilienfeld, A. M. (1962a). Effects of errors in classification and diagnosis in various type of epidemiological studies. *Am. J. Public Health*, **52**, 1137–1144.

Diamond, E. L. and Lilienfeld, A. M. (1962b). Misclassification errors in 2×2 tables with one margin fixed: Some further comments. *Am. J. Public Health*, **52**, 2106–2110.

Duffy, S. W., Rohan, T. E., and Day, N. E. (1989). Misclassification in more than one factor in a case-control study: A combination of Mantel-Haenszel and maximum likelihood approaches. *Statist. in Med.*, **8**, 1529–1536.

Elton, R. A. and Duffy, S. W. (1983). Correcting for the effect of misclassification bias in a case-control study using data from two different questionnaires. *Biometrics*, **39**, 659–663.

Endicott, J. and Spitzer, R. (1978). A diagnostic interview: The schedule for affective disorders and schizophrenia. *Arch. Gen. Psychiatry*, **35**, 837–844.

Espeland, M. A. and Hui, S. L. (1987). A general approach to analyzing epidemiologic data that contain misclassification errors. *Biometrics*, **43**, 1001–1012.

Espeland, M. A. and Odoroff, C. L. (1985). Log-linear models for doubly sampled categorical data fitted by the EM algorithm. *J. Am. Statist. Assoc.*, **80**, 663–670.

Feighner, J. P., Robins, E., Guze, S. B., Woodruff, R. A., Winokur, G., and Munoz, R. (1972). Diagnostic criteria for use in psychiatric research. *Arch. Gen. Psychiatry*, **26**, 57–63.

Fieve, R. R., Brauninger, G., Fleiss, J. L., and Cohen, G. (1965). Glucose-6-phosphate dehydrogenase deficiency and schizophrenic behavior. *J. Psychiatr. Res.*, **3**, 255–262.

Finkelstein, M. O. and Levin, B. (2001). *Statistics for Lawyers*, 2nd ed. New York: Springer-Verlag.

First, M. B., Spitzer, R. L., Gibbon, M., and Williams, J. (1996). *Structured clinical interview for DSM-IV axis I disorders—Patient edition (SCID-I/P, version 2.0)*. Biometrics Research Department. New York: New York State Psychiatric Institute.

Fletcher, C. M. (1952) Clinical diagnosis of pulmonary emphysema—an experimental study. *Proc. R. Soc. Med.*, **45**, 577–584.

Ganz, V. H., Gurland, B. J., Deming, W. E., and Fisher, B. (1972). The study of the psychiatric symptoms of systemic lupus erythematosus: A biometric study. *Psychosom. Med.*, **34**, 199–206.

Garland, L. H. (1960). The problem of observer error. *Bull. N.Y. Acad. Med.*, **36**, 570–584.

Goldberg, J. D. (1975). The effects of misclassification on the bias in the difference between two proportions and the relative odds in the fourfold table. *J. Am. Statist. Assoc.*, **70**, 561–567.

Greenland, S. (1982). The effect of misclassification in matched-pair case-control studies. *Am. J. Epidemiol.*, **116**, 402–406.

Greenland, S. (1988). Variance estimation for epidemiologic effect estimates under misclassification. *Statist. in Med.*, **7**, 745–757.

Greenland, S. and Brenner, H. (1993). Correcting for non-differential misclassification in ecologic analyses. *Appl. Statist.*, **42**, 117–126.

Greenland, S. and Robins, J. M. (1985). Confounding and misclassification. *Am. J. Epidemiol.*, **122**, 495–506.

Harper, D. (1964). Misclassification in epidemiological surveys. *Am. J. Public Health*, **54**, 1882–1886.

Hasin, D. and Miele, G. (1997). *Psychiatric research interview for substance and mental disorders*. New York: New York State Psychiatric Institute.

Hochberg, Y. (1977). On the use of double sampling schemes in analyzing categorical data with misclassification errors. *J. Am. Statist. Assoc.*, **72**, 914–921.

Horwitz, O. and Lysgaard-Hansen, B. (1975). Medical observations and bias. *Am. J. Epidemiol.*, **101**, 391–399.

Hsieh, C.-C. (1991). The effect of non-differential outcome misclassification on estimates of the attributable and prevented fraction. *Statist. in Med.*, **10**, 361–373.

Hsieh, C.-C. and Walter, S. D. (1988). The effect of non-differential exposure misclassification on estimates of the attributable and prevented fraction. *Statist. in Med.*, **7**, 1073–1085.

Keys, A. and Kihlberg, J. K. (1963). The effect of misclassification on estimated relative prevalence of a characteristic. *Am. J. Public Health*, **53**, 1656–1665.

Klerman, G. L. (1983). The significance of DSM-III in American psychiatry. Pp. 3–25 in Spitzer, R. L., Williams, J. B., and Skodol, A. (Eds.), *International Perspectives on DSM-III*. Washington, DC: American Psychiatric Press.

Koch, G. G. (1969). The effect of non-sampling errors on measures of association in 2×2 contingency tables. *J. Am. Statist. Assoc.*, **64**, 852–863.

Koran, L. M. (1975a). The reliability of clinical methods, data and judgments, part 1. *New Engl. J. Med.*, **293**, 642–646.

Koran, L. M. (1975b). The reliability of clinical methods, data and judgments, part 2. *New Engl. J. Med.*, **293**, 695–701.

Kosinski, A. S. and Flanders, W. D. (1999). Evaluating the exposure and disease relationship with adjustment for different types of exposure misclassification: A regression approach. *Statist. in Med.*, **18**, 2795–2808.

Lagakos, S. W. (1988). Effects of mismodelling and mismeasuring explanatory variables on tests of their association with a response variable. *Statist. in Med.*, **7**, 257–274.

Lee, P. N. and Forey, B. A. (1996). Misclassification of smoking habits as a source of bias in the study of environmental tobacco smoke and lung cancer. *Statist. in Med.*, **15**, 581–605.

Levin, M. L. (1954). Etiology of lung cancer: Present status. *N.Y. State J. Med.*, **54**, 769–777.

Lilienfeld, A. M. and Graham, S. (1958). Validity of determining circumcision status by questionnaire as related to epidemiological studies of cancer of the cervix. *J. Natl. Cancer Inst.*, **21**, 713–720.

Liu, X. and Liang, K.-Y. (1991). Adjustment for non-differential misclassification error in the generalized linear model. *Statist. in Med.*, **10**, 1197–1211.

Liu, X. and Liang, K.-Y. (1992). Efficiency of repeated measures in regression models with measurement error. *Biometrics*, **48**, 645–654.

Magder, L. S. and Hughes, J. P. (1997). Logistic regression when the outcome is measured with uncertainty. *Am. J. Epidemiol.*, **146**, 195–203.

Markush, R. E., Schaaf, W. E., and Seigel, D. G. (1967). The influence of the death certifier on the results of epidemiologic studies. *J. Natl. Med. Assoc.*, **59**, 105–113.

Medical Research Council (1966). *Questionnaire on respiratory diseases.* Dawlish, Devon, England: W.J. Holman, Ltd.

Mote, V. L. and Anderson, R. L. (1965). An investigation of the effect of misclassification on the properties of chi square tests in the analysis of categorical data. *Biometrika*, **52**, 95–109.

Nathan, P. and Langenbucher, J. (1999). Psychopathology: Description and classification. *Annual Review of Psychology*, **50**, 79–107.

Newell, D. J. (1962). Errors in the interpretation of errors in epidemiology. *Am. J. Public Health*, **52**, 1925–1928.

Palmgren, J. (1987). Precision of double sampling estimators for comparing two probabilities. *Biometrika*, **74**, 687–694.

Pepe, M. S. (1992). Inference using surrogate outcome data and a validation sample. *Biometrika*, **79**, 687–694.

Pfeffermann, D., Skinner, C., and Humphreys, K. (1988). The estimation of gross flows in the presence of measurement error using auxiliary variables. *J. R. Statist. Soc., Ser. A*, **161**, 13–32.

Prentice, R. L. (1989). Surrogate endpoints in clinical trials: Definition and operational criteria. *Statist. in Med.*, **8**, 431–440.

Press, S. J. (1968). Estimating from misclassified data. *J. Am. Statist. Assoc.*, **63**, 123–133.

Reade-Christopher, S. J. and Kupper, L. L. (1991). Effects of exposure misclassification on regression analyses of epidemiologic follow-up study data. *Biometrics*, **47**, 535–548.

Riskind, J. H., Beck, A. T., Berchick, R. J., Brown, G., and Steer, R. A. (1987). Reliability of DSM-III diagnoses for major depression and generalized anxiety disorder using the structured clinical interview for DSM-III. *Arch. Gen. Psychiatry*, **44**, 817–820.

Robbins, H. and Levin, B. (1983). A note on the underadjustment phenomenon. *Statist. Probab. Lett.*, **1**, 137–139.

Rogot, E. (1961). A note on measurement errors and detecting real differences. *J. Am. Statist. Assoc.*, **56**, 314–319.

Rubin, T., Rosenbaum, J., and Cobb, S. (1956). The use of interview data for the detection of association in field studies. *J. Chronic Dis.*, **4**, 253–266.

Selen, J. (1986). Adjusting for errors in classification and measurement in the analysis of partly and purely categorical data. *J. Am. Statist. Assoc.*, **81**, 75–81.

Skre, I., Onstad, S., Torgersen, S., and Kringlen, E. (1991). High interrater reliability for the structured clinical interview for DSM-III-R axis I (SCID-I). *Acta Psychiat. Scand.*, **84**, 167–173.

Spiegelman, D. (1994). Cost-efficient study designs for relative risk modeling with covariate measurement error. *J. Statist. Plann. Inference*, **42**, 187–208.

Spiegelman, D. and Casella, M. (1997). Fully parametric and semi-parametric regression models for common events with covariate measurement error in main study/validation study designs. *Biometrics*, **53**, 395–409.

Spitzer, R. L., Endicott, J., Fleiss, J. L., and Cohen, J. (1970). Psychiatric Status Schedule: A technique for evaluating psychopathology and impairment in role functioning. *Arch. Gen. Psychiatry*, **23**, 41–55.

Spitzer, R., Endicott, J., and Robins, E. (1978). Research diagnostic criteria: rationale and reliability. *Arch. Gen. Psychiatry*, **35**, 773–782.

Spitzer, R. L. and Fleiss, J. L. (1974). A re-analysis of the reliability of psychiatric diagnosis. *Brit. J. Psychiatry*, **125**, 341–347.

Spitzer, R. L., Fleiss, J. L., Endicott, J., and Cohen, J. (1967). Mental Status Schedule: Properties of factor analytically derived scales. *Arch. Gen. Psychiatry*, **16**, 479–493.

Spitzer, R., Williams, J., Gibbon, M., and First, M. B. (1990). *Structured clinical interview for DSM-III-R—patient edition (SCID-P)*. Washington DC: American Psychiatric Press.

Spitzer, R., Williams, J., Gibbon, M., and First, M. B. (1992). The structured clinical interview for DSM-III-R (SCID): History, rationale, and description. *Arch. Gen. Psychiatry*, **49**, 624–629.

Stefanski, L. A. (1985). The effects of measurement error on parameter estimation. *Biometrika*, **72**, 583–592.

Stewart, S. L., Swallen, K. C., Glaser, S. L., Horn-Ross, P. L., and West, D. W. (1998). Adjustment of cancer incidence rates for ethnic misclassification. *Biometrics*, **54**, 774–781.

Tenenbein, A. (1970). A double sampling scheme for estimating from binomial data with misclassifications. *J. Am. Statist. Assoc.*, **65**, 1350–1361.

Tenenbein, A. (1971). A double sampling scheme for estimating from binomial data with misclassifications: Sample size determination. *Biometrics*, **27**, 935–944.

Ventura, J., Liberman, R. P., Green, M. F., Shaner, A., and Mintz, J. (1998). Training and quality assurance with the structured clinical interview for DSM-IV (SCID-I/P). *Psychiatry Res.*, **79**, 163–173.

Wacholder, S., Armstrong, B., and Hartge, P. (1993). Validation studies using an alloyed gold standard. *Am. J. Epidemiol.*, **137**, 1251–1258.

Wang, C. Y. and Pepe, M. S. (2000). Expected estimating equations to accommodate covariate measurement error. *J. R. Statist. Soc.*, *Ser. B*, **62**, 509–524.

Wang, N., Carroll, R. J., and Liang, K.-Y. (1996). Quasilikelihood estimation in measurement error models with correlated replicates. *Biometrics*, **52**, 401–411.

Williams, J. B., Gibbon, M., First, M. B., Spitzer, R. L., Davies, M., Borus, J., Howes, M. J., Kane, J., Pope, H. G., Roundsaville, B., and Wittchen, H. U. (1992). The structured clinical interview for DSM-III-R (SCID). *Arch. Gen. Psychiatry*, **49**, 630–636.

Wilson, M. (1993). DSM III and the transformation of American psychiatry. *Am. J. Psychiatry*, **150**, 399–410.

Wing, J. K., Birley, J. L. T., Cooper, J. E., Graham, P., and Isaacs, A. D. (1967). Reliability of a procedure for measuring and classifying "present psychiatric state." *Brit. J. Psychiatry*, **113**, 499–515.

Yerushalmy, J. (1947). Statistical problems in assessing methods of medical diagnosis, with special reference to X-ray techniques. *Public Health Rep.*, **62**, 1432–1449.

Zelen, M. and Haitovsky, Y. (1991). Testing hypotheses with binary data subject to misclassification errors: Analysis and experimental designs. *Biometrika*, **78**, 857–865.

Zubin, J. (1967). Classification of the behavior disorders. Pp. 373–406 in P. R. Farnsworth, O. McNemar, and Q. McNemar (Eds.), *Annual Review of Psychology*. Palo Alto, Calif.: Annual Reviews.

CHAPTER 18

The Measurement of Interrater Agreement

The statistical methods described in the preceding chapter for controlling for error are applicable only when the rates of misclassification are known from external sources or are estimable by applying a well-defined standard classification procedure to a subsample of the group under study. For some variables of importance, however, no such standard is readily apparent.

To assess the extent to which a given characterization of a subject is reliable, it is clear that we must have a number of subjects classified more than once, for example by more than one rater. The degree of agreement among the raters provides no more than an upper bound on the degree of accuracy present in the ratings, however. If agreement among the raters is good, then there is a possibility, but by no means a guarantee, that the ratings do in fact reflect the dimension they are purported to reflect. If their agreement is poor, on the other hand, then the usefulness of the ratings is severely limited, for it is meaningless to ask what is associated with the variable being rated when one cannot even trust those ratings to begin with.

In this chapter we consider the measurement of interrater agreement when the ratings are on categorical scales. Section 18.1 is devoted to the case of the same two raters per subject. Section 18.2 considers weighted kappa to incorporate a notion of distance between rating categories. Section 18.3 is devoted to the case of multiple ratings per subject with different sets of raters. Applications to other problems are indicated in Section 18.4. Section 18.5* relates the results of the preceding sections to the theory presented in Chapter 15 on correlated binary variables.

Statistical Methods for Rates and Proportions, Third Edition
By Joseph L. Fleiss, Bruce Levin, and Myunghee Cho Paik
ISBN 0-471-52629-0   Copyright © 2003 John Wiley & Sons, Inc.

Table 18.1. *Diagnoses on n = 100 subjects by two raters*

| | Rater B | | | |
Rater A	Psychotic	Neurotic	Organic	Total
Psychotic	0.75	0.01	0.04	0.80
Neurotic	0.05	0.04	0.01	0.10
Organic	0	0	0.10	0.10
Total	0.80	0.05	0.15	1.00

18.1. THE SAME PAIR OF RATERS PER SUBJECT

Suppose that each of a sample of n subjects is rated independently by the same two raters, with the ratings being on a categorical scale consisting of k categories. Consider the hypothetical example of Table 18.1, in which each cell entry is the proportion of all subjects classified into one of $k = 3$ diagnostic categories by rater A and into another by rater B. Thus, for example, 5% of all subjects were diagnosed neurotic by rater A and psychotic by rater B.

Suppose it is desired to measure the degree of agreement on each category separately as well as across all categories. The analysis begins by collapsing the original $k \times k$ table into a 2×2 table in which all categories other than the one of current interest are combined into a single "all others" category. Table 18.2 presents the results in general, as well as for neurosis from Table 18.1 in particular. It must be borne in mind that the entries a, b, c, and d in the general table refer to *proportions* of subjects, not to their numbers.

The simplest and most frequently used index of agreement is the overall proportion of agreement, say

$$p_o = a + d. \tag{18.1}$$

Table 18.2. *Data for measuring agreement on a single category*

| | General | | | | For Neurosis | | | |
| | Rater B | | | | | Rater B | | |
Rater A	Given Category	All Others	Total	Rater A	Neurosis	All Others	Total
Given category	a	b	p_1	Neurosis	0.04	0.06	0.10
All others	c	d	q_1	All others	0.01	0.89	0.90
Total	p_2	q_2	1	Total	0.05	0.95	1.00

Table 18.3. *Values of several indices of agreement from data of Table 18.1*

Category	p_o	p_s	λ_r	p_s'	A	κ
Psychotic	0.90	0.94	0.88	0.75	0.84	0.69
Neurotic	0.93	0.53	0.06	0.96	0.75	0.50
Organic	0.95	0.80	0.60	0.97	0.89	0.77

p_o, or a simple variant of it such as $2p_o - 1$, has been proposed as the agreement index of choice by Holley and Guilford (1964) and by Maxwell (1977). For neurosis, the overall proportion of agreement is

$$p_o = 0.04 + 0.89 = 0.93.$$

This value, along with the overall proportions of agreement for the other two categories, is given in the column labeled p_o in Table 18.3. The conclusion that might be drawn from these values is that agreement is, effectively, equally good on all three categories, with agreement on organic disorders being somewhat better than on neurosis, and agreement on neurosis being somewhat better than on psychosis.

Suppose the category under study is rare, so that the proportion d, representing agreement on absence, is likely to be large and thus to inflate the value of p_o. A number of indices of agreement have been proposed that are based only on the proportions a, b, and c. Of all of them, only the so-called proportion of specific agreement, say

$$p_s = \frac{2a}{2a + b + c} = \frac{a}{\bar{p}}, \tag{18.2}$$

where $\bar{p} = (p_1 + p_2)/2$, has a sensible probabilistic interpretation. Let one of the two raters be selected at random, and let attention be focused on the subjects assigned to the category of interest. The quantity p_s is the conditional probability that the second rater will also make an assignment to that category, given that the randomly selected first rater did. This index was first proposed by Dice (1945) as a measure of similarity.

The proportion of specific agreement on neurosis is

$$p_s = \frac{2 \times 0.04}{2 \times 0.04 + 0.06 + 0.01} = 0.53,$$

and the values for all three categories are presented in the column headed p_s in Table 18.3. The conclusions based on p_s are rather different from those based on p_o. Agreement now seems best on psychosis, rather less good on organic disorders, and much poorer than either on neurosis.

Define $\bar{q} = 1 - \bar{p}$, or

$$\bar{q} = \frac{1}{2}(q_1 + q_2) = d + \frac{b+c}{2}, \tag{18.3}$$

and suppose that $\bar{q} > \bar{p}$. Goodman and Kruskal (1954) proposed

$$\lambda_r = \frac{(a+d) - \bar{q}}{1 - \bar{q}} = \frac{2a - (b+c)}{2a + (b+c)} \tag{18.4}$$

as an index of agreement; it is motivated less by notions of agreement than by a consideration of the frequencies of correct predictions of a subject's category when predictions are made with and without knowledge of the joint ratings. λ_r assumes its maximum value of $+1$ when there is complete agreement, but assumes its minimum value of -1 whenever $a = 0$, irrespective of the value of d [not, as Goodman and Kruskal (1954, p. 758) imply, only when $a + d = 0$].

For neurosis,

$$\lambda_r = \frac{2 \times 0.04 - (0.06 + 0.01)}{2 \times 0.04 + (0.06 + 0.01)} = 0.06,$$

and the values of λ_r for all three categories are listed under the indicated column of Table 18.3. Because of the identity

$$\lambda_r = 2p_s - 1, \tag{18.5}$$

the categories are ordered on λ_r exactly as on p_s.

The proportion of specific agreement ignores the proportion d. If, instead, we choose to ignore a, we would calculate the corresponding index, say

$$p'_s = \frac{d}{\bar{q}} = \frac{2d}{2d + b + c}, \tag{18.6}$$

where $\bar{q} = 1 - \bar{p}$. For neurosis

$$p'_s = \frac{2 \times 0.89}{2 \times 0.89 + 0.06 + 0.01} = 0.96,$$

and this value and the other two are presented in the indicated column of Table 18.3. Yet a different picture emerges from these values than from earlier ones. Agreement (with respect to absence) on organic disorders and on neurosis seems to be equally good and apparently substantially better than on psychosis.

Rather than having to choose between p_s and p'_s, Rogot and Goldberg (1966) proposed simply taking their mean, say

$$A = \frac{1}{2}(p_s + p'_s) = \frac{a}{p_1 + p_2} + \frac{d}{q_1 + q_2}, \qquad (18.7)$$

as an index of agreement. For neurosis,

$$A = \frac{0.04}{0.10 + 0.05} + \frac{0.89}{0.90 + 0.95} = 0.75.$$

As seen in the indicated column of Table 18.3, the index A orders the three categories in yet a new way: agreement on organic disorders is better than on psychosis, and agreement on organic disorders and on psychosis is better than on neurosis.

Yet other indices of agreement between two raters have been proposed (e.g., Fleiss, 1965; Armitage, Blendis, and Smyllie, 1966; Rogot and Goldberg, 1966; and Bennett, 1972), but it should already be clear that there must be more to the measurement of interrater agreement than the arbitrary selection of an index of agreement.

The new dimension is provided by a realization that, except in the most extreme circumstances (either $p_1 = q_2 = 0$ or $p_2 = q_1 = 0$), some degree of agreement is to be expected by chance alone (see Table 18.4). For example, if rater A employs one set of criteria for distinguishing between the presence and the absence of a condition, and if rater B employs an entirely different and independent set of criteria, then *all* the observed agreement is explainable by chance.

Different opinions have been stated on the need to incorporate chance-expected agreement into the assessment of interrater reliability. Rogot and Goldberg (1966), for example, emphasize the importance of contrasting observed with expected agreement when comparisons are to be made between different pairs of raters or different kinds of subjects. Goodman and

Table 18.4. *Chance-expected proportions of joint judgments by two raters, for data of Table 18.2*

	General				For Neurosis		
	Rater B				Rater B		
Rater A	Given Category	All Others	Total	Rater A	Neurosis	All Others	Total
Given category	$p_1 p_2$	$p_1 q_2$	p_1	Neurosis	0.005	0.095	0.10
All others	$q_1 p_2$	$q_1 q_2$	q_1	All others	0.045	0.855	0.90
Total	p_2	q_2	1	Total	0.05	0.95	1

Kruskal (1954, p. 758), on the other hand, contend that chance-expected agreement need not cause much concern, that the observed degree of agreement may usually be assumed to be in excess of chance. (Even if one is willing to grant this assumption, one should nevertheless check whether the excess is trivially small or substantially large.)

Armitage, Blendis, and Smyllie (1966, p. 102) occupy a position between that of Rogot and Goldberg and that of Goodman and Kruskal. They appreciate the necessity for introducing chance-expected agreement whenever different sets of data are being compared, but claim that too much uncertainty exists as to how the correction for chance is to be incorporated into the measure of agreement.

There does exist, however, a natural means for correcting for chance. Consider any index that assumes the value 1 when there is complete agreement. Let I_o denote the observed value of the index (calculated from the proportions in Table 18.2), and let I_e denote the value expected on the basis of chance alone (calculated from the proportions in Table 18.4).

The obtained excess beyond chance is $I_o - I_e$, whereas the maximum possible excess is $1 - I_e$. The ratio of these two differences is called *kappa*,

$$\hat{\kappa} = \frac{I_o - I_e}{1 - I_e}. \tag{18.8}$$

Kappa is a measure of agreement with desirable properties. If there is complete agreement, $\hat{\kappa} = +1$. If observed agreement is greater than or equal to chance agreement, $\hat{\kappa} \geq 0$, and if observed agreement is less than or equal to chance agreement, $\hat{\kappa} \leq 0$. The minimum value of $\hat{\kappa}$ depends on the marginal proportions. If they are such that $I_e = 0.5$, then the minimum equals -1. Otherwise, the minimum is between -1 and 0.

It may be checked by simple algebra that, *for each of the indices of agreement defined above*, the same value of $\hat{\kappa}$ results after the chance-expected value is incorporated as in (18.8) (see Problem 18.1):

$$\hat{\kappa} = \frac{2(ad - bc)}{p_1 q_2 + p_2 q_1}. \tag{18.9}$$

An important unification of various approaches to the indexing of agreement is therefore achieved by introducing a correction for chance-expected agreement.

For neurosis,

$$\hat{\kappa} = \frac{2(0.04 \times 0.89 - 0.06 \times 0.01)}{0.10 \times 0.95 + 0.05 \times 0.90} = 0.50.$$

This value and the other two are presented in the final column of Table 18.3. They are close to those found by Spitzer and Fleiss (1974) in a review of the literature on the reliability of psychiatric diagnosis. Agreement is best on organic disorders, less good on psychosis, and poorest on neurosis.

The kappa statistic was first proposed by Cohen (1960). Variants of kappa have been proposed by Scott (1955) and by Maxwell and Pilliner (1968). All have interpretations as *intraclass correlation coefficients* (see Ebel, 1951). The intraclass correlation coefficient is a widely used measure of interrater reliability for the case of quantitative ratings. As shown by Fleiss (1975) and Krippendorff (1970), only kappa is identical (except for a term involving the factor $1/n$, where n is the number of subjects) to that version of the intraclass correlation coefficient due to Bartko (1966) in which a difference between the raters in their base rates (i.e., a difference between p_1 and p_2) is considered a source of unwanted variability.

Landis and Koch (1977a) have characterized different ranges of values for kappa with respect to the degree of agreement they suggest. For most purposes, values greater than 0.75 or so may be taken to represent excellent agreement beyond chance, values below 0.40 or so may be taken to represent poor agreement beyond chance, and values between 0.40 and 0.75 may be taken to represent fair to good agreement beyond chance.

Often, a composite measure of agreement across all categories is desired. An overall value of kappa may be defined as a weighted average of the individual kappa values, where the weights are the denominators of the individual kappas [i.e., the quantities $p_1 q_2 + p_2 q_1$ in (18.9)]. An equivalent and more suggestive formula is based on arraying the data as in Table 18.5.

The overall proportion of observed agreement is, say,

$$p_o = \sum_{i=1}^{k} p_{ii}, \qquad (18.10)$$

and the overall proportion of chance-expected agreement is, say,

$$p_e = \sum_{i=1}^{k} p_{i.} p_{.i}. \qquad (18.11)$$

Table 18.5. *Joint proportions of ratings by two raters on a scale with k categories*

Rater A	Rater B				
	1	2	$\cdots$	k	Total
1	p_{11}	p_{12}	$\cdots$	p_{1k}	$p_{1.}$
2	p_{21}	p_{22}	$\cdots$	p_{2k}	$p_{2.}$
$\vdots$	$\vdots$	$\vdots$		$\vdots$	$\vdots$
k	p_{k1}	p_{k2}	$\cdots$	p_{kk}	$p_{k.}$
Total	$p_{.1}$	$p_{.2}$	$\cdots$	$p_{.k}$	1

The overall value of kappa is then, say,

$$\hat{\kappa} = \frac{p_o - p_e}{1 - p_e}. \tag{18.12}$$

For the data of Table 18.1,

$$p_o = 0.75 + 0.04 + 0.10 = 0.89$$

and

$$p_e = 0.80 \times 0.80 + 0.10 \times 0.05 + 0.10 \times 0.15 = 0.66,$$

so that

$$\hat{\kappa} = \frac{0.89 - 0.66}{1 - 0.66} = 0.68.$$

For testing the hypothesis that the ratings are independent (so that the underlying value of kappa is zero), Fleiss, Cohen, and Everitt (1969) showed that the appropriate standard error of kappa is estimated by

$$\widehat{se}_0(\hat{\kappa}) = \frac{1}{(1 - p_e)\sqrt{n}} \sqrt{p_e + p_e^2 - \sum_{i=1}^{k} p_{i.} p_{.i} (p_{i.} + p_{.i})}, \tag{18.13}$$

where p_e is defined in (18.11). The hypothesis may be tested against the alternative that agreement is better than chance would predict by referring the quantity

$$z = \frac{\hat{k}}{\widehat{se}_0(\hat{\kappa})} \tag{18.14}$$

to tables of the standard normal distribution and rejecting the hypothesis if z is sufficiently large (a one-sided test is more appropriate here than a two-sided test).

For the data at hand,

$$\widehat{se}_0(\hat{\kappa}) = \frac{1}{(1 - 0.66)\sqrt{100}} \sqrt{0.66 + 0.66^2 - 1.0285} = 0.076$$

and

$$z = \frac{0.68}{0.076} = 8.95.$$

The overall value of kappa is therefore statistically highly significant, and, by virtue of its magnitude, it indicates a good degree of agreement beyond chance.

Table 18.6. *Kappas for individual categories and across all categories of Table 18.1*

Category	p_o	p_e	$\hat{\kappa}$	$\widehat{se}_0(\hat{\kappa})$	z
Psychotic	0.90	0.68	0.69	0.100	6.90
Neurotic	0.93	0.86	0.50	0.093	5.38
Organic	0.95	0.78	0.77	0.097	7.94
Overall	0.89	0.66	0.68	0.076	8.95

Formulas (18.10)–(18.14) apply even when k, the number of categories, is equal to two. They may therefore be applied to the study of each category's reliability, as shown in Table 18.6 for the data of Table 18.1.

Note that the overall value of kappa is equal to the sum of the individual differences $p_o - p_e$ (i.e., of the numerators of the individual kappas) divided by the sum of the individual differences $1 - p_e$ (i.e., of the denominators of the individual kappas),

$$\hat{\bar{\kappa}} = \frac{(0.90 - 0.68) + (0.93 - 0.86) + (0.95 - 0.78)}{(1 - 0.68) + (1 - 0.86) + (1 - 0.78)} = \frac{0.46}{0.68} = 0.68,$$

confirming that $\hat{\bar{\kappa}}$ is a weighted average of the individual $\hat{\kappa}$'s.

For testing the hypothesis that the underlying value of kappa (either overall or for a single category) is equal to a prespecified value κ *other than zero*, Fleiss, Cohen, and Everitt (1969) showed that the appropriate standard error of $\hat{\kappa}$ is estimated by

$$\widehat{se}(\hat{\kappa}) = \frac{\sqrt{A + B - C}}{(1 - p_e)\sqrt{n}}, \tag{18.15}$$

where

$$A = \sum_{i=1}^{k} p_{ii}\left[1 - (p_{i.} + p_{.i})(1 - \hat{\kappa})\right]^2, \tag{18.16}$$

$$B = (1 - \hat{\kappa})^2 \sum\sum_{i \neq j} p_{ij}(p_{.i} + p_{j.})^2, \tag{18.17}$$

$$C = \left[\hat{\kappa} - p_e(1 - \hat{\kappa})\right]^2. \tag{18.18}$$

The hypothesis that κ is the underlying value would be rejected if the critical ratio

$$z = \frac{|\hat{\kappa} - \kappa|}{\widehat{se}(\hat{\kappa})} \tag{18.19}$$

were found to be significantly large from tables of the normal distribution.

An approximate $100(1-\alpha)\%$ confidence interval for κ is

$$\hat{\kappa} - z_{\alpha/2}\,\widehat{se}(\hat{\kappa}) \le \kappa \le \hat{\kappa} + z_{\alpha/2}\,\widehat{se}(\hat{\kappa}). \tag{18.20}$$

Consider testing the hypothesis that the overall value of kappa underlying the data in Table 18.1 is 0.80. The three quantities (18.16)–(18.18) needed to determine the standard error of $\hat{\bar{\kappa}}$ are

$$A = 0.75\big[1 - (0.80 + 0.80)(1 - 0.68)\big]^2$$

$$+ 0.04\big[1 - (0.10 + 0.05)(1 - 0.68)\big]^2$$

$$+ 0.10\big[1 - (0.10 + 0.15)(1 - 0.68)\big]^2$$

$$= 0.2995,$$

$$B = (1 - 0.68)^2\big[0.01(0.80 + 0.10)^2 + 0.04(0.80 + 0.10)^2$$

$$+ 0.05(0.05 + 0.80)^2 + 0.01(0.05 + 0.10)^2$$

$$+ 0(0.15 + 0.80)^2 + 0(0.15 + 0.10)^2\big]$$

$$= 0.0079,$$

$$C = \big[0.68 - 0.66(1 - 0.68)\big]^2 = 0.2198.$$

Thus

$$\widehat{se}(\hat{\bar{\kappa}}) = \frac{\sqrt{0.2995 + 0.0079 - 0.2198}}{(1 - 0.66)\sqrt{100}} = 0.087$$

and

$$z = \frac{|0.68 - 0.80|}{0.087} = 1.38,$$

so the hypothesis that $\bar{\kappa} = 0.80$ is not rejected.

Suppose one wishes to compare and combine g (≥ 2) independent estimates of kappa. The theory of Section 10.1 applies. Define, for the mth estimate, $V_m(\hat{\kappa}_m)$ to be the squared standard error of $\hat{\kappa}_m$, that is, the square of the expression in (18.15). The combined estimate of the supposed common value of kappa is, say,

$$\hat{\kappa}_{\text{overall}} = \frac{\displaystyle\sum_{m=1}^{g} \frac{\hat{\kappa}_m}{V_m(\hat{\kappa}_m)}}{\displaystyle\sum_{m=1}^{g} \frac{1}{V_m(\hat{\kappa}_m)}}. \tag{18.21}$$

To test the hypothesis that the g underlying values of kappa are equal, the value of

$$\chi^2_{\text{equal } \kappa \text{'s}} = \sum_{m=1}^{g} \frac{\left(\hat{\kappa}_m - \hat{\kappa}_{\text{overall}}\right)^2}{V_m(\hat{\kappa}_m)} \tag{18.22}$$

may be referred to tables of chi squared with $g - 1$ df. The hypothesis is rejected if the value is significantly large. The limits of an approximate $100(1 - \alpha)\%$ confidence interval for the supposed common underlying value are given by

$$\hat{\kappa}_{\text{overall}} \pm z_{\alpha/2} \sqrt{\frac{1}{\displaystyle\sum_{m=1}^{g} \frac{1}{V_m(\hat{\kappa}_m)}}} . \tag{18.23}$$

18.2. WEIGHTED KAPPA

Cohen (1968) (see also Spitzer et al. 1967) generalized his kappa measure of interrater agreement to the case where the relative seriousness of each possible disagreement could be quantified. Suppose that, independently of the data actually collected, agreement weights, say w_{ij} ($i = 1, \ldots, k$; $j = 1, \ldots, k$), are assigned on rational or clinical grounds to the k^2 cells (see Cicchetti, 1976). The weights are restricted to lie in the interval $0 \le w_{ij} \le 1$ and to be such that

$$w_{ii} = 1 \tag{18.24}$$

(i.e., exact agreement is given maximal weight),

$$0 \le w_{ij} < 1 \qquad \text{for} \quad i \ne j \tag{18.25}$$

(i.e., all disagreements are given less than maximal weight), and

$$w_{ij} = w_{ji} \tag{18.26}$$

(i.e., the two raters are considered symmetrically).

The observed weighted proportion of agreement is, say,

$$P_{o(w)} = \sum_{i=1}^{k} \sum_{j=1}^{k} w_{ij} p_{ij}, \tag{18.27}$$

where the proportions p_{ij} are arrayed as in Table 18.5, and the chance-expected weighted proportion of agreement is, say,

$$P_{e(w)} = \sum_{i=1}^{k} \sum_{j=1}^{k} w_{ij} p_{i.} p_{.j}. \tag{18.28}$$

Weighted kappa is then given by

$$\hat{\kappa}_w = \frac{p_{o(w)} - p_{e(w)}}{1 - p_{e(w)}}. \qquad (18.29)$$

Note that, when $w_{ij} = 0$ for all $i \neq j$ (i.e., when all disagreements are considered as being equally serious), then weighted kappa becomes identical to the overall kappa given in (18.12).

The interpretation of the magnitude of weighted kappa is like that of unweighted kappa: $\hat{\kappa}_w \geq 0.75$ or so signifies excellent agreement, for most purposes, and $\hat{\kappa}_w \leq 0.40$ or so signifies poor agreement.

Suppose that the k categories are ordered and that the decision is made to apply a two-way analysis of variance to the data resulting from taking the numerals $1, 2, \ldots, k$ as bona fide measurements. Bartko (1966) gives a formula for the intraclass correlation coefficient derived from this analysis of variance, and Fleiss and Cohen (1973) have shown that, aside from a term involving the factor $1/n$, the intraclass correlation coefficient is identical to weighted kappa provided the weights are taken as

$$w_{ij} = 1 - \frac{(i-j)^2}{(k-1)^2}. \qquad (18.30)$$

Independently of Cohen (1968), Cicchetti and Allison (1971) proposed a statistic for measuring interrater reliability that is formally identical to weighted kappa. They suggested that the weights be taken as

$$w_{ij} = 1 - \frac{|i-j|}{k-1}. \qquad (18.31)$$

The sampling distribution of weighted kappa was derived by Fleiss, Cohen, and Everitt (1969) and confirmed by Cicchetti and Fleiss (1977), Landis and Koch (1977a), Fleiss and Cicchetti (1978), and Hubert (1978). For testing the hypothesis that the underlying value of weighted kappa is zero, the appropriate estimated standard error of $\hat{\kappa}_w$ is

$$\widehat{\mathrm{se}}_0(\hat{\kappa}_w) = \frac{1}{(1 - p_{e(w)})\sqrt{n}} \sqrt{\sum_{i=1}^{k} \sum_{j=1}^{k} p_{i.}p_{.j}\left[w_{ij} - \left(\bar{w}_{i.} + \bar{w}_{.j}\right)\right]^2 - p_{e(w)}^2}, \quad (18.32)$$

where

$$\bar{w}_{i.} = \sum_{j=1}^{k} p_{.j}w_{ij} \qquad (18.33)$$

and

$$\bar{w}_{.j} = \sum_{i=1}^{k} p_{i.}w_{ij}, \qquad (18.34)$$

The hypothesis may be tested by referring the value of the critical ratio

$$z = \frac{\hat{\kappa}_w}{\widehat{se}_0(\hat{\kappa}_w)} \tag{18.35}$$

to tables of the standard normal distribution.

For testing the hypothesis that the underlying value of weighted kappa is equal to a prespecified κ_w *other than zero*, the appropriate formula for the estimated standard error of $\hat{\kappa}_w$ is

$$\widehat{se}(\hat{\kappa}_w) = \frac{1}{(1 - p_{e(w)})\sqrt{n}}$$

$$\times \sqrt{\sum_{i=1}^{k} \sum_{j=1}^{k} p_{ij} \left[w_{ij} - (\bar{w}_{i.} + \bar{w}_{.j})(1 - \hat{\kappa}_w) \right]^2 - \left[\hat{\kappa}_w - p_{e(w)}(1 - \hat{\kappa}_w) \right]^2}.$$

$$\tag{18.36}$$

The hypothesis may be tested by referring the value of the critical ratio

$$z = \frac{|\hat{\kappa}_w - \kappa_w|}{\widehat{se}(\hat{\kappa}_w)} \tag{18.37}$$

to tables of the standard normal distribution and rejecting the hypothesis if the critical ratio is too large.

It may be shown (see Problem 18.4) that the standard errors of un-weighted kappa given in (18.13) and (18.15) are special cases of the standard errors of weighted kappa given in (18.32) and (18.36) when $w_{ii} = 1$ for all i and $w_{ij} = 0$ for all $i \neq j$.

Some attempts have been made to generalize kappa to the case where each subject is rated by each of the same set of more than two raters (Light, 1971; Landis and Koch, 1977a). Kairam et al. (1993) use the multivariate multiple noncentral hypergeometric distribution to study kappa in the case of $m \geq 2$ fixed raters with a prespecified interview schedule of subjects. Their analysis allows some subjects not to be seen by some raters. We consider in the next section the problem of different raters for different subjects when (i) $k = 2$ with varying m_i, or (ii) $k > 2$ with $m_i = m$ for all i. Kraemer (1980) considered the case in which $k > 2$ with varying m_i.

18.3. MULTIPLE RATINGS PER SUBJECT WITH DIFFERENT RATERS

Suppose that a sample of n subjects has been studied, with m_i being the number of ratings on the ith subject. The raters responsible for rating one subject are not assumed to be same as those responsible for rating another. Suppose, further, that $k = 2$, that is, that the ratings consist of classifications into one of two categories; the case $k > 2$ will be considered later in this section. Finally, let x_i denote the number of (arbitrarily defined) positive ratings on subject i, so that $m_i - x_i$ is the number of negative ratings on him.

Identities between intraclass correlation coefficients and kappa statistics will be exploited to derive a kappa statistic by starting with an analysis of variance applied to the data (forming a one-way layout) obtained by coding a positive rating as 1 and a negative rating as 0. This was precisely the approach taken by Landis and Koch (1977b), except that they took the number of degrees of freedom for the mean square between subjects to be $n - 1$ instead of, as below, n.

Define the overall proportion of positive ratings to be

$$\bar{p} = \frac{\sum_{i=1}^{n} x_i}{n\bar{m}}, \tag{18.38}$$

where

$$\bar{m} = \frac{\sum_{i=1}^{n} m_i}{n}, \tag{18.39}$$

the mean number of ratings per subject. If the number of subjects is large (say, $n \geq 20$), the mean square between subjects (BMS) is approximately equal to

$$\text{BMS} = \frac{1}{n} \sum_{i=1}^{n} \frac{(x_i - m_i\bar{p})^2}{m_i} \tag{18.40}$$

and the mean square within subjects (WMS) is equal to

$$\text{WMS} = \frac{1}{n(\bar{m} - 1)} \sum_{i=1}^{n} \frac{x_i(m_i - x_i)}{m_i}. \tag{18.41}$$

Technically, the intraclass correlation coefficient should be estimated as

$$r = \frac{\text{BMS} - \text{WMS}}{\text{BMS} + (m_0 - 1)\text{WMS}}, \tag{18.42}$$

where

$$m_0 = \bar{m} - \frac{\sum_{i=1}^{n}(m_i - \bar{m})^2}{n(n-1)\bar{m}}. \tag{18.43}$$

If n is at all large, though, m_0 and $\bar{m}$ will be very close in magnitude. If m_0 is replaced by $\bar{m}$ in (18.42), the resulting expression for the intraclass correlation coefficient, and therefore for kappa, is

$$\hat{\kappa} = \frac{\text{BMS} - \text{WMS}}{\text{BMS} + (\overline{m} - 1)\text{WMS}}$$

$$= 1 - \frac{\displaystyle\sum_{i=1}^{n} \frac{x_i(m_i - x_i)}{m_i}}{n(\overline{m} - 1)\overline{p}\overline{q}}, \tag{18.44}$$

where $\overline{q} = 1 - \overline{p}$.

$\hat{\kappa}$ has the following properties. If there is no subject-to-subject variation in the proportion of positive ratings (i.e., if $x_i/m_i = \overline{p}$ for all i, with $\overline{p}$ not equal to either 0 or 1), then there is more disagreement within subjects than between subjects. In this case $\hat{\kappa}$ may be seen to assume its minimum value of $-1/(\overline{m} - 1)$.

If the several proportions x_i/m_i vary exactly as binomial proportions with parameters m_i and a common probability $\overline{p}$, then there is as much similarity within subjects as between subjects. In this case, the value of $\hat{\kappa}$ is equal to 0.

If each proportion x_i/m_i assumes either the values 0 or 1, then there is perfect agreement within subjects. In this case, $\hat{\kappa}$ may be seen to assume the value 1.

Consider the hypothetical data of Table 18.7 on $n = 25$ subjects. For these data, the mean number of ratings per subject is

$$\overline{m} = \frac{81}{25} = 3.24,$$

Table 18.7. *Hypothetical ratings by different sets of raters on $n = 25$ subjects*

Subject i	Number of Raters, m_i	Number of Positive Ratings, x_i	i	m_i	x_i
1	2	2	14	4	3
2	2	0	15	2	0
3	3	2	16	2	2
4	4	3	17	3	1
5	3	3	18	2	1
6	4	1	19	4	1
7	3	0	20	5	4
8	5	0	21	3	2
9	2	0	22	4	0
10	4	4	23	3	0
11	5	5	24	3	3
12	3	3	25	2	2
13	4	4	Total	81	46

the overall proportion of positive ratings is

$$\bar{p} = \frac{46}{25 \times 3.24} = 0.568,$$

and the value of $\Sigma x_i(m_i - x_i)/m_i$ is

$$\sum_{i=1}^{25} \frac{x_i(m_i - x_i)}{m_i} = 6.30.$$

The value of kappa in (18.44) for these ratings is therefore

$$\hat{\kappa} = 1 - \frac{6.30}{25(3.24 - 1) \times 0.568 \times 0.432}$$

$$= 0.54,$$

indicating only a modest degree of interrater agreement.

Fleiss and Cuzick (1979) derived the standard error of $\hat{\kappa}$ appropriate for testing the hypothesis that the underlying value of kappa is 0. Define $\bar{m}_H$ to be the *harmonic mean* of the number of ratings per subject, that is,

$$\bar{m}_H = \frac{n}{\sum_{i=1}^{n} 1/m_i}. \tag{18.45}$$

The standard error of $\hat{\kappa}$ is estimated by

$$\widehat{se}_0(\hat{\kappa}) = \frac{1}{(\bar{m} - 1)\sqrt{n\bar{m}_H}} \sqrt{2(\bar{m}_H - 1) + \frac{(\bar{m} - \bar{m}_H)(1 - 4\bar{p}\bar{q})}{\bar{m}\bar{p}\bar{q}}}, \tag{18.46}$$

and the hypothesis may be tested by referring the value of the critical ratio

$$z = \frac{\hat{\kappa}}{\widehat{se}_0(\hat{\kappa})} \tag{18.47}$$

to tables of the standard normal distribution.

For the data of Table 18.7,

$$\bar{m}_H = \frac{25}{8.5167} = 2.935$$

and

$$\widehat{se}_0(\hat{\kappa}) = \frac{1}{(3.24 - 1)\sqrt{25 \times 2.935}}$$

$$\times \sqrt{2(2.935 - 1) + \frac{(3.24 - 2.935)(1 - 4 \times 0.568 \times 0.432)}{3.24 \times 0.568 \times 0.432}}$$

$$= 0.103.$$

The value of the critical ratio in (18.47) is then

$$z = \frac{0.54}{0.103} = 5.24,$$

indicating that $\hat{\kappa}$ is significantly greater than zero.

Suppose, now, that the number of categories into which ratings are made is $k \geq 2$. Denote by $\bar{p}_j$ the overall proportion of ratings in category j and by $\hat{\kappa}_j$ the value of kappa for category, $j, j = 1, \ldots, k$. Landis and Koch (1977b) proposed taking the weighted average

$$\hat{\bar{\kappa}} = \frac{\sum_{j=1}^{k} \bar{p}_j \bar{q}_j \hat{\kappa}_j}{\sum_{j=1}^{k} \bar{p}_j \bar{q}_j} \tag{18.48}$$

as an overall measure of interrater agreement, where $\bar{q}_j = 1 - \bar{p}_j$. The standard error of $\hat{\bar{\kappa}}$ has yet to be derived, when the numbers of ratings per subject vary, to test the hypothesis that the underlying value is zero.

When, however, the number of ratings per subject is constant and equal to m, simple expressions for $\hat{\kappa}_j$, $\hat{\bar{\kappa}}$, and their standard errors are available. Define x_{ij} to be the number of ratings on subject i $(i = 1, \ldots, n)$ into category j $(j = 1, \ldots, k)$; note that

$$\sum_{j=1}^{k} x_{ij} = m \tag{18.49}$$

for all i. The value of $\hat{\kappa}_j$ is then

$$\hat{\kappa}_j = 1 - \frac{\sum_{i=1}^{n} x_{ij}(m - x_{ij})}{nm(m - 1)\bar{p}_j \bar{q}_j}, \tag{18.50}$$

and the value of $\hat{\bar{\kappa}}$ is

$$\hat{\bar{\kappa}} = 1 - \frac{nm^2 - \sum_{i=1}^{n}\sum_{j=1}^{k} x_{ij}^2}{nm(m - 1)\sum_{j=1}^{k} \bar{p}_j \bar{q}_j}. \tag{18.51}$$

Table 18.8. *Five ratings on each of ten subjects into one of three categories*

Subject	Number of Ratings into Category			$\sum_{j=1}^{3} x_{ij}^2$
	1	2	3	
1	1	4	0	17
2	2	0	3	13
3	0	0	5	25
4	4	0	1	17
5	3	0	2	13
6	1	4	0	17
7	5	0	0	25
8	0	4	1	17
9	1	0	4	17
10	3	0	2	13
Total	20	12	18	174

Algebraically equivalent versions of these formulas were first presented by Fleiss (1971), who showed explicitly how they represent chance-corrected measures of agreement.

Table 18.8 presents hypothetical data representing, for each of $n = 10$ subjects, $m = 5$ ratings into one of $k = 3$ categories.

The three overall proportions are $\bar{p}_1 = 20/50 = 0.40$, $\bar{p}_2 = 12/50 = 0.24$, and $\bar{p}_3 = 18/50 = 0.36$. For category 1, the numerator in expression (18.50) for $\hat{\kappa}_1$ is

$$\sum_{i=1}^{10} x_{i1}(5 - x_{i1}) = 1 \times (5 - 1) + 2 \times (5 - 2) + \cdots + 3 \times (5 - 3) = 34,$$

and thus

$$\hat{\kappa}_1 = 1 - \frac{34}{10 \times 5 \times 4 \times 0.40 \times 0.60} = 0.29.$$

Similarly, $\hat{\kappa}_2 = 0.67$ and $\hat{\kappa}_3 = 0.35$. The overall value of $\hat{\bar{\kappa}}$ is, by (18.51),

$$\hat{\bar{\kappa}} = 1 - \frac{10 \times 25 - 174}{10 \times 5 \times 4 \times (0.40 \times 0.60 + 0.24 \times 0.76 + 0.36 \times 0.64)} = 0.42.$$

Alternatively,

$$\hat{\bar{\kappa}} = \frac{(0.40 \times 0.60) \times 0.29 + (0.24 \times 0.76) \times 0.67 + (0.36 \times 0.64) \times 0.35}{0.40 \times 0.60 + 0.24 \times 0.76 + 0.36 \times 0.64}$$

$$= 0.42.$$

When the numbers of ratings per subject are equal, Fleiss, Nee, and Landis (1979) derived and confirmed the following formulas for the approximate standard errors of $\hat{\bar{\kappa}}$ and $\hat{\kappa}_j$, each appropriate for testing the hypothesis that the underlying value is zero:

$$\widehat{se}_0(\hat{\bar{\kappa}}) = \frac{\sqrt{2}}{\sum_{j=1}^{k} \bar{p}_j \bar{q}_j \sqrt{nm(m-1)}}$$

$$\times \sqrt{\left(\sum_{j=1}^{k} \bar{p}_j \bar{q}_j\right)^2 - \sum_{j=1}^{k} \bar{p}_j \bar{q}_j (\bar{q}_j - \bar{p}_j)}, \qquad (18.52)$$

and

$$se_0(\hat{\kappa}_j) = \sqrt{\frac{2}{nm(m-1)}}. \qquad (18.53)$$

Note that $se_0(\hat{\kappa}_j)$ is independent of $\bar{p}_j$ and $\bar{q}_j$! Further, it is easily checked that formula (18.53) is a special case of (18.46) when the m_i's are all equal, because then $\bar{m} = \bar{m}_H = m$.

For the data of Table 18.8,

$$\sum_{j=1}^{3} \bar{p}_j \bar{q}_j = 0.40 \times 0.60 + 0.24 \times 0.76 + 0.36 \times 0.64 = 0.6528$$

and

$$\sum_{j=1}^{3} \bar{p}_j \bar{q}_j (\bar{q}_j - \bar{p}_j) = 0.40 \times 0.60 \times (0.60 - 0.40) + 0.24 \times 0.76 \times (0.76 - 0.24)$$

$$+ 0.36 \times 0.64 \times (0.64 - 0.36)$$

$$= 0.2074,$$

so that

$$\widehat{se}_0(\hat{\bar{\kappa}}) = \frac{\sqrt{2}}{0.6528\sqrt{10 \times 5 \times 4}} \sqrt{0.6528^2 - 0.2074} = 0.072.$$

Because

$$z = \frac{\hat{\bar{\kappa}}}{\widehat{se}_0(\hat{\bar{\kappa}})} = \frac{0.42}{0.072} = 5.83,$$

the overall value of kappa is significantly different from zero (although its magnitude indicates only mediocre reliability).

The approximate standard error of each $\hat{\kappa}_j$ is, by (18.53),

$$\text{se}_0(\hat{\kappa}_j) = \sqrt{\frac{2}{10 \times 5 \times 4}} = 0.10.$$

Each individual kappa is significantly different ($p < 0.01$) from zero, but only $\hat{\kappa}_2$ approaches a value suggestive of fair reliability.

Various approaches have been taken to obtain the standard error of κ. Fleiss and Davies (1982) and Bloch and Kraemer (1989) obtain an asymptotic variance, and a jackknife technique is proposed by Fleiss and Davies (1982), Schouten (1986), and Flack (1987). Flack (1987) proposes a skewness-corrected confidence interval using a jackknife estimate of the third moment of the distribution of delete-one κ statistics. Donner and Eliasziw (1992) obtain a standard error with a method based on a goodness-of-fit test statistic frequently used for clustered binary data. Lee and Tu (1994) propose yet another confidence interval for κ in the case of two raters with binary ratings, by reparameterizing κ as a monotone function of p_{11}. Garner (1991) obtains the standard error conditioning on the margins. Hale and Fleiss (1993) give two variance estimates of κ depending on whether the rater effect is treated as fixed or random. Lipsitz, Laird, and Brennan (1994) provide an asymptotic variance of κ statistics based on the theory of estimating equations.

18.4. FURTHER APPLICATIONS

Even though the various kappa statistics were originally developed and were illustrated here for the measurement of interrater agreement, their applicability extends far beyond this specific problem. In fact, they are useful for measuring, on categorical data, such constructs as "similarity," "concordance," and "clustering." Some examples will be given.

1. In a study of the correlates or determinants of drug use among teenagers, it may be of interest to determine how concordant the attitudes toward drug use are between each subject's same-sex parent and the subject's best friend. Either unweighted kappa or weighted kappa (Section 18.1) may be used, with rater A replaced by parent and rater B by best friend.

2. Suppose that m monitoring stations are set up in a city to measure levels of various pollutants and that, on each of n days, each station is characterized by whether or not the level of a specified pollutant (e.g., sulfur dioxide) exceeds an officially designated threshold. The version of kappa presented in Section 18.3 may be applied to describe how well (or poorly) the several stations agree.

3. Consider a study of the role of familial factors in the development of a condition such as adolescent hypertension. Suppose that n sibships are

studied and that m_i is the number of siblings in the ith sibship. The version of kappa presented in Section 18.3 may be applied to describe the degree to which there is familial aggregation in the condition.

4. Many of the indices of agreement cited in Section 18.1 are used in numerical taxonomy (Sneath and Sokal, 1973) to describe the degree of similarity between different study units; in fact, p_s (18.2) was originally proposed for this purpose by Dice (1945). Suppose that two units (people, languages, or whatever) are being compared with respect to whether they possess or do not possess each of n dichotomous characteristics. The proportions $a-d$ in the left-hand part of Table 18.2 then refer to the proportion of all n characteristics that both units possess, the proportion that one possesses but the other does not, and so on. Corrections for chance-expected similarity in this kind of problem are as important as corrections for chance-expected agreement in the case of interrater reliability. Bloch and Kraemer (1989) discuss kappa as a measure of agreement and association.

5. Studies in which several controls are matched with each case or each experimental unit were discussed in Section 13.3. If the several controls in each matched set were successfully matched, the responses by the controls from the same set should be more similar than the responses by controls from different sets. The version of kappa presented in Section 18.2 may be used to describe how successful the matching was.

6. Although κ is widely used in psychology and educational research, its application extends to periodontal research (Boushka et al., 1990), econometrics (Hirschberg and Slottje, 1989), veterinary epidemiology (Shourkri, Martin, and Mian, 1995), anesthesiology (Posner et al., 1990), neurology (Kairam et al., 1993), and radiology (Musch et al., 1984).

Whether used to measure agreement, or, more generally, similarity, kappa in effect treats all the raters or units symmetrically. When one or more of the sources of ratings may be viewed as a standard, however (two of $m = 5$ raters, e.g., may be senior to the others, or one of the air pollution monitoring stations in example 2 may employ more precise measuring instruments than the others), kappa may no longer be appropriate, and the procedures described by Light (1971), Williams (1976), and Wackerley, McClave, and Rao (1978) should be employed instead.

18.5.* INTERRATER AGREEMENT AS ASSOCIATION IN A MULTIVARIATE BINARY VECTOR

Many problems of interrater agreement can be solved in the framework of clustered categorical data (see Chapter 15). For a binary rating, the notion of interrater agreement is closely related to the correlation among the binary ratings clustered within a subject. Specifically, suppose there are m_i raters, each of whom gives a two-category rating to subject i for $i = 1, \ldots, n$. Let the binary indicator Y_{ij} be 1 if rater j judges subject i positive, and 0 if negative, for $j = 1, \ldots, m_i$. Then $Y_i = (Y_{i1}, \ldots, Y_{im_i})'$ constitutes a vector of binary outcomes, and the dependence among its components can be characterized by the intraclass correlation coefficient (ICC) or kappa, among many other measures. When m_i is the same for all i, the ICC and κ are identical.

One way to specify the distribution of the Y_{ij}'s is to consider all possible 2^{m_i} mutually exclusive response profiles and assume a 2^{m_i}-variate multinomial distribution. Some authors specify the multivariate distribution of Y_i this way, while some focus on the distribution of the total number of positive ratings for subject i, Y_{i+}, and assume it has a beta-binomial distribution; in either case they express kappa in terms of the parameters of the chosen distribution and obtain the maximum likelihood estimate (mle). See Verducci, Mack, and DeGroot (1988), Shoukri, Martin, and Mian (1995), Shoukri and Mian (1995), and Barlow (1996). Other authors construct a multivariate distribution using a latent class model; see Aickin (1990), Agresti and Lang (1993), and Uebersax (1993).

In a different approach, the pairwise association between Y_{ij} and Y_{ik} can be expressed as a function of kappa without making a full distributional assumption. Landis and Koch (1977b) structure the correlation using a random effects model. They assume

$$Y_{ij} = P + s_i + e_{ij},$$

where P is the probability of a positive rating, the s_i's are independent and identically distributed with mean 0 and variance σ_s^2, the e_{ij}'s are similarly distributed with mean 0 and variance σ_e^2, and the s_i's and e_{ij}'s are mutually independent. Then Y_{ij} and Y_{ik} are conditionally independent given the random effect s_i which is unique to subject i, but are marginally correlated, because they share the random effect s_i. See Section 15.5.2 at expression (15.42). The intraclass correlation coefficient is

$$\rho = \frac{\sigma_s^2}{\sigma_s^2 + \sigma_e^2}.$$

The authors use a moment estimator to estimate ρ and derive its standard error.

Lipsitz, Laird, and Brennan (1994) propose a class of estimators for kappa using an estimating-equation approach (see Section 15.5.1). Assuming that each subject has the same probability of a positive rating, say $P = P(Y_{ij} = 1)$, and the same joint probability of being rated positive by a pair of raters for all pairs of raters, $P_{11} = E(Y_{ij}Y_{ik}) = P(Y_{ij} = 1, Y_{ik} = 1)$, kappa can be written as a function of the probability of agreement under two assumptions: nonindependence among the elements of Y_i, and independence. The probability of agreement without assuming independence, P_a, is

$$P_a = P(Y_{ij} = 1, Y_{ik} = 1) + P(Y_{ij} = 0, Y_{ik} = 0)$$
$$= P_{11} + \{(1 - P) - (P - P_{11})\} = P_{11} + 1 - 2P + P_{11}. \quad (18.54)$$

The chance-expected probability of agreement, P_e, is the probability of agreement under marginal independence among the elements in Y_i:

$$P_e = P^2 + (1 - P)^2. \tag{18.55}$$

With

$$\kappa = \frac{P_a - P_e}{1 - P_e} = 1 - \frac{1 - P_a}{1 - P_e},$$

after substitution of (18.54) and (18.55) we have

$$\kappa = 1 - \frac{P - P_{11}}{P(1 - P)}. \tag{18.56}$$

We can rewrite P_{11} in terms of P and κ thus:

$$P_{11} = P^2 + \kappa P(1 - P).$$

Lipsitz, Laird, and Brennan (1994) construct a class of estimating equations each of whose solutions becomes an estimate of kappa. Based on the identities $E(Y_{i+}) = m_i P$ and $E\{Y_{i+}(Y_{i+} - 1)\} = P_{11} m_i (m_i - 1)$, the authors construct a joint estimating equation,

$$\begin{pmatrix} U_1(P) \\ U_2(\kappa, P) \end{pmatrix} = 0$$

with

$$U_1(P) = \sum_{i=1}^{n} \frac{Y_{i+} - m_i P}{v_i},$$

and

$$U_2(\kappa, P) = \sum_{i=1}^{n} \frac{Y_{i+}(Y_{i+} - 1) - P_{11} m_i (m_i - 1)}{w_i},$$

where v_i and w_i are weights to be chosen. The estimating equation is unbiased, that is, $E\{U_1(P)\} = E\{U_2(\kappa, P)\} = 0$ for all κ and P, and, as explained in Section 15.5.1, the solution is consistent and asymptotically normal. Applying further results from the standard theory of estimating equations, the variance of $\hat{\kappa}$ has a sandwich-type estimator which can be obtained easily. A convenience of this approach is that on choosing the weights v_i and w_i appropriately, the solution of the estimating equation coincides with existing kappa statistics, including the kappa statistic of Fleiss

(1971) and the weighted kappa statistic of Schouten (1986). For example, Fleiss' kappa can be obtained by solving

$$U_1(\hat{P}) = \sum_{i=1}^{n} U_{i1} = \sum_{i=1}^{n} \left(Y_{i+} - m_i\hat{P}\right) = 0 \qquad (18.57)$$

and

$$-U_2(\hat{\kappa}, \hat{P}) = \sum_{i=1}^{n} U_{2i} = \sum_{i=1}^{n} \left\{ \frac{Y_{i+}(m_i - Y_{i+})}{m_i - 1} - (1 - \hat{\kappa})\hat{P}(1 - \hat{P})m_i \right\}$$

$$= 0. \qquad (18.58)$$

The sandwich-type variance of Lipsitz, Laird, and Brennan (1994) is asymptotically equivalent to the jackknife variance estimate proposed by Schouten (1986). The sandwich variance of Fleiss' kappa statistic has the form $\text{Var}(\hat{\kappa}) = \Sigma_i V_i^2$, where

$$V_i = \frac{U_{2i} - \dfrac{(1 - \kappa)(1 - 2P)}{\overline{m}} U_{1i}}{nP(1 - P)}.$$

The authors also show that the asymptotic relative efficiency against the mle assuming a beta-binomial distribution (Verducci, Mack, and DeGroot, 1988) is highest for Fleiss' kappa, lower for weighted kappa (Schouten, 1986), and lowest for unweighted kappa, where both v_i and w_i are constants.

The estimating-equation approach can be extended to the regression case in which kappa is modeled as a function of covariates. Alternative ways of incorporating covariates and testing homogeneity of kappa across covariate levels are discussed by Barlow, Lai, and Azen (1991), Barlow (1996), and Donner, Eliasziew, and Klar (1996).

Both mle and estimating-equation estimators require a large sample size for inferences to be valid. Small-sample properties of kappa estimates have been studied by Koval and Blackman (1996) and Gross (1986). Lau (1993) provides higher-order kappa-type statistics for a dichotomous attribute with multiple raters.

Several authors investigate alternative measures of agreement. Kupper and Hafner (1989) discuss correcting for chance agreement when the raters' attribute selection probabilities are equal, and use a hypergeometric distribution. O'Connell and Dobson (1984) describe a class of agreement measures in which kappa is a special case. Uebersax (1993) considers a measure of agreement based on a latent-class model. Aickin (1990) uses a mixture of distributions assuming independent ratings and perfect agreement, and takes the mixing probability as a measure of agreement. He finds that his measure of agreement has a kappa-like form, but tends to be larger than Cohen's kappa except in the case of uniform margins. Agresti (1992) and Banerjee, Capozzoli, and McSweeney (1999) give a review of measures of agreement, and Smeeton (1985) describes the early history of kappa.

PROBLEMS

18.1. Prove that, when each of the indices of agreement given by (18.1), (18.2), (18.4), (18.6), and (18.7) is corrected for chance-expected agreement using formula (18.8), the same formula for kappa (18.9) is obtained.

18.2. Prove that, when $k = 2$, the square of the critical ratio given in (18.14) is identical to the standard chi squared statistic without the continuity correction.

18.3. Suppose that $g = 3$ independent reliability studies of a given kind of rating have been conducted, with results as follows:

	Study 1 ($n = 20$)			Study 2 ($n = 20$)			Study 3 ($n = 30$)	
	Rater B			Rater D			Rater F	
Rater A	+	−	Rater C	+	−	Rater E	+	−
+	0.60	0.05	+	0.75	0.10	+	0.50	0.20
−	0.20	0.15	−	0.05	0.10	−	0.10	0.20

(a) What are the three values of kappa? What are their standard errors [see (18.15)]? What is the overall value of kappa [see (18.21)]?

(b) Are the three estimates of kappa significantly different? [Refer the value of the statistic in (18.22) to tables of chi squared with 2 df.]

(c) Using (18.23), find an approximate 95% confidence interval for the common value of kappa.

18.4. Prove that, when $w_{ii} = 1$ for all i and $w_{ij} = 0$ for all $i \neq j$, the standard-error formulas (18.13) and (18.32) are identical. Prove that, with this same system of agreement weights, the standard-error formulas (18.15) and (18.36) are identical.

18.5. Prove that, when $k = 2$, formulas (18.52) and (18.53) are identical.

REFERENCES

Agresti, A. (1992). Modeling patterns of agreement and disagreement. *Statist. Methods Med. Res.*, **1**, 201–218.

Agresti, A. and Lang, J. B. (1993). Quasi-symmetrical latent class models, with application to rater agreement. *Biometrics*, **49**, 131–139.

Aickin, M. (1990). Maximum likelihood estimation of agreement in the constant predictive probability model, and its relation to Cohen's kappa. *Biometrics*, **46**, 293–302.

Armitage, P., Blendis, L. M., and Smyllie, H. C. (1966). The measurement of observer disagreement in the recording of signs. *J. R. Statist. Soc., Ser. A*, **129**, 98–109.

Armstrong, B. (1985). Measurement error in the generalised linear model. *Comm. Statist.*, **B14**, 529–544.

Banerjee, M., Capozzoli, M., and McSweeney, L. (1999). Beyond kappa: A review of interrater agreement measures. *Canad. J. Statist.*, **27**, 3–23.

Barlow, W. (1996). Measurement of interrater agreement with adjustment for covariates. *Biometrics*, **52**, 695–702.

Barlow, W., Lai, M.-Y., and Azen, S. P. (1991). A comparison of methods for calculating a stratified kappa. *Statist. in Med.*, **10**, 1465–1472.

Bartko, J. J. (1966). The intraclass correlation coefficient as a measure of reliability. *Psychol. Rep.*, **19**, 3–11.

Bennett, B. M. (1972). Measures for clinicians' disagreements over signs. *Biometrics*, **28**, 607–612.

Bloch, D. A. and Kraemer, H. C. (1989). 2×2 kappa coefficients: Measures of agreement or association (C/R: pp. 1329–1330). *Biometrics*, **45**, 269–287.

Boushka, W. M., Martinez, Y. N., Prihoda, T. J., Dunford, R., and Barnwell, G. M. (1990). A computer program for calculating kappa: Application to interexaminer agreement in periodontal research. *Computer Methods Programs Biomed.*, **33**, 35–41.

Cicchetti, D. V. (1976). Assessing inter-rater reliability for rating scales: Resolving some basic issues. *Brit. J. Psychiatry*, **129**, 452–456.

Cicchetti, D. V. and Allison, T. (1971). A new procedure for assessing reliability of scoring EEG sleep recordings. *Am. J. EEG Technol.*, **11**, 101–109.

Cicchetti, D. V. and Fleiss, J. L. (1977). Comparison of the null distributions of weighted kappa and the C ordinal statistic. *Appl. Psychol. Meas.*, **1**, 195–201.

Cohen, J. (1960). A coefficient of agreement for nominal scales. *Educ. Psychol. Meas.*, **20**, 37–46.

Cohen, J. (1968). Weighted kappa: Nominal scale agreement with provision for scaled disagreement or partial credit. *Psychol. Bull.*, **70**, 213–220.

Dice, L. R. (1945). Measures of the amount of ecologic association between species. *Ecology*, **26**, 297–302.

Donner, A. and Eliasziw, M. (1992). A goodness-of-fit approach to inference procedures for the kappa statistic: Confidence interval construction, significance-testing, and sample size estimation. *Statist. in Med.*, **11**, 1511–1519.

Donner, A., Eliasziew, M., and Klar, N. (1996). Testing the homogeneity of kappa statistics. *Biometrics*, **52**, 176–183.

Ebel, R. L. (1951). Estimation of the reliability of ratings. *Psychometrika*, **16**, 407–424.

Flack, V. F. (1987). Confidence intervals for the interrater agreement measure kappa. *Comm. Statist.*, **A16**, 953–968.

Fleiss, J. L. (1965). Estimating the accuracy of dichotomous judgments. *Psychometrika*, **30**, 469–479.

Fleiss, J. L. (1971). Measuring nominal scale agreement among many raters. *Psychol. Bull.*, **76**, 378–382.

Fleiss, J. L. (1975). Measuring agreement between two judges on the presence or absence of a trait. *Biometrics*, **31**, 651–659.

Fleiss, J. L. and Cicchetti, D. V. (1978). Inference about weighted kappa in the non-null case. *Appl. Psychol. Meas.*, **2**, 113–117.

Fleiss, J. L. and Cohen, J. (1973). The equivalence of weighted kappa and the intraclass correlation coefficient as measures of reliability. *Educ. Psychol. Meas.*, **33**, 613–619.

Fleiss, J. L., Cohen, J., and Everitt, B. S. (1969). Large sample standard errors of kappa and weighted kappa. *Psychol. Bull.*, **72**, 323–327.

Fleiss, J. L. and Cuzick, J. (1979). The reliability of dichotomous judgments: Unequal numbers of judges per subject. *Appl. Psychol. Meas.*, **3**, 537–542.

Fleiss, J. L. and Davies, M. (1982). Jackknifing functions of multinomial frequencies, with an application to a measure of concordance. *Am. J. Epidemiol.*, **115**, 841–845.

Fleiss, J. L., Nee, J. C. M., and Landis, J. R. (1979). The large sample variance of kappa in the case of different sets of raters. *Psychol. Bull.*, **86**, 974–977.

Garner, J. B. (1991). The standard error of Cohen's kappa. *Statist. in Med.*, **10**, 767–775.

Goodman, L. A. and Kruskal, W. H. (1954). Measures of association for cross classifications. *J. Am. Statist. Assoc.*, **49**, 732–764.

Gross, S. T. (1986). The kappa coefficient of agreement for multiple observers when the number of subjects is small. *Biometrics*, **42**, 883–893.

Hale, C. A. and Fleiss, J. L. (1993). Interval estimation under two study designs for kappa with binary classifications. *Biometrics*, **49**, 523–533.

Hirschberg, J. G. and Slottje, D. J. (1989). Remembrance of things past the distribution of earnings across occupations and the kappa criterion. *J. Econometrics*, **42**, 121–130.

Holley, J. W. and Guilford, J. P. (1964). A note on the *G* index of agreement. *Educ. Psychol. Meas.*, **32**, 281–288.

Hubert, L. J. (1978). A general formula for the variance of Cohen's weighted kappa. *Psychol. Bull.*, **85**, 183–184.

Kairam, R., Kline, J., Levin, B., Brambilla, D., Coulter, D., Kuban, K., Lansky, L., Marshall, P., Velez-Borras, J., and Rodriguez, E. (1993). Reliability of neurologic assessment in a collaborative study of HIV infection in children. *Ann. N.Y. Acad. Sci.*, **693**, 123–140.

Koval, J. J. and Blackman, N. J.-M. (1996). Estimators of kappa—exact small sample properties. *J. Statist. Comput. Simul.* **55**, 315–336.

Kraemer, H. C. (1980). Extension of the kappa coefficient. *Biometrics*, **36**, 207–216.

Krippendorff, K. (1970). Bivariate agreement coefficients for reliability of data. Pp. 139–150 in E. F. Borgatta (Ed.). *Sociological methodology 1970*. San Francisco: Jossey-Bass.

Kupper, L. L. and Hafner, K. B. (1989). On assessing interrater agreement for multiple attribute responses. *Biometrics*, **45**, 957–967.

Landis, J. R. and Koch, G. G. (1977a). The measurement of observer agreement for categorical data. *Biometrics*, **33**, 159–174.

Landis, J. R. and Koch, G. G. (1977b). A one-way components of variance model for categorical data. *Biometrics*, **33**, 671–679.

Lau, T.-S. (1993). Higher-order kappa-type statistics for a dichotomous attribute in multiple ratings. *Biometrics*, **49**, 535–542.

Lee, J. J. and Tu, Z. N. (1994). A better confidence interval for kappa (κ) on measuring agreement between two raters with binary outcomes. *J. Comput. Graph. Statist.*, **3**, 301–321.

Light, R. J. (1971). Measures of response agreement for qualitative data: Some generalizations and alternatives. *Psychol. Bull.*, **76**, 365–377.

Lipsitz, S. R., Laird, N. M., and Brennan, T. A. (1994). Simple moment estimates of the κ-coefficient and its variance. *Appl. Statist.*, **43**, 309–323.

Maxwell, A. E. (1977). Coefficients of agreement between observers and their interpretation. *Brit. J. Psychiatry*, **130**, 79–83.

Maxwell, A. E. and Pilliner, A. E. G. (1968). Deriving coefficients of reliability and agreement for ratings. *Brit. J. Math. Statist. Psychol.*, **21**, 105–116.

Musch, D. C., Landis, J. R., Higgins, I. T. T., Gilson, J. C., and Jones, R. N. (1984). An application of kappa-type analysis to interobserver variation in classifying chest radiographs for pneumoconiosis. *Statist. in Med.*, **3**, 73–83.

O'Connell, D. L. and Dobson, A. J. (1984). General observer-agreement measures on individual subjects and groups of subjects. *Biometrics*, **40**, 973–983.

Posner, K. L., Sampson, P. D., Caplan, R. A., Ward, R. J., and Cheney, F. W. (1990). Measuring interrater reliability among multiple raters: An example of methods for nominal data. *Statist. in Med.*, **9**, 1103–1115.

Rogot, E. and Goldberg, I. D. (1966). A proposed index for measuring agreement in test-retest studies. *J. Chronic Dis.*, **19**, 991–1006.

Schouten, H. J. A. (1986). Nominal scale agreement among observers. *Psychometrika*, **51**, 453–466.

Scott, W. A. (1955). Reliability of content analysis: The case of nominal scale coding. *Public Opinion Quart.*, **19**, 321–325.

Shoukri, M. M., Martin, S. W., and Mian, I. U. H. (1995). Maximum likelihood estimation of the kappa coefficient from models of matched binary responses. *Statist. in Med.*, **14**, 83–99.

Shoukri, M. M. and Mian, I. U. H. (1995). Maximum likelihood estimation of the kappa coefficient from logistic regression. *Statist. in Med.*, **15**, 1409–1419.

Smeeton, N. C. (1985). Early history of the kappa statistic. *Biometrics*, **41**, 795.

Sneath, P. H. A. and Sokal, R. R. (1973). *Numerical Taxonomy*. San Francisco: W. H. Freeman.

Spitzer, R. L., Cohen, J., Fleiss, J. L., and Endicott, J. (1967). Quantification of agreement in psychiatric diagnosis. *Arch. Gen. Psychiatry*, **17**, 83–87.

Spitzer, R. L. and Fleiss, J. L. (1974). A reanalysis of the reliability of psychiatric diagnosis. *Brit. J. Psychiatry*, **125**, 341–347.

Uebersax, J. S. (1993). Statistical modeling of expert ratings on medical-treatment appropriateness. *J. Am. Statist. Assoc.*, **88**, 421–427.

Verducci, J. S., Mack, M. E., and DeGroot, M. H. (1988). Estimating multiple rater agreement for a rare diagnosis. *J. Multivariate Anal.*, **27**, 512–535.

Wackerley, D. D., McClave, J. T., and Rao, P. V. (1978). Measuring nominal scale agreement between a judge and a known standard. *Psychometrika*, **43**, 213–223.

Williams, G. W. (1976). Comparing the joint agreement of several raters with another rater. *Biometrics*, **32**, 619–627.

CHAPTER 19

The Standardization of Rates

One of the most frequently occurring problems in epidemiology and vital statistics is the comparison of the rate for some event or characteristic across different populations or for the same population over time. If the populations were similar with respect to factors associated with the event under study—factors such as age, sex, race, or marital status—there would be no problem in comparing the *overall* rates (synonyms are *total* and *crude* rates) as they stand.

If the populations are not similarly constituted, however, the direct comparison of the overall rates may be misleading. Algebraically, the problem with such a comparison is as follows. Let $p_1, \ldots, p_I$ denote the proportions of all members of one of the populations being compared who fall into the various strata (age intervals, socioeconomic groups, etc.), there being I strata in all. Thus $\Sigma_i p_i = 1$. If c_i denotes the rate specific to the ith stratum of this population, then the overall or crude rate for it is

$$c = \sum_{i=1}^{I} c_i p_i. \tag{19.1}$$

If the distribution for the second population across the I strata is represented by the proportions $P_1, \ldots, P_I$, so that $\Sigma_i P_i = 1$, and if C_i denotes the rate specific to the ith stratum in the second population, then the crude rate for this population is

$$C = \sum_{i=1}^{I} C_i p_i. \tag{19.2}$$

Statistical Methods for Rates and Proportions, Third Edition
By Joseph L. Fleiss, Bruce Levin, and Myunghee Cho Paik
ISBN 0-471-52629-0   Copyright © 2003 John Wiley & Sons, Inc.

The difference between the two crude rates is

$$d = c - C, \tag{19.3}$$

and it is easy to check that

$$d = \sum_{i=1}^{I} \frac{p_i + P_i}{2}(c_i - C_i) + \sum_{i=1}^{I} \frac{c_i + C_i}{2}(p_i - P_i) \tag{19.4}$$

(see Kitagawa, 1955; Hemphill and Ament, 1970). Miettinen (1972) conducted a similar analysis for the ratio of two crude rates.

It is thus seen that the difference between the two crude rates has two
components. One of them,

$$d_1 = \sum_{i=1}^{I} \frac{p_i + P_i}{2}(c_i - C_i), \tag{19.5}$$

is a true summarization of the differences between the two schedules of
specific rates, differences that are usually of major interest. However, the
second component,

$$d_2 = \sum_{i=1}^{I} \frac{c_i + C_i}{2}(p_i - P_i), \tag{19.6}$$

is a summarization of the differences between the two sets of population
distributions, differences that are of little if any interest.

A number of conclusions can be drawn from the representation (19.4):

1. If the two population distributions are equal, that is, if $p_1 = P_1, \ldots,$
$p_I = P_I$, then $d_2 = 0$ and the difference between the crude rates indeed
summarizes the differences between the schedules of specific rates.

2. If the two schedules of specific rates are equal, that is, if $c_1 = C_1, \ldots,$
$c_I = C_I$, then $d_1 = 0$ and the difference between the crude rates measures
only the difference in population distributions across the strata, a difference
usually of no importance.

3. For any given value of d_1, that is, for a given summarization of the
differences between two schedules of specific rates, the apparent difference
between the two populations measured by d may be unaltered, increased,
decreased, or even changed in sign depending on the differences between the
two population distributions. The effect of d_2 is an additive one if the first
population has a larger proportion of its members in the strata where the
rates are high than does the second—that is, if $p_i > P_i$ in those strata where
$(c_i + C_i)/2$ is large—and the effect of d_2 is a subtractive one if the reverse
holds. It is these kinds of effects that explain why, when each of one

population's specific rates is greater than another's, the first population's crude rate may nevertheless be lower than the second's.

Section 19.1 presents some reasons for standardization, and some warnings against its uncritical use. Section 19.2 defines two types of standardization, direct and indirect, and sets the stage for a comparison of the two. Section 19.3 describes the indirect method of standardization, and Section 19.4 illustrates how it can give misleading results. Section 19.5 describes the direct method of standardization, Section 19.6 presents some other methods of standardization, and Section 19.7 discusses techniques for standardizing on two correlated dimensions.

19.1. REASONS FOR AND WARNINGS AGAINST STANDARDIZATION

It is to prevent anomalies of the sort described in conclusions 2 and 3 above that resort is made to *standardization* (synonymously, *adjustment*) in the comparison of two or more schedules of specific rates. Standardization should, never, however, substitute for a comparison of the specific rates themselves. It is these that characterize the experience (morbidity, mortality, or whatever the rate refers to) of the population being studied.

Woolsey has pointed out that "The specific rates are essential (because) it is only through the analysis of specific rates that an accurate and detailed study can be made of the variation (of the phenomenon under study) among population classes" (1959, p. 60). Elveback (1966), too, stresses the importance of studying the specific rates and strongly criticizes the calculation of adjusted rates.

One criticism of the adjustment of rates is that if the specific rates vary in different ways across the various strata, then no single method of standardization will indicate that these differences exist. Standardization will, on the contrary, tend to mask these differences. As one example (see Kitagawa, 1966), there is the contrast between the age-specific death rates for white males resident in metropolitan counties of the United States in 1960 and those for white males resident in nonmetropolitan counties. Up to age 40, the rates in metropolitan counties are lower than in nonmetropolitan counties; after age 40, the reverse is true. No single summary comparison will reveal this information. On the contrary, at least two summary comparisons are needed.

Another example is provided by data reported by El-Badry (1969). He points out that in Ceylon, India, and Pakistan, mortality among males occurs at a lower rate than among females in many age categories. Single summary indices for males and females might mask this phenomenon and thus fail to reveal data suggestive of further research. Doll and Cook (1967), in addition, cite the inadequacy of a single index for summarizing age- and sex-specific incidence rates.

Bearing in mind that there is no substitute for examining the specific rates themselves, we may consider some of the reasons for standardization.

1. A single summary index for a population is more easily compared with other summary indices than are entire schedules of specific rates.

2. If some strata are composed of small numbers of people, the associated specific rates may be too imprecise and unreliable for use in detailed comparisons.

3. For small populations, or for some groups of especial interest, specific rates may not exist. This may be the case for selected occupational groups and for populations from geographic areas especially demarcated for a single study. In such cases, only the total number of events (e.g., deaths) may be available and not their subdivision by strata.

Other reasons for standardization are given by Woolsey (1959), Kalton (1968), and Cochran (1968), who in addition studied the effects of varying the number of strata, I. Mausner and Bahn (1974, p. 138) give an elegant summary of the advantages and disadvantages of analyzing crude, specific, and adjusted rates.

19.2. TWO TYPES OF STANDARDIZATION: DIRECT AND INDIRECT

There are two types of standardization, *direct* and *indirect*. Both types express the standardized rate as a product of two terms, the crude rate of the standard population, say c_S, and a ratio which determines whether the standardization is direct or indirect:

$$c_{\text{indirect}} = c_S \, \text{Ratio}_{\text{indirect}} = c_S \frac{\sum_{i=1}^{I} c_i p_i}{\sum_{i=1}^{I} c_{Si} p_i}$$

and

$$c_{\text{direct}} = c_S \, \text{Ratio}_{\text{direct}} = c_S \frac{\sum_{i=1}^{I} c_i p_{Si}}{\sum_{i=1}^{I} c_{Si} p_{Si}},$$

where c_i and p_i denote, respectively, the specific rate and the proportion of the population in stratum i of the study population, and where c_{Si} and p_{Si} denote their counterparts in the standard population. In both ratios, the numerator and denominator use, respectively, the rates of the study population and those of the standard population. In the ratio for indirect standardization, the rates are multiplied (adjusted) by the study-population distribution, whereas in the ratio for direct standardization, the rates are multiplied by the standard-population distribution.

The above two expressions can be simplified. The numerator of $c_{indirect}$ reduces to the crude rate of the study population, say c. Let the number of events in the study population in stratum i be Y_i and the total study population size be N. Then $c_i = Y_i/(Np_i)$, and

$$c = \sum_{i=1}^{I} c_i p_i = \frac{\sum_{i=1}^{I} Y_i}{N}.$$

Then

$$c_{indirect} = c_S \, \text{Ratio}_{indirect} = c_S \frac{\sum_{i=1}^{I} Y_i}{N \sum_{i=1}^{I} c_{Si} p_i}. \tag{19.7}$$

Thus $\text{Ratio}_{indirect}$ is the ratio of the total observed number of events to that which would be expected if the standard population rates were applied to the study population's strata.

Simplification also occurs in c_{direct}. The denominator of c_{direct} is nothing but the crude rate of the standard population:

$$c_S = \sum_{i=1}^{I} c_{Si} p_{Si},$$

so that c_{direct} reduces to

$$c_{direct} = c_S \frac{\sum_{i=1}^{I} c_i p_{Si}}{c_S} = \sum_{i=1}^{I} c_i p_{Si} = \frac{\sum_{i=1}^{I} Y_i p_{Si}}{N}. \tag{19.8}$$

Standard errors of the standardized rates can be obtained assuming p_i, p_{Si}, and c_{Si} are known constants, and the Y_i's are independent Poisson random variables. Equation (19.7) shows that the indirect rate is a multiple of $\sum_i Y_i$, which is a sum of independent Poisson random variables, and therefore a Poisson random variable itself. We can set an exact confidence interval using the method of Section 12.1 at (12.5) (see also Ulm, 1990). Specifically, an exact $100(1 - \alpha)\%$ confidence interval by the equal-tail method for $c_{indirect}$ is

$$\left(c_S \frac{\chi^2_{2t, \alpha/2}}{2E}, c_S \frac{\chi^2_{2t+2, 1-\alpha/2}}{2E} \right),$$

where $t = \sum_i Y_i$ is the total number of events in the study population, and where $E = N \sum_i c_{Si} p_i$ is the expected number of events in the standard population, and also the denominator of (19.7).

Alternatively, an approximate confidence interval can be constructed based on the square-root transformation (Vandenbroucke, 1982). Swift (1995)

applied the approximate bootstrap method of DiCiccio and Efron (1992) to
set a skewness-corrected confidence interval. As shown in equation (19.8),
c_{direct} has the form of a weighted sum of Poisson random variables. Dobson
et al. (1991) propose an exact confidence interval for weighted Poisson
parameters. Approximate confidence intervals are also given in Fay and
Feuer (1997) and Fay (1999).

19.3. INDIRECT STANDARDIZATION

The second and third reasons just given for standardization, the unreliability
and possibly even the unavailability of some specific rates, lead to perhaps
the most frequently adopted method of standardization, the so-called indirect
method. The ingredients necessary for its implementation are:

1. The crude rate for the population being studied, c.
2. The distribution across the various strata for that population, $p_1, \ldots, p_I$.
3. The schedule of specific rates for a selected standard population,
   $c_{S1}, \ldots, c_{SI}$.
4. The crude rate for the standard population, c_S.

The first calculation in indirect standardization is of the overall rate that
would obtain if the schedule of specific rates for the standard population
were applied to the given population. It is

$$c' = \sum_{i=1}^{I} c_{Si} p_i. \tag{19.9}$$

The indirect adjusted rate is then

$$c_{\text{indirect}} = c_S \frac{c}{c'}; \tag{19.10}$$

that is, the crude rate for the standard population, c_S, multiplied by the ratio
of the actual crude rate for the given population, c, to the crude rate, c', that
would exist if the given population were subject to the standard population's
schedule of rates.

As an example, consider the following data from Stark and Mantel (1966).
In the state of Michigan, from 1950 to 1964, 731,177 infants were the first-
born to their mothers; of these, 412 had Down's syndrome (trisomy 21), giving
a crude rate of $c = 56.3$ Down's births, per 100,000 first-born live births. In
the same 15-year interval, 442,811 infants were the fifth-born or later to their
mothers; of these, 740 were Down's births, giving a crude rate of $C = 167.1$
Down's births, per 100,000 fifth-born or later live births.

Table 19.1. *An example of indirect standardization*

| Maternal Age | Specific Rates for All Michigan per 100,000, c_{Si} | Birth Order | | | |
| | | First | | Fifth or Later | |
		p_i	$c_{Si}p_i$	P_i	$c_{Si}P_i$
Under 20	42.5	0.315	13.4	0.001	0.0
20–24	42.5	0.451	19.2	0.069	2.9
25–29	52.3	0.157	8.2	0.279	14.6
30–34	87.7	0.054	4.7	0.339	29.7
35–39	264.0	0.019	5.0	0.235	62.0
40 and over	864.4	0.004	3.5	0.078	67.4
Sum			54.0 $(= c')$		176.6 $(= C')$

The comparison as it stands is not a fair one, because maternal age is known to be associated with both birth order and Down's syndrome. Some method has therefore to be applied to adjust for possible differences between the first-born and later-born in maternal age distributions. Table 19.1 illustrates indirect adjustment.

The selected standard population was all the live births in Michigan during the years 1950–1964. The crude rate of Down's syndrome for the state as a whole was $c_S = 89.5$ per 100,000 live births, and the rates specific for maternal age are given in the column headed c_{Si} in the table. For the infants born first and born fifth or later, the maternal age distributions are given in the columns headed p_i and P_i. The results of applying formula (19.9) are shown in the bottom row of the table.

To review, we are given the crude rates

$$c = 56.3 \text{ Down's births per 100,000 first-borns} \qquad (19.11)$$

and

$$C = 167.1 \text{ Down's births per 100,000 fifth- or later-borns.} \qquad (19.12)$$

By applying the rates of Down's syndrome specific to maternal age for the state of Michigan as a whole, we would have expected

$$c' = 54.0 \text{ Down's syndrome per 100,000 first-borns,}$$

and

$$C' = 176.6 \text{ Down's syndrome per 100,000 fifth- or later-borns.}$$

Given the crude rate for the entire state,

$$c_S = 89.5 \text{ Down's syndrome per 100,000 live births,}$$

we find, by (14.8), the indirect adjusted rates

$$c_{\text{indirect}} = 89.5 \times \frac{56.3}{54.0}$$

$$= 93.3 \text{ Down's syndrome per } 100{,}000 \text{ first-borns} \qquad (19.13)$$

and

$$C_{\text{indirect}} = 89.5 \times \frac{167.1}{176.6}$$

$$= 84.7 \text{ Down's syndrome per } 100{,}000 \text{ fifth- or later-borns.} \quad (19.14)$$

By just comparing the crude rates given in (19.11) and (19.12), we would conclude that there was a threefold increase in the risk of Down's syndrome from first-borns to infants born fifth or later. By comparing the adjusted rates given by (19.13) and (19.14), on the other hand, we would conclude that there was no effective difference in the risk of Down's syndrome.

It seems that the apparent greater risk of Down's syndrome for later births, suggested by a comparison of the crude rates in (19.11) and (19.12), is a reflection of differences in maternal age distribution. Proportionately more mothers of later-born infants are in the older age categories, where the specific rates are higher, than are mothers of first-born infants. After adjustment for differences in the maternal age distributions, it appears that, if anything, the rate of Down's syndrome in later-born infants is somewhat less than the rate in first-born infants.

19.4. A FEATURE OF INDIRECT STANDARDIZATION

Consider the data of Table 19.2, giving hypothetical sex-specific mortality rates (per 1000) in each of two groups. The two sets of sex-specific rates are equal, but the unequal sex distributions in the two groups yield unequal overall rates. For group 1, the crude rate is

$$c = 2.0 \times 0.60 + 1.0 \times 0.40 = 1.6 \text{ deaths}/1000, \qquad (19.15)$$

and for group 2 the crude rate is

$$C = 2.0 \times 0.80 + 1.0 \times 0.20 = 1.8 \text{ deaths}/1000. \qquad (19.16)$$

Table 19.2. *Sex-specific mortality rates in two groups*

Sex	Group 1		Group 2	
	p_i	Rate/1000	P_i	Rate/1000
Male	0.60	2.0	0.80	2.0
Female	0.40	1.0	0.20	1.0

Suppose, now, that the two sets of sex-specific rates could have been obtained only with the greatest difficulty, so that the only data actually available were the two sex distributions and the two crude rates. Indirect adjustment would therefore have to be resorted to. For the population chosen as the standard, suppose that the crude rate is

$$c_S = 1.5 \text{ deaths}/1000, \tag{19.17}$$

and that the sex-specific rates are

$$c_{S1} = 2.2 \text{ deaths}/1000 \text{ males} \tag{19.18}$$

and

$$c_{S2} = 0.9 \text{ deaths}/1000 \text{ females}. \tag{19.19}$$

The expected crude rate in group 1 is

$$c' = 2.2 \times 0.60 + 0.9 \times 0.40 = 1.68 \text{ deaths}/1000, \tag{19.20}$$

yielding an indirect adjusted rate of

$$c_{\text{indirect}} = 1.5 \times \frac{1.6}{1.68} = 1.43 \text{ deaths}/1000. \tag{19.21}$$

The expected crude rate in group 2 is

$$C' = 2.2 \times 0.80 + 0.9 \times 0.20 = 1.94 \text{ deaths}/1000, \tag{19.22}$$

so that, for group 2,

$$C_{\text{indirect}} = 1.5 \times \frac{1.8}{1.94} = 1.39 \text{ deaths}/1000. \tag{19.23}$$

The two adjusted rates given by (19.21) and (19.23) are more nearly equal than the two unadjusted rates given by (19.15) and (19.16), reflecting more accurately the equality of sex-specific rates indicated in Table 19.2. It is a bit disquieting, however, that equality of the two schedules of specific rates has not been reflected in precise equality of the two indirect adjusted rates. This is a defect of indirect adjustment that does not afflict direct adjustment, the method to be considered next. Neither in this example nor in most other instances is the distortion great, however. Furthermore, such distortion will not occur if the standard population is the composite of the two populations studied.

It is clear that indirect standardization does not completely adjust for differences in population composition. Thus when attempting to explain variability across groups of indirect adjusted rates, one should bear in mind that, whereas variation of schedules of specific rates accounts for most of it, variation in population composition may still account for some of it. Additional criticisms of indirect adjustment are given by Yule (1934) and Kilpatrick (1963). Breslow and Day (1975), however, present a particular mathematical model for the specific rates (each specific rate is assumed to be the product of two terms, one descriptive of the stratum and the other of the population) under which indirect standardization is appropriate.

19.5. DIRECT STANDARDIZATION

The method of standardization used second most frequently is the so-called direct method. Direct standardization may be applied only when the schedule of specific rates for a given population is available. The data necessary for its implementation are:

1. The schedule of specific rates for the population being studied, say $c_1, \ldots, c_I$.
2. The distribution across the various strata for a selected standard population, say $p_{S1}, \ldots, p_{SI}$.

The direct adjusted rate is then simply

$$c_{\text{direct}} = \sum_{i=1}^{I} c_i p_{Si}. \tag{19.24}$$

The term direct refers to working directly with the specific rates of the population being studied, in distinction to what was done in the method previously presented.

As an example, let us consider the same event, Down's syndrome studied in Section 19.3. Table 19.3 gives the maternal age distribution for all infants

Table 19.3. *An example of direct standardization (rates per 100,000)*

Maternal Age	Distribution for All of Michigan, p_{Si}	Birth Order			
		First		Fifth or Later	
		c_i	$c_i p_{Si}$	C_i	$C_i p_{Si}$
Under 20	0.113	46.5	5.3	0	0.0
20–24	0.330	42.8	14.1	26.1	8.6
25–29	0.278	52.2	14.5	51.0	14.2
30–34	0.173	101.3	17.5	74.7	12.9
35–39	0.084	274.5	23.1	251.7	21.1
40 and over	0.022	819.1	18.0	857.8	18.9
Sum			$92.5\ (= c_{\text{direct}})$		$75.7\ (= C_{\text{direct}})$

born in the state of Michigan from 1950 to 1964 (the standard distribution), and the rates of Down's syndrome specific to maternal age for first-borns and for infants born fifth or later (data from Stark and Mantel, 1966).

The conclusion drawn from a comparison of these direct adjusted rates is the same as that drawn before from the indirect adjusted rates: the rates of Down's syndrome are about the same for infants born first and for infants born fifth or later. Such concordance between the conclusions drawn from comparisons of indirect and direct adjusted rates is usually, although not invariably, the case.

Given the consistent contrast between the specific rates shown in Table 19.3—in five of the six maternal age categories, the rate of Down's syndrome among first-borns was slightly greater than the rate among infants born fifth or later—there was clearly no compelling reason for any standardization at all. The specific rates spoke for themselves. The only legitimate reason for standardization in such a case is the one cited first at the conclusion of Section 19.1, namely, the greater simplicity of working with a single summary index than of working with an entire schedule of specific rates.

There is one decided advantage to direct over indirect standardization. If, stratum by stratum, the specific rate in one group is equal to the specific rate in a second group, then, no matter which population is chosen as standard, the direct adjusted rates will be equal. Consider, for example, the specific rates presented in Table 19.2. The direct adjusted rate for group 1 is

$$c_{\text{direct}} = 2.0 \times p_{S1} + 1.0 \times p_{S2}, \tag{19.25}$$

and that for group 2 is obviously the same.

Direct standardization has a more general property. Consistent inequalities among specific rates, stratum by stratum, yield direct adjusted rates bearing the same inequalities. Thus if each specific rate in group 1 is greater than the corresponding rate in group 2, the direct adjusted rate for group 1 will be greater than that for group 2, no matter what the composition of the standard population.

These features of direct adjusted rates are actually quite trivial, for the circumstances leading to them are fully described by the specific rates themselves. Here the adjusted rates serve merely as convenient summarizations.

An important point to bear in mind is that an adjusted rate, no matter which method of adjustment is used, has meaning only when compared with a similarly adjusted rate. Its magnitude means little in and of itself. For the rates of Table 19.2, for example, the direct adjusted rate varies from 1.25 through 1.50 to 1.75 as the standard sex distribution varies from $(0.25, 0.75)$ through $(0.50, 0.50)$ to $(0.75, 0.25)$. No matter which standard is used, the direct adjusted rates for the two groups will be identical. The magnitude of the rate, however, is seen to depend strongly on the composition of the standard population. Spiegelman and Marks (1966) have shown that, in the direct standardization of mortality rates, the choice of a standard population generally has little effect on the differences between adjusted rates, and tends to affect only their individual magnitudes.

When the specific rates in the groups being compared do not bear consistent relations across the strata, then any kind of overall standardization is questionable. Problem 19.1 is concerned with the comparison of two groups for which the specific rates of one are higher than those for the other in some strata but are lower in other strata. It is shown that, depending on the strata in which the standard population is concentrated, either of the two groups can end up with the larger adjusted rate. The standard population may even be chosen to give equal adjusted rates. In addition, the phenomenon of a crossover in specific rates is lost by the usual methods of standardization.

A compromise calls for the calculation of a number of adjusted rates, one for each contiguous set of strata in which the specific rates bear consistent relations over the groups being compared. This device is illustrated in Problem 19.1, where two such sets of strata may be constituted. The division of the strata into such sets is not always easy, and sometimes may have to be forced. Nevertheless, working with a number of adjusted rates is preferable to working with one overall adjusted rate that may be more of a distortion than a summarization.

19.6. SOME OTHER SUMMARY INDICES

Woolsey (1959) and Kitagawa (1964) have reviewed a number of approaches to the standardization of rates. Formulas for determining standard errors have been given by Chiang (1961) and Keyfitz (1966).

One sometimes encounters variations of the two kinds of adjusted rates considered so far. With respect to indirect standardization, the quantity

$$\text{SMR} = \frac{c}{c'} = \frac{c_{\text{indirect}}}{c_S} \tag{19.26}$$

may be used, where c_S is the rate for the standard population. This quantity, called the *standardized mortality ratio* (or the *standard mortality figure*) when the event studied is mortality, is merely the ratio of the actual to the expected crude rate. This is the quantity $\text{Ratio}_{\text{indirect}}$ defined in Section 19.2. The SMR can be calculated for deaths from all causes or for deaths from a specific cause. Kupper et al. (1978) have shown how, under some modest assumptions, inferences about the SMR for a specific cause of death can be based on an analysis of proportional mortality rates, that is, the ratios of numbers of deaths from a specific cause to the number of deaths from all causes. Gail (1978) presents methods for analyzing variations in the SMR across different populations.

The corresponding ratio for direct adjustment,

$$\text{CMF} = \frac{c_{\text{direct}}}{c_S},\qquad(19.27)$$

is dubbed the *comparative mortality figure* when applied to mortality. This is the quantity $\text{Ratio}_{\text{direct}}$ defined in Section 19.2.

Some other methods of adjustment exist but are less frequently used than the ones so far studied. One is a simple average of the crude and the direct adjusted rates,

$$\text{CMR} = \tfrac{1}{2}(c + c_{\text{direct}}) = \sum_{i=1}^{I} \tfrac{1}{2}(p_{Si} + p_i)c_i,\qquad(19.28)$$

and is referred to as the *comparative mortality rate* when mortality is studied. Its infrequent use is testimony to its virtual uninterpretability.

Two indices are available for use with age-specific rates that in effect give equal weight to each year of age. Let n_i denote the number of years in the ith age interval, so that if, for example, the first age interval is 0–4 years, then $n_1 = 5$. The first such index (see Yule, 1934) is

$$\text{EADR} = \frac{\sum_{i=1}^{I} n_i c_i}{\sum_{i=1}^{I} n_i},\qquad(19.29)$$

named the *equivalent average death rate* when applied to mortality. This index may be viewed as a direct adjusted rate where each year of age is assumed to have the same number of people.

The second such index (see Yerushalmy, 1951, and Elveback, 1966) is

$$\text{MI} = \frac{\displaystyle\sum_{i=1}^{I} n_i \frac{c_i}{c_{Si}}}{\displaystyle\sum_{i=1}^{I} n_i},\qquad(19.30)$$

named the *mortality index* when applied to mortality. The mortality index is a simple average of the ratios of specific rates, with weights given by the numbers of years in the varous age intervals.

The usefulness of these two indices is limited because of the questionable validity of assigning equal importance to each year of age.

An index similar to (19.30) is

$$\text{RMI} = \sum_{i=1}^{I} p_i \frac{c_i}{c_{Si}},\qquad(19.31)$$

named the *relative mortality index* when applied to mortality. The relative mortality index is also an average of the ratios of the actual specific rates to the standard population's specific rates, but is weighted by the given population's actual age distribution.

An equivalent expression is

$$\text{RMI} = \frac{\sum_{i=1}^{I} e_i/c_{Si}}{N},\tag{19.32}$$

where e_i is the observed *number* of deaths (in general, of events) in the ith stratum and N is the total number of people in the given population. It is thus seen that one only needs, for the given population, its total size and the distribution over its strata of its total number of events in order to calculate the relative mortality index. An implication is that the relative mortality index may be calculated in years between censuses when, say, the age distribution of the population is not available but when the age distribution of deaths may be determined from registration data.

19.7. ADJUSTMENT FOR TWO FACTORS

Table 19.4 presents data on the incidence of Down's syndrome specific both to birth order and to maternal age. The two methods to be described, the first based on direct and the second on indirect standardization, are useful

Table 19.4. *Distribution of discovered Down's syndrome and of total live births by maternal age and birth order, Michigan, 1950–1964*[a]

Maternal Age	Birth Order					Total
	1	2	3	4	5 +	
Under 20	107 / 230,061	25 / 72,202	3 / 15,050	1 / 2,293	0 / 327	136 / 319,933
20–24	141 / 329,449	150 / 326,701	71 / 175,702	26 / 68,800	8 / 30,666	396 / 931,318
25–29	60 / 114,920	110 / 208,667	114 / 207,081	64 / 132,424	63 / 123,419	411 / 786,511
30–34	40 / 39,487	84 / 83,228	103 / 117,300	89 / 98,301	112 / 149,919	428 / 488,235
35–39	39 / 14,208	82 / 28,466	108 / 45,026	137 / 46,075	262 / 104,088	628 / 237,863
40 and over	25 / 3,052	39 / 5,375	75 / 8,660	96 / 9,834	295 / 34,392	530 / 61,312
Total	412 / 731,177	490 / 724,639	474 / 568,819	413 / 357,727	740 / 442,811	2,529 / 2,825,173

[a] Values in cells are numbers of Down's births found per live birth. Data from Stark and Mantel (1966).

Table 19.5. *Incidence rates of discovered Down's syndrome (number of Down's births found per 100,000 live births) by maternal age and birth order*

Maternal Age	Birth Order					Crude Rate	Adjusted Rate[a]
	1	2	3	4	5 +		
Under 20	46.5	34.6	19.9	43.6	0	42.5	30.4
20–24	42.8	45.9	40.4	37.8	26.1	42.5	39.9
25–29	52.2	52.7	55.1	48.3	51.0	52.3	52.2
30–34	101.3	100.9	87.8	90.5	74.7	87.7	92.9
35–39	274.5	288.1	239.9	297.3	251.7	264.0	270.3
40 and over	819.1	725.6	866.1	976.2	857.8	864.4	830.4
Crude rate	56.3	67.6	83.3	115.5	167.1	89.5	
Adjusted rate[b]	92.3	91.2	85.1	92.7	75.5		88.0[c]

[a]The last column contains rates specific for maternal age and directly adjusted for birth order, with the standard birth-order distribution being that of the total sample.
[b]The last row contains rates specific for birth order and directly adjusted for maternal age, with the standard maternal age distribution being that of the total sample.
[c]Whenever the two standard distributions are those of the total sample, the overall rates based on the two series of directly adjusted rates will be equal to each other, but not necessarily to the overall crude rate.

when two factors are both associated with some disorder and with each other, and when one wishes to identify and measure their separate effects.

Simultaneous Direct Adjustment

Table 19.5 presents the various specific rates, the crude rates, and the direct adjusted rates.

In this case the specific rates speak for themselves. Within none of the maternal age categories is there any appreciable variation in the rates of Down's syndrome specific to birth order. The increasing gradient with birth order of the crude rates is therefore likely to be only a reflection of the association between birth order and maternal age, and not of any direct relationship between birth order and the incidence of Down's syndrome.

Maternal age, on the other hand, is seen to be strongly associated with the incidence of Down's syndrome. Within each birth-order category, there is a clear increase in the incidence rate with increasing maternal age.

The direct adjusted rates shown in the last row and last column of Table 19.5 serve only to summarize the information provided by the 30 specific rates: little effect of birth order but a strong effect of maternal age on the incidence of Down's syndrome. In fact, direct adjustment is appropriate only because of the consistency found both within maternal age categories (rather little variability among the birth-order-specific rates) and within birth-order categories (a clear gradient with increasing maternal age).

Simultaneous Indirect Adjustment

If all the specific rates are available, and all are based on samples of sufficient size to possess adequate precision, then simultaneous direct adjust-

Table 19.6. *Distribution of total live births by maternal age and birth order, overall crude rates, and indirectly adjusted rates*

Maternal	Birth Order					Crude	Adjusted
Age	1	2	3	4	5 +	Rate	Rate[a]
Under 20	230,061	72,202	15,050	2,293	327	42.5	62.7
20–24	329,449	326,701	175,702	68,800	30,666	42.5	51.9
25–29	114,920	208,667	207,081	132,424	123,419	52.3	49.9
30–34	39,487	83,228	117,300	98,301	149,919	87.7	70.9
35–39	14,208	28,466	45,026	46,075	104,088	264.0	192.6
40 and over	3,052	5,375	8,660	9,834	34,392	864.4	582.9
Crude rate	56.3	67.6	83.3	115.5	167.1	89.5	79.2[c]
Adjusted rate[b]	93.0	92.7	87.3	94.3	84.8	90.7[c]	

The last column contains rates specific for maternal age and indirectly adjusted for birth order, with the standard set of rates specific for birth order being that of the total sample. Thus, for example,

$$c_{20-24(\text{indirect})} = 51.9 = 89.5 \times \frac{42.5 \times 9.31318}{56.3 \times 3.29449 + \cdots + 167.1 \times 0.30666}.$$

[b]The last row contains rates specific for birth order and indirectly adjusted for maternal age, with the standard set of rates specific for maternal age being that of the total sample. Thus, for example,

$$c_{2(\text{indirect})} = 92.7 = 89.5 \times \frac{67.6 \times 7.24639}{42.5 \times 0.72202 + \cdots + 864.4 \times 0.05375}.$$

[c]The overall rates based on the two series of indirectly adjusted rates will almost never equal each other, nor will either of them equal the overall crude rate.

ment, the method just described, may be applied. If the specific rates are not available or are based on small sample sizes, then a method due to Mantel and Stark (1968), based on indirect adjustment, may be applied.

It might have happened that the data required to calculate rates specific for maternal age and birth order simultaneously did not exist. In fact, the only data available might have been those in Table 19.6, together with the crude rates for birth order and for maternal age.

In contrast to the summarizing role played by the direct adjusted rates, the indirect adjusted rates, presented in the last row and last column of Table 19.6, must almost of necessity be calculated when the schedules of specific rates do not exist. They must be interpreted with a great deal of caution, however.

Two awkward features of the indirectly adjusted rates can be seen. For one thing, they do not yield equal overall rates. For another, the indirectly adjusted rates for some of the maternal age categories are totally out of the range of the specific rates (compare, e.g., the indirect adjusted rate of 62.7

for the first maternal age category with the specific rates ranging from 0 to 46.5, as seen in Table 19.5).

As a means of correcting these and possibly other anomalies, Mantel and Stark (1968) recommend the following procedure.

1. Beginning with the schedule of crude rates specific to maternal age, obtain the indirect adjusted rates specific for birth order. These have already been calculated and appear in the final row of Table 19.6.

2. Using *these latter rates* as the standard schedule, calculate the indirect adjusted rates specific for maternal age. Multiply the obtained rates by the ratio of the expected total crude rate (90.7) to the actual crude rate (89.5):

Maternal age	Under 20	20–24	25–29	30–34	35–39	40 and Over
Adjusted rate	41.6	42.0	52.4	89.0	270.3	892.9

For example, 41.6 is calculated as

$$41.6 = \frac{42.5}{92.7} \times 89.5 \times \frac{90.7}{89.5} = \frac{42.5 \times 90.7}{92.7},$$

where 42.5 is the crude rate in the first maternal age category, 90.7 is the overall expected crude rate, and

$$92.7 = \frac{93.0 \times 2.30061 + 92.7 \times 0.72202 + \cdots + 84.8 \times 0.00327}{3.19933}.$$

3. Continue in the same manner, each time using the previous set of indirect adjusted rates for one of the two variables to generate a new set for the other variable. Multiply each rate in the new set by the ratio of the expected total crude rate based on the previous set to the actual total crude rate.

4. Stop the process when successive sets of rates are unchanged. Here, about four cycles were necessary.

5. The sets of rates we end up with are

Maternal age	Under 20	20–24	25–29	30–34	35–39	40 and Over
Adjusted rate	41.0	41.8	52.6	89.7	273.3	904.5

for maternal age, and

Birth order	1	2	3	4	5 +
Adjusted rate	95.2	93.7	87.3	93.6	83.6

for birth order.

6. These two schedules of rates have the property that either, when used as the standard, implies the other. Furthermore, each of these rates happens for these data to lie within the range of the specific rates. This need not always occur with the Mantel-Stark adjustment method. Finally, their adjusted rates both yield the same expected total rate, 91.2. This final property would not have held had we not, at every step, multiplied the general set of rates by the ratio of the total expected rate based on the preceding set of rates to the total observed rate.

The inferences from these adjusted rates are the same as were drawn previously: a strong effect of maternal age and little if any effect of birth order. Recall, however, that here we have made no use at all of the specific rates.

The Mantel-Stark procedure has the property that it will yield the same results no matter what set of rates one starts with, although the number of steps will vary with the starting set.

Several authors consider regression models for the standardized mortality/morbidity ratio (SMR) (Berry, 1970; Breslow and Day, 1975; Gail, 1978; Fay, 1999). The approach of Gail (1978) is typical. For example, let Y_{ij} be the number of deaths or events in stratum i of population j ($i = 1, \ldots, I$, $j = 1, \ldots, J$). Y_{ij} is assumed to be a Poisson random variable with mean $N_j p_{ij} c_{ij}$, where N_j is the total size of population j, p_{ij} is the proportion of population j in stratum i, and c_{ij} is the event rate in stratum i in study population j. It is further assumed that $c_{ij} = c_{Si} \theta_j$, where c_{Si} is the event rate of stratum i for the standard population and θ_j is the rate ratio comparing the study population with the standard population. Note that θ_j is the estimand of the SMR. The mean of the Poisson random variable Y_{ij} is $\mu_{ij} = N_j p_{ij} c_{Si} \theta_j$, or

$$\ln \mu_{ij} = \ln(N p_{ij} c_{Si}) + \ln \theta_j.$$

The maximum likelihood estimate of θ_j can be obtained by maximizing the likelihood function

$$\prod_{i=1}^{I} \prod_{j=1}^{J} \frac{e^{-\mu_{ij}} \mu_{ij}^{Y_{ij}}}{Y_{ij}!}.$$

This is a Poisson regression problem which can be solved by the methods of Chapter 12. Note that because the number of people at risk, Np_{ij}, and the event rate of the standard population are assumed known, $\ln(Np_{ij} c_{Si})$ should be declared as an offset in standard programs for Poisson regression.

Testing equality of SMRs across different populations can be accomplished using the standard likelihood ratio, Wald, or score tests, and regression models of the form $\ln \theta_j = \beta_0 + \beta_X X_j$ for population-level covariates are straightforward to fit. McCullagh and Nelder (1989, ch. 5) show how Poisson regression models can be used to draw inferences about θ_j. Clayton and Kaldor (1987) considered the case in which Y_{ij} are not independent. When the strata represent geographical areas, the number of events may be correlated due to spatial proximity. The authors assume the Y_{ij}'s are conditionally independent given θ_j, with θ_j distributed as gamma variates. This is a random effects model for Poisson outcomes (see Section 12.3).

PROBLEMS

19.1. The following data are from Table 2 of Discher and Feinberg (1969).

Age-Specific Rates of Abnormal Lung Functioning in Males
Employed in Manufacturing or Service Industries

	Manufacturing		Services	
Age Interval	Number	% Abnormal	Number	% Abnormal
20–29	403	2.2	256	4.8
30–39	688	3.2	525	3.2
40–49	683	2.2	599	2.8
50–59	539	6.9	453	6.6
60 +	133	12.8	155	9.0

(a) Comparing the age-specific rates for the two kinds of industries, what conclusions would you be willing to draw?

(b) What do you think would be gained by calculating an age-adjusted rate for each kind of industry and then comparing the adjusted rates? What do you think might be lost?

(c) Consider the three following standard age distributions:

	Standard		
Age Interval	1	2	3
20–29	0.25	0.05	0.07
30–39	0.25	0.05	0.75
40–49	0.30	0.10	0.06
50–59	0.10	0.40	0.06
60 +	0.10	0.40	0.06

(1) The first standard distribution is concentrated below age 49. What are the values of the two direct adjusted rates using this standard? What are the direction and magnitude of the difference between them?

(2) The second standard distribution is concentrated above age 50. What are the values of the two direct adjusted rates using this standard? What are the direction and magnitude of the difference between them?

(3) The third standard distribution is concentrated in the age interval 30–39. What are the values of the two direct adjusted rates using this standard? What are the direction and magnitude of the difference between them?

(d) Using the age distribution of the total sample as a standard, calculate two direct adjusted rates for both kinds of industries, one for the age interval 20–49 and the other for the interval 50 and over. Do the comparisons now seem fair to the data?

REFERENCES

Berry, G. (1970). Parametric analysis of disease incidences in multiway tables. *Biometrics*, **26**, 572–579.

Breslow, N. E. and Day, N. E. (1975). Indirect standardization and multiplicative models for rates, with reference to the age adjustment of cancer incidence and relative frequency data. *J. Chronic Dis.*, **28**, 289–303.

Chiang, C. L. (1961). Standard error of the age-adjusted death rate. *U.S. Dept. of Health, Education and Welfare: Vital Statist.—Special Rep.*, **47**, 271–285.

Clayton, D. and Kaldor, J. (1987). Empirical Bayes estimates of age-standardized relative risks for use in disease mapping. *Biometrics*, **43**, 671–681.

Cochran, W. G. (1968). The effectiveness of adjustment by subclassification in removing bias in observational studies. *Biometrics*, **24**, 295–313.

DiCiccio, T. and Efron, B. (1992). More accurate confidence intervals in exponential families. *Biometrika*, **79**, 231–245.

Discher, D. P. and Feinberg, H. C. (1969). Screening for chronic pulmonary disease: Survey of 10,000 industrial workers. *Am. J. Public Health*, **59**, 1857–1867.

Dobson, A. J., Kuulasmaa, K., Eberle, E., and Scherer, J. (1991). Confidence intervals for weighted sums of Poisson parameters. *Statist. in Med.*, **10**, 457–462.

Doll, R. and Cook, P. (1967). Summarizing indices for comparison of cancer incidence data. *Int. J. Cancer*, **2**, 269–279.

El-Badry, M. A. (1969). Higher female than male mortality in some countries of south Asia: A digest. *J. Am. Statist. Assoc.*, **64**, 1234–1244.

Elveback, L. R. (1966). Discussion of "Indices of mortality and tests of their statistical significance." *Hum. Biol.*, **38**, 322–324.

Fay, M. P. (1999). Approximate confidence intervals for rate ratios from directly standardized rates with sparse data. *Comm. Statist.*, **A28**, 2141–2160.

Fay, M. P. and Feuer, E. J. (1997). Confidence intervals for directly standardized rates: A method based on the gamma distribution. *Statist. in Med.*, **16**, 791–801.

Gail, M. (1978). The analysis of heterogeneity for indirect standardized mortality ratios. *J. R. Statist. Soc., Ser. A*, **141**, 224–234.

Hemphill, F. M. and Ament, R. P. (1970). Quantitative assessment of subcategory contributions to observed change in relative frequencies. Paper read at annual meeting of American Public Health Association, Houston.

Kalton, G. (1968). Standardization: A technique to control for extraneous variables. *Appl. Statist.*, **17**, 118–136.

Keyfitz, N. (1966). Sampling variance of standardized mortality rates. *Hum. Biol.*, **38**, 309–317.

Kilpatrick, S. J. (1963). Mortality comparisons in socio-economic groups. *Appl. Statist.*, **12**, 65–86.

Kitagawa, E. M. (1955). Components of a difference between two rates. *J. Am. Statist. Assoc.*, **50**, 1168–1194.

Kitagawa, E. M. (1964). Standardized comparisons in population research. *Demography*, **1**, 296–315.

Kitagawa, E. M. (1966). Theoretical considerations in the selection of a mortality index, and some empirical comparisons. *Hum. Biol.*, **38**, 293–308.

Kupper, L. L., McMichael, A. J., Symons, M. J., and Most, B. M. (1978). On the utility of proportional mortality analysis. *J. Chronic Dis.*, **31**, 15–22.

Mantel, N. and Stark, C. R. (1968). Computation of indirect-adjusted rates in the presence of confounding. *Biometrics*, **24**, 997–1005.

Mausner, J. S. and Bahn, A. K. (1974). *Epidemiology: An introductory text*. Philadelphia: W. B. Saunders.

McCullagh, P. and Nelder, J. A. (1989). *Generalized linear models*, 2nd ed. New York: Chapman & Hall.

Miettienen, O. S. (1972). Components of the crude risk ratio. *Am. J. Epidemiol.*, **96**, 168–172.

Spiegelman, M. and Marks, H. H. (1966). Empirical testing of standards for the age adjustment of death rates by the direct method. *Hum. Biol.*, **38**, 280–292.

Stark, C. R. and Mantel, N. (1966). Effects of maternal age and birth order on the risk of mongolism and leukemia. *J. Natl. Cancer Inst.*, **37**, 687–698.

Swift, M. B. (1995). Simple confidence intervals for standardized rates based on the approximate bootstrap method. *Statist. in Med.*, **14**, 1875–1888.

Ulm, K. (1990). A simple method to calculate the confidence interval of a standardized mortality ratio (SMR). *Am. J. Epidemiol.*, **131**, 373–375.

Vandenbroucke, J. P. (1982). A shortcut method for calculating the 95 percent confidence interval of the standardized mortality ratio. *Am. J. Epidemiol.*, **115**, 303–304.

Woolsey, T. D. (1959). Adjusted death rates and other indices of mortality. Chapter 4 in F. E. Linder and R. D. Grove (Eds.), *Vital statistics rates in the United States, 1900–1940*. Washington, D.C.: U.S. Government Printing Office.

Yerushalmy, J. (1951). A mortality index for use in place of the age-adjusted death rate. *Am. J. Public Health*, **41**, 907–922.

Yule, G. U. (1934). On some points relating to vital statistics, more especially statistics of occupation mortality. *J. R. Statist. Soc.*, **97**, 1–72.

APPENDIX A

Numerical Tables

Statistical Methods for Rates and Proportions, Third Edition
By Joseph L. Fleiss, Bruce Levin, and Myunghee Cho Paik
ISBN 0-471-52629-0   Copyright © 2003 John Wiley & Sons, Inc.

Table A.1. *Critical values of the normal distribution*

Z	P	Z	P	Z	P
0.0	1.0000	1.2	0.2301	2.4	0.0164
0.1	0.9203	1.282	0.20	2.5	0.0124
0.126	0.90	1.3	0.1936	2.576	0.01
0.2	0.8415	1.4	0.1615	2.6	0.0093
0.3	0.7642	1.440	0.15	2.7	0.0069
0.385	0.70	1.5	0.1336	2.8	0.0051
0.4	0.6892	1.6	0.1096	2.813	0.005
0.5	0.6171	1.645	0.10	2.9	0.0037
0.524	0.60	1.7	0.0891	3.0	0.0027
0.6	0.5485	1.8	0.0719	3.090	0.002
0.674	0.50	1.9	0.0574	3.1	0.0019
0.7	0.4839	1.960	0.05	3.2	0.0014
0.8	0.4237	2.0	0.0455	3.3	0.0010
0.842	0.40	2.1	0.0357	3.4	0.0007
0.9	0.3681	2.2	0.0278	3.5	0.0005
1.0	0.3173	2.242	0.025	3.6	0.0003
1.036	0.30	2.3	0.0214	3.7	0.0002
1.1	0.2713	2.326	0.02	3.8	0.0001

P = area in the tails of the normal curve below $-Z$ and above $+Z$. In a test of significance, P is the significance level associated with the obtained value of Z.

The total area under the normal curve to the right of Z is $1 - P/2$ if Z is negative, and is $P/2$ if Z is positive.

Suppose one must find that value of Z such that the total area under the normal curve to the right of Z is $1 - B$. If $1 - B$ is greater than 0.50, take the value of Z corresponding to $P = 2B$, and affix a minus sign to it. If $1 - B$ is less than 0.50, take the value of Z corresponding to $P = 2(1 - B)$.

Source. Adapted from Tables 1 and 4 of *Biometrika tables for statisticians*, Vol. I, 2nd ed. E. S. Pearson and H. O. Hartley (Eds.), Cambridge University Press, 1958.

Table A.2. *Critical values of the chi squared distribution (cutting off probability α in upper tail)*

Degrees of Freedom	Critical Value					
	$\alpha = 0.10$	0.05	0.025	0.01	0.005	0.001
1	2.706	3.841	5.024	6.635	7.879	10.83
2	4.605	5.991	7.378	9.210	10.60	13.82
3	6.251	7.815	9.348	11.34	12.84	16.27
4	7.779	9.488	11.14	13.28	14.86	18.47
5	9.236	11.07	12.83	15.09	16.75	20.52
6	10.64	12.59	14.45	16.81	18.55	22.46
7	12.02	14.07	16.01	18.48	20.28	24.32
8	13.36	15.51	17.53	20.09	21.95	26.12
9	14.68	16.92	19.02	21.67	23.59	27.88
10	15.99	18.31	20.48	23.21	25.19	29.59
11	17.28	19.68	21.92	24.72	26.76	31.26
12	18.55	21.03	23.34	26.22	28.30	32.91
13	19.81	22.36	24.74	27.69	29.82	34.53
14	21.06	23.68	26.12	29.14	31.32	36.12
15	22.31	25.00	27.49	30.58	32.80	37.70
16	23.54	26.30	28.85	32.00	34.27	39.25
17	24.77	27.59	30.19	33.41	35.72	40.79
18	25.99	28.87	31.53	34.81	37.16	42.31
19	27.20	30.14	32.85	36.19	38.58	43.82
20	28.41	31.41	34.17	37.57	40.00	45.32
25	34.38	37.65	40.65	44.31	46.93	52.62
30	40.26	43.77	46.98	50.89	53.67	59.70
40	51.81	55.76	59.34	63.69	66.77	73.40
60	74.40	79.08	83.30	88.38	91.95	99.61
100	118.5	124.3	129.6	135.8	140.2	149.4

Table A.2. (*Concluded*)

Degrees of Freedom	Critical Value					
	$\alpha = 0.90$	0.95	0.975	0.99	0.995	0.999
1	0.01579	0.003932	0.0009821	0.0001571	0.00003927	0.000001571
2	0.2107	0.1026	0.0506	0.02010	0.01003	0.002001
3	0.5844	0.3518	0.2158	0.1148	0.07172	0.02430
4	1.064	0.7107	0.4844	0.2971	0.2070	0.09080
5	1.610	1.145	0.8312	0.5543	0.4117	0.2102
6	2.204	1.635	1.237	0.8721	0.6757	0.3811
7	2.833	2.167	1.690	1.239	0.9893	0.5985
8	3.490	2.733	2.180	1.646	1.344	0.8571
9	4.168	3.325	2.700	2.088	1.735	1.152
10	4.865	3.940	3.247	2.558	2.156	1.479
11	5.578	4.575	3.816	3.053	2.603	1.834
12	6.304	5.226	4.404	3.571	3.074	2.214
13	7.042	5.892	5.009	4.107	3.565	2.617
14	7.790	6.571	5.629	4.660	4.075	3.041
15	8.547	7.261	6.262	5.229	4.601	3.483
16	9.312	7.962	6.908	5.812	5.142	3.942
17	10.09	8.672	7.564	6.408	5.697	4.416
18	10.86	9.390	8.231	7.015	6.265	4.905
19	11.65	10.12	8.907	7.633	6.844	5.407
20	12.44	10.85	9.591	8.260	7.434	5.921
25	16.47	14.61	13.12	11.52	10.52	8.649
30	20.60	18.49	16.79	14.95	13.79	11.59
40	29.05	26.51	24.43	22.16	20.71	17.92
60	46.46	43.19	40.48	37.48	35.53	31.74
100	82.36	77.93	74.22	70.06	67.33	61.92

Table A.3. *Percentage points of the F distribution[a]*

$$P[F > F_{\nu_1, \nu_2; 0.05}] = 0.05$$

ν_2	Numerator df (ν_1)													
	1	2	3	4	5	6	8	12	15	20	30	60	∞
1	161.45	199.50	215.71	224.58	230.16	233.99	238.88	243.91	245.95	248.01	250.10	252.20	254.31
2	18.51	19.00	19.16	19.25	19.30	19.33	19.37	19.41	19.43	19.45	19.46	19.48	19.50
3	10.13	9.55	9.28	9.12	9.01	8.94	8.85	8.74	8.70	8.66	8.62	8.57	8.53
4	7.71	6.94	6.59	6.39	6.26	6.16	6.04	5.91	5.86	5.80	5.75	5.69	5.63
5	6.61	5.79	5.41	5.19	5.05	4.95	4.82	4.68	4.62	4.56	4.50	4.43	4.36
6	5.99	5.14	4.76	4.53	4.39	4.28	4.15	4.00	3.94	3.87	3.81	3.74	3.67
7	5.59	4.74	4.35	4.12	3.97	3.87	3.73	3.57	3.51	3.44	3.38	3.30	3.23
8	5.32	4.46	4.07	3.84	3.69	3.58	3.44	3.28	3.22	3.15	3.08	3.01	2.93
9	5.12	4.26	3.86	3.63	3.48	3.37	3.23	3.07	3.01	2.94	2.86	2.79	2.71
10	4.96	4.10	3.71	3.48	3.33	3.22	3.07	2.91	2.85	2.77	2.70	2.62	2.54
11	4.84	3.98	3.59	3.36	3.20	3.09	2.95	2.79	2.72	2.65	2.57	2.49	2.40
12	4.75	3.89	3.49	3.26	3.11	3.00	2.85	2.69	2.62	2.54	2.47	2.38	2.30
13	4.67	3.81	3.41	3.18	3.03	2.92	2.77	2.60	2.53	2.46	2.38	2.30	2.21
14	4.60	3.74	3.34	3.11	2.96	2.85	2.70	2.53	2.46	2.39	2.31	2.22	2.13
15	4.54	3.68	3.29	3.06	2.90	2.79	2.64	2.48	2.40	2.33	2.25	2.16	2.07

Denominator df (ν_2)

Denominator df (v_2)													
16	4.49	3.63	3.24	3.01	2.85	2.74	2.59	2.42	2.35	2.28	2.19	2.11	2.01
17	4.45	3.59	3.20	2.96	2.81	2.70	2.55	2.38	2.31	2.23	2.15	2.06	1.96
18	4.41	3.55	3.16	2.93	2.77	2.66	2.51	2.34	2.27	2.19	2.11	2.02	1.92
19	4.38	3.52	3.13	2.90	2.74	2.63	2.48	2.31	2.23	2.16	2.07	1.98	1.88
20	4.35	3.49	3.10	2.87	2.71	2.60	2.45	2.28	2.20	2.12	2.04	1.95	1.84
21	4.32	3.47	3.07	2.84	2.68	2.57	2.42	2.25	2.18	2.10	2.01	1.92	1.81
22	4.30	3.44	3.05	2.82	2.66	2.55	2.40	2.23	2.15	2.07	1.98	1.89	1.78
23	4.28	3.42	3.03	2.80	2.64	2.53	2.37	2.20	2.13	2.05	1.96	1.86	1.76
24	4.26	3.40	3.01	2.78	2.62	2.51	2.36	2.18	2.11	2.03	1.94	1.84	1.73
25	4.24	3.39	2.99	2.76	2.60	2.49	2.34	2.16	2.09	2.01	1.92	1.82	1.71
26	4.23	3.37	2.98	2.74	2.59	2.47	2.32	2.15	2.07	1.99	1.90	1.80	1.69
27	4.21	3.35	2.96	2.73	2.57	2.46	2.31	2.13	2.06	1.97	1.88	1.79	1.67
28	4.20	3.34	2.95	2.71	2.56	2.45	2.29	2.12	2.04	1.96	1.87	1.77	1.65
29	4.18	3.33	2.93	2.70	2.55	2.43	2.28	2.10	2.03	1.94	1.85	1.75	1.64
30	4.17	3.32	2.92	2.69	2.53	2.42	2.27	2.09	2.01	1.93	1.84	1.74	1.62
40	4.08	3.23	2.84	2.61	2.45	2.34	2.18	2.00	1.92	1.84	1.74	1.64	1.51
60	4.00	3.15	2.76	2.53	2.37	2.25	2.10	1.92	1.84	1.75	1.65	1.53	1.39
120	3.92	3.07	2.68	2.45	2.29	2.18	2.02	1.83	1.75	1.66	1.55	1.43	1.25
∞	3.84	3.00	2.60	2.37	2.21	2.10	1.94	1.75	1.67	1.57	1.46	1.32	1.00

[a]The tables give values of $F_{v_1, v_2; p}$ such that an F variable with v_1 and v_2 df exceeds $F_{v_1, v_2; p}$ with probability p, that is, $P[F > F_{v_1, v_2; p}] = p$. The first table gives critical values for $p = 0.05$, and the next tables give critical values for $p = 0.025$, 0.01, and 0.005.

Table A.3. (*Continued*)

$$P[F > F_{\nu_1, \nu_2; 0.025}] = 0.025$$

ν_2	Numerator df (ν_1)												
	1	2	3	4	5	6	8	12	15	20	30	60	∞
1	647.79	799.50	864.16	899.58	921.85	937.11	956.66	976.71	984.87	993.10	1001.41	1009.80	1018.26
2	38.51	39.00	39.17	39.25	39.30	39.33	39.37	39.41	39.43	39.45	39.46	39.48	39.50
3	17.44	16.04	15.44	15.10	14.88	14.73	14.54	14.34	14.25	14.17	14.08	13.99	13.90
4	12.22	10.65	9.98	9.60	9.36	9.20	8.98	8.75	8.66	8.56	8.46	8.36	8.26
5	10.01	8.43	7.76	7.39	7.15	6.98	6.76	6.52	6.43	6.33	6.23	6.12	6.02
6	8.81	7.26	6.60	6.23	5.99	5.82	5.60	5.37	5.27	5.17	5.07	4.96	4.85
7	8.07	6.54	5.89	5.52	5.29	5.12	4.90	4.67	4.57	4.47	4.36	4.25	4.14
8	7.57	6.06	5.42	5.05	4.82	4.65	4.43	4.20	4.10	4.00	3.89	3.78	3.67
9	7.21	5.71	5.08	4.72	4.48	4.32	4.10	3.87	3.77	3.67	3.56	3.45	3.33
10	6.94	5.46	4.83	4.47	4.24	4.07	3.85	3.62	3.52	3.42	3.31	3.20	3.08
11	6.72	5.26	4.63	4.28	4.04	3.88	3.66	3.43	3.33	3.23	3.12	3.00	2.88
12	6.55	5.10	4.47	4.12	3.89	3.73	3.51	3.28	3.18	3.07	2.96	2.85	2.72
13	6.41	4.97	4.35	4.00	3.77	3.60	3.39	3.15	3.05	2.95	2.84	2.72	2.60
14	6.30	4.86	4.24	3.89	3.66	3.50	3.29	3.05	2.95	2.84	2.73	2.61	2.49
15	6.20	4.77	4.15	3.80	3.58	3.41	3.20	2.96	2.86	2.76	2.64	2.52	2.40

Denominator df (ν_2)

654

Denominator df (ν_2)													
16	6.12	4.69	4.08	3.73	3.50	3.34	3.12	2.89	2.79	2.68	2.57	2.45	2.32
17	6.04	4.62	4.01	3.66	3.44	3.28	3.06	2.82	2.72	2.62	2.50	2.38	2.25
18	5.98	4.56	3.95	3.61	3.38	3.22	3.01	2.77	2.67	2.56	2.44	2.32	2.19
19	5.92	4.51	3.90	3.56	3.33	3.17	2.96	2.72	2.62	2.51	2.39	2.27	2.13
20	5.87	4.46	3.86	3.51	3.29	3.13	2.91	2.68	2.57	2.46	2.35	2.22	2.09
21	5.83	4.42	3.82	3.48	3.25	3.09	2.87	2.64	2.53	2.42	2.31	2.18	2.04
22	5.79	4.38	3.78	3.44	3.22	3.05	2.84	2.60	2.50	2.39	2.27	2.14	2.00
23	5.75	4.35	3.75	3.41	3.18	3.02	2.81	2.57	2.47	2.36	2.24	2.11	1.97
24	5.72	4.32	3.72	3.38	3.15	2.99	2.78	2.54	2.44	2.33	2.21	2.08	1.94
25	5.69	4.29	3.69	3.35	3.13	2.97	2.75	2.51	2.41	2.30	2.18	2.05	1.91
26	5.66	4.27	3.67	3.33	3.10	2.94	2.73	2.49	2.39	2.28	2.16	2.03	1.88
27	5.63	4.24	3.65	3.31	3.08	2.92	2.71	2.47	2.36	2.25	2.13	2.00	1.85
28	5.61	4.22	3.63	3.29	3.06	2.90	2.69	2.45	2.34	2.23	2.11	1.98	1.83
29	5.59	4.20	3.61	3.27	3.04	2.88	2.67	2.43	2.32	2.21	2.09	1.96	1.81
30	5.57	4.18	3.59	3.25	3.03	2.87	2.65	2.41	2.31	2.20	2.07	1.94	1.79
40	5.42	4.05	3.46	3.13	2.90	2.74	2.53	2.29	2.18	2.07	1.94	1.80	1.64
60	5.29	3.93	3.34	3.01	2.79	2.63	2.41	2.17	2.06	1.94	1.82	1.67	1.48
120	5.15	3.80	3.23	2.89	2.67	2.52	2.30	2.05	1.94	1.82	1.69	1.53	1.31
∞	5.02	3.69	3.12	2.79	2.57	2.41	2.19	1.94	1.83	1.71	1.57	1.39	1.00

[a] The tables give values of $F_{\nu_1, \nu_2; p}$ such that an F variable with ν_1 and ν_2 df exceeds $F_{\nu_1, \nu_2; p}$ with probability p, that is, $P[F > F_{\nu_1, \nu_2; p}] = p$. The first table gives critical values for $p = 0.05$, and the next tables give critical values for $p = 0.025$, 0.01, and 0.005.

Table A.3. (Continued)

$$P[F > F_{\nu_1, \nu_2; 0.01}] = 0.01$$

ν_2	Numerator df (ν_1)												
	1	2	3	4	5	6	8	12	15	20	30	60	∞
1	4052.18	4999.50	5403.35	5624.58	5763.65	5858.99	5981.07	6106.32	6157.28	6208.73	6260.65	6313.03	6365.86
2	98.50	99.00	99.17	99.25	99.30	99.33	99.37	99.42	99.43	99.45	99.47	99.48	99.50
3	34.12	30.82	29.46	28.71	28.24	27.91	27.49	27.05	26.87	26.69	26.50	26.32	26.13
4	21.20	18.00	16.69	15.98	15.52	15.21	14.80	14.37	14.20	14.02	13.84	13.65	13.46
5	16.26	13.27	12.06	11.39	10.97	10.67	10.29	9.89	9.72	9.55	9.38	9.20	9.02
6	13.75	10.92	9.78	9.15	8.75	8.47	8.10	7.72	7.56	7.40	7.23	7.06	6.88
7	12.25	9.55	8.45	7.85	7.46	7.19	6.84	6.47	6.31	6.16	5.99	5.82	5.65
8	11.26	8.65	7.59	7.01	6.63	6.37	6.03	5.67	5.52	5.36	5.20	5.03	4.86
9	10.56	8.02	6.99	6.42	6.06	5.80	5.47	5.11	4.96	4.81	4.65	4.48	4.31
10	10.04	7.56	6.55	5.99	5.64	5.39	5.06	4.71	4.56	4.41	4.25	4.08	3.91
11	9.65	7.21	6.22	5.67	5.32	5.07	4.74	4.40	4.25	4.10	3.94	3.78	3.60
12	9.33	6.93	5.95	5.41	5.06	4.82	4.50	4.16	4.01	3.86	3.70	3.54	3.36
13	9.07	6.70	5.74	5.21	4.86	4.62	4.30	3.96	3.82	3.66	3.51	3.34	3.17
14	8.86	6.51	5.56	5.04	4.69	4.46	4.14	3.80	3.66	3.51	3.35	3.18	3.00
15	8.68	6.36	5.42	4.89	4.56	4.32	4.00	3.67	3.52	3.37	3.21	3.05	2.87

Denominator df (ν_2)

Denominator df (ν_2)

ν_2													
16	8.53	6.23	5.29	4.77	4.44	4.20	3.89	3.55	3.41	3.26	3.10	2.93	2.75
17	8.40	6.11	5.18	4.67	4.34	4.10	3.79	3.46	3.31	3.16	3.00	2.83	2.65
18	8.29	6.01	5.09	4.58	4.25	4.01	3.71	3.37	3.23	3.08	2.92	2.75	2.57
19	8.18	5.93	5.01	4.50	4.17	3.94	3.63	3.30	3.15	3.00	2.84	2.67	2.49
20	8.10	5.85	4.94	4.43	4.10	3.87	3.56	3.23	3.09	2.94	2.78	2.61	2.42
21	8.02	5.78	4.87	4.37	4.04	3.81	3.51	3.17	3.03	2.88	2.72	2.55	2.36
22	7.95	5.72	4.82	4.31	3.99	3.76	3.45	3.12	2.98	2.83	2.67	2.50	2.31
23	7.88	5.66	4.76	4.26	3.94	3.71	3.41	3.07	2.93	2.78	2.62	2.45	2.26
24	7.82	5.61	4.72	4.22	3.90	3.67	3.36	3.03	2.89	2.74	2.58	2.40	2.21
25	7.77	5.57	4.68	4.18	3.85	3.63	3.32	2.99	2.85	2.70	2.54	2.36	2.17
26	7.72	5.53	4.64	4.14	3.82	3.59	3.29	2.96	2.81	2.66	2.50	2.33	2.13
27	7.68	5.49	4.60	4.11	3.78	3.56	3.26	2.93	2.78	2.63	2.47	2.29	2.10
28	7.64	5.45	4.57	4.07	3.75	3.53	3.23	2.90	2.75	2.60	2.44	2.26	2.06
29	7.60	5.42	4.54	4.04	3.73	3.50	3.20	2.87	2.73	2.57	2.41	2.23	2.03
30	7.56	5.39	4.51	4.02	3.70	3.47	3.17	2.84	2.70	2.55	2.39	2.21	2.01
40	7.31	5.18	4.31	3.83	3.51	3.29	2.99	2.66	2.52	2.37	2.20	2.02	1.80
60	7.08	4.98	4.13	3.65	3.34	3.12	2.82	2.50	2.35	2.20	2.03	1.84	1.60
120	6.85	4.79	3.95	3.48	3.17	2.96	2.66	2.34	2.19	2.03	1.86	1.66	1.38
∞	6.63	4.61	3.78	3.32	3.02	2.80	2.51	2.18	2.04	1.88	1.70	1.47	1.00

[a]The tables give values of $F_{\nu_1, \nu_2; p}$ such that an F variable with ν_1 and ν_2 df exceeds $F_{\nu_1, \nu_2; p}$ with probability p, that is, $P[F > F_{\nu_1, \nu_2; p}] = p$. The first table gives critical values for p = 0.05, and the next tables give critical values for p = 0.025, 0.01, and 0.005.

Table A.3. (*Concluded*)

$$P[F > F_{\nu_1, \nu_2; 0.005}] = 0.005$$

ν_2	Numerator df (ν_1)												
	1	2	3	4	5	6	8	12	15	20	30	60	∞
1	16210.72	19999.50	21614.74	22499.58	23055.80	23437.11	23925.41	24426.37	24630.21	24835.97	25043.63	25253.60	25464.46
2	198.50	199.00	199.17	199.25	199.30	199.33	199.37	199.42	199.43	199.45	199.47	199.48	199.50
3	55.55	49.80	47.47	46.19	45.39	44.84	44.13	43.39	43.08	42.78	42.47	42.15	41.83
4	31.33	26.28	24.26	23.15	22.46	21.97	21.35	20.70	20.44	20.17	19.89	19.61	19.32
5	22.78	18.31	16.53	15.56	14.94	14.51	13.96	13.38	13.15	12.90	12.66	12.40	12.14
6	18.63	14.54	12.92	12.03	11.46	11.07	10.57	10.03	9.81	9.59	9.36	9.12	8.88
7	16.24	12.40	10.88	10.05	9.52	9.16	8.68	8.18	7.97	7.75	7.53	7.31	7.08
8	14.69	11.04	9.60	8.81	8.30	7.95	7.50	7.01	6.81	6.61	6.40	6.18	5.95
9	13.61	10.11	8.72	7.96	7.47	7.13	6.69	6.23	6.03	5.83	5.62	5.41	5.19
10	12.83	9.43	8.08	7.34	6.87	6.54	6.12	5.66	5.47	5.27	5.07	4.86	4.64
11	12.23	8.91	7.60	6.88	6.42	6.10	5.68	5.24	5.05	4.86	4.65	4.45	4.23
12	11.75	8.51	7.23	6.52	6.07	5.76	5.35	4.91	4.72	4.53	4.33	4.12	3.90
13	11.37	8.19	6.93	6.23	5.79	5.48	5.08	4.64	4.46	4.27	4.07	3.87	3.65
14	11.06	7.92	6.68	6.00	5.56	5.26	4.86	4.43	4.25	4.06	3.86	3.66	3.44
15	10.80	7.70	6.48	5.80	5.37	5.07	4.67	4.25	4.07	3.88	3.69	3.48	3.26

Denominator df (ν_2)

Denominator df (ν_2)													
16	10.58	7.51	6.30	5.64	5.21	4.91	4.52	4.10	3.92	3.73	3.54	3.33	3.11
17	10.38	7.35	6.16	5.50	5.07	4.78	4.39	3.97	3.79	3.61	3.41	3.21	2.98
18	10.22	7.21	6.03	5.37	4.96	4.66	4.28	3.86	3.68	3.50	3.30	3.10	2.87
19	10.07	7.09	5.92	5.27	4.85	4.56	4.18	3.76	3.59	3.40	3.21	3.00	2.78
20	9.94	6.99	5.82	5.17	4.76	4.47	4.09	3.68	3.50	3.32	3.12	2.92	2.69
21	9.83	6.89	5.73	5.09	4.68	4.39	4.01	3.60	3.43	3.24	3.05	2.84	2.61
22	9.73	6.81	5.65	5.02	4.61	4.32	3.94	3.54	3.36	3.18	2.98	2.77	2.55
23	9.63	6.73	5.58	4.95	4.54	4.26	3.88	3.47	3.30	3.12	2.92	2.71	2.48
24	9.55	6.66	5.52	4.89	4.49	4.20	3.83	3.42	3.25	3.06	2.87	2.66	2.43
25	9.48	6.60	5.46	4.84	4.43	4.15	3.78	3.37	3.20	3.01	2.82	2.61	2.38
26	9.41	6.54	5.41	4.79	4.38	4.10	3.73	3.33	3.15	2.97	2.77	2.56	2.33
27	9.34	6.49	5.36	4.74	4.34	4.06	3.69	3.28	3.11	2.93	2.73	2.52	2.29
28	9.28	6.44	5.32	4.70	4.30	4.02	3.65	3.25	3.07	2.89	2.69	2.48	2.25
29	9.23	6.40	5.28	4.66	4.26	3.98	3.61	3.21	3.04	2.86	2.66	2.45	2.21
30	9.18	6.35	5.24	4.62	4.23	3.95	3.58	3.18	3.01	2.82	2.63	2.42	2.18
40	8.83	6.07	4.98	4.37	3.99	3.71	3.35	2.95	2.78	2.60	2.40	2.18	1.93
60	8.49	5.79	4.73	4.14	3.76	3.49	3.13	2.74	2.57	2.39	2.19	1.96	1.69
120	8.18	5.54	4.50	3.92	3.55	3.28	2.93	2.54	2.37	2.19	1.98	1.75	1.43
∞	7.88	5.30	4.28	3.72	3.35	3.09	2.74	2.36	2.19	2.00	1.79	1.53	1.00

[a] The tables give values of $F_{\nu_1, \nu_2; p}$ such that an F variable with ν_1 and ν_2 df exceeds $F_{\nu_1, \nu_2; p}$ with probability p, that is, $P[F > F_{\nu_1, \nu_2; p}] = p$. The first table gives critical values for $p = 0.05$, and the next tables give critical values for $p = 0.025$, 0.01, and 0.005.

Table A.4. *Sample sizes per group for a two-tailed test of two proportions*

| | | $P_1 = 0.05$ | | | | | | | | |
| | | Power | | | | | | | | |
P_2	α	0.99	0.95	0.90	0.85	0.80	0.75	0.70	0.65	0.50
0.10	0.01	1368	1025	863	762	686	624	572	525	407
	0.02	1235	911	760	665	595	538	489	446	339
	0.05	1054	758	621	536	474	423	381	344	252
	0.10	910	637	513	437	381	336	299	267	188
	0.20	758	512	402	336	288	250	219	192	128
0.15	0.01	447	337	285	253	228	209	192	177	139
	0.02	404	300	252	221	199	180	165	151	117
	0.05	345	251	207	179	160	143	130	118	88
	0.10	299	212	172	147	130	115	103	93	67
	0.20	250	171	136	115	99	87	77	68	47
0.20	0.01	241	183	155	138	125	115	106	98	77
	0.02	218	163	137	121	109	99	91	84	65
	0.05	187	136	113	99	88	79	72	66	50
	0.10	162	115	94	81	72	64	58	52	38
	0.20	135	94	75	64	55	49	44	39	28
0.25	0.01	157	120	102	91	83	76	70	65	52
	0.02	142	107	90	80	72	66	61	56	44
	0.05	122	90	75	65	58	53	48	44	34
	0.10	106	76	62	54	48	43	39	35	26
	0.20	88	62	50	42	37	33	29	26	19
0.30	0.01	113	87	74	66	60	55	51	48	38
	0.02	102	77	66	58	53	48	44	41	33
	0.05	88	65	54	48	43	39	35	32	25
	0.10	76	55	45	39	35	32	29	26	20
	0.20	64	45	36	31	27	24	22	20	14
0.35	0.01	86	66	57	51	46	43	40	37	30
	0.02	78	59	50	45	41	37	34	32	25
	0.05	67	50	42	37	33	30	28	25	20
	0.10	58	42	35	30	27	25	22	20	16
	0.20	48	34	28	24	21	19	17	16	12
0.40	0.01	68	53	45	41	37	34	32	30	24
	0.02	62	47	40	36	33	30	28	26	21
	0.05	53	39	33	29	27	24	22	21	16
	0.10	46	34	28	24	22	20	18	17	13
	0.20	38	27	22	19	17	15	14	13	10
0.45	0.01	55	43	37	33	31	28	26	25	20
	0.02	50	38	33	29	27	25	23	21	17
	0.05	43	32	27	24	22	20	18	17	14
	0.10	37	27	23	20	18	16	15	14	11
	0.20	31	22	18	16	14	13	12	11	8
0.50	0.01	46	36	31	28	26	24	22	21	17
	0.02	41	32	27	25	23	21	19	18	15
	0.05	35	27	23	20	18	17	16	14	12
	0.10	31	23	19	17	15	14	13	12	9
	0.20	26	19	15	13	12	11	10	9	7

Table A.4. (*Continued*)

P_2	α	$P_1 = 0.05$ (*Continued*) Power								
		0.99	0.95	0.90	0.85	0.80	0.75	0.70	0.65	0.50
0.55	0.01	38	30	26	24	22	20	19	18	15
	0.02	35	27	23	21	19	18	17	16	13
	0.05	30	23	19	17	16	14	13	12	10
	0.10	26	19	16	14	13	12	11	10	8
	0.20	21	16	13	11	10	9	9	8	6
0.60	0.01	32	26	22	20	19	18	16	16	13
	0.02	29	23	20	18	17	15	14	13	11
	0.05	25	19	16	15	14	12	12	11	9
	0.10	22	16	14	12	11	10	9	9	7
	0.20	18	13	11	10	9	8	7	7	5
0.65	0.01	28	22	19	18	16	15	14	14	11
	0.02	25	20	17	16	14	13	13	12	10
	0.05	21	16	14	13	12	11	10	9	8
	0.10	18	14	12	11	10	9	8	8	6
	0.20	15	11	10	9	8	7	7	6	5
0.70	0.01	23	19	17	15	14	13	13	12	10
	0.02	21	17	15	14	13	12	11	10	9
	0.05	18	14	12	11	10	10	9	8	7
	0.10	16	12	10	9	9	8	7	7	6
	0.20	13	10	8	7	7	6	6	5	4
0.75	0.01	20	16	15	13	13	12	11	11	9
	0.02	18	15	13	12	11	10	10	9	8
	0.05	15	12	11	10	9	8	8	7	6
	0.10	13	10	9	8	7	7	7	6	5
	0.20	11	8	7	6	6	5	5	5	4
0.80	0.01	17	14	13	12	11	10	10	9	8
	0.02	15	13	11	10	10	9	9	8	7
	0.05	13	10	9	8	8	7	7	7	6
	0.10	11	9	8	7	7	6	6	5	5
	0.20	9	7	6	6	5	5	5	4	4
0.85	0.01	15	12	11	10	10	9	9	8	7
	0.02	13	11	10	9	8	8	8	7	6
	0.05	11	9	8	7	7	7	6	6	5
	0.10	9	8	7	6	6	5	5	5	4
	0.20	8	6	5	5	5	4	4	4	3
0.90	0.01	12	10	9	9	8	8	8	7	7
	0.02	11	9	8	8	7	7	7	7	6
	0.05	9	8	7	6	6	6	6	5	5
	0.10	8	6	6	5	5	5	5	4	4
	0.20	6	5	5	4	4	4	4	3	3
0.95	0.01	10	9	8	8	7	7	7	7	6
	0.02	9	8	7	7	7	6	6	6	5
	0.05	8	6	6	6	5	5	5	5	4
	0.10	6	5	5	5	4	4	4	4	4
	0.20	5	4	4	4	4	3	3	3	3

Table A.4. (*Continued*)

P_2	α	0.99	0.95	0.90	0.85	0.80	0.75	0.70	0.65	0.50
						$P_1 = 0.10$				
						Power				
0.15	0.01	2137	1595	1340	1179	1060	963	880	806	620
	0.02	1928	1416	1176	1027	916	826	749	682	513
	0.05	1642	1174	957	823	725	646	579	520	375
	0.10	1415	984	787	667	579	509	450	399	275
	0.20	1175	787	613	508	433	373	324	281	182
0.20	0.01	627	471	397	351	316	288	264	243	189
	0.02	566	419	349	306	274	248	226	206	157
	0.05	483	348	286	247	219	196	176	159	117
	0.10	417	293	236	201	176	156	139	124	88
	0.20	347	236	185	155	133	116	102	89	60
0.25	0.01	316	238	202	179	162	147	136	125	98
	0.02	285	212	178	156	140	127	116	107	82
	0.05	244	177	146	127	113	101	91	83	62
	0.10	211	149	121	104	91	81	73	65	47
	0.20	176	120	96	81	70	61	54	48	33
0.30	0.01	196	149	126	112	102	93	86	79	63
	0.02	178	133	112	98	89	81	74	68	53
	0.05	152	111	92	80	71	64	58	53	40
	0.10	131	94	76	66	58	52	47	42	31
	0.20	110	76	61	51	45	39	35	31	22
0.35	0.01	136	104	88	79	72	66	61	56	45
	0.02	123	93	78	69	62	57	52	48	38
	0.05	105	77	64	56	50	45	41	38	29
	0.10	91	65	54	46	41	37	33	30	22
	0.20	76	53	43	36	32	28	25	22	16
0.40	0.01	101	77	66	59	54	49	46	42	34
	0.02	91	69	58	52	47	43	39	36	29
	0.05	78	58	48	42	38	34	31	29	22
	0.10	68	49	40	35	31	28	25	23	17
	0.20	56	40	32	27	24	21	19	17	13
0.45	0.01	78	60	51	46	42	39	36	33	27
	0.02	71	54	46	41	37	34	31	29	23
	0.05	60	45	38	33	30	27	25	23	18
	0.10	52	38	31	27	24	22	20	18	14
	0.20	44	31	25	22	19	17	15	14	10
0.50	0.01	62	48	41	37	34	31	29	27	22
	0.02	56	43	37	33	30	27	25	23	19
	0.05	48	36	30	27	24	22	20	19	15
	0.10	42	30	25	22	20	18	16	15	12
	0.20	35	25	20	18	16	14	13	11	9

Table A.4. (*Continued*)

					$P_1 = 0.10$ (*Continued*)					
					Power					
P_2	α	0.99	0.95	0.90	0.85	0.80	0.75	0.70	0.65	0.50
0.55	0.01	51	39	34	31	28	26	24	23	19
	0.02	46	35	30	27	25	23	21	20	16
	0.05	39	29	25	22	20	18	17	16	12
	0.10	34	25	21	18	16	15	14	13	10
	0.20	28	20	17	15	13	12	11	10	7
0.60	0.01	42	33	28	26	24	22	20	19	16
	0.02	38	29	25	23	21	19	18	17	14
	0.05	32	24	21	18	17	15	14	13	11
	0.10	28	21	17	15	14	13	12	11	8
	0.20	23	17	14	12	11	10	9	8	6
0.65	0.01	35	27	24	22	20	19	17	16	14
	0.02	31	24	21	19	18	16	15	14	12
	0.05	27	20	18	16	14	13	12	11	9
	0.10	23	17	15	13	12	11	10	9	7
	0.20	19	14	12	10	9	8	8	7	6
0.70	0.01	29	23	20	19	17	16	15	14	12
	0.02	26	21	18	16	15	14	13	12	10
	0.05	22	17	15	13	12	11	11	10	8
	0.10	19	15	13	11	10	9	9	8	7
	0.20	16	12	10	9	8	7	7	6	5
0.75	0.01	25	20	17	16	15	14	13	12	11
	0.02	22	18	15	14	13	12	11	11	9
	0.05	19	15	13	12	11	10	9	9	7
	0.10	16	13	11	10	9	8	8	7	6
	0.20	14	10	9	8	7	6	6	6	4
0.80	0.01	21	17	15	14	13	12	11	11	9
	0.02	19	15	13	12	11	11	10	9	8
	0.05	16	13	11	10	9	9	8	8	6
	0.10	14	11	9	8	8	7	7	6	5
	0.20	11	9	7	7	6	6	5	5	4
0.85	0.01	18	14	13	12	11	11	10	10	8
	0.02	16	13	11	11	10	9	9	8	7
	0.05	13	11	9	9	8	8	7	7	6
	0.10	11	9	8	7	7	6	6	6	5
	0.20	10	7	6	6	5	5	5	4	4
0.90	0.01	15	12	11	10	10	9	9	8	7
	0.02	13	11	10	9	9	8	8	7	6
	0.05	11	9	8	7	7	7	6	6	5
	0.10	10	8	7	6	6	5	5	5	4
	0.20	8	6	6	5	5	4	4	4	3
0.95	0.01	12	10	9	9	8	8	8	7	7
	0.02	11	9	8	8	7	7	7	7	6
	0.05	9	8	7	6	6	6	6	5	5
	0.10	8	6	6	5	5	5	5	4	4
	0.20	6	5	5	4	4	4	4	3	3

Table A.4. (*Continued*)

		$P_1 = 0.15$								
		Power								
P_2	α	0.99	0.95	0.90	0.85	0.80	0.75	0.70	0.65	0.50
0.20	0.01	2810	2094	1756	1545	1388	1259	1149	1052	806
	0.02	2534	1858	1541	1343	1198	1078	977	888	664
	0.05	2157	1538	1252	1075	945	840	751	674	483
	0.10	1856	1287	1027	868	753	660	582	515	351
	0.20	1539	1027	797	659	559	480	415	360	228
0.25	0.01	783	586	494	435	392	357	326	300	232
	0.02	707	521	434	380	340	307	279	254	193
	0.05	603	433	354	305	270	241	216	195	142
	0.10	520	363	292	248	216	191	169	151	106
	0.20	432	291	228	190	163	141	123	108	71
0.30	0.01	380	286	241	213	193	176	161	148	116
	0.02	343	254	213	187	167	152	138	126	97
	0.05	293	212	174	151	134	120	108	98	72
	0.10	253	178	144	123	108	95	85	76	54
	0.20	211	143	113	95	82	71	63	55	38
0.35	0.01	229	173	147	130	118	108	99	91	72
	0.02	207	154	130	114	102	93	85	78	60
	0.05	177	129	106	92	82	74	67	61	45
	0.10	153	109	88	76	67	59	53	48	35
	0.20	128	88	70	59	51	45	39	35	24
0.40	0.01	155	118	100	89	81	74	68	63	50
	0.02	140	105	89	78	70	64	59	54	42
	0.05	120	88	73	63	57	51	46	42	32
	0.10	104	74	60	52	46	41	37	33	25
	0.20	87	60	48	41	35	31	28	25	18
0.45	0.01	113	86	73	65	60	55	50	47	37
	0.02	102	77	65	57	52	47	44	40	32
	0.05	87	64	53	47	42	38	34	32	24
	0.10	75	54	44	39	34	31	28	25	19
	0.20	63	44	35	30	26	23	21	19	14
0.50	0.01	86	66	56	50	46	42	39	36	29
	0.02	78	59	50	44	40	37	34	31	25
	0.05	66	49	41	36	32	29	27	25	19
	0.10	57	42	34	30	26	24	22	20	15
	0.20	48	34	27	23	21	18	16	15	11
0.55	0.01	67	52	45	40	37	34	31	29	24
	0.02	61	46	39	35	32	29	27	25	20
	0.05	52	39	33	29	26	24	22	20	16
	0.10	45	33	27	24	21	19	17	16	12
	0.20	38	27	22	19	17	15	13	12	9

Table A.4. (*Continued*)

		\multicolumn{9}{c}{$P_1 = 0.15$ (*Continued*)}								
		\multicolumn{9}{c}{Power}								
P_2	α	0.99	0.95	0.90	0.85	0.80	0.75	0.70	0.65	0.50
0.60	0.01	54	42	36	33	30	28	26	24	20
	0.02	49	37	32	29	26	24	22	21	17
	0.05	42	31	26	23	21	19	18	16	13
	0.10	36	27	22	19	17	16	14	13	10
	0.20	30	22	18	15	14	12	11	10	8
0.65	0.01	44	34	30	27	25	23	21	20	16
	0.02	40	31	26	24	22	20	19	17	14
	0.05	34	26	22	19	18	16	15	14	11
	0.10	29	22	18	16	15	13	12	11	9
	0.20	25	18	15	13	11	10	9	9	7
0.70	0.01	36	29	25	23	21	19	18	17	14
	0.02	33	26	22	20	18	17	16	15	12
	0.05	28	21	18	16	15	14	13	12	9
	0.10	24	18	15	14	12	11	10	10	8
	0.20	20	15	12	11	10	9	8	7	6
0.75	0.01	30	24	21	19	18	16	15	15	12
	0.02	27	21	19	17	16	14	13	13	11
	0.05	23	18	15	14	13	12	11	10	8
	0.10	20	15	13	11	10	10	9	8	7
	0.20	17	12	10	9	8	8	7	6	5
0.80	0.01	25	20	18	16	15	14	13	13	11
	0.02	23	18	16	14	13	12	12	11	9
	0.05	19	15	13	12	11	10	9	9	7
	0.10	17	13	11	10	9	8	8	7	6
	0.20	14	10	9	8	7	7	6	6	4
0.85	0.01	21	17	15	14	13	12	12	11	9
	0.02	19	15	13	12	11	11	10	10	8
	0.05	16	13	11	10	9	9	8	8	6
	0.10	14	11	9	8	8	7	7	6	5
	0.20	12	9	8	7	6	6	5	5	4
0.90	0.01	18	14	13	12	11	11	10	10	8
	0.02	16	13	11	11	10	9	9	8	7
	0.05	13	11	9	9	8	8	7	7	6
	0.10	11	9	8	7	7	6	6	6	5
	0.20	10	7	6	6	5	5	5	4	4
0.95	0.01	15	12	11	10	10	9	9	8	7
	0.02	13	11	10	9	8	8	8	7	6
	0.05	11	9	8	7	7	7	6	6	5
	0.10	9	8	7	6	6	5	5	5	4
	0.20	8	6	5	5	5	4	4	4	3

Table A.4. (*Continued*)

						$P_1 = 0.20$				
						Power				
P_2	α	0.99	0.95	0.90	0.85	0.80	0.75	0.70	0.65	0.50
0.25	0.01	3386	2522	2114	1858	1668	1512	1379	1262	965
	0.02	3053	2236	1853	1615	1438	1294	1172	1064	794
	0.05	2597	1850	1504	1290	1134	1007	900	806	575
	0.10	2235	1547	1233	1041	901	789	695	614	417
	0.20	1852	1232	955	788	668	572	494	426	268
0.30	0.01	915	685	576	507	456	415	379	348	268
	0.02	826	608	506	442	395	356	324	295	222
	0.05	704	504	412	355	313	279	250	225	163
	0.10	607	423	339	288	250	220	195	174	121
	0.20	504	339	265	220	188	162	141	123	80
0.35	0.01	433	325	274	242	219	199	183	168	131
	0.02	391	289	242	212	190	172	156	143	109
	0.05	334	240	197	171	151	135	122	110	81
	0.10	288	202	163	139	122	107	96	85	61
	0.20	240	162	128	107	92	80	70	62	41
0.40	0.01	256	193	164	145	131	120	110	101	79
	0.02	232	172	144	127	114	103	94	86	66
	0.05	198	143	118	102	91	82	74	67	50
	0.10	171	121	98	84	74	65	58	52	38
	0.20	142	97	77	65	56	49	43	38	26
0.45	0.01	171	129	110	98	88	81	74	69	54
	0.02	154	115	97	85	77	70	64	59	46
	0.05	132	96	79	69	62	56	50	46	35
	0.10	114	81	66	57	50	45	40	36	26
	0.20	95	65	52	44	38	34	30	27	19
0.50	0.01	122	93	79	71	64	59	54	50	40
	0.02	110	83	70	62	56	51	47	43	34
	0.05	94	69	57	50	45	41	37	34	26
	0.10	82	58	48	41	37	33	29	27	20
	0.20	68	47	38	32	28	25	22	20	14
0.55	0.01	92	70	60	54	49	45	41	38	31
	0.02	83	63	53	47	43	39	36	33	26
	0.05	71	52	44	38	34	31	28	26	20
	0.10	61	44	36	32	28	25	23	21	16
	0.20	51	36	29	25	22	19	17	15	11

Table A.4. (*Continued*)

		$P_1 = 0.20$ (*Continued*)								
		Power								
P_2	α	0.99	0.95	0.90	0.85	0.80	0.75	0.70	0.65	0.50
0.60	0.01	71	55	47	42	38	35	33	31	25
	0.02	64	49	42	37	34	31	28	26	21
	0.05	55	41	34	30	27	25	23	21	16
	0.10	47	35	29	25	22	20	18	17	13
	0.20	40	28	23	20	17	15	14	13	9
0.65	0.01	56	44	38	34	31	29	27	25	20
	0.02	51	39	33	30	27	25	23	21	17
	0.05	44	33	27	24	22	20	18	17	13
	0.10	38	28	23	20	18	16	15	14	11
	0.02	31	22	18	16	14	13	11	10	8
0.70	0.01	46	36	31	28	25	24	22	21	17
	0.02	41	32	27	24	22	21	19	18	14
	0.05	35	26	22	20	18	17	15	14	11
	0.10	30	22	19	17	15	14	12	11	9
	0.20	25	18	15	13	12	11	10	9	7
0.75	0.01	37	29	25	23	21	20	18	17	14
	0.02	34	26	23	20	19	17	16	15	12
	0.05	29	22	19	17	15	14	13	12	10
	0.10	25	18	16	14	12	11	10	10	8
	0.20	21	15	12	11	10	9	8	7	6
0.80	0.01	31	24	21	19	18	17	16	15	12
	0.02	28	22	19	17	16	15	14	13	11
	0.05	23	18	16	14	13	12	11	10	8
	0.10	20	15	13	12	11	10	9	8	7
	0.20	17	12	10	9	8	8	7	6	5
0.85	0.01	25	20	18	16	15	14	13	13	11
	0.02	23	18	16	14	13	12	12	11	9
	0.05	19	15	13	12	11	10	9	9	7
	0.10	17	13	11	10	9	8	8	7	6
	0.20	14	10	9	8	7	7	6	6	4
0.90	0.01	21	17	15	14	13	12	11	11	9
	0.02	19	15	13	12	11	11	10	9	8
	0.05	16	13	11	10	9	9	8	8	6
	0.10	14	11	9	8	8	7	7	6	5
	0.20	11	9	7	7	6	6	5	5	4
0.95	0.01	17	14	13	12	11	10	10	9	8
	0.02	15	13	11	10	10	9	9	8	7
	0.05	13	10	9	8	8	7	7	7	6
	0.10	11	9	8	7	7	6	6	5	5
	0.20	9	7	6	6	5	5	5	4	4

Table A.4. (*Continued*)

						Power				
P_2	α	0.99	0.95	0.90	0.85	0.80	0.75	0.70	0.65	0.50
0.30	0.01	3867	2878	2411	2119	1902	1723	1572	1438	1098
	0.02	3486	2552	2114	1841	1639	1474	1334	1211	902
	0.05	2965	2110	1714	1470	1291	1145	1023	916	652
	0.10	2550	1764	1404	1185	1025	897	789	696	471
	0.20	2112	1404	1087	895	758	649	559	482	301
0.35	0.01	1023	765	643	566	509	462	423	387	298
	0.02	923	679	564	493	440	397	360	328	247
	0.05	786	563	459	395	348	310	278	250	181
	0.10	678	472	378	320	278	245	217	192	133
	0.20	562	377	294	244	208	179	156	136	88
0.40	0.01	476	357	301	266	240	218	200	183	142
	0.02	430	317	265	232	207	188	171	156	118
	0.05	366	264	216	187	165	147	133	120	88
	0.10	316	221	178	152	133	117	104	93	65
	0.20	263	178	140	117	100	87	76	67	44
0.45	0.01	278	209	177	156	141	129	118	109	85
	0.02	251	186	156	137	123	111	101	93	71
	0.05	214	155	127	110	98	88	79	72	53
	0.10	185	130	105	90	79	70	63	56	40
	0.20	154	105	83	70	60	52	46	41	28
0.50	0.01	182	138	117	104	94	86	79	73	57
	0.02	165	123	103	91	82	74	68	62	48
	0.05	141	102	85	74	65	59	53	48	36
	0.10	121	86	70	60	53	47	42	38	28
	0.20	101	70	55	47	41	36	31	28	20
0.55	0.01	129	98	83	74	67	62	57	53	42
	0.02	117	87	74	65	59	53	49	45	35
	0.05	99	73	60	53	47	43	39	35	27
	0.10	86	61	50	43	38	34	31	28	21
	0.20	72	50	40	34	29	26	23	21	15
0.60	0.01	96	73	62	56	51	47	43	40	32
	0.02	86	65	55	49	44	40	37	34	27
	0.05	74	54	45	40	36	32	29	27	21
	0.10	64	46	38	33	29	26	24	21	16
	0.20	53	37	30	26	22	20	18	16	12

$P_1 = 0.25$

Table A.4. (*Continued*)

		$P_1 = 0.25$ (*Continued*)							
		Power							
P_2	α	0.99	0.95	0.90	0.85	0.80	0.75	0.70	0.65	0.50
0.65	0.01	73	56	48	43	39	36	34	31	25
	0.02	66	50	43	38	34	32	29	27	21
	0.05	57	42	35	31	28	25	23	21	17
	0.10	49	36	29	26	23	21	19	17	13
	0.20	41	29	23	20	18	16	14	13	9
0.70	0.01	58	45	38	34	32	29	27	25	21
	0.02	52	40	34	30	28	25	23	22	17
	0.05	44	33	28	25	22	20	19	17	14
	0.10	38	28	23	20	18	17	15	14	11
	0.20	32	23	19	16	14	13	12	10	8
0.75	0.01	46	36	31	28	26	24	22	21	17
	0.02	42	32	27	25	22	21	19	18	15
	0.05	35	27	23	20	18	17	15	14	11
	0.10	31	23	19	17	15	14	12	11	9
	0.20	26	18	15	13	12	11	10	9	7
0.80	0.01	37	29	25	23	21	20	18	17	14
	0.02	34	26	23	20	19	17	16	15	12
	0.05	29	22	19	17	15	14	13	12	10
	0.10	25	18	16	14	12	11	10	10	8
	0.20	21	15	12	11	10	9	8	7	6
0.85	0.01	30	24	21	19	18	16	15	15	12
	0.02	27	21	19	17	16	14	13	13	11
	0.05	23	18	15	14	13	12	11	10	8
	0.10	20	15	13	11	10	10	9	8	7
	0.20	17	12	10	9	8	8	7	6	5
0.90	0.01	25	20	17	16	15	14	13	12	11
	0.02	22	18	15	14	13	12	11	11	9
	0.05	19	15	13	12	11	10	9	9	7
	0.10	16	13	11	10	9	8	8	7	6
	0.20	14	10	9	8	7	6	6	6	4
0.95	0.01	20	16	15	13	13	12	11	11	9
	0.02	18	15	13	12	11	10	10	9	8
	0.05	15	12	11	10	9	8	8	7	6
	0.10	13	10	9	8	7	7	7	6	5
	0.20	11	8	7	6	6	5	5	5	4

Table A.4. (*Continued*)

		$P_1 = 0.30$								
		Power								
P_2	α	0.99	0.95	0.90	0.85	0.80	0.75	0.70	0.65	0.50
0.35	0.01	4251	3163	2650	2328	2089	1892	1726	1578	1204
	0.02	3832	2804	2322	2022	1800	1618	1464	1329	989
	0.05	3259	2318	1882	1613	1416	1256	1122	1004	714
	0.10	2803	1937	1541	1300	1124	983	865	762	514
	0.20	2320	1541	1192	981	830	710	611	527	327
0.40	0.01	1108	827	695	612	550	499	456	418	322
	0.02	999	734	610	532	475	428	389	354	266
	0.05	851	608	496	427	376	334	300	269	194
	0.10	733	510	408	345	300	264	233	207	142
	0.20	608	407	317	263	224	193	167	145	94
0.45	0.01	508	381	321	283	255	232	213	195	151
	0.02	459	338	282	247	221	200	182	166	126
	0.05	391	281	230	199	175	157	141	127	93
	0.10	337	236	190	161	141	124	110	98	69
	0.20	280	189	148	124	106	92	80	70	47
0.50	0.01	293	220	186	165	149	135	124	114	89
	0.02	264	196	164	144	129	117	106	97	75
	0.05	225	163	134	116	103	92	83	75	56
	0.10	194	137	111	95	83	73	66	59	42
	0.20	162	110	87	73	63	55	48	42	29
0.55	0.01	190	144	122	108	98	89	82	76	60
	0.02	172	128	107	94	85	77	71	65	50
	0.05	147	106	88	76	68	61	55	50	38
	0.10	127	90	73	63	55	49	44	39	29
	0.20	105	72	57	48	42	37	33	29	20
0.60	0.01	133	101	86	76	69	63	59	54	43
	0.02	120	90	76	67	60	55	50	46	36
	0.05	103	75	62	54	48	44	40	36	27
	0.10	89	63	52	45	39	35	32	29	21
	0.20	74	51	41	35	30	27	24	21	15

Table A.4. (*Continued*)

					$P_1 = 0.30$ (*Continued*)					
					Power					
P_2	α	0.99	0.95	0.90	0.85	0.80	0.75	0.70	0.65	0.50
0.65	0.01	98	75	64	57	52	47	44	41	32
	0.02	88	66	56	50	45	41	38	35	27
	0.05	75	55	46	40	36	33	30	27	21
	0.10	65	47	38	33	30	27	24	22	16
	0.20	54	38	31	26	23	20	18	16	12
0.70	0.01	74	57	49	44	40	37	34	32	25
	0.02	67	51	43	38	35	32	29	27	22
	0.05	57	42	36	31	28	26	23	21	17
	0.10	49	36	30	26	23	21	19	17	13
	0.20	41	29	24	20	18	16	14	13	9
0.75	0.01	58	45	38	34	32	29	27	25	21
	0.02	52	40	34	30	28	25	23	22	17
	0.05	44	33	28	25	22	20	19	17	14
	0.10	38	28	23	20	18	17	15	14	11
	0.20	32	23	19	16	14	13	12	10	8
0.80	0.01	46	36	31	28	25	24	22	21	17
	0.02	41	32	27	24	22	21	19	18	14
	0.05	35	26	22	20	18	17	15	14	11
	0.10	30	22	19	17	15	14	12	11	9
	0.20	25	18	15	13	12	11	10	9	7
0.85	0.01	36	29	25	23	21	19	18	17	14
	0.02	33	26	22	20	18	17	16	15	12
	0.05	28	21	18	16	15	14	13	12	9
	0.10	24	18	15	14	12	11	10	10	8
	0.20	20	15	12	11	10	9	8	7	6
0.90	0.01	29	23	20	19	17	16	15	14	12
	0.02	26	21	18	16	15	14	13	12	10
	0.05	22	17	15	13	12	11	11	10	8
	0.10	19	15	13	11	10	9	9	8	7
	0.20	16	12	10	9	8	7	7	6	5
0.95	0.01	23	19	17	15	14	13	13	12	10
	0.02	21	17	15	14	13	12	11	10	9
	0.05	18	14	12	11	10	10	9	8	7
	0.10	16	12	10	9	9	8	7	7	6
	0.20	13	10	8	7	7	6	6	5	4

Table A.4. (*Continued*)

		\multicolumn{9}{c}{$P_1 = 0.35$}
		\multicolumn{9}{c}{Power}
P_2	α	0.99	0.95	0.90	0.85	0.80	0.75	0.70	0.65	0.50
0.40	0.01	4540	3377	2828	2484	2229	2019	1841	1683	1284
	0.02	4092	2993	2478	2157	1920	1726	1562	1417	1054
	0.05	3479	2474	2008	1721	1511	1340	1196	1070	760
	0.10	2992	2067	1644	1386	1198	1047	921	812	547
	0.20	2476	1644	1271	1046	885	756	650	560	347
0.45	0.01	1168	872	732	644	579	526	480	440	338
	0.02	1053	774	642	561	500	451	409	372	279
	0.05	897	641	522	449	395	352	315	283	204
	0.10	772	537	429	363	316	277	245	217	149
	0.20	640	429	334	276	235	202	176	152	98
0.50	0.01	530	397	334	295	265	241	221	203	157
	0.02	478	352	294	257	230	208	189	172	131
	0.05	407	293	239	207	182	163	146	132	96
	0.10	351	246	197	168	146	129	115	102	71
	0.20	292	197	154	128	110	95	83	73	48
0.55	0.01	302	227	192	169	153	139	128	118	92
	0.02	272	202	169	148	133	120	110	100	77
	0.05	232	168	138	119	106	95	85	77	57
	0.10	200	141	114	97	85	75	67	60	43
	0.20	167	113	89	75	65	56	49	43	29
0.60	0.01	194	147	124	110	100	91	84	77	61
	0.02	175	130	109	96	87	79	72	66	51
	0.05	149	109	90	78	69	62	56	51	38
	0.10	129	91	74	64	56	50	45	40	29
	0.20	108	74	59	49	43	37	33	29	20
0.65	0.01	134	102	87	77	70	64	59	55	43
	0.02	121	91	76	68	61	55	51	47	36
	0.05	104	76	63	55	49	44	40	36	28
	0.10	89	64	52	45	40	35	32	29	21
	0.20	75	52	41	35	30	27	24	21	15

Table A.4. (*Continued*)

					Power				
P_2	α	0.99	0.95	0.90	0.85	0.80	0.75	0.70	0.65	0.50
0.70	0.01	98	75	64	57	52	47	44	41	32
	0.02	88	66	56	50	45	41	38	35	27
	0.05	75	55	46	40	36	33	30	27	21
	0.10	65	47	38	33	30	27	24	22	16
	0.20	54	38	31	26	23	20	18	16	12
0.75	0.01	73	56	48	43	39	36	34	31	25
	0.02	66	50	43	38	34	32	29	27	21
	0.05	57	42	35	31	28	25	23	21	17
	0.10	49	36	29	26	23	21	19	17	13
	0.20	41	29	23	20	18	16	14	13	9
0.80	0.01	56	44	38	34	31	29	27	25	20
	0.02	51	39	33	30	27	25	23	21	17
	0.05	44	33	27	24	22	20	18	17	13
	0.10	38	28	23	20	18	16	15	14	11
	0.20	31	22	18	16	14	13	11	10	8
0.85	0.01	44	34	30	27	25	23	21	20	16
	0.02	40	31	26	24	22	20	19	17	14
	0.05	34	26	22	19	18	16	15	14	11
	0.10	29	22	18	16	15	13	12	11	9
	0.20	25	18	15	13	11	10	9	9	7
0.90	0.01	35	27	24	22	20	19	17	16	14
	0.02	31	24	21	19	18	16	15	14	12
	0.05	27	20	18	16	14	13	12	11	9
	0.10	23	17	15	13	12	11	10	9	7
	0.20	19	14	12	10	9	8	8	7	6
0.95	0.01	28	22	19	18	16	15	14	14	11
	0.02	25	20	17	16	14	13	13	12	10
	0.05	21	16	14	13	12	11	10	9	8
	0.10	18	14	12	11	10	9	8	8	6
	0.20	15	11	10	9	8	7	7	6	5

$P_1 = 0.35$ (*Continued*)

Table A.4. (*Continued*)

		$P_1 = 0.40$								
		Power								
P_2	α	0.99	0.95	0.90	0.85	0.80	0.75	0.70	0.65	0.50
0.45	0.01	4732	3520	2947	2589	2322	2104	1918	1753	1337
	0.02	4265	3119	2582	2248	2001	1798	1627	1476	1097
	0.05	3626	2578	2093	1793	1573	1395	1245	1114	791
	0.10	3118	2153	1713	1444	1248	1090	959	845	568
	0.20	2581	1712	1323	1089	921	787	677	582	360
0.50	0.01	1204	898	754	664	597	542	495	453	348
	0.02	1086	797	662	578	515	464	421	383	287
	0.05	924	660	538	463	407	362	324	291	210
	0.10	796	553	442	374	325	285	252	223	153
	0.20	660	441	343	284	242	208	180	157	100
0.55	0.01	540	405	341	301	271	246	225	207	160
	0.02	488	359	299	262	234	212	192	175	133
	0.05	415	298	244	211	186	166	149	134	98
	0.10	358	250	201	171	149	131	117	104	73
	0.20	298	201	157	131	112	97	85	74	49
0.60	0.01	305	229	193	171	154	141	129	119	93
	0.02	275	204	170	149	134	121	111	101	77
	0.05	235	169	139	120	107	96	86	78	58
	0.10	202	142	115	98	86	76	68	61	43
	0.20	168	114	90	76	65	57	50	44	30
0.65	0.01	194	147	124	110	100	91	84	77	61
	0.02	175	130	109	96	87	79	72	66	51
	0.05	149	109	90	78	69	62	56	51	38
	0.10	129	91	74	64	56	50	45	40	29
	0.20	108	74	59	49	43	37	33	29	20
0.70	0.01	133	101	86	76	69	63	59	54	43
	0.02	120	90	76	67	60	55	50	46	36
	0.05	103	75	62	54	48	44	40	36	27
	0.10	89	63	52	45	39	35	32	29	21
	0.20	74	51	41	35	30	27	24	21	15

Table A.4. (*Continued*)

						Power				
						$P_1 = 0.40$ (*Continued*)				
P_2	α	0.99	0.95	0.90	0.85	0.80	0.75	0.70	0.65	0.50
0.75	0.01	96	73	62	56	51	47	43	40	32
	0.02	86	65	55	49	44	40	37	34	27
	0.05	74	54	45	40	36	32	29	27	21
	0.10	64	46	38	33	29	26	24	21	16
	0.20	53	37	30	26	22	20	18	16	12
0.80	0.01	71	55	47	42	38	35	33	31	25
	0.02	64	49	42	37	34	31	28	26	21
	0.05	55	41	34	30	27	25	23	21	16
	0.10	47	35	29	25	22	20	18	17	13
	0.20	40	28	23	20	17	15	14	13	9
0.85	0.01	54	42	36	33	30	28	26	24	20
	0.02	49	37	32	29	26	24	22	21	17
	0.05	42	31	26	23	21	19	18	16	13
	0.10	36	27	22	19	17	16	14	13	10
	0.20	30	22	18	15	14	12	11	10	8
0.90	0.01	42	33	28	26	24	22	20	19	16
	0.02	38	29	25	23	21	19	18	17	14
	0.05	32	24	21	18	17	15	14	13	11
	0.10	28	21	17	15	14	13	12	11	8
	0.20	23	17	14	12	11	10	9	8	6
0.95	0.01	32	26	22	20	19	18	16	16	13
	0.02	29	23	20	18	17	15	14	13	11
	0.05	25	19	16	15	14	12	12	11	9
	0.10	22	16	14	12	11	10	9	9	7
	0.20	18	13	11	10	9	8	7	7	5

Table A.4. (*Continued*)

| | | $P_1 = 0.45$ | | | | | | | | |
| | | Power | | | | | | | | |
P_2	α	0.99	0.95	0.90	0.85	0.80	0.75	0.70	0.65	0.50
0.50	0.01	4828	3591	3007	2641	2369	2146	1956	1788	1364
	0.02	4352	3182	2635	2293	2041	1834	1659	1505	1119
	0.05	3700	2630	2135	1829	1605	1423	1270	1136	806
	0.10	3181	2197	1747	1472	1273	1112	978	861	579
	0.20	2633	1747	1350	1110	939	802	690	593	367
0.55	0.01	1216	907	762	670	603	547	499	458	352
	0.02	1097	805	668	583	520	469	425	387	290
	0.05	933	667	543	467	411	366	328	294	212
	0.10	804	558	446	378	328	288	254	255	155
	0.20	667	446	347	287	244	210	182	158	101
0.60	0.01	540	405	341	301	271	246	225	207	160
	0.02	488	359	299	262	234	212	192	175	133
	0.05	415	298	244	211	186	166	149	134	98
	0.10	358	250	201	171	149	131	117	104	73
	0.20	298	201	157	131	112	97	85	74	49
0.65	0.01	302	227	192	169	153	139	128	118	92
	0.02	272	202	169	148	133	120	110	100	77
	0.05	232	168	138	119	106	95	85	77	57
	0.10	200	141	114	97	85	75	67	60	43
	0.20	167	113	89	75	65	56	49	43	29
0.70	0.01	190	144	122	108	98	89	82	76	60
	0.02	172	128	107	94	85	77	71	65	50
	0.05	147	106	88	76	68	61	55	50	38
	0.10	127	90	73	63	55	49	44	39	29
	0.20	105	72	57	48	42	37	33	29	20
0.75	0.01	129	98	83	74	67	62	57	53	42
	0.02	117	87	74	65	59	53	49	45	35
	0.05	99	73	60	53	47	43	39	35	27
	0.10	86	61	50	43	38	34	31	28	21
	0.20	72	50	40	34	29	26	23	21	15
0.80	0.01	92	70	60	54	49	45	41	38	31
	0.02	83	63	53	47	43	39	36	33	26
	0.05	71	52	44	38	34	31	28	26	20
	0.10	61	44	36	32	28	25	23	21	16
	0.20	51	36	29	25	22	19	17	15	11
0.85	0.01	67	52	45	40	37	34	31	29	24
	0.02	61	46	39	35	32	29	27	25	20
	0.05	52	39	33	29	26	24	22	20	16
	0.10	45	33	27	24	21	19	17	16	12
	0.20	38	27	22	19	17	15	13	12	9
0.90	0.01	51	39	34	31	28	26	24	23	19
	0.02	46	35	30	27	25	23	21	20	16
	0.05	39	29	25	22	20	18	17	16	12
	0.10	34	25	21	18	16	15	14	13	10
	0.20	28	20	17	15	13	12	11	10	7
0.95	0.01	38	30	26	24	22	20	19	18	15
	0.02	35	27	23	21	19	18	17	16	13
	0.05	30	23	19	17	16	14	13	12	10
	0.10	26	19	16	14	13	12	11	10	8
	0.20	21	16	13	11	10	9	9	8	6

Table A.4. (*Continued*)

		$P_1 = 0.50$								
		Power								
P_2	α	0.99	0.95	0.90	0.85	0.80	0.75	0.70	0.65	0.50
0.55	0.01	4828	3591	3007	2641	2369	2146	1956	1788	1364
	0.02	4352	3182	2635	2293	2041	1834	1659	1505	1119
	0.05	3700	2630	2135	1829	1605	1423	1270	1136	806
	0.10	3181	2197	1747	1472	1273	1112	978	861	579
	0.20	2633	1747	1350	1110	939	802	690	593	367
0.60	0.01	1204	898	754	664	597	542	495	453	348
	0.02	1086	797	662	578	515	464	421	383	287
	0.05	924	660	538	463	407	362	324	291	210
	0.10	796	553	442	374	325	285	252	223	153
	0.20	660	441	343	284	242	208	180	157	100
0.65	0.01	530	397	334	295	265	241	221	203	157
	0.02	478	352	294	257	230	208	189	172	131
	0.05	407	293	239	207	182	163	146	132	96
	0.10	351	246	197	168	146	129	115	102	71
	0.20	292	197	154	128	110	95	83	73	48
0.70	0.01	293	220	186	165	149	135	124	114	89
	0.02	264	196	164	144	129	117	106	97	75
	0.05	225	163	134	116	103	92	83	75	56
	0.10	194	137	111	95	83	73	66	59	42
	0.20	162	110	87	73	63	55	48	42	29
0.75	0.01	182	138	117	104	94	86	79	73	57
	0.02	165	123	103	91	82	74	68	62	48
	0.05	141	102	85	74	65	59	53	48	36
	0.10	121	86	70	60	53	47	42	38	28
	0.20	101	70	55	47	41	36	31	28	20
0.80	0.01	122	93	79	71	64	59	54	50	40
	0.02	110	83	70	62	56	51	47	43	34
	0.05	94	69	57	50	45	41	37	34	26
	0.10	82	58	48	41	37	33	29	27	20
	0.20	68	47	38	32	28	25	22	20	14
0.85	0.01	86	66	56	50	46	42	39	36	29
	0.02	78	59	50	44	40	37	34	31	25
	0.05	66	49	41	36	32	29	27	25	19
	0.10	57	42	34	30	26	24	22	20	15
	0.20	48	34	27	23	21	18	16	15	11
0.90	0.01	62	48	41	37	34	31	29	27	22
	0.02	56	43	37	33	30	27	25	23	19
	0.05	48	36	30	27	24	22	20	19	15
	0.10	42	30	25	22	20	18	16	15	12
	0.20	35	25	20	18	16	14	13	11	9
0.95	0.01	46	36	31	28	26	24	22	21	17
	0.02	41	32	27	25	23	21	19	18	15
	0.05	35	27	23	20	18	17	16	14	12
	0.10	31	23	19	17	15	14	13	12	9
	0.20	26	19	15	13	12	11	10	9	7

Table A.4. (*Continued*)

		$P_1 = 0.55$								
		Power								
P_2	α	0.99	0.95	0.90	0.85	0.80	0.75	0.70	0.65	0.50
0.60	0.01	4732	3520	2947	2589	2322	2104	1918	1753	1337
	0.02	4265	3119	2582	2248	2001	1798	1627	1476	1097
	0.05	3626	2578	2093	1793	1573	1395	1245	1114	791
	0.10	3118	2153	1713	1444	1248	1090	959	845	568
	0.20	2581	1712	1323	1089	921	787	677	582	360
0.65	0.01	1168	872	732	644	579	526	480	440	338
	0.02	1053	774	642	561	500	451	409	372	279
	0.05	897	641	522	449	395	352	315	283	204
	0.10	772	537	429	363	316	277	245	217	149
	0.20	640	429	334	276	235	202	176	152	98
0.70	0.01	508	381	321	283	255	232	213	195	151
	0.02	459	338	282	247	221	200	182	166	126
	0.05	391	281	230	199	175	157	141	127	93
	0.10	337	236	190	161	141	124	110	98	69
	0.20	280	189	148	124	106	92	80	70	47
0.75	0.01	278	209	177	156	141	129	118	109	85
	0.02	251	186	156	137	123	111	101	93	71
	0.05	214	155	127	110	98	88	79	72	53
	0.10	185	130	105	90	79	70	63	56	40
	0.20	154	105	83	70	60	52	46	41	28
0.80	0.01	171	129	110	98	88	81	74	69	54
	0.02	154	115	97	85	77	70	64	59	46
	0.05	132	96	79	69	62	56	50	46	35
	0.10	114	81	66	57	50	45	40	36	26
	0.20	95	65	52	44	38	34	30	27	19
0.85	0.01	113	86	73	65	60	55	50	47	37
	0.02	102	77	65	57	52	47	44	40	32
	0.05	87	64	53	47	42	38	34	32	24
	0.10	75	54	44	39	34	31	28	25	19
	0.20	63	44	35	30	26	23	21	19	14
0.90	0.01	78	60	51	46	42	39	36	33	27
	0.02	71	54	46	41	37	34	31	29	23
	0.05	60	45	38	33	30	27	25	23	18
	0.10	52	38	31	27	24	22	20	18	14
	0.20	44	31	25	22	19	17	15	14	10
0.95	0.01	55	43	37	33	31	28	26	25	20
	0.02	50	38	33	29	27	25	23	21	17
	0.05	43	32	27	24	22	20	18	17	14
	0.10	37	27	23	20	18	16	15	14	11
	0.20	31	22	18	16	14	13	12	11	8

Table A.4. (*Continued*)

						$P_1 = 0.60$				
						Power				
P_2	α	0.99	0.95	0.90	0.85	0.80	0.75	0.70	0.65	0.50
0.65	0.01	4540	3377	2828	2484	2229	2019	1841	1683	1284
	0.02	4092	2993	2478	2157	1920	1726	1562	1417	1054
	0.05	3479	2474	2008	1721	1511	1340	1196	1070	760
	0.10	2992	2067	1644	1386	1198	1047	921	812	547
	0.20	2476	1644	1271	1046	885	756	650	560	347
0.70	0.01	1108	827	695	612	550	499	456	418	322
	0.02	999	734	610	532	475	428	389	354	266
	0.05	851	608	496	427	376	334	300	269	194
	0.10	733	510	408	345	300	264	233	207	142
	0.20	608	407	317	263	224	193	167	145	94
0.75	0.01	476	357	301	266	240	218	200	183	142
	0.02	430	317	265	232	207	188	171	156	118
	0.05	366	264	216	187	165	147	133	120	88
	0.10	316	221	178	152	133	117	104	93	65
	0.20	263	178	140	117	100	87	76	67	44
0.80	0.01	256	193	164	145	131	120	110	101	79
	0.02	232	172	144	127	114	103	94	86	66
	0.05	198	143	118	102	91	82	74	67	50
	0.10	171	121	98	84	74	65	58	52	38
	0.20	142	97	77	65	56	49	43	38	26
0.85	0.01	155	118	100	89	81	74	68	63	50
	0.02	140	105	89	78	70	64	59	54	42
	0.05	120	88	73	63	57	51	46	42	32
	0.10	104	74	60	52	46	41	37	33	25
	0.20	87	60	48	41	35	31	28	25	18
0.90	0.01	101	77	66	59	54	49	46	42	34
	0.02	91	69	58	52	47	43	39	36	29
	0.05	78	58	48	42	38	34	31	29	22
	0.10	68	49	40	35	31	28	25	23	17
	0.20	56	40	32	27	24	21	19	17	13
0.95	0.01	68	53	45	41	37	34	32	30	24
	0.02	62	47	40	36	33	30	28	26	21
	0.05	53	39	33	29	27	24	22	21	16
	0.10	46	34	28	24	22	20	18	17	13
	0.20	38	27	22	19	17	15	14	13	10

Table A.4. (*Continued*)

P_2	α	0.99	0.95	0.90	0.85	0.80	0.75	0.70	0.65	0.50
0.70	0.01	4251	3163	2650	2328	2089	1892	1726	1578	1204
	0.02	3833	2804	2322	2022	1800	1618	1464	1329	989
	0.05	3259	2318	1882	1613	1416	1256	1122	1004	714
	0.10	2803	1937	1541	1300	1124	983	865	762	514
	0.20	2320	1541	1192	981	830	710	611	527	327
0.75	0.01	1023	765	643	566	509	462	423	387	298
	0.02	923	679	564	493	440	397	360	328	247
	0.05	786	563	459	395	348	310	278	250	181
	0.10	678	472	378	320	278	245	217	192	133
	0.20	562	377	294	244	208	179	156	136	88
0.80	0.01	433	325	274	242	219	199	183	168	131
	0.02	391	289	242	212	190	172	156	143	109
	0.05	334	240	197	171	151	135	122	110	81
	0.10	288	202	163	139	122	107	96	85	61
	0.20	240	162	128	107	92	80	70	62	41
0.85	0.01	229	173	147	130	118	108	99	91	72
	0.02	207	154	130	114	102	93	85	78	60
	0.05	177	129	106	92	82	74	67	61	45
	0.10	153	109	88	76	67	59	53	48	35
	0.20	128	88	70	59	51	45	39	35	24
0.90	0.01	136	104	88	79	72	66	61	56	45
	0.02	123	93	78	69	62	57	52	48	38
	0.05	105	77	64	56	50	45	41	38	29
	0.10	91	65	54	46	41	37	33	30	22
	0.20	76	53	43	36	32	28	25	22	16
0.95	0.01	86	66	57	51	46	43	40	37	30
	0.02	78	59	50	45	41	37	34	32	25
	0.05	67	50	42	37	33	30	28	25	20
	0.10	58	42	35	30	27	25	22	20	16
	0.20	48	34	28	24	21	19	17	16	12

$P_1 = 0.65$

Power

Table A.4. (*Continued*)

						Power				
						$P_1 = 0.70$				
P_2	α	0.99	0.95	0.90	0.85	0.80	0.75	0.70	0.65	0.50
0.75	0.01	3867	2878	2411	2119	1902	1723	1572	1438	1098
	0.02	3486	2552	2114	1841	1639	1474	1334	1211	902
	0.05	2965	2110	1714	1470	1291	1145	1023	916	652
	0.10	2550	1764	1404	1185	1025	897	789	696	471
	0.20	2112	1404	1087	895	758	649	559	482	301
0.80	0.01	915	685	576	507	456	415	379	348	268
	0.02	826	608	506	442	395	356	324	295	222
	0.05	704	504	412	355	313	279	250	225	163
	0.10	607	423	339	288	250	220	195	174	121
	0.20	504	339	265	220	188	162	141	123	80
0.85	0.01	380	286	241	213	193	176	161	148	116
	0.02	343	254	213	187	167	152	138	126	97
	0.05	293	212	174	151	134	120	108	98	72
	0.10	253	178	144	123	108	95	85	76	54
	0.20	211	143	113	95	82	71	63	55	38
0.90	0.01	196	149	126	112	102	93	86	79	63
	0.02	178	133	112	98	89	81	74	68	53
	0.05	152	111	92	80	71	64	58	53	40
	0.10	131	94	76	66	58	52	47	42	31
	0.20	110	76	61	51	45	39	35	31	22
0.95	0.01	113	87	74	66	60	55	51	48	38
	0.02	102	77	66	58	53	48	44	41	33
	0.05	88	65	54	48	43	39	35	32	25
	0.10	76	55	45	39	35	32	29	26	20
	0.20	64	45	36	31	27	24	22	20	14

Table A.4. (*Continued*)

		$P_1 = 0.75$								
		Power								
P_2	α	0.99	0.95	0.90	0.85	0.80	0.75	0.70	0.65	0.50
0.80	0.01	3386	2522	2114	1858	1668	1512	1379	1262	965
	0.02	3053	2236	1853	1615	1438	1294	1172	1064	794
	0.05	2597	1850	1504	1290	1134	1007	900	806	575
	0.10	2235	1547	1233	1041	901	789	695	614	417
	0.20	1852	1232	955	788	668	572	494	426	268
0.85	0.01	783	586	494	435	392	357	326	300	232
	0.02	707	521	434	380	340	307	279	254	193
	0.05	603	433	354	305	270	241	216	195	142
	0.10	520	363	292	248	216	191	169	151	106
	0.20	432	291	228	190	163	141	123	108	71
0.90	0.01	316	238	202	179	162	147	136	125	98
	0.02	285	212	178	156	140	127	116	107	82
	0.05	244	177	146	127	113	101	91	83	62
	0.10	211	149	121	104	91	81	73	65	47
	0.20	176	120	96	81	70	61	54	48	33
0.95	0.01	157	120	102	91	83	76	70	65	52
	0.02	142	107	90	80	72	66	61	56	44
	0.05	122	90	75	65	58	53	48	44	34
	0.10	106	76	62	54	48	43	39	35	26
	0.20	88	62	50	42	37	33	29	26	19

Table A.4. (*Continued*)

$P_1 = 0.80$

Power

P_2	α	0.99	0.95	0.90	0.85	0.80	0.75	0.70	0.65	0.50
0.85	0.01	2810	2094	1756	1545	1388	1259	1149	1052	806
	0.02	2534	1858	1541	1343	1198	1078	977	888	664
	0.05	2157	1538	1252	1075	945	840	751	674	483
	0.10	1856	1287	1027	868	753	660	582	515	351
	0.20	1539	1027	797	659	559	480	415	360	228
0.90	0.01	627	471	397	351	316	288	264	243	189
	0.02	566	419	349	306	274	248	226	206	157
	0.05	483	348	286	247	219	196	176	159	117
	0.10	417	293	236	201	176	156	139	124	88
	0.20	347	236	185	155	133	116	102	89	60
0.95	0.01	241	183	155	138	125	115	106	98	77
	0.02	218	163	137	121	109	99	91	84	65
	0.05	187	136	113	99	88	79	72	66	50
	0.10	162	115	94	81	72	64	58	52	38
	0.20	135	94	75	64	55	49	44	39	28

$P_1 = 0.85$

Power

P_2	α	0.99	0.95	0.90	0.85	0.80	0.75	0.70	0.65	0.50
0.90	0.01	2137	1595	1340	1179	1060	963	880	806	620
	0.02	1928	1416	1176	1027	916	826	749	682	513
	0.05	1642	1174	957	823	725	646	579	520	375
	0.10	1415	984	787	667	579	509	450	399	275
	0.20	1175	787	613	508	433	373	324	281	182
0.95	0.01	447	337	285	253	228	209	192	177	139
	0.02	404	300	252	221	199	180	165	151	117
	0.05	345	251	207	179	160	143	130	118	88
	0.10	299	212	172	147	130	115	103	93	67
	0.20	250	171	136	115	99	87	77	68	47

$P_1 = 90$

Power

P_2	α	0.99	0.95	0.90	0.85	0.80	0.75	0.70	0.65	0.50
0.95	0.01	1368	1025	863	762	686	624	572	525	407
	0.02	1235	911	760	665	595	538	489	446	339
	0.05	1054	758	621	536	474	423	381	344	252
	0.10	910	637	513	437	381	336	299	267	188
	0.20	758	512	402	336	288	250	219	192	128

Table A.5. *20,000 random digits*

08939	53632	41345	65379	20165	32576	13967	90616	17995	92422
92578	23668	08801	39792	59541	99117	58830	60923	36068	68101
83994	91054	90377	22776	23263	34593	98191	77811	83144	98563
43080	71414	40760	01831	44145	48387	93018	22618	98547	87716
39372	46789	26381	37186	85684	79426	05395	17538	56671	82181
83046	58644	04452	98912	53406	30224	00687	32099	86414	29590
99808	32539	96961	88917	60847	64826	41332	64557	15354	11111
28478	70870	68912	75644	33648	21097	23745	52593	01849	37760
09916	19651	28659	95093	12626	19919	05879	56003	83100	94572
19537	66067	20569	28808	87722	67059	12851	73573	25776	92500
23013	05574	26320	07754	09642	88068	41626	57139	68199	94938
55838	80585	80967	60540	34528	62310	63106	17843	39104	74036
92279	87344	93556	75233	09394	79265	91047	32891	77925	71530
27850	23332	89336	26026	52130	78544	02090	05645	15060	39550
01760	54605	11794	79312	69728	04554	99775	57659	47981	68954
81889	70751	87501	88247	41966	57574	67745	88304	20118	25964
74722	14654	15425	60665	25162	04987	03467	75915	24282	62456
56196	75068	44643	92240	51651	79743	13598	63901	61020	91003
96842	62021	00543	45073	65545	87612	35765	26079	34589	72821
25619	98328	59393	71401	93871	20611	78830	87477	15390	05044
91746	05084	04781	82933	54564	80986	94843	40178	87483	63288
92384	84706	76778	98313	98875	08427	60687	88272	83448	06237
86390	62208	95735	14535	25591	22730	06059	31786	36181	31016
60458	83606	57510	92609	38061	94881	26736	06489	98303	31419
03783	39922	05489	73630	92379	91602	18193	84741	44704	05558
31011	36035	37113	98362	56149	51634	04468	62096	32361	35301
20555	05621	48728	41776	12101	96615	70781	55151	93876	66892
56466	36766	12400	43510	49456	05140	85736	68155	37306	10438
26875	67304	61950	65962	38223	35676	70043	99178	64677	95457
90648	84770	92791	93814	27760	22232	83545	01183	55188	20482
26197	72840	01264	52019	00739	36259	10905	39097	36437	66743
72522	34445	53975	13840	97262	59007	78685	41044	38103	59216
12370	41270	36290	46307	51230	90614	82613	80148	37371	02895
81028	60112	31415	47478	02131	85480	93699	92876	13958	47867
61573	38634	77650	18189	10283	97999	95442	90657	84963	93863
98511	46300	91199	30492	62159	98525	31710	03540	35844	83200
76606	10834	75548	55779	54744	26450	66001	57949	53685	00567
20237	16311	15733	47599	43998	35594	17577	85113	52487	48900
21022	86025	26951	87480	82317	06580	98627	32536	07573	52612
47512	11564	41777	46581	03492	01722	78900	57901	37307	02727
80598	59041	28861	41793	91007	69907	00376	73086	35132	53014
01892	34226	88327	21926	36607	22307	04376	25491	13563	51955
89657	70349	15176	57916	10911	44218	67108	04678	24097	02476
97983	65616	11841	80504	76452	34176	16986	94328	13091	29592
59727	92033	14654	59622	25844	18460	78162	02832	13528	55683
12340	72894	26303	01771	73895	27432	99536	50328	06141	83886
48049	33318	67463	04914	22316	89663	37132	15825	60759	22131
85953	16537	25639	05004	99269	50577	10036	05022	39800	93605
03426	78111	37828	23967	03350	04397	96227	37787	60680	23993
97837	71085	45973	36073	02680	91425	24425	23725	22521	21601

Table A.5. (*Continued*)

26916	67086	60270	57846	04646	07258	01734	45079	54869	23505
47205	71678	05222	86233	70398	46287	44139	48247	92230	19157
84869	36794	56943	10512	50582	08884	98068	08447	68071	32397
81740	98868	57546	55461	14850	89946	06024	26626	05543	93616
11808	28306	63559	26600	87569	86007	27922	93468	09509	15841
09464	14219	00130	72813	35704	58905	32091	62397	85560	51783
40656	77886	01411	07490	32240	26028	66002	61762	76551	03442
31693	59176	69817	86317	89547	60424	56618	95888	65770	31622
97799	02197	32987	78146	71992	28633	23868	85504	98216	19756
34590	29732	67082	34899	05654	19830	68088	30054	67535	34721
00504	90537	38681	17248	55362	76935	63352	87699	56022	46835
76814	39363	44851	14836	85357	78617	03482	13336	48678	72047
94171	16606	52092	63096	09752	90644	56092	20751	19678	31311
10758	82747	99662	53243	22501	55820	32406	92052	60659	35477
66933	82305	91425	07804	24003	73777	26634	95806	35126	48503
74883	12771	02671	01090	82498	85176	68569	44827	51844	07616
79102	06066	24478	92267	33300	69392	16652	75381	02415	36065
94649	43308	08005	58253	77473	40559	46096	11540	54375	22388
44952	68217	04728	14414	43931	33854	07744	41771	80933	09655
29531	90289	75949	43091	75005	62207	98196	29316	92128	88918
04355	25867	16008	63243	35388	43138	40330	53741	59469	73144
03640	63541	48488	19060	77959	96217	75666	88042	47261	91184
21749	09836	63276	91133	77308	43654	66146	03991	28629	35848
57425	21919	14688	90852	12918	59833	42736	17916	22868	75963
49962	16108	46986	36939	98761	60113	71822	89915	93090	49299
57985	04214	03417	82576	64699	45011	87770	21525	39212	41547
96374	04318	58540	12375	47382	72917	11063	10129	61201	76044
05457	48338	40916	10453	94473	72759	86299	62959	01064	39749
28918	15769	34348	64162	75841	77582	82921	99286	49425	02973
73010	11300	10710	62560	78969	10771	53899	26454	73627	03681
59435	23480	05967	24479	93169	38697	93658	13676	39128	11680
17929	02455	53366	98097	08284	66830	26423	57062	04563	13822
41862	26768	83848	62175	18414	50906	39708	80097	23206	18358
01294	42540	43590	78681	79771	70501	05062	95860	29602	14866
22775	02858	12165	47273	74148	19427	49227	20518	80065	95722
53747	60983	82171	44180	25536	55599	03762	22186	99253	95841
81766	28025	32247	41257	57319	72602	19740	65016	12435	89463
24862	44004	40269	45574	11018	55941	36479	15404	64110	46027
99169	80770	92093	25630	24942	18977	89382	65496	88534	41734
53600	45992	93546	47348	42169	26882	81774	48703	56244	99137
88627	39523	39496	81268	32137	61411	79234	22696	23073	34171
97367	76657	83638	11912	18723	05129	62265	27431	04195	78294
32005	87382	36246	31037	60009	80722	44244	38968	35608	62938
57154	76478	44478	78561	71064	19331	76406	84452	19058	54278
54146	36375	30932	58210	70875	01355	70257	09341	23730	58309
36283	92917	30953	49460	18185	63965	20121	45041	89156	29563
74973	83767	27843	13152	28328	51597	54624	63371	88603	61277
70237	69924	87413	95159	84237	48986	35781	73808	20817	60630
76426	12882	89455	20792	19655	30803	07915	70264	50346	69701
65088	63220	93521	92145	11180	37773	26018	16150	62735	31062

Table A.5. (*Continued*)

21755	50969	10016	01373	18088	96168	14217	19786	90759	66476
82024	93860	24943	04919	05019	85844	69890	46740	51431	87922
64649	96595	97725	16988	22404	81529	87537	91453	60886	42239
05455	52581	66391	25111	53143	92863	78886	37547	15306	53911
85711	29066	02999	56394	11372	60689	61784	24499	90934	25106
32230	67428	14496	80119	50249	80419	30275	57878	74784	27806
93773	12383	30343	70604	50537	67783	51863	01132	40022	29939
19436	47161	08039	23786	70362	08094	15302	18963	76059	85683
29564	06230	71308	71770	88850	87166	23344	55564	23287	39647
28294	12945	23018	21604	22457	40306	39721	75568	95922	95419
09211	96490	96042	07837	82647	25343	08236	21325	53823	31010
01652	30822	70058	42947	27160	76437	14177	97132	55193	56972
45091	57793	40937	25483	84462	77419	04356	29363	36969	57549
12567	57462	31667	72844	52056	56741	71936	20944	78241	80949
81524	60599	29872	33841	34193	00587	95783	69415	54442	01910
21482	11696	76840	55775	43085	56535	51444	99849	36099	17950
82810	35306	66543	81499	90106	07145	31914	27172	75808	10295
79498	84331	90497	84000	89528	81166	81247	56983	10673	51195
11109	05896	35392	59285	37186	89548	02607	09712	34804	21413
15244	98745	55271	42923	60096	74268	04743	60039	17547	64932
31666	05605	48629	41332	10329	89982	46927	71723	07996	02466
42826	34764	23143	25983	47607	51791	82282	27570	24876	01128
82881	87130	76850	76921	69879	26981	32973	55008	33291	04669
28391	28322	14413	31579	59754	74317	08112	79815	05879	16938
48719	39869	00739	45610	67010	91567	46312	53765	05780	50798
52763	59397	81517	54521	93475	70156	79661	46562	62420	55458
70967	26680	21377	88141	36450	25424	24495	18149	88435	67268
07692	40737	75193	84524	30406	21722	56673	44542	57189	42256
38832	52688	66638	25632	54050	93604	75178	08625	75145	73248
63182	19854	50484	24217	90941	27692	47680	36849	91973	20190
93388	78611	31175	79544	96694	64262	15325	13587	43599	39302
43423	06816	50091	39199	84373	53446	61320	86900	69517	35003
84358	91122	87506	04936	42059	07924	69016	42775	35505	28060
48808	40305	02561	52614	92636	82287	60001	19417	76491	84195
16750	42742	05696	49496	45709	28786	61339	08953	01668	29427
61552	04467	72828	96765	25138	79942	53404	00946	25034	41690
24829	73764	19122	50857	33043	40546	45884	10391	49390	02819
72401	09034	02594	34257	82193	84846	69338	52408	90406	70765
10932	28706	73841	84692	43581	99260	03325	26610	29737	38927
65930	45238	78052	61167	64536	36708	39425	06176	82227	37781
86639	79801	99050	76091	65094	05740	48597	39918	02130	53520
01947	29996	62454	04755	66442	55854	37146	20187	86811	39179
53770	70012	36138	86720	95077	89978	84171	95222	13796	25774
30475	50884	31026	28195	89935	85855	05715	61588	18092	54261
62739	88081	63832	90260	67072	90095	36914	10629	31549	93630
77844	24386	45720	54845	17591	11938	13307	72402	14648	36263
85747	88110	56936	48625	79327	38333	16052	51315	63422	18693
41361	79928	07316	24546	81431	67669	73127	29744	20315	54192
42317	66171	16169	01470	63300	66571	29722	79191	07644	33148
30088	82194	22366	94453	65418	42430	65820	13046	85896	97958

Table A.5. (*Continued*)

14679	06451	06588	81467	29514	43874	97618	90837	66459	81223
89204	04220	22479	96891	79032	02169	01727	90834	29465	59280
90491	09422	42113	67877	28245	58572	97229	56225	62283	67668
45465	63773	73453	66756	39456	35932	60485	39521	92761	00876
70407	14550	53641	90888	62562	57373	81180	70722	93714	25780
11254	35507	11749	50931	99843	40677	45472	06738	31180	26435
77992	30030	78254	99249	91207	54003	03149	32871	68881	17444
84733	51402	45811	12247	61182	56872	90592	31698	74858	63867
09476	82052	07023	03671	58821	19882	89900	60456	53637	77719
83577	01987	59725	40464	05258	67372	56907	35085	98351	74336
60855	96100	28905	08526	91010	69331	96888	57348	72097	16448
49813	50842	56729	82794	86204	72075	56610	90983	36404	99578
69832	22786	08230	44306	91759	51802	84976	43633	97016	89399
63245	74878	80059	06446	18147	50861	41846	93322	83316	59991
10105	20707	33291	13385	80687	63653	55732	61518	67517	51439
00977	42906	48644	05707	96448	27318	95873	29376	13401	16019
75501	08838	73515	61548	07645	91940	82831	69523	71658	04241
80525	44978	45143	66055	90038	45735	64065	72771	60040	05302
91446	00959	82739	87803	82164	02753	77038	37448	31342	51018
24031	85017	93826	97797	42345	73895	62266	08538	90827	68122
91285	34606	86074	04984	55238	86574	22300	54630	27078	70794
81062	49226	65798	51749	18313	44134	99983	02693	16310	73623
94945	07061	87861	63618	90956	73170	20417	63972	00075	24697
47508	62774	49067	29437	35021	45184	55918	28848	69823	59308
27440	30866	38231	51593	65475	28517	81818	34260	69189	06796
18072	47268	20958	00335	13388	77308	43355	64352	95916	96329
14722	21374	95744	82090	30844	46254	99924	83255	00209	51956
09853	91508	60367	38631	88481	83202	02881	68468	84877	93045
94373	28832	23632	82309	81160	46174	46608	64077	64988	13237
94526	48016	37362	92027	15906	67185	59957	55076	90844	49373
78640	27483	57136	95467	58574	92235	26245	27355	27918	21312
76610	67852	17624	95070	11800	15172	84826	72409	71016	74412
07321	74221	79429	08584	36645	42613	25865	71671	97244	38423
55337	86213	19237	39510	63919	27925	92274	02322	83458	79852
27987	49253	43638	18546	18533	44280	98884	94782	78736	19373
07610	71301	59319	14196	51309	80085	18726	91587	80992	61663
41047	91314	78463	48950	87529	84618	19947	58119	69184	92035
29552	48994	27991	27000	10082	17489	14188	27732	38692	82566
47166	39897	14884	30234	47445	12559	48351	77069	27255	69909
74159	15772	27203	21269	82781	05262	86541	71890	52467	67787
34518	97021	71462	55582	90333	41760	37564	49543	59181	09194
22533	52449	11893	99313	88836	39198	35665	61203	46236	26586
43385	21033	35736	25113	29055	48307	28348	35323	56803	22908
26224	51169	70990	65422	53620	32916	14914	93239	25205	12074
45601	64938	79216	90857	32195	75453	62960	98682	25443	64524
58151	68188	85768	00919	33595	93299	57440	04948	12724	31809
76340	71754	43465	15001	98816	57885	57961	26798	39138	93645
09625	14943	03037	83731	75049	96716	04849	58650	08254	21673
55746	39415	34777	53925	10558	78021	73106	36443	60700	36211
70966	99897	60680	65010	43936	78523	75711	47553	03918	95528

Table A.5. (*Continued*)

37906	67684	64945	80515	98580	66844	13841	81451	64133	51736
33214	33660	03036	15271	64298	48348	11405	33299	97141	83158
24673	99616	75635	57261	62852	61758	04883	73473	96889	20071
48424	09907	23621	52564	02788	43652	36819	28046	36901	68989
81824	70042	83835	72632	81280	33986	72398	28508	19464	60208
86072	74558	72701	65183	36787	34078	73381	33580	41052	44089
95065	73583	85914	53236	46186	97991	72273	51718	59845	93607
23036	95754	67198	41400	43613	89077	41942	49956	22261	83956
03385	64705	57768	64255	65622	15430	01983	73023	20295	64558
04689	47109	40454	18734	48321	21315	93002	66173	60023	64576
47246	02296	88556	10674	67034	06143	33545	45982	73986	30075
14570	16742	69321	65249	67601	18364	01776	45378	56279	29273
69122	51274	85540	51772	40770	78669	05078	22446	88971	31817
90157	54589	16114	05382	87269	75173	65610	17102	12127	18837
03879	53737	87508	41417	60925	92795	08442	15497	17004	62546
22236	70503	22890	02810	10852	39816	41230	89031	63119	77428
96497	82130	24298	06620	21037	66636	10484	63177	84701	39611
75355	95630	95584	12836	16760	85032	59349	90801	10663	46768
84645	86953	59912	76888	22124	40748	45370	05479	24547	97967
66878	19564	15482	16818	61566	18034	54106	62327	87010	61112
83586	51499	56724	76848	50567	11768	15509	87138	83245	15223
42133	15790	15539	51120	66864	41105	44854	99171	91340	55499
10936	66119	98287	94653	83328	48089	38583	98693	44910	81224
83154	67905	59041	43101	27232	75480	07791	67427	34439	99786
88765	34520	08226	38677	58026	00065	78152	68330	06605	24659
88509	09116	58112	66633	76782	60996	74937	00650	29469	70960
60539	24597	02726	94980	45345	17247	95374	17014	43723	09207
61732	87526	69563	29647	51811	44040	97946	91308	66335	76237
60406	76296	14122	98066	61291	85153	59295	89395	02711	11708
45845	69699	05584	06215	87034	66264	14275	89270	07145	39440
72327	79003	23073	27408	56790	94062	53259	72995	58638	94869
41471	95004	96783	25663	82927	66588	53186	19823	40260	63150
16553	30969	36833	42272	22134	52349	14887	18182	75107	87002
46044	93244	45068	31210	81646	08985	19099	33722	30442	79154
00942	93267	51118	67305	43765	56843	47168	71421	04014	81289
51611	78061	03866	20642	89054	48544	89778	01766	02593	99660
74620	50774	33064	41415	50910	32721	38133	34307	62641	67084
38731	28630	23199	81522	80336	48317	66878	66416	96592	81803
21487	92695	62781	42431	89552	55433	26629	60878	25607	05738
03962	72124	97090	33420	26704	59442	16319	62932	30719	17924
31070	25105	70997	00037	61248	67153	51682	05715	69150	63466
58445	79472	50823	89685	80704	77058	36012	22548	11179	64137
84211	28033	10300	09500	64296	00270	22957	35313	05259	13737
35087	86887	05537	51242	57611	84488	88429	70179	25215	19675
91108	69575	97474	58666	74734	20403	49813	15245	43150	21696
41824	55683	57679	44922	50418	98213	35513	29157	55322	69516
19196	89530	64420	80747	04696	01452	66444	85596	15581	23122
98495	82872	10780	18824	15923	26125	13436	45495	52042	02791
48367	65082	55187	45381	75601	45172	90624	37190	07520	10413
94793	75039	97093	07207	69403	51555	84698	44192	02867	19475

Table A.5. (*Continued*)

91046	70999	06579	00484	43692	57795	53540	01085	24645	38105
06824	97998	26567	77415	25388	55594	05067	30055	34726	37855
14595	46870	49867	77370	15416	96161	38219	63861	39195	60419
09751	14737	00661	71330	22026	90185	42872	45571	87570	15285
03574	83877	71094	71667	90150	95901	64049	21185	50667	13340
24033	24135	28513	53860	66540	14499	88130	98287	96551	94717
99341	43590	67468	12497	67768	94135	54895	82151	98848	53733
32760	12964	82939	80956	39285	07097	89021	70247	20290	89516
54491	21296	37353	32456	58553	59215	28308	36913	66700	67981
07583	33673	33787	99662	93888	66367	53206	21934	52744	19057
39647	66364	41356	50860	32955	39987	43329	00091	10580	62660
80732	20453	96128	92692	90996	11743	51493	03267	56168	07600
40090	72135	71999	82780	48686	47093	44383	42461	55315	49745
00632	56081	30796	80045	03103	98211	61335	84114	52662	58949
79731	47847	69497	86357	92669	78799	38769	23422	91608	38848
08614	02049	34765	90145	27982	56589	87690	16839	11823	19391
09935	85090	21118	60897	75323	03859	45248	36755	13296	48981
74216	04471	58876	13015	48205	72092	98703	43385	71982	41419
00677	31291	81644	08248	14690	13905	51216	82150	31951	52357
26580	88272	90406	41986	74259	13682	13754	59388	32537	60731
71552	82733	52426	69959	47917	57872	15979	75022	06320	62721
19442	52160	37978	58426	08753	26686	81330	47810	54884	99014
00122	09604	56525	52716	07567	70954	57616	07110	24118	80713
67216	76877	56318	46014	69224	01212	84256	94624	09438	05009
45110	25576	47459	54570	00287	10586	60938	70350	73650	08754
89671	59232	48355	57037	07029	28837	09759	99012	06245	46358
21941	14417	89031	04431	25308	11970	44044	56533	42796	47979
02705	84418	82163	33219	59841	60076	21881	90604	46695	64728
68115	26133	43759	27355	70302	75614	20963	45249	82820	89682
92707	49102	60251	19581	75228	75131	73738	66245	33821	06721
35939	55142	07399	48110	22069	99420	97897	92602	74539	13811
12019	47810	78689	41839	42832	80434	97117	58792	78698	43063
50092	12981	27059	45518	29575	67789	40553	33217	34323	06982
32986	35078	13588	65822	72642	43450	06917	50448	40435	88575
67536	08040	40407	70084	56838	10269	50074	08019	97450	12526
98106	75894	72414	51431	56860	78280	57941	43121	37253	35425
77276	44827	73475	37404	63144	42226	85056	30301	16297	25073
03764	96921	47652	13621	52855	94537	91525	98316	66168	12161
77455	55276	34556	09855	48125	00049	67169	02566	10876	42160
55073	50995	10314	02925	24721	22000	09511	59060	68761	81026
67299	74565	41692	79065	99163	83388	07859	96658	09217	85375
29298	07412	80784	17996	80921	23560	13066	66357	80544	86050
91407	73988	21260	61665	78651	16919	93657	09667	15090	03532
85379	80488	14514	62693	45528	08934	43846	82672	01415	64436
73877	63341	15148	20821	88589	44145	67572	08120	40576	70372
57044	08909	40062	60187	00559	61672	65001	34955	24717	33706
79784	75348	34030	26050	50030	65726	44081	72952	40980	89306
67019	98358	86971	36607	36901	91939	19522	89680	62379	67151
41496	44616	94227	63819	34868	34838	95217	57756	89580	17676
99834	39917	40995	86715	51336	27577	03438	72434	03659	70046

Table A.5. (*Continued*)

87340	93621	75668	11412	87464	22069	45241	72818	29736	23057
70713	16765	64165	34106	27152	55954	91352	44525	44980	69154
10102	38228	38442	86601	73625	62341	11417	07431	41828	84087
28072	11642	17204	98450	35856	29088	51820	49122	28351	28007
12884	25234	35447	85574	94423	96364	28378	02991	62542	48328
27094	27605	21783	82254	97475	44559	90078	39433	25896	00475
69789	14454	58626	21664	02351	19124	93582	89374	94004	59659
11915	34559	00117	89667	36950	14694	55609	01408	07963	35106
38964	17831	56305	77347	57337	47900	71366	97092	40254	67697
43892	54073	29411	89805	74131	36540	52057	83475	32340	42757
65481	08075	59117	82023	60088	22314	93095	57736	08564	31758
13466	94974	48647	37115	84859	75118	86979	45810	92049	40000
11558	09341	52027	28088	00284	48909	90897	05195	13099	31837
73126	52226	55216	61265	70639	72451	98949	41632	59251	80815
51628	82433	29946	37772	57118	02761	02502	90157	18424	99129
28958	81585	28890	39072	74422	94883	99498	43036	62730	89054
69755	17039	74438	93269	89674	98623	84667	20393	60353	78578
28290	62543	20640	60954	79960	31174	67404	23853	36480	04202
96886	43500	89025	42647	54653	44096	72699	39322	81643	35955
80940	62044	43802	04416	32270	53875	32820	12044	76883	52900
25451	76608	30584	94033	88940	87339	23568	55358	20032	21972
51540	11490	05081	27069	16685	56486	88750	24122	45978	58768
38809	03936	74336	10590	94518	71798	80119	34531	86118	05922
60470	09522	12897	91680	34003	78900	67368	94108	58328	02998
93030	31200	49927	18762	63223	10480	93871	68905	68583	91355
30880	63084	00584	35748	09225	33618	18680	09517	88981	48227
88533	97152	86114	42311	78843	92251	43919	33256	04265	26280
19299	79270	01925	98119	71388	45254	29028	66878	40017	38202
69054	70503	01526	74633	34061	32661	89417	42554	50565	20407
67352	20450	16530	15129	41996	15818	16940	59277	03202	85715
85468	41376	79039	01850	99744	81812	93169	22705	97709	81907
12057	35180	02566	98772	69539	28280	43827	08444	56220	61323
61951	19798	61229	89189	84075	01746	53801	07092	58342	86217
92224	77389	34320	09414	47608	00915	77016	53859	30015	95353
01982	53711	04423	43139	19021	25871	84038	71386	71973	89367
88443	26351	62114	35523	54106	04932	42631	11399	84712	05686
71700	79026	28855	61893	11658	12915	72563	19139	61766	98345
34173	19937	12062	92936	49051	57880	05821	14005	31644	63815
98089	14200	02395	86565	97833	07913	66981	30666	81164	10981
35414	13649	63167	56163	68467	05339	15824	46897	38963	11698
19522	11849	95389	65695	35664	22725	15372	87703	87868	37883
36480	77931	39265	34212	51883	03389	53384	89802	58350	41882
26138	79888	44088	45532	76396	48583	03931	86340	82657	18881
69367	46269	53313	03455	40910	14365	18002	78724	10321	53409
27566	84710	60165	98597	50090	13172	28217	50750	50546	46520
24208	26566	41518	10015	86420	28387	92538	99744	65618	96011
85497	48885	23833	03027	03664	94744	35480	60186	41792	09076
78331	88300	24816	54195	01822	23175	22655	27351	60205	15074
48594	55901	98052	85207	28770	05754	75593	01764	30247	65604
21400	37964	35184	69430	99920	74647	48604	19798	81347	09895

Table A.5. (*Concluded*)

27247	74427	01337	38176	17021	58543	98070	61531	86549	65516
14156	95285	44308	08275	50878	30794	26858	84002	62289	17713
45673	14618	76646	28312	80058	25534	32686	66307	03660	25200
18256	82731	32083	47921	98771	61337	79083	22463	23032	36026
08862	28939	93878	02811	71963	06475	91182	88814	12247	74153
34694	40786	32471	27744	74229	95669	05957	74718	94691	95680
21859	70031	23453	10432	51516	15202	27567	28584	23404	83160
88328	81523	94184	31389	40680	61577	03337	65833	64959	97256
98901	18100	18490	48034	21791	98440	94518	81149	36224	87001
95993	92944	93729	25874	11685	37237	18258	74414	82159	23219
99886	90343	43080	45388	84604	99135	33371	08008	47709	14181
55707	06608	38286	70240	76861	29006	82287	32662	55387	38363
31696	44902	84149	00774	47296	76811	35197	19884	02527	36204
94480	41042	95933	06218	73908	87481	59713	70946	88258	91030
51854	91851	84421	79859	19367	97465	10491	85755	20110	48867
12205	33427	90714	43441	44220	74345	48089	19423	83736	27611
12035	23714	33964	90354	36447	05492	04934	80168	36601	98093
59152	72070	00051	51676	09597	92497	68607	79172	57563	32830
78914	78012	57844	44952	49118	90138	98763	81334	99134	62792
84548	42156	91999	72590	07545	91955	83829	75373	97778	08310
69856	44345	37359	25052	14076	58986	27231	32509	49973	07253
93760	97283	39850	63554	22674	64053	80248	05012	07838	01917
40959	28502	02379	57758	25133	30976	59655	79147	37982	15567
51562	69272	51570	85970	51690	36403	53207	91615	70820	00385
64929	86104	32268	18664	21571	61451	74567	94342	94943	20582
69002	28768	51591	50633	39475	81155	31652	59516	72230	97730
36308	38281	02907	72917	11332	11740	68452	05049	14222	39893
11359	09112	52439	32620	23768	49023	80229	40159	18894	51933
41544	81869	17314	67064	46558	75767	35582	31585	69270	31356
64702	06004	53711	68222	25934	41607	16231	22923	91454	42414
31398	06654	57345	84180	88969	76195	56445	52913	09476	80635
98527	65438	05890	46391	25333	34481	78886	62987	67946	40786
33203	32139	94004	74772	02591	42598	32264	10207	70859	33289
62005	72426	76511	07230	54774	63575	88484	58723	55982	07384
40465	76337	93835	75973	11321	84168	03118	61194	39104	83876
51313	52998	56165	60010	54571	87333	32852	11115	71019	26079
17303	69107	58913	31510	58840	69451	87141	97787	02447	34599
85562	01985	41848	33221	22690	37149	18677	77720	98226	89880
55239	22513	37930	24957	08372	25614	78337	39488	31896	35980
28818	49087	35155	69148	98487	68591	25162	33651	75444	49804
19825	70717	45870	38769	19778	69745	40464	15079	26297	22066
95718	75713	92817	75483	17542	25903	97538	52096	34734	39538
24624	91901	29784	51594	41504	84679	34535	45096	59754	52661
78177	95113	67082	46472	75090	32286	17907	16865	40027	88378
70022	24726	18150	86370	54867	51867	17396	37574	68877	75099
30696	08284	73441	66084	35537	18463	90940	79472	58367	34949
84393	91813	91338	21704	08183	53759	48903	09586	17386	18038
51751	48159	23192	05719	25583	02027	81915	73246	02237	54207
05106	42768	10657	79027	78247	58237	45199	47058	75553	29795
98790	24578	58358	28940	48422	30065	44593	96972	80495	10221

Table A.6. *Natural logarithm of x* (**ln** *x*)

x	0.00	0.01	0.02	0.03	0.04	0.05	0.06	0.07	0.08	0.09
1.0	0.00000	0.00995	0.01980	0.02956	0.03922	0.04879	0.05827	0.06766	0.07696	0.08618
1.1	0.09531	0.10436	0.11333	0.12222	0.13103	0.13976	0.14842	0.15700	0.16551	0.17395
1.2	0.18232	0.19062	0.19885	0.20701	0.21511	0.22314	0.23111	0.23902	0.24686	0.25464
1.3	0.26236	0.27003	0.27763	0.28518	0.29267	0.30010	0.30748	0.31481	0.32208	0.32930
1.4	0.33647	0.34359	0.35066	0.35767	0.36464	0.37156	0.37844	0.38526	0.39204	0.39878
1.5	0.40546	0.41211	0.41871	0.42527	0.43178	0.43825	0.44468	0.45107	0.45742	0.46373
1.6	0.47000	0.47623	0.48243	0.48858	0.49470	0.50077	0.50682	0.51272	0.51879	0.52473
1.7	0.53063	0.53649	0.54232	0.54812	0.55388	0.55961	0.56531	0.57098	0.57661	0.58221
1.8	0.58779	0.59333	0.59884	0.60432	0.60977	0.61518	0.62058	0.62594	0.63127	0.63658
1.9	0.64185	0.64710	0.65232	0.65752	0.66269	0.66783	0.67294	0.67803	0.68310	0.68813
2.0	0.69315	0.69813	0.70310	0.70804	0.71295	0.71784	0.72271	0.72755	0.73237	0.73716
2.1	0.74194	0.74669	0.75142	0.75612	0.76081	0.76547	0.77011	0.77473	0.77932	0.78390
2.2	0.78846	0.79299	0.79751	0.80200	0.80648	0.81093	0.81536	0.81978	0.82417	0.82855
2.3	0.83291	0.83725	0.84157	0.84587	0.85015	0.85441	0.85866	0.86289	0.86710	0.87129
2.4	0.87547	0.87963	0.88377	0.88789	0.89200	0.89609	0.90016	0.90422	0.90826	0.91228
2.5	0.91629	0.92028	0.92426	0.92822	0.93216	0.93609	0.94001	0.94391	0.94779	0.95166
2.6	0.95551	0.95935	0.96317	0.96698	0.97078	0.97456	0.97833	0.98208	0.98582	0.98954
2.7	0.99325	0.99695	1.00063	1.00430	1.00796	1.01160	1.01523	1.01885	1.02245	1.02604
2.8	1.02962	1.03318	1.03674	1.04028	1.04380	1.04732	1.05082	1.05431	1.05779	1.06126
2.9	1.06471	1.06815	1.07158	1.07500	1.07841	1.08180	1.08519	1.08856	1.09192	1.09527
3.0	1.09861	1.10194	1.10526	1.10856	1.11186	1.11514	1.11841	1.12168	1.12493	1.12817
3.1	1.13140	1.13462	1.13783	1.14103	1.14422	1.14740	1.15057	1.15373	1.15688	1.16002
3.2	1.16315	1.16627	1.16938	1.17248	1.17557	1.17865	1.18173	1.18479	1.18784	1.19089
3.3	1.19392	1.19695	1.19996	1.20297	1.20597	1.20896	1.21194	1.21491	1.21787	1.22083
3.4	1.22377	1.22671	1.22964	1.23256	1.23547	1.23837	1.24127	1.24415	1.24703	1.24990
3.5	1.25276	1.25562	1.25846	1.26130	1.26413	1.26695	1.26976	1.27256	1.27536	1.27815
3.6	1.28093	1.28371	1.28647	1.28923	1.29198	1.29473	1.29746	1.30019	1.30291	1.30563
3.7	1.30833	1.31103	1.31372	1.31641	1.31908	1.32175	1.32442	1.32707	1.32972	1.33237
3.8	1.33500	1.33763	1.34025	1.34286	1.34547	1.34807	1.35067	1.35325	1.35583	1.35841
3.9	1.36098	1.36354	1.36609	1.36864	1.37118	1.37371	1.37624	1.37877	1.38128	1.38379
4.0	1.38629	1.38879	1.39128	1.39377	1.39624	1.39872	1.40118	1.40364	1.40610	1.40854
4.1	1.41099	1.41342	1.41585	1.41828	1.42070	1.42311	1.42551	1.42792	1.43031	1.43270
4.2	1.43508	1.43746	1.43983	1.44220	1.44456	1.44692	1.44927	1.45161	1.45395	1.45629
4.3	1.45861	1.46094	1.46325	1.46557	1.46787	1.47017	1.47247	1.47476	1.47705	1.47933
4.4	1.48160	1.48387	1.48614	1.48840	1.49065	1.49290	1.49515	1.49739	1.49962	1.50185
4.5	1.50408	1.50630	1.50851	1.51072	1.51293	1.51513	1.51732	1.51951	1.52170	1.52388
4.6	1.52606	1.52823	1.53039	1.53256	1.53471	1.53687	1.53901	1.54116	1.54330	1.54543
4.7	1.54756	1.54969	1.55181	1.55392	1.55604	1.55814	1.56025	1.56235	1.56444	1.56653
4.8	1.56861	1.57070	1.57277	1.57485	1.57691	1.57898	1.58104	1.58309	1.58514	1.58719
4.9	1.58923	1.59127	1.59331	1.59534	1.59736	1.59939	1.60141	1.60342	1.60543	1.60744
5.0	1.60944	1.61143	1.61343	1.61542	1.61741	1.61939	1.62137	1.62334	1.62531	1.62728
5.1	1.62924	1.63120	1.63315	1.63511	1.63705	1.63900	1.64094	1.64287	1.64480	1.64673
5.2	1.64866	1.65058	1.65250	1.65441	1.65632	1.65823	1.66013	1.66203	1.66393	1.66582
5.3	1.66771	1.66959	1.67147	1.67335	1.67523	1.67710	1.67896	1.68083	1.68269	1.68454
5.4	1.68640	1.68825	1.69009	1.69194	1.69378	1.69561	1.69745	1.69928	1.70110	1.70293
5.5	1.70475	1.70656	1.70838	1.71019	1.71199	1.71380	1.71560	1.71739	1.71919	1.72098
5.6	1.72277	1.72455	1.72633	1.72811	1.72988	1.73166	1.73342	1.73519	1.73695	1.73871
5.7	1.74047	1.74222	1.74397	1.74572	1.74746	1.74920	1.75094	1.75267	1.75440	1.75613
5.8	1.75786	1.75958	1.76130	1.76302	1.76473	1.76644	1.76815	1.76985	1.77156	1.77326
5.9	1.77495	1.77664	1.77834	1.78002	1.78171	1.78339	1.78507	1.78675	1.78842	1.79009

Table A.6. (*Concluded*)

x	0.00	0.01	0.02	0.03	0.04	0.05	0.06	0.07	0.08	0.09
6.0	1.79176	1.79342	1.79509	1.79675	1.79840	1.80006	1.80171	1.80336	1.80500	1.80665
6.1	1.80829	1.80993	1.81156	1.81319	1.81482	1.81645	1.81808	1.81970	1.82132	1.82293
6.2	1.82455	1.82616	1.82777	1.82938	1.83098	1.83258	1.83418	1.83578	1.83737	1.83896
6.3	1.84055	1.84213	1.84372	1.84530	1.84688	1.84845	1.85003	1.85160	1.85317	1.85473
6.4	1.85630	1.85786	1.85942	1.86097	1.86253	1.86408	1.86563	1.86718	1.86872	1.87026
6.5	1.87180	1.87334	1.87487	1.87641	1.87794	1.87946	1.88099	1.88251	1.88403	1.88555
6.6	1.88707	1.88858	1.89009	1.89160	1.89311	1.89462	1.89612	1.89762	1.89912	1.90061
6.7	1.90211	1.90360	1.90509	1.90657	1.90806	1.90954	1.91102	1.91250	1.91398	1.91545
6.8	1.91692	1.91839	1.91986	1.92132	1.92279	1.92425	1.92571	1.92716	1.92862	1.93007
6.9	1.93152	1.93297	1.93441	1.93586	1.93730	1.93874	1.94018	1.94162	1.94305	1.94448
7.0	1.94591	1.94734	1.94876	1.95019	1.95161	1.95303	1.95444	1.95586	1.95727	1.95868
7.1	1.96009	1.96150	1.96291	1.96431	1.96571	1.96711	1.96851	!.96990	1.97130	1.97269
7.2	1.97408	1.97547	1.97685	1.97824	1.97962	1.98100	1.98238	1.98376	1.98513	1.98650
7.3	1.98787	1.98924	1.99061	1.99197	1.99334	1.99470	1.99606	1.99742	1.99877	2.00013
7.4	2.00148	2.00283	2.00418	2.00553	2.00687	2.00821	2.00955	2.01089	2.01223	2.01357
7.5	2.01490	2.01623	2.01757	2.01889	2.02022	2.02155	2.02287	2.02419	2.02551	2.02683
7.6	2.02815	2.02946	2.03078	2.03209	2.03340	2.03471	2.03601	2.03732	2.03862	2.03992
7.7	2.04122	2.04252	2.04381	2.04511	2.04640	2.04769	2.04898	2.05027	2.05156	2.05284
7.8	2.05412	2.05540	2.05668	2.05796	2.05924	2.06051	2.06179	2.06306	2.06433	2.06560
7.9	2.06686	2.06813	2.06939	2.07065	2.07191	2.07317	2.07443	2.07568	2.07694	2.07819
8.0	2.07944	2.08069	2.08194	2.08318	2.08443	2.08567	2.08691	2.08815	2.08939	2.09063
8.1	2.09186	2.09310	2.09433	2.09556	2.09679	2.09802	2.09924	2.10047	2.10169	2.10291
8.2	2.10413	2.10535	2.10657	2.10779	2.10900	2.11021	2.11142	2.11263	2.11384	2.11505
8.3	2.11625	2.11746	2.11866	2.11986	2.12106	2.12226	2.12346	2.12465	2.12585	2.12704
8.4	2.12823	2.12942	2.13061	2.13180	2.13298	2.13417	2.13535	2.13653	2.13771	2.13889
8.5	2.14007	2.14124	2.14242	2.14359	2.14476	2.14593	2.14710	2.14827	2.14943	2.15060
8.6	2.15176	2.15292	2.15408	2.15524	2.15640	2.15756	2.15871	2.15987	2.16102	2.16217
8.7	2.16332	2.16447	2.16562	2.16677	2.16791	2.16905	2.17020	2.17134	2.17248	2.17361
8.8	2.17475	2.17589	2.17702	2.17815	2.17929	2.18042	2.18155	2.18267	2.18380	2.18493
8.9	2.18605	2.18717	2.18830	2.18942	2.19053	2.19165	2.19277	2.19388	2.19500	2.19611
9.0	2.19722	2.19833	2.19944	2.20055	2.20166	2.20276	2.20387	2.20497	2.20607	2.20717
9.1	2.20827	2.20937	2.21047	2.21157	2.21266	2.21375	2.21485	2.21594	2.21703	2.21812
9.2	2.21920	2.22029	2.22137	2.22246	2.22354	2.22462	2.22570	2.22678	2.22786	2.22894
9.3	2.23001	2.23109	2.23216	2.23323	2.23431	2.23538	2.23644	2.23751	2.23858	2.23965
9.4	2.24071	2.24177	2.24283	2.24390	2.24496	2.24601	2.24707	2.24813	2.24918	2.25024
9.5	2.25129	2.25234	2.25339	2.25444	2.25549	2.25654	2.25759	2.25863	2.25968	2.26072
9.6	2.26176	2.26280	2.26384	2.26488	2.26592	2.26696	2.26799	2.26903	2.27006	2.27109
9.7	2.27213	2.27316	2.27419	2.27521	2.27624	2.27727	2.27829	2.27932	2.28034	2.28136
9.8	2.28238	2.28340	2.28442	2.28544	2.28646	2.28747	2.28849	2.28950	2.29051	2.29152
9.9	2.29253	2.29354	2.29455	2.29556	2.29657	2.29757	2.29858	2.29958	2.30058	2.30158

$\ln 10 = 2.30259$.

If $x > 10$, express x as $y \times 10^n$, where $1 < y < 10$ and n is an integer. Then $\ln x = \ln y + n \ln 10$. For example, $974 = 9.74 \times 10^2$, so that $y = 9.74$ and $n = 2$. Therefore, $\ln 974 = \ln 9.74 + 2 \ln 10 = 2.27624 + 2 \times 2.30259 = 6.88142$.

If $x < 1$, express x as $y/10^n$, where $1 < y < 10$ and n is an integer. Then $\ln x = \ln y - n \ln 10$. For example, $0.974 = 9.74/10$, so that $y = 9.74$ and $n = 1$. Therefore, $\ln 0.974 = \ln 9.74 - \ln 10 = 2.27624 - 2.30259 = -0.02635$.

Table A.7. *Percentage points of Bartholomew's test for order when*
m = 3 proportions are compared

c	α				
	0.10	0.05	0.025	0.01	0.005
0.0	2.952	4.231	5.537	7.289	8.628
0.1	2.885	4.158	5.459	7.208	8.543
0.2	2.816	4.081	5.378	7.122	8.455
0.3	2.742	4.001	5.292	7.030	8.360
0.4	2.664	3.914	5.200	6.932	8.258
0.5	2.580	3.820	5.098	6.822	8.146
0.6	2.486	3.715	4.985	6.700	8.016
0.7	2.379	3.593	4.852	6.556	7.865
0.8	2.251	3.446	4.689	6.377	7.677
0.9	2.080	3.245	4.465	6.130	7.413
1.0	1.642	2.706	3.841	5.413	6.635

Source: Reproduced from Table A.1 of Barlow, R. E., Bartholomew, D. J., Bremner, J. M., and Brunk, H. D., *Statistical inference under order restrictions*, New York: Wiley, 1972.

Table A.8. *Percentage points of Bartholomew's test for order when m = 4 proportions are compared*

c_2	α	c_1 0.0	0.1	0.2	0.3	0.4	0.5	0.6	0.7
0.0	0.10	4.010							
	0.05	5.435							
	0.025	6.861							
	0.01	8.746							
	0.005	10.171							
0.1	0.10	3.952	3.891						
	0.05	5.372	5.305						
	0.025	6.794	6.724						
	0.01	8.676	8.601						
	0.005	10.098	10.020						
0.2	0.10	3.893	3.827	3.758					
	0.05	5.307	5.235	5.160					
	0.025	6.725	6.649	6.570					
	0.01	8.602	8.522	8.437					
	0.005	10.022	9.939	9.851					
0.3	0.10	3.831	3.760	3.685	3.606				
	0.05	5.239	5.162	5.080	4.993				
	0.025	6.653	6.571	6.484	6.391				
	0.01	8.525	8.438	8.346	8.246				
	0.005	9.942	9.852	9.756	9.653				
0.4	0.10	3.765	3.688	3.607	3.519	3.423			
	0.05	5.166	5.083	4.994	4.898	4.791			
	0.025	6.575	6.486	6.392	6.289	6.174			
	0.01	8.442	8.348	8.247	8.137	8.014			
	0.005	9.855	9.758	9.653	9.539	9.411			
0.5	0.10	3.695	3.610	3.521	3.423	3.313	3.187		
	0.05	5.088	4.997	4.898	4.791	4.670	4.528		
	0.025	6.491	6.394	6.289	6.173	6.043	5.891		
	0.01	8.352	8.246	8.136	8.013	7.873	7.709		
	0.005	9.761	9.654	9.537	9.409	9.264	9.092		
0.6	0.10	3.617	3.523	3.422	3.310	3.183	3.031	2.837	
	0.05	5.002	4.900	4.789	4.665	4.524	4.354	4.135	
	0.025	6.398	6.289	6.170	6.038	5.886	5.702	5.462	
	0.01	8.251	8.135	8.008	7.867	7.703	7.504	7.244	
	0.005	9.656	9.535	9.404	9.256	9.085	8.877	8.604	
0.7	0.10	3.530	3.422	3.305	3.172	3.017	2.822	2.550	1.987
	0.05	4.904	4.787	4.657	4.510	4.337	4.118	3.805	3.137
	0.025	6.291	6.166	6.027	5.870	5.682	5.443	5.100	4.346
	0.01	8.135	8.002	7.854	7.684	7.482	7.223	6.846	6.000
	0.005	9.534	9.395	9.242	9.065	8.853	8.581	8.183	7.279
0.8	0.10	3.427	3.296	3.151	2.981	2.770	2.473	1.642	
	0.05	4.787	4.644	4.483	4.294	4.056	3.715	2.706	
	0.025	6.163	6.011	5.838	5.634	5.375	4.999	3.841	
	0.01	7.994	7.832	7.647	7.427	7.146	6.734	5.412	
	0.005	9.385	9.217	9.025	8.795	8.500	8.064	6.635	
0.9	0.10	3.291	3.110	2.897	2.621	2.166			
	0.05	4.631	4.432	4.195	3.883	3.353			
	0.025	5.990	5.778	5.523	5.182	4.591			
	0.01	7.804	7.577	7.303	6.933	6.277			
	0.005	9.183	8.948	8.661	8.273	7.576			
1.0	0.10	2.952							
	0.05	4.231							
	0.025	5.537							
	0.01	7.289							
	0.005	8.628							

The table is symmetric in c_1 and c_2.

Source: Reproduced from Table A.2 of Barlow, R. E., Bartholomew, D. J., Bremner, J. M., and Brunk, H. D., *Statistical inference under order restrictions*, New York: Wiley, 1972.

Table A.9. *Percentage points of Bartholomew's test for order when up to m = 12 proportions based on equal sample sizes are compared*

			α		
m	0.10	0.05	0.025	0.01	0.005
3	2.580	3.820	5.098	6.822	8.146
4	3.187	4.528	5.891	7.709	9.092
5	3.636	5.049	6.471	8.356	9.784
6	3.994	5.460	6.928	8.865	10.327
7	4.289	5.800	7.304	9.284	10.774
8	4.542	6.088	7.624	9.639	11.153
9	4.761	6.339	7.901	9.946	11.480
10	4.956	6.560	8.145	10.216	11.767
11	5.130	6.758	8.363	10.458	12.025
12	5.288	6.937	8.561	10.676	12.257

Source: Reproduced from Table A.3 of Barlow, R. E., Bartholomew, D. J. Bremner, J. M., and Brunk, H. D., *Statistical inference under order restrictions*, New York: Wiley, 1972.

Table A.10. *The logit transformation*

P	$1 - P$	$\lambda = \ln\{P/(1-P)\}$	$\lambda = \ln\{P/(1-P)\}$	P	$1 - P$
0.999	0.001	6.9068	9.0	0.9999	0.0001
0.99	0.01	4.5951	8.5	0.9998	0.0002
0.98	0.02	3.8918	8.0	0.9997	0.0003
0.97	0.03	3.4761	7.5	0.9994	0.0006
0.96	0.04	3.1781	7.0	0.9991	0.0009
0.95	0.05	2.9444	6.5	0.9985	0.0015
0.94	0.06	2.7515	6.0	0.9975	0.0025
0.93	0.07	2.5867	5.5	0.9959	0.0041
0.92	0.08	2.4423	5.0	0.9933	0.0067
0.91	0.09	2.3136	4.5	0.9890	0.0110
0.90	0.10	2.1972	4.0	0.9820	0.0180
0.89	0.11	2.0907	3.9	0.9802	0.0198
0.88	0.12	1.9924	3.8	0.9781	0.0219
0.87	0.13	1.9010	3.7	0.9759	0.0241
0.86	0.14	1.8153	3.6	0.9734	0.0266
0.85	0.15	1.7346	3.5	0.9707	0.0293
0.84	0.16	1.6582	3.4	0.9677	0.0323
0.83	0.17	1.5856	3.3	0.9644	0.0356
0.82	0.18	1.5163	3.2	0.9608	0.0392
0.81	0.19	1.4500	3.1	0.9569	0.0431
0.80	0.20	1.3863	3.0	0.9526	0.0474
0.79	0.21	1.3249	2.9	0.9478	0.0522
0.78	0.22	1.2657	2.8	0.9427	0.0573
0.77	0.23	1.2083	2.7	0.9370	0.0630
0.76	0.24	1.1527	2.6	0.9309	0.0691
0.75	0.25	1.0986	2.5	0.9241	0.0759
0.74	0.26	1.0460	2.4	0.9168	0.0832
0.73	0.27	0.9946	2.3	0.9089	0.0911
0.72	0.28	0.9445	2.2	0.9002	0.0998
0.71	0.29	0.8954	2.1	0.8909	0.1091
0.70	0.30	0.8473	2.0	0.8808	0.1192
0.69	0.31	0.8001	1.9	0.8699	0.1301
0.68	0.32	0.7538	1.8	0.8581	0.1419
0.67	0.33	0.7082	1.7	0.8455	0.1545
0.66	0.34	0.6633	1.6	0.8320	0.1680
0.65	0.35	0.6190	1.5	0.8176	0.1824
0.64	0.36	0.5754	1.4	0.8022	0.1978
0.63	0.37	0.5322	1.3	0.7858	0.2142
0.62	0.38	0.4895	1.2	0.7685	0.2315
0.61	0.39	0.4473	1.1	0.7503	0.2497
0.60	0.40	0.4055	1.0	0.7311	0.2689
0.59	0.41	0.3640	0.9	0.7109	0.2891
0.58	0.42	0.3228	0.8	0.6900	0.3100
0.57	0.43	0.2819	0.7	0.6682	0.3318
0.56	0.44	0.2412	0.6	0.6457	0.3543
0.55	0.45	0.2007	0.5	0.6225	0.3775
0.54	0.46	0.1603	0.4	0.5987	0.4013
0.53	0.47	0.1201	0.3	0.5744	0.4256
0.52	0.48	0.0800	0.2	0.5498	0.4502
0.51	0.49	0.0400	0.1	0.5250	0.4750
0.50	0.50	0.0000	0.0	0.5000	0.5000

Values of λ require a minus sign for $P < \frac{1}{2}$.

APPENDIX B

The Basic Theory of Maximum Likelihood Estimation

This appendix contains a synopsis of the basic properties of maximum likelihood estimation. Suppose $Y_1, \ldots, Y_n$ are statistically independent random variables with distribution governed by $f(Y_i | \theta)$, where θ is an unknown parameter indexing a parametric family of distributions. For absolutely continuous random variables, $f(Y_i | \theta)$ denotes the probability density function of Y_i; for discrete random variables, $f(Y_i | \theta)$ denotes the point probability function $P(Y_i | \theta)$. The *likelihood function*, denoted by $L(\theta)$, is simply the joint probability of observing values $Y_1 = y_1, \ldots, Y_n = y_n$ when viewed as a function of the parameter θ:

$$L_n(\theta) = \prod_{i=1}^{n} f(y_i | \theta).$$

Any value of θ that maximizes the likelihood function is called a *maximum likelihood estimate* (mle), $\hat{\theta}_n$, and satisfies

$$L(\hat{\theta}_n) \geq L(\theta)$$

for all θ. The subscript n in $L_n(\theta)$ and $\hat{\theta}_n$ reminds us that the likelihood function and mle depend on the sample size n. There need not be a unique value of θ that maximizes the likelihood function (see, e.g., Sections 16.8 and 16.9), but for the most part the likelihood functions considered in this book have at most one local maximum, which is a global maximum, and a unique θ that achieves that maximum value.

Statistical Methods for Rates and Proportions, Third Edition
By Joseph L. Fleiss, Bruce Levin, and Myunghee Cho Paik
ISBN 0-471-52629-0   Copyright © 2003 John Wiley & Sons, Inc.

Because it is simpler to deal with sums than products, the natural logarithm of the likelihood function is most convenient to use, and if $\hat{\theta}_n$ maximizes the log likelihood function, it also maximizes the likelihood function. The derivative of the log likelihood function is called the *score function*, $U_n(\theta)$:

$$U_n(\theta) = \frac{d}{d\theta} \ln L_n(\theta) = \sum_{i=1}^{n} \frac{d}{d\theta} \ln f(y_i|\theta).$$

Usually we can find the maximum likelihood estimate by solving the *likelihood equation*, $U_n(\hat{\theta}_n) = 0$ for $\hat{\theta}_n$. Since $U_n(\theta)$ depends on the observations $Y_1, \ldots, Y_n$, $U_n(\theta)$ is a random variable for each θ, that is, is a random function of θ, and thus its root $\hat{\theta}_n$ is a random variable as well.

The negative second derivative of the log likelihood function is the *observed information*, $I_n(\theta)$:

$$I_n(\theta) = -\frac{d^2}{d\theta^2} \ln L_n(\theta) = -\sum_{i=1}^{n} \frac{d^2}{d\theta^2} \ln f(y_i|\theta) = -\frac{d}{d\theta} U_n(\theta).$$

Generally, the observed information depends on the data, and so is also a random variable. The expected value of $I_n(\theta)$, say $i_n(\theta)$, is called the *expected information* or *Fisher information*, after R. A. Fisher, who first investigated the properties of the log likelihood function and its derivatives. In some special cases (e.g., an exponential family of distributions with natural parameterization), $I_n(\theta)$ does not depend on the observations Y_i, in which case the observed information and expected information are the same.

It turns out that the expected value of $U_n(\theta)$ is 0 and the variance of $U_n(\theta)$ is $i_n(\theta)$. The proof is as follows. Because $f(Y|\theta)$ is a density (or probability) function, it integrates (or sums) to 1 over all values of Y in the sample space for each value of θ. We write this with the single notation

$$1 = \int f(y|\theta)\, dy \qquad \text{for all } \theta.$$

Differentiating this identity with respect to θ yields

$$0 = \frac{d}{d\theta} \int f(y|\theta)\, dy = \int \frac{d}{d\theta} f(y|\theta)\, dy = \int \left\{ \frac{d}{d\theta} \ln f(y|\theta) \right\} f(y|\theta)\, dy$$

$$= E\left\{ \frac{d}{d\theta} \ln f(Y|\theta) \right\} = E U_n(\theta)/n. \tag{B.1}$$

For the second equality in (B.1), we have assumed that one can express the derivative of the integral as the integral of the derivative; mild regularity conditions on the parametric family of densities $f(Y|\theta)$ allow this interchange of operations. Differentiating (B.1) with respect to θ we have

$$
0 = \frac{d}{d\theta} \int \left\{ \frac{d}{d\theta} \ln f(y|\theta) \right\} f(y|\theta)\, dy
$$

$$
= \int \left\{ \frac{d^2}{d\theta^2} \ln f(y|\theta) \right\} f(y|\theta)\, dy
$$

$$
+ \int \left\{ \frac{d}{d\theta} \ln f(y|\theta) \right\} \left\{ \frac{d}{d\theta} \ln f(y|\theta) \right\} f(y|\theta)\, dy.
$$

It follows that

$$
\int \left\{ -\frac{d^2}{d\theta^2} \ln f(y|\theta)\, dy \right\} f(y|\theta)\, dy = \int \left\{ \frac{d}{d\theta} \ln f(y|\theta) \right\}^2 f(y|\theta)\, dy. \quad \text{(B.2)}
$$

Summing (B.2) over each value y_i, and using the statistical independence of the components $(d/d\theta) \ln f(Y_i|\theta)$ of the score function, we find

$$
i_n(\theta) = E\left\{ \sum_{i=1}^{n} -\frac{d^2}{d\theta^2} \ln f(Y_i|\theta) \right\} = \sum_{i=1}^{n} \int \left\{ -\frac{d^2}{d\theta^2} \ln f(y_i|\theta) \right\} f(y_i|\theta)\, dy_i
$$

$$
= \sum_{i=1}^{n} \int \left\{ \frac{d}{d\theta} \ln f(y_i|\theta) \right\}^2 f(y_i|\theta)\, dy_i = \sum_{i=1}^{n} \mathrm{Var}\left\{ \frac{d}{d\theta} \ln f(Y_i|\theta) \right\}
$$

$$
= \mathrm{Var}\left\{ \sum_{i=1}^{n} \frac{d}{d\theta} \ln f(Y_i|\theta) \right\} = \mathrm{Var}\{U_n(\theta)\}.
$$

Now let θ_0 denote the true value of θ. The maximum likelihood estimate of θ has three important statistical properties. First, it is *consistent*, that is, $\hat{\theta}_n$ converges to θ_0 as $n \to \infty$, both in probability and almost surely (weak and strong convergence). This result is remarkably subtle to prove rigorously, and instead we give only a heuristic argument. Let $A_0(\theta)$ be defined as the function of θ equal to $1/n$ times the expected value of the score function, where the expectation is taken with respect to the true value θ_0 of θ:

$$
A_0(\theta) = E_0\left\{ \frac{1}{n} U_n(\theta) \right\} = \frac{1}{n} \sum_{i=1}^{n} \int \left\{ \frac{d}{d\theta} \ln f(y_i|\theta) \right\} f(y_i|\theta_0)\, dy_i.
$$

The subscript 0 on $A_0(\theta)$ and $E_0\{\cdot\}$ reminds us that the expectation is taken with respect to θ_0, for any value of θ in the function $U_n(\theta)$. Now for θ near θ_0, $A_0(\theta)$ is a decreasing function of θ (do you see why?), and takes value 0 at $\theta = \theta_0$, because by (B.1), $A_0(\theta_0) = E_0\{U_n(\theta_0)/n\} = 0$. On the other hand, $U_n(\theta)/n$ is a random decreasing function of θ, and takes value 0 at $\theta = \hat{\theta}_n$, because $U(\hat{\theta}_n) = 0$, by definition of $\hat{\theta}_n$. As n increases, the random function $U_n(\theta)/n$ converges to its expected value $A_0(\theta)$ for each θ by the strong law of large numbers. Because the two curves merge as n increases, the root $\hat{\theta}_n$ of $U_n(\theta)/n$ (where it crosses the x axis) is forced to approach the root θ_0 of $A_0(\theta)$.

Second, the maximum likelihood estimator is *asymptotically normally distributed*, that is, with increasing accuracy as n increases, the mle has an approximate normal distribution. To see this, use a Taylor expansion about θ_0 to write

$$0 = U_n(\hat{\theta}_n) = U_n(\theta_0) + (\hat{\theta}_n - \theta_0)\frac{d}{d\theta}U_n(\theta_n^*)$$

$$= U_n(\theta_0) - (\hat{\theta}_n - \theta_0)I_n(\theta_n^*), \tag{B.3}$$

where θ_n^* is some number that lies between $\hat{\theta}_n$ and θ_0. Rewrite (B.3) as follows:

$$\frac{U_n(\theta_0)/\sqrt{i_n(\theta_0)}}{I_n(\theta_n^*)/i_n(\theta_0)} = \sqrt{i_n(\theta_0)}\,(\hat{\theta}_n - \theta_0). \tag{B.4}$$

Since $U_n(\theta_0)$ has mean 0, has variance $i_n(\theta_0)$, and is a sum of independent and identically distributed random variables, the numerator of (B.4) is distributed asymptotically as standard normal. By consistency of $\hat{\theta}_n$ and the strong law of large numbers, the denominator of (B.4) approaches 1. Thus by Slutsky's theorem, the right-hand side of (B.4) also has an asymptotic standard normal distribution. We use this conclusion to justify the approximation most often used in practice, that $\hat{\theta}_n$ is approximately normally distributed in large samples with mean θ_0 and variance $i_n(\theta_0)^{-1}$. Furthermore, the variance may be consistently estimated by $i_n(\hat{\theta}_n)^{-1}$ and used to find the standard error of the mle, if $i_n(\theta)$ can be easily calculated. Most often in practice, one uses $I_n(\hat{\theta}_n)^{-1}$, the reciprocal of the observed information evaluated at the mle of θ, to consistently estimate Var($\hat{\theta}_n$). Thus, a large-sample $100(1 - \alpha)\%$ confidence interval for θ_0 is given by $\hat{\theta}_n \pm z_{\alpha/2}/I_n(\hat{\theta}_n)^{1/2}$.

Third, under mild regularity conditions, the maximum likelihood estimator is *asymptotically efficient*, meaning that the large-sample variance of any other estimator of θ will be no smaller than that of the mle. Thus in large samples, the mle makes the fullest use possible of the information contained in the data.

When the parameter θ is a vector in p dimensions, the above relations generalize as follows. The score function $U_n(\theta)$ is defined as the p-vector of partial derivatives of the log likelihood function with respect to $\theta_1, \ldots, \theta_p$. The observed information is the $p \times p$ matrix of negative second partial derivatives of the log likelihood function, $I_n(\theta) = [(-\partial^2/\partial\theta_i\partial\theta_j)\ln L_n(\theta)]$. The maximum likelihood estimate of θ is then asymptotically multivariate normally distributed in p dimensions, with mean θ_0 and variance-covariance matrix consistently estimated by the inverse observed information matrix, $I_n(\hat{\theta}_n)^{-1}$.

Except in simple cases, the likelihood equation $U_n(\hat{\theta}_n) = 0$ does not have a closed form solution, and one must solve for $\hat{\theta}_n$ iteratively. The *Newton-Raphson algorithm* may be used to calculate $\hat{\theta}_n$ when p is not too large (say $p < 100$). Starting from some initial value $\theta^{(0)}$, one iteratively updates the approximation to the mle via

$$\theta^{(\nu+1)} = \theta^{(\nu)} + I_n(\theta^{(\nu)})^{-1} U_n(\theta^{(\nu)})$$

for $\nu = 0, 1, \ldots$. When the update becomes sufficiently small, e.g., $|\theta^{(\nu+1)} - \theta^{(\nu)}| < 10^{-8}$, convergence is declared and $\theta^{(\nu+1)}$ is taken as the mle $\hat{\theta}_n$. In order for the Newton-Raphson algorithm to converge, the initial estimate should not be too far from the actual mle. Often a consistent, but not necessarily efficient, estimate of θ_0, such as a weighted least-squares estimate, is used for the initial estimate of $\hat{\theta}_n$. The Newton-Raphson algorithm is quadratically convergent, meaning that after a few iterations, the number of correct decimal places doubles after each successive iteration. Typically only four or five iterations suffice for double-precision accuracy.

Example 1 (The Binomial Distribution). Suppose that Y_i has the binomial distribution, $\text{Bin}(N_i, \theta)$, for $i = 1, \ldots, n$. Let $Y_+ = \sum_{i=1}^n Y_i$ and $N_+ = \sum_{i=1}^n N_i$. The likelihood function is

$$L_n(\theta) = \prod_{i=1}^n \left\{ \binom{N_i}{Y_i} \theta^{Y_i}(1-\theta)^{N_i-Y_i} \right\} = \left\{ \prod_{i=1}^n \binom{N_i}{Y_i} \right\} \left(\frac{\theta}{1-\theta} \right)^{Y_+} (1-\theta)^{N_+}.$$

Although the Y_i are not identically distributed, $L(\theta)$ is equivalent to the likelihood function that would arise from N_+ binary observations $Z_1, \ldots, Z_{N_+}$ identically distributed as $\text{Bin}(1, \theta)$ with $\sum_{i=1}^{N_+} Z_i = Y_+$:

$$L_n(\theta) = \left(\frac{\theta}{1-\theta} \right)^{Y_+} (1-\theta)^{N_+}.$$

Note that two likelihood functions are said to be *equivalent* if their ratio does not depend on the parameter θ. Equivalent likelihood functions have identical score functions, mle's, and information.

The score function is

$$U_n(\theta) = \sum_{i=1}^n \left(\frac{Y_i}{\theta} - \frac{N_i - Y_i}{1-\theta} \right) = \frac{Y_+}{\theta} - \frac{N_+ - Y_+}{1-\theta},$$

the observed information is

$$I_n(\theta) = \sum_{i=1}^{n} \left\{ \frac{Y_i}{\theta^2} + \frac{N_i - Y_i}{(1-\theta)^2} \right\} = \frac{Y_+}{\theta^2} + \frac{N_+ - Y_+}{(1-\theta)^2},$$

and the expected information is

$$i_n(\theta) = \sum_{i=1}^{n} \left\{ \frac{N_i\theta}{\theta^2} + \frac{N_i - N_i\theta}{(1-\theta)^2} \right\} = \frac{N_+}{\theta(1-\theta)}.$$

In this case the maximum likelihood estimate can be obtained noniteratively: $\hat{\theta}_n = Y_+/N_+$. The variance of $\hat{\theta}_n$ is $i_n(\theta)^{-1} = \theta(1-\theta)/N_+$. If we define the likelihood as a function of the log odds parameter $\beta = \ln\{\theta/(1-\theta)\}$ instead of θ, then the likelihood function is

$$L_n(\beta) = \exp\{\beta Y_+ - N_+ \ln(1 + e^\beta)\},$$

the score function is

$$U_n(\beta) = Y_+ - \frac{N_+ e^\beta}{1 + e^\beta},$$

the mle of β is

$$\hat{\beta}_n = \ln \frac{Y_+}{N_+ - Y_+},$$

and the observed information is

$$I_n(\beta) = \frac{N_+ e^\beta}{(1 + e^\beta)^2},$$

which does not depend on Y_i. Therefore $i_n(\beta) = I_n(\beta)$. The asymptotic variance of $\hat{\beta}_n$ is $i_n(\beta)^{-1} = I_n(\beta)^{-1}$, and is consistently estimated by $\{1/Y_+\} + \{1/(N_+ - Y_+)\}$. The log-odds parameter β is called the natural parameter, because it multiplies the sufficient statistic Y_+ in the likelihood function, and this example illustrates an exponential family distribution with natural parameterization (a so-called canonical exponential family distribution).

Example 2 (Simple Linear Logistic Regression). Suppose that, given covariate values $X_1, \ldots, X_n$, the conditional distribution of Y_i given X_i is binomial, Bin$(1, \theta_i)$, for $i = 1, \ldots, n$, with

$$\ln \frac{\theta_i}{1 - \theta_i} = \alpha + \beta X_i, \quad \text{so that} \quad \theta_i = \frac{e^{\alpha + \beta X_i}}{1 + e^{\alpha + \beta X_i}}.$$

The unknown parameter is now the vector (α, β). Even though the binary variables are not identically distributed, the main properties of maximum likelihood estimation continue to hold so long as the information grows without bound as n becomes large. The likelihood function is now the product of the conditional probabilities given X_i,

$$L_n(\alpha, \beta) = \prod_{i=1}^{n} \theta_i^{Y_i}(1 - \theta_i)^{1-Y_i} = \prod_{i=1}^{n} \frac{\exp\{Y_i(\alpha + \beta X_i)\}}{1 + \exp(\alpha + \beta X_i)}$$

$$= \frac{\exp\left(\alpha Y_+ + \beta \sum_{i=1}^{n} X_i Y_i\right)}{\prod_{i=1}^{n}\{1 + \exp(\alpha + \beta X_i)\}},$$

and the score function is the vector

$$U_n(\alpha, \beta) = \begin{pmatrix} \dfrac{\partial}{\partial \alpha} \ln L_n(\alpha, \beta) \\ \dfrac{\partial}{\partial \beta} \ln L_n(\alpha, \beta) \end{pmatrix} = \sum_{i=1}^{n} \begin{pmatrix} 1 \\ X_i \end{pmatrix} \left(Y_i - \frac{e^{\alpha + \beta X_i}}{1 + e^{\alpha + \beta X_i}} \right)$$

$$= \begin{pmatrix} \Sigma(Y_i - \theta_i) \\ \Sigma X_i(Y_i - \theta_i) \end{pmatrix}.$$

Again, in this natural parameterization, the observed information and the expected information are the same because the observed information does not depend on Y_i:

$$I_n(\alpha, \beta) = \begin{pmatrix} -\dfrac{\partial^2}{\partial \alpha^2} \ln L_n & -\dfrac{\partial^2}{\partial \alpha\, \partial \beta} \ln L_n \\ -\dfrac{\partial^2}{\partial \beta\, \partial \alpha} \ln L_n & -\dfrac{\partial^2}{\partial \beta^2} \ln L_n \end{pmatrix}$$

$$= \begin{pmatrix} \displaystyle\sum_{i=1}^{n} \theta_i(1 - \theta_i) & \displaystyle\sum_{i=1}^{n} X_i \theta_i(1 - \theta_i) \\ \displaystyle\sum_{i=1}^{n} X_i \theta_i(1 - \theta_i) & \displaystyle\sum_{i=1}^{n} X_i^2 \theta_i(1 - \theta_i) \end{pmatrix}.$$

The maximum likelihood estimates of α and β may be calculated iteratively by the Newton-Raphson algorithm. The reader may verify that the square roots of the diagonal elements of $I_n(\alpha, \beta)^{-1}$ evaluated at the mle's $\hat{\alpha}$ and $\hat{\beta}$ are the estimated standard errors of $\hat{\alpha}$ and $\hat{\beta}$ shown in (11.6) and (11.7), respectively, and the off-diagonal element of the inverse information matrix is the covariance of $\hat{\alpha}$ and $\hat{\beta}$ shown in (11.8).

APPENDIX C

Answers to Selected Problems

Problem 1.2. We are given the value $P(B) = 0.001$.

(a) $P(A|B) = 0.99$ and $P(A|\bar{B}) = 0.01$. By (1.11),

$$\text{PPV} = 0.99(0.001)/\{0.99(0.001) + 0.01(1 - 0.001)\} = 0.0902.$$

By (1.12),

$$\text{NPV} = (1 - 0.01)(1 - 0.001)/\{(1 - 0.01)(1 - 0.001) + (1 - 0.99)0.001\}$$
$$= 0.99999$$

(so that one per 100,000 of those found negative have the disease). The positive predictive value is too low for most purposes.

(b) Now, $P(A|B) = 0.98$ and $P(A|\bar{B}) = 0.0001$. For the new definition of a positive result,

$$\text{PPV} = 0.98(0.001)/\{0.98(0.001) + 0.0001(1 - 0.001)\} = 0.9075$$

and

$$\text{NPV} = (1 - 0.0001)(1 - 0.001)/\{(1 - 0.0001)(1 - 0.001) + (1 - 0.98)0.001\}$$
$$= 0.99998$$

(so that two per 100,000 of those found negative have the disease).

The positive predictive value is ten times larger than it was in part (a), and the negative predictive value is still very close to 1.0.

Statistical Methods for Rates and Proportions, Third Edition
By Joseph L. Fleiss, Bruce Levin, and Myunghee Cho Paik
ISBN 0-471-52629-0   Copyright © 2003 John Wiley & Sons, Inc.

(c) The proportion who are positive on the first test is, by (1.8), $P(A) = 0.99 \times 0.001 + 0.01 \times 0.999 = 0.01098$, or 1,098 individuals per 100,000 tested. Therefore, 98,902 per 100,000 will be negative on the first test and will not have to be retested.

Problem 1.3

(a) (1) 40,000 of the neurotics live alone. (2) 200 of them will be hospitalized. (3) 60,000 of the neurotics live with their families. (4) 360 of them will be hospitalized. (5) $p_1 = 200/(200 + 360) = 0.357$. (6) $p_1 < P(A|B)$.

(b) (1) 200,000 nonneurotics live alone. (2) 1000 of them will be hospitalized. (3) 800,000 nonneurotics live with their families. (4) 1800 of them will be hospitalized. (5) $p_2 = 1000/(1000 + 1800) = 0.357$. (6) $p_2 > P(A|\bar{B})$.

(c) p_1 is equal to p_2 even though $P(A|B)$ is much larger than $P(A|\bar{B})$.

Problem 2.5 We are given the values of $n = 100$ and $p = 0.05$.

(a) By (2.17), $P_L = 0.01$. By (2.18), $P_U = 0.15$.

(b) The value of $z_{\alpha/2}\sqrt{pq/n} + 1/(2n)$ is 0.06, so the lower and upper 99% confidence limits on P using (2.19) are -0.01 and 0.11.

(c) The interval in (b) is narrower than the interval in (a), but the fact that the lower limit is negative in (b) raises doubts about its validity. If the continuity correction in (2.19) were ignored, the limits of the interval would be the same to two decimal places as in (b). The fault does not lie in the continuity correction.

Problem 4.4 We would like to distinguish between $P_1 = 0.45$ for placebo and $P_2 = 0.65$ for an active drug with a one-tailed test.

(a) For a one-tailed test with a significant level of 0.01, we use $z_{0.01} = 2.326$ in (4.14); for a power of 0.95, we use $z_{0.05} = 1.645$. The value of $\bar{P}$ is 0.55. Thus $n' = [2.326(2 \times 0.55 \times 0.45)^{1/2} + 1.645(0.45 \times 0.55 + 0.65 \times 0.35)^{1/2}]^2/0.2^2 = 191.85$. By (4.15), $n = 201.73$, or 202 patients per treatment. Alternatively, look in Table A.4 under $P_1 = 0.45$, $P_2 = 0.65$, $\alpha = 0.02$ (recall that we are considering a one-tailed test), and power $= 0.95$.

(b) If $\alpha = 0.05$ (still for a one-tailed test) and $1 - \beta = 0.80$, then 85 patients per group will be needed.

(c) If $n = 52$, the value of z_β from (4.17) is 0.20. The corresponding power is 0.58. (Table A.1 gives the value $P = 0.8415$ as corresponding to $z = 0.2$. The area under the normal curve above the value 0.20 is $P/2 = 0.42$, and the power is $1 - P/2 = 0.58$.)

Problem 4.5 We wish to distinguish between the probabilities $P_1 = 0.25$ and $P_2 = 0.40$.

(a), (b) We apply (4.19) and (4.18) for each value of r, using $z_\alpha = 2.576$ and $z_\beta = 1.645$, to find the value of $n_1 = m$. The value of n_2 is then rm, so that the total sample size is $n_1 + n_2 = m(r + 1)$. The total cost is $10n_1 + 12n_2$ $= 10m + 12rm = m(10 + 12r)$. The complete table is

Ratio of Sample Sizes (r)	n_1	n_2	Total Sample Size	Total Cost
0.5	530	265	795	$8,480
0.6	473	284	757	8,138
0.7	432	302	734	7,944
0.8	401	321	722	7,862
0.9	377	339	716	7,838
1	357	357	714	7,854

The total cost is minimized when $r = 0.9$ (i.e., when $n_1 = 377$ and $n_2 = 0.9(377) = 339$).

(c) If the total cost must be $6,240 and if the investigator decides to employ the value $r = 0.9$, the value of m is $m = 6240/(10 + 12 \times 0.9) = 300$. The value of m', from (4.20), is $m' = 300 - (0.9 + 1)/(0.9 \times 0.15) = 285.93$. To solve (4.19) for z_β, note that, for $r = 0.9$ we have $\bar{P} = 0.32$ and $\bar{P}\bar{Q} = 0.2176$. Therefore,

$$z_\beta = \frac{0.15\sqrt{0.9 \times 285.93} - 2.576\sqrt{(0.9 + 1) \times 0.2176}}{\sqrt{0.9 \times 0.25 \times 0.75 + 0.40 \times 0.60}} = 1.17.$$

The power of the test is found, by interpolating in Table A.1, to be approximately 0.88.

Problem 6.4

(a)

Hospital Diagnosis

	Schizophrenia	Affective	Total
New York	82	24	106
London	51	67	118
Total	133	91	224

Project Diagnosis

	Schizophrenia	Affective	Total
New York	43	53	96
London	33	85	118
Total	76	138	214

| | Computer Diagnosis | | |
	Schizophrenia	Affective	Total
New York	67	27	94
London	56	37	93
Total	123	64	187

(b)

	Odds Ratio from (6.16)
Source	
Hospital	4.49
Project	2.09
Computer	1.64

The odds ratio for the project and computer diagnoses are close, and both differ substantially from the odds ratio for the hospital diagnosis.

(c)

Source	o	o'
Hospital	4.49	4.41
Project	2.09	2.08
Computer	1.63	1.63

Problem 6.9 For the values of n_{ij} in Table 6.1 and of N_{ij} in Table 6.6, the value of $\chi^2 = \Sigma\Sigma(n_{ij} - N_{ij})^2/N_{ij}$ is 3.32, which is close to the value 3.25 found in (6.65).

Problem 6.10 For an initial approximation of $\omega_U^{(1)} = 5.37$, the value of X is 527.75, and that of Y is 401.48; the value of N_{11} is therefore 14.45, and that of W is 0.1993. The value of F, with the continuity correction taken as $+\frac{1}{2}$, is -0.73, so the iterative process must be undertaken.

The value of T is 0.9345, that of U is 0.0049, and that of V, with $+\frac{1}{2}$ replacing $-\frac{1}{2}$, is 1.5428. The second approximation to the upper limit on the odds ratio is therefore, from (6.72),

$$\omega_U^{(2)} = 5.37 - \frac{-0.73}{1.5428} = 5.84.$$

For this value of the odds ratio, $N_{11} = 14.87$ and $W = 0.2016$. The value of F is 0.01, which is sufficiently close to zero to stop the iterative procedure. The upper 95% confidence limit for the odds ratio underlying the data of Table 6.1 is $\omega_U = 5.84$.

Problem 6.12

(a) For nonwhite live births, the estimated risk of infant mortality attributable to low birthweight is

$$r_A = \frac{0.0140 \times 0.8625 - 0.1147 \times 0.0088}{0.0228 \times 0.8713} = 0.557,$$

which is equal, to two decimal places, to the value for white live births.

(b) By (6.99), the standard error of $\ln(1 - r_A)$ is

$$\widehat{se}[\ln(1 - r_A)] = \sqrt{\frac{0.1147 + 0.557(0.0140 + 0.8625)}{37{,}840 \times 0.0088}} = 0.043.$$

A 95% confidence interval for the parameter is the interval from 0.518 to 0.593. It overlaps well with the interval found in (6.105) for white live births, but is somewhat wider. The number of nonwhite live births is less than the number of white live births, however, so the difference in interval lengths is expected.

Problem 6.15.

(a) The exact two-sided 95% confidence interval for the blindness/O_2 odds ratio using the point probability method is $(0, 0.887)$. At $\omega_U = 0.88747$, the noncentral hypergeometric distribution for the reference cell (low O_2, blind) is as follows:

x	$P(X = x \mid T = 64, m = 6,$ $n = 28, \ \omega = \omega_U)$
0	0.0352
1	0.1693
2	0.3169
3	0.2955
4	0.1446
5	0.0352
6	0.0033

At ω_U, the p-value is $\text{pval}(0, \omega_U) = 0.0352 + 0.0352 + 0.0033 = 0.0737 > 0.05$. Slightly larger values of ω_U cause the point probability at $x = 5$ to exceed that at $x = 0$, thus causing $x = 5$ to be excluded from the tail region, resulting in p-values less than 0.05. $\omega_U = 0.88747$ is the least upper bound of odds ratios with $\text{pval}(0, \omega) > 0.05$.

(b) An approximate 95% confidence interval for $L = \ln \omega$ is $l' \pm 1.96\, \widehat{se}(l')$, where

$$l' = \ln \frac{(0.5)(30.5)}{(6.5)(28.5)} = -2.497$$

(corresponding to $o' = 0.0823$), and

$$\widehat{se}(l') = \sqrt{\frac{1}{0.5} + \frac{1}{30.5} + \frac{1}{6.5} + \frac{1}{28.5}} = 1.4905.$$

The approximate confidence interval for L is $-2.497 \pm 1.96(1.4905) = (-5.418, 0.4244)$. Exponentiating, the confidence interval for ω is $(0.0044, 1.53)$. This is not satisfactory. The lower limit excludes values close to

$\omega = 0$ that are obviously supported by the data. More importantly, the interval includes $\omega = 1$, in contradiction to the exact test.

(c) For the mortality table,

$$l' = \ln \frac{(12.5)(36.5)}{(9.5)(28.5)} = 0.5218$$

(corresponding to $o' = 1.685$). This compares reasonably well with

$$l = \ln \frac{(12)(36)}{(9)(28)} = 0.5390$$

and $o = 1.714$. The standard error is estimated to be

$$\widehat{se}(l') = \sqrt{\frac{1}{12.5} + \frac{1}{28.5} + \frac{1}{9.5} + \frac{1}{36.5}} = 0.4977.$$

The approximate confidence interval is

$$0.5218 \pm 1.96(0.4977) = (-0.4537, 1.497),$$

and exponentiating, we have $(0.6353, 4.468)$. This compares reasonably well with the exact $(0.6146, 4.730)$ although it is too narrow.

Problem 7.3.

(a)

	Smokers	Nonsmokers	Total
Cases	26	9	34
Controls	73	141	214
Total	99	149	248

Uncorrected $\chi^2 = 21.95$
$\varphi = 0.30$

(b)

	Smokers	Nonsmokers	Total
Cases	163	51	214
Controls	12	22	34
Total	175	73	248

Uncorrected $\chi^2 = 23.60$
$\varphi = 0.31$

The phi coefficients in (a) and (b) are close.

(c)

	Smokers	Nonsmokers	Total
Cases	94	30	124
Controls	42	82	124
Total	136	112	248

$$\text{Uncorrected } \chi^2 = 44.03$$
$$\varphi = 0.42$$

The phi coefficient in (c) differs appreciably from those in (a) and (b). The percentage difference between the coefficients in (a) and (c) is $100(0.42 - 0.30)/0.30 = 40\%$.

Problem 7.4.

(a) The required value of $n_{..}$ is 807.

(b) The required value of N_P is 702. The percentage reduction from $n_{..}$ to N_P is $100(807 - 702)/807 = 13\%$.

(c) The required value of N_R is 398. The percentage reduction from $n_{..}$ to N_R is $100(807 - 398)/807 = 51\%$. The percentage reduction from N_P to N_R is $100(702 - 398)/702 = 43\%$.

Problem 7.5.

$$R_A = \left\{ \frac{P(B|A) - P(B|\bar{A})}{P(B|A)} \right\} P(A|B)$$

$$= \left\{ \frac{P(A|B)P(B)}{P(A)} - \frac{P(\bar{A}|B)P(B)}{P(\bar{A})} \right\} \frac{P(A)}{P(B)}$$

$$= P(A|B) - P(\bar{A}|B) \frac{P(A)}{P(\bar{A})} = \frac{P(A|B)P(\bar{A}) - P(\bar{A}|B)P(A)}{1 - P(A)}$$

$$= \frac{P(A|B) - \{P(A|B) + P(\bar{A}|B)\}P(A)}{1 - P(A)} = \frac{P(A|B) - P(A)}{1 - P(A)}.$$

Problem 7.7.

$$(7.23) = \frac{P(A|B) - P(A|\bar{B})}{1 - P(A|\bar{B})} = \frac{\dfrac{P_{11}}{P_{11} + P_{12}} - \dfrac{P_{21}}{P_{21} + P_{22}}}{1 - \dfrac{P_{21}}{P_{21} + P_{22}}}$$

$$= \frac{P_{11}P_{22} - P_{12}P_{21}}{P_{22}(P_{11} + P_{12})},$$

using the representation $P(A|B) = P_{11}/P_{1.}$ and $P(A|\bar{B}) = P_{21}/P_{2.}$. At the same time,

$$(7.32) = \left(1 - \frac{1}{o}\right) P(A|B) = \left(1 - \frac{P_{12}P_{21}}{P_{11}P_{22}}\right)\frac{P_{11}}{P_{1.}}$$

$$= \frac{P_{11}P_{22} - P_{12}P_{21}}{P_{11}P_{22}} \cdot \frac{P_{11}}{P_{11} + P_{12}} = \frac{P_{11}P_{22} - P_{12}P_{21}}{P_{22}(P_{11} + P_{12})}.$$

Problem 7.8. Sens $= 50/50 = 1.0$, Spec $= 63/66 = 0.9545$, $1 - $ Spec $=$ $P(+|\overline{D}) = 0.0455$.

(a) $\dfrac{\text{PPV}}{1 - \text{PPV}} = \dfrac{\text{Sens}}{1 - \text{Spec}} \cdot \dfrac{P(D)}{P(\overline{D})}$, which is estimated by

$$\frac{1}{0.0455} \cdot \frac{40}{99,960} = 0.00879,$$

so

$$\widehat{\text{PPV}} = \frac{0.00879}{1 + 0.00879} = 0.00872 \quad \text{and} \quad \ln \frac{\widehat{\text{PPV}}}{1 - \widehat{\text{PPV}}} = -4.734.$$

(b) $\ln \dfrac{\text{PPV}}{1 - \text{PPV}} = \ln \text{RR} + \ln \dfrac{40}{99,960}$. Using $\dfrac{n - x + \frac{1}{2}}{x + \frac{1}{2}}$ to estimate Q/P, we have

$$\widehat{\text{se}}\left(\ln \frac{\widehat{\text{PPV}}}{1 - \widehat{\text{PPV}}}\right) = \widehat{\text{se}}\{\ln \widehat{\text{RR}}\} = \sqrt{\frac{0.5}{50(50.5)} + \frac{63.5}{66(3.5)}}$$

$$= 0.5245.$$

Thus an approximate 95% confidence interval for $\ln \text{RR}$ and thus $\ln \text{PPV}$ odds is

$$-4.734 \pm 1.96(0.5245) = (-5.762, -3.706),$$

and exponentiating gives $(0.00314, 0.0246)$ for the PPV odds, and using PPV $=$ odds$/(1 + $ odds$)$ yields an approximate 95% confidence interval for PPV of $(0.003, 0.024)$.

Problem 8.1

(a) The value of the critical ratio (with continuity correction) is 5.54. The difference between improvement rates is significant in the second hospital.

(b) The simple difference between the two improvement rates is $d_2 = 0.75 - 0.35 = 0.40$. Its estimated standard error is $\widehat{\text{se}}(d_2) = 0.06$. The critical ratio for testing the significance of the difference between $d_1 = 0.20$ and $d_2 = 0.40$ is $z = 2.17$. The two are significantly different at the 0.05 level.

(c) The relative difference between the two improvement rates in the second hospital is $p_{e(2)} = (0.75 - 0.35)/(1 - 0.35) = 0.62$. The value of L_2 is -0.97, and the estimated standard error of L_2 is 0.19. The critical ratio for comparing L_1 and L_2 is

$$z = \frac{|-0.69 - (-0.97)|}{\sqrt{0.28^2 + 0.19^2}} = 0.83,$$

so that the two relative differences do not differ significantly.

Problem 8.2

(a) For the sample of patients given the treatments in the order AB, we have $n = 20$ and $p_1 = 15/20 = 0.75$.

(b) For the sample of patients given the treatments in the order BA, we have $m = 15$ and $p_2 = 5/15 = 0.33$. (Recall that p_2 is the proportion out of m who had a good response to the treatment given first, i.e., to B.)

(c) The value of the critical ratio for comparing p_1 and p_2, with the continuity correction, is 2.14. The effects of treatments A and B are significantly different.

Problem 9.3.

(a)

Sample	n	Proportion Affective
1	105	0.019
2	192	0.068
3	145	0.166
Overall	442	0.088

The value of chi squared is 18.18 with 2 df. The proportions diagnosed affective differ significantly at better than the 0.01 level.

(b) $\bar{p}_{1,2} = 0.051$ and $n_{1,2} = 297$. The value of chi squared for the difference between $\bar{p}_{1,2}$ and p_3 is 16.06; the difference is significant at better than the 0.01 level. The value of chi squared for the difference between p_1 and p_2 is 2.03, so the difference is not significant.

(c) $\bar{\chi}^2 = \chi^2 = 18.18$, and

$$c = \sqrt{\frac{105 \times 145}{297 \times 337}} = 0.39.$$

The hypothesized ordering is significant at better than the 0.01 level.

Problem 9.5.

(a) The mean ridit for group B, with A as the reference, is 0.963. The probability is 0.963 that a randomly selected member of group B will experience an injury at least as serious as that experienced by a randomly selected member of group A.

(b) The mean ridit for group A, with B as the reference, is 0.037, exactly the complement of the value found in (a).

(c) The standard error of the mean ridit from (9.40) is equal to 0.040.

(d) The standard error of the mean ridit from (9.45) is equal to 0.041, only slightly larger than the value found in (c).

Problem 9.6.

(a) There are mutually exclusive events that constitute the event $[X_2 > X_0]$, so

$$P(X_2 > X_0) = P(X_1 > X_2 > X_0) + P(X_2 > X_1 > X_0) + P(X_2 > X_0 > X_1).$$

Similarly,

$$P(X_2 > X_1) = P(X_0 > X_2 > X_1) + P(X_2 > X_0 > X_1) + P(X_2 > X_1 > X_0)$$

and

$$P(X_1 > X_0) = P(X_2 > X_1 > X_0) + P(X_1 > X_2 > X_0) + P(X_1 > X_0 > X_2).$$

Subtracting the first expression from the sum of the other two expressions yields

$$P(X_2 > X_1) + P(X_1 > X_0) - P(X_2 > X_0)$$
$$= P(X_1 > X_0 > X_2) + P(X_0 > X_2 > X_1) + P(X_2 > X_1 > X_0),$$

which gives the result.

(b) If X_0, X_1, and X_2 are identically distributed, then the six events $[X_2 > X_1 > X_0]$, $[X_2 > X_0 > X_1]$, $[X_1 > X_2 > X_0]$, $[X_1 > X_0 > X_2]$, $[X_0 > X_2 > X_1]$, and $[X_0 > X_1 > X_2]$ are equally likely and exhaust the possibilities (ignoring ties, which occur with zero probability). Thus the probability of each event is $\frac{1}{6}$, and so

$$P(X_1 > X_0 > X_2) + P(X_0 > X_2 > X_1) + P(X_2 > X_1 > X_0) = \frac{1}{2},$$

leading to no bias.

Problem 9.7.*

(a)

$$\ln \frac{P_{i1}}{P_{11}} = \ln \frac{P_{i1}}{P_{(i-1),1}} + \ln \frac{P_{(i-1),1}}{P_{(i-2),1}} + \cdots + \ln \frac{P_{21}}{P_{11}} = L_{i-1}^{(1)} + \cdots + L_1^{(1)}.$$

Similarly,

$$\ln \frac{P_{i2}}{P_{12}} = L_{i-1}^{(2)} + \cdots + L_1^{(2)} = (i-1)\Delta + L_{i-1}^{(1)} + \cdots + L_1^{(1)}.$$

Thus

$$\lambda_i = \ln \frac{P_{i2}/P_{12}}{P_{i1}/P_{11}} = (i-1)\Delta.$$

Substituting this in the noncentral multiple hypergeometric probability function yields

$$P(n_{12},\ldots,n_{k2}|n_1,n_1.,\ldots,n_k.,\Delta) = \frac{\binom{n_1.}{n_{12}} \cdots \binom{n_k.}{n_{k2}} \exp\left\{\Delta \sum_{i=2}^{k} (i-1)n_{i2}\right\}}{\sum_{u \in D} \binom{n_1.}{u_1} \cdots \binom{n_k.}{u_k} \exp\left\{\Delta \sum_{i=2}^{k} (i-1)u_i\right\}}.$$

Multiplying numerator and denominator by the constant $\exp(\Delta n_{..})$ $= \exp(\Delta n_1. + \cdots + \Delta n_k.)$ yields the equivalent expression

$$P(n_{12},\ldots,n_{k2}|n_1,n_1.,\ldots,n_k.,\Delta) = \frac{\binom{n_1.}{n_{12}} \cdots \binom{n_k.}{n_{k2}} \exp\left\{\Delta \sum_{i=1}^{k} in_{i2}\right\}}{\sum_{u \in D} \binom{n_1.}{u_1} \cdots \binom{n_k.}{u_k} \exp\left\{\Delta \sum_{i=1}^{k} iu_i\right\}}.$$

(b) The derivative of the log of the above expression with respect to Δ at $\Delta = 0$ is

$$\sum_{i=1}^{k} in_{i2} - \frac{\sum_{u \in D} \binom{n_1.}{u_1} \cdots \binom{n_k.}{u_k} \sum_{i=1}^{k} iu_i}{\sum_{u \in D} \binom{n_1.}{u_1} \cdots \binom{n_k.}{u_k}} = \sum_{i=1}^{k} i(n_{i2} - EU_i)$$

$$= \sum_{i=1}^{k} i(n_{i2} - n_2\bar{p}_i),$$

where $U_1, \ldots, U_k$ has a central multiple hypergeometric distribution given sample size n_2 and margins $n_1, \ldots, n_k$, with mean $EU_i = n_2 n_i / n_{..} = n_2 \bar{p}_i$ and covariance matrix $[n_2 n_1 / (n_{..} - 1)](\text{Diag}_{\bar{p}} - \bar{p}\bar{p}')$.

(c)

$$n_{i2} - n_2 \bar{p}_i = n_{i2} - n_2 \left(\frac{n_1 p_{i1} + n_2 p_{i2}}{n_1 + n_2} \right) = n_2 \left\{ p_{i2} - \left(\frac{n_1 p_{i1} + n_2 p_{i2}}{n_1 + n_2} \right) \right\}$$

$$= \frac{n_1 n_2}{n_1 + n_2} (p_{i2} - p_{i1}).$$

Thus

$$S = \sum_{i=1}^{k} a_i (n_{i2} - n_2 \bar{p}_i) = \frac{n_1 n_2}{n_{..}} \sum_{i=1}^{k} a_i (p_{i2} - p_{i1}).$$

Also,

$$\text{Var}_0(S) = \text{Var}(S|n_2, n_1, \ldots, n_k, \Delta = 0) = \frac{n_1 n_2}{n_{..} - 1} \left\{ \sum_{i=1}^{k} \bar{p}_i a_i^2 - \left(\sum_{i=1}^{k} \bar{p}_i a_i \right)^2 \right\}$$

$$= \frac{n_1 n_2}{n_{..} - 1} \sum_{i=1}^{k} \bar{p}_i (a_i - \bar{a}_w)^2 = \frac{n_1 n_2}{n_{..} - 1} s_a^2 \quad \text{with } \bar{a}_w = \sum_{i=1}^{k} \bar{p}_i a_i.$$

Thus

$$\frac{|S| - \frac{1}{2}}{\sqrt{\text{Var}_0 S}} = \frac{\left| \dfrac{n_1 n_2}{n_{..}} \sum\limits_{i=1}^{k} a_i (p_{i2} - p_{i1}) \right| - \dfrac{1}{2}}{\sqrt{\dfrac{n_1 n_2}{n_{..} - 1} s_a^2}}$$

$$= \frac{\left| \sum\limits_{i=1}^{k} a_i (p_{i2} - p_{i1}) \right| - \dfrac{1}{2} \left(\dfrac{1}{n_1} + \dfrac{1}{n_2} \right)}{s_a \sqrt{\dfrac{1}{n_1} + \dfrac{1}{n_2}}} \sqrt{\frac{n_{..} - 1}{n_{..}}}.$$

Problem 10.1

(a) The value of $\chi^2_{2 \text{ vs } 3}$ is 0.02, confirmation, if any was needed, of the virtual equality of the odds ratios in studies 2 and 3.

(b) The weighted average of L'_2 and L'_3 is $\bar{L}_{2,3} = 0.862$. The value of $\chi^2_{1 \text{ vs } (2, 3)}$ is 9.40, indicating that L'_1 is significantly different from $\bar{L}_{2,3}$ at the 0.01 level (the appropriate critical value for chi squared is 9.21).

(c) The sum of the chi squared values in (a) and (b) is 9.42, equal except for rounding errors to the value of χ^2_{homog} found in (10.18).

Problem 10.2.

(a) The mean log odds ratio for groups 2 and 3 is $\bar{L}_{2,3} = 0.862$ [see Problem 10.1(b)], with an estimated standard error of

$$\widehat{se}(\bar{L}_{2,3}) = \frac{1}{\sqrt{w_2' + w_3'}} = 0.160.$$

The value of χ^2_{assoc} for these two groups is

$$\chi^2_{assoc} = \left(\frac{\bar{L}_{2,3}}{\widehat{se}(\bar{L}_{2,3})}\right)^2 = 29.03,$$

so the mean log odds ratio is significantly different from zero.

(b) An approximate 95% confidence interval for the underlying log odds ratio is

$$\bar{L}_{2,3} \pm 1.96\,\widehat{se}(\bar{L}_{2,3}),$$

or the interval from 0.548 to 1.176.

(c) The mean odds ratio is equal to antilog $(0.862) = 2.37$. An approximate 95% confidence interval is the interval from antilog(0.548) to antilog(1.176), that is, from 1.73 to 3.24.

Problem 10.3. The sum of $k + 1$ hypergeometric variables with minimum value $\max(l_h, 0)$ and maximum value $\min(m_h, n_{h1})$ for $h = 1, \ldots, k + 1$ can be no less than $\sum_{h=1}^{k+1} \max(l_h, 0)$ and no greater than $\sum_{h=1}^{k+1} \min(m_k, n_{h1})$. Thus c_j is nonzero only if $\sum_{h=1}^{k+1} \max(l_h, 0) \leq j \leq \sum_{h=1}^{k+1} \min(m_h, n_{h1})$. Since a_i in (10.28) is nonzero only if

$$i \leq \sum_{h=1}^{k} \min(m_h, n_{h1}) \quad \text{and} \quad i \geq \sum_{h=1}^{k} \max(l_h, 0)$$

and b_{j-i} is nonzero only if $j - i \geq \max(l_{k+1}, 0)$ and $j - i \leq \min(m_{k+1}, n_{k+1,1})$, it follows that i must be no greater than the smaller of $\sum_{h=1}^{k} \min(m_h, n_{h1})$ and $j - \max(l_{k+1}, 0)$, and must be no smaller than the larger of $\sum_{h=1}^{k} \max(l_h, 0)$ and $j - \min(m_{k+1}, n_{k+1,1})$.

Problem 10.4. The probability that $X_1 + X_2 = 6$ is obtained from the convolution of $(\frac{1}{70}, \frac{16}{70}, \frac{36}{70}, \frac{16}{70}, \frac{1}{70})$ with itself:

$$c_6 = \frac{36}{70} \cdot \frac{1}{70} + \frac{16}{70} \cdot \frac{16}{70} + \frac{1}{70} \cdot \frac{36}{70} = \frac{328}{70^2} \approx 0.0669.$$

The probabilities of observing $(X_1, X_2) = (4, 2), (3, 3)$, or $(2, 4)$, given $X_1 + X_2 = 6$, are, from (10.31), respectively,

$$\left(\frac{\frac{1}{70} \cdot \frac{36}{70}}{\frac{328}{70^2}}, \frac{\frac{16}{70} \cdot \frac{16}{70}}{\frac{328}{70^2}}, \frac{\frac{36}{70} \cdot \frac{1}{70}}{\frac{328}{70^2}} \right) = \left(\frac{36}{328}, \frac{256}{328}, \frac{36}{328} \right).$$

The two-tailed p-value is $(36 + 36)/328 = 0.22$.

Problem 10.8. From (10.97),

$$P(X_i = j + 1 | n_{i \cdot}, n_{i1}, m_i, \omega_i) = \frac{C(j + 1 | n_{i \cdot}, n_{i1}, m_i)}{C(j | n_{i \cdot}, n_{i1}, m_i)} \omega_i P(X_i = j | n_{i \cdot}, n_{i1}, m_i, \omega_i).$$

Suppressing $n_{i \cdot}$ and n_{i1} from the notation, let $G_\omega(\omega | m_i)$ denote the posterior distribution of ω given m_i. Integrating both sides against dG_ω yields

$$P(X_i = j + 1 | m_i) = \int_0^\infty P(X_i = j + 1 | m_i, \omega_i) \, dG_\omega(\omega_i | m_i)$$

$$= \frac{C(j + 1 | m_i)}{C(j | m_i)} \int_0^\infty \omega_i P(X_i = j | m_i, \omega_i) \, dG_\omega(\omega_i | m_i)$$

$$= \frac{C(j + 1 | m_i)}{C(j | m_i)} \frac{\int_0^\infty \omega_i P(X_i = j | m_i, \omega_i) \, dG_\omega(\omega_i | m_i)}{\int_0^\infty P(X_i = j | m_i, \omega_i) \, dG_\omega(\omega_i | m_i)}$$

$$\times \int_0^\infty P(X_i = j | m_i, \omega_i) \, dG_\omega(\omega_i | m_i)$$

$$= \frac{C(j + 1 | m_i)}{C(j | m_i)} E(\omega_i | X_i = j, m_i) \cdot P(X_i = j | m_i),$$

since the posterior density of ω_i given $X_i = j$ and $X_i + Y_i = m_i$ is

$$\frac{P(X_i = j | m_i, \omega_i) \, dG_\omega(\omega_i | m_i)}{\int_0^\infty P(X_i = j | m_i, \omega_i) \, dG_\omega(\omega_i | m_i)}.$$

Problem 12.2.*

(a) $\zeta_Y(t) = E(1 + t)^Y = \sum_{y=0}^\infty p_y(1 + t)^y$, where $p_y = P(Y = y)$. Thus $\zeta_Y'(t) = \sum_{y=1}^\infty y p_y(1 + t)^{y-1}$, and evaluating at $t = 0$ gives $\sum_{y=0}^\infty y p_y = EY$. The reader should note that term-by-term differentiation in the series is justified by the convergence of $\zeta_Y(t)$ in a neighborhood of $t = 0$. To see this, note that for $|h| \le \delta$,

$$\left| \frac{(1+h)^y - 1}{h} \right| = \left| \sum_{i=1}^{y} \binom{y}{i} h^{i-1} \right| \le \sum_{i=1}^{y} \binom{y}{i} |h|^{i-1}$$

$$\le \sum_{i=1}^{y} \binom{y}{i} \delta^{i-1} = \frac{(1+\delta)^y - 1}{\delta}.$$

Therefore, the series $[\zeta_Y(h) - \zeta_Y(0)]/h = \sum_{y=0}^{\infty} p_y[(1+h)^y - 1]/h$ is absolutely convergent if $\zeta_Y(t)$ exists for $|t| \le \delta$, and the limit as $h \to 0$ exists by the dominated convergence theorem. Repeating the argument shows $\zeta_Y^{(r)}(t) = \sum_{y=r}^{\infty} y(y-1)\cdots(y-r+1)(1+t)^{y-r} p_y$, and evaluating at $t = 0$ yields $\zeta_Y^{(r)}(0) = EY^{(r)}$.

(b) $Y \sim$ Poisson(μ), and we have

$$\zeta_Y(t) = E(1+t)^Y = \sum_{y=0}^{\infty} \frac{(1+t)^y e^{-\mu} \mu^y}{y!} = e^{-\mu} \sum_{y=0}^{\infty} \frac{\{(1+t)\mu\}^y}{y!}$$

$$= e^{-\mu + (1+t)\mu} = e^{t\mu}.$$

It follows that $\zeta_Y^{(r)}(t) = \mu^r e^{t\mu}$ and $EY^{(r)} = \mu^r$.

(c) $y^{(2)} = y(y-1)$ implies $y^2 = y^{(2)} + y$;

$$y^{(3)} = y(y-1)(y-2) = y^3 - 3y^2 + 2y = y^3 - 3(y^{(2)} + y) + 2y$$

$$= y^3 - 3y^{(2)} - y$$

implies $y^3 = y^{(3)} + 3y^{(2)} + y$; and

$$y^{(4)} = y(y-1)(y-2)(y-3) = y^4 - 6y^3 + 11y^2 - 6y$$

$$= y^4 - 6(y^{(3)} + 3y^{(2)} + y) + 11(y^{(2)} + y) - 6y = y^4 - 6y^{(3)} - 7y^{(2)} - y$$

implies $y^4 = y^{(4)} + 6y^{(3)} + 7y^{(2)} + y$.

(d) Similar to (b).

(e) We have

$$\zeta_{\underline{X}}(t) = \sum_{\underline{x}} \binom{m}{\underline{x}} P_1^{x_1} \cdots P_n^{x_n} (1 + t_1)^{x_1} \cdots (1 + t_n)^{x_n}$$

$$= \{ P_1(1 + t_1) + \cdots + P_n(1 + t_n) \}^m$$

$$= \left(1 + \sum_{i=1}^{n} P_i t_i \right)^m.$$

Then

$$\left(\partial^{r_1 \cdots + r_n}/\partial^{r_1}t_1 \cdots \partial^{r_n}t_n\right)\zeta_{\underline{X}}(t)$$
$$= m^{r_1 + \cdots + r_n}\prod_{i=1}^{n}P_i^{r_i}\left(1 + \sum_{i=1}^{n}P_i t_i\right)^{m - (r_1 + \cdots + r_n)}$$

implies $EX_1^{(r_1)} \cdots X_n^{(r_n)} = m^{(r_1 + \cdots + r_n)}\prod_{i=1}^{n}P_i^{r_i}$.

(f) $T = \sum_{i=1}^{n}(Y_i - \overline{Y}_n)^2 = \sum_{i=1}^{n}Y_i^2 - (m^2/n)$, where $\overline{Y}_n = S/n = m/n$. Thus

$$E(T|S = m) = \sum_{i=1}^{n}E(Y_i^2|S = m) - \frac{m^2}{n} = \sum_{i=1}^{n}EX_i^2 - \frac{m^2}{n},$$

where $\underline{X} \sim \text{Mult}_n(m, (1/n, \ldots, 1/n))$. Now $EX_i^2 = EX_i^{(2)} + EX_i = (m^{(2)}/n^2) + (m/n)$, whence

$$E(T|S = m) = n\left(\frac{m^{(2)}}{n^2} + \frac{m}{n}\right) - \frac{m^2}{n} = \frac{m(m-1)}{n} + m - \frac{m^2}{n}$$
$$= m\left(1 - \frac{1}{n}\right) = m\left(\frac{n-1}{n}\right).$$

(g) We have

$$\text{Var}(T|S = m) = \text{Var}\left\{\sum_{i=1}^{n}Y_i^2 - \frac{m^2}{n}\bigg| S = m\right\} = \text{Var}\left(\sum_{i=1}^{n}Y_i^2 \bigg| S = m\right)$$
$$= \text{Var}\left(\sum_{i=1}^{n}X_i^2\right),$$

where $\underline{X} \sim \text{Mult}_n(m, (1/n, \ldots, 1/n))$. Then

$$\text{Var}(T|S = m) = E\left(\sum_i X_i^2\right)^2 - \left\{E\left(\sum_i X_i^2\right)\right\}^2$$
$$= \sum_i EX_i^4 + 2\sum_{i<j}E\left(X_i^2 X_j^2\right) - \sum_i \left(EX_i^2\right)^2 - 2\sum_{i<j}EX_i^2 EX_j^2$$
$$= n\left\{EX_1^4 - \left(EX_1^2\right)^2\right\} + n(n-1)\left\{E\left(X_1^2 X_2^2\right) - \left(EX_1^2\right)\left(EX_2^2\right)\right\}$$
$$= n\left\{EX_1^{(4)} + 6EX_1^{(3)} + 7EX_1^{(2)} + EX_1 - \left(EX_1^2\right)^2\right\}$$
$$+ n(n-1)\left\{E\left(X_1^{(2)} + X_1\right)\left(X_2^{(2)} + X_2\right) - \left(EX_1^2\right)^2\right\}$$
$$= n\left\{\frac{m^{(4)}}{n^4} + 6\frac{m^{(3)}}{n^3} + 7\frac{m^{(2)}}{n^2} + \frac{m}{n}\right\} + n(n-1)$$
$$\times \left\{\frac{m^{(4)}}{n^4} + 2\frac{m^{(3)}}{n^3} + \frac{m^{(2)}}{n^2}\right\} - n^2\left\{\frac{m^{(2)}}{n^2} + \frac{m}{n}\right\}^2$$

$$= \frac{m^{(4)}}{n^4} - \frac{m^{(3)}}{n^3} + \frac{m^{(4)} - m^{(2)}m^{(2)}}{n^2} + 6\frac{m^{(3)}}{n^3} - 2\frac{m^{(3)}}{n^2}$$

$$+ \frac{2m^{(3)} - 2mm^{(2)}}{n} + 7\frac{m^{(2)}}{n} - \frac{m^{(2)}}{n} + m^{(2)} - m^2 + m$$

$$= \frac{m(m-1)}{n^2}\{(m-2)(m-3) - m(m-1)\} + 4\frac{m^{(3)}}{n^2}$$

$$+ \frac{2}{n}m(m-1)(m-2-m) + 6\frac{m^{(2)}}{n}$$

$$= \frac{m(m-1)}{n^2}\{-4(m-2) - 2\} + 4\frac{m^{(3)}}{n^2} - 4\frac{m^{(2)}}{n} + 6\frac{m^{(2)}}{n}$$

$$= -4\frac{m^{(3)}}{n^2} - 2\frac{m^{(2)}}{n^2} + 4\frac{m^{(3)}}{n^2} - 4\frac{m^{(2)}}{n} + 6\frac{m^{(2)}}{n}$$

$$= -2\frac{m^{(2)}}{n^2} + 2\frac{m^{(2)}}{n} = 2\frac{m^{(2)}}{n}\left(1 - \frac{1}{n}\right) = 2\frac{m^{(2)}}{n^2}(n-1).$$

(h) $S = Y_1 + \cdots + Y_n \sim$ Poisson$(n\mu)$, which implies $ES^{(2)} = (n\mu)^2$ by part (b), and Var $S = n\mu$. Then

$$\text{Var } T = E\{\text{Var}(T|S)\} + \text{Var}\{E(T|S)\}$$

$$= E\left\{\frac{2S^{(2)}}{n^2}(n-1)\right\} + \text{Var}\left\{\frac{S(n-1)}{n}\right\}$$

$$= \frac{2(n-1)}{n^2}ES^{(2)} + \left(\frac{n-1}{n}\right)^2 \text{Var } S$$

$$= \frac{2(n-1)}{n^2}(n\mu)^2 + \left(\frac{n-1}{n}\right)^2(n\mu)$$

$$= \frac{\mu}{n}\{n - 1 + 2n\mu\}(n-1)$$

and

$$\text{Var}(S_n^2) = \text{Var}\left(\frac{T}{n-1}\right) = \frac{\text{Var}(T)}{(n-1)^2} = \frac{\mu}{n}\left\{1 + \frac{2n\mu}{n-1}\right\} > \frac{\mu}{n}.$$

Problem 13.1. For comparing the proportions of patients diagnosed affectively ill, the value of McNemar's statistic is $(|20 - 10| - 1)^2/(20 + 10) = 2.70$. The difference is not statistically significant.

For comparing the proportions diagnosed something other than schizophrenic or affectively ill, the value of McNemar's statistic is $(|15 - 5| - 1)^2/(15 + 5) = 4.05$. Because this fails to exceed 5.99, the difference is not statistically significant.

Problem 13.2.

(a) The value of the Stuart-Maxwell chi squared statistic is 10.43 with 2 df. The two outcome distributions differ significantly.

(b) The value of d_1 is $70 - 50 = +20$, that of d_3 is $10 - 20 = -10$, and that of $d_1 - d_3$ is $+30$. The new treatment seems to be superior to the standard in that it is associated with a greater net improvement. The value of the test statistic in (13.20) is 9.57, so that the new treatment is significantly better than the standard.

Problem 14.3. By Bayes' theorem,

$$\frac{P(Y=1|X,Z,S=1)}{P(Y=0|X,Z,S=1)} = \frac{P(S=1|Y=1,X,Z)}{P(S=1|Y=0,X,Z)}$$

$$\cdot \frac{P(Y=1|X,Z)}{P(Y=0|X,Z)} \Big/ \frac{P(S=1|X,Z)}{P(S=1|X,Z)},$$

and by unbiased sampling,

$$\frac{P(S=1|Y=1,X,Z)}{P(S=1|Y=0,X,Z)} = \frac{P(S=1|Y=1,Z)}{P(S=1|Y=0,Z)};$$

then take logs. For the second equality,

$$\frac{P(S=1|Y=1,Z)}{P(S=1|Y=0,Z)} = \frac{P(Y=1|S=1,Z)P(S=1|Z)}{P(Y=0|S=1,Z)P(S=1|Z)} \Big/ \frac{P(Y=1|Z)}{P(Y=0|Z)};$$

but for matched pairs, $P(Y=1|S=1,Z) = P(Y=0|S=1,Z) = \frac{1}{2}$, whence

$$\ln \frac{P(S=1|Y=1,Z)}{P(S=1|Y=0,Z)} = -\ln \frac{P(Y=1|Z)}{P(Y=0|Z)}.$$

Problem 16.10. First note that

(A) $P(R_Y|X,Z) = P(R_Y|Y,Z) = P(R_Y|X,Y,Z) = P(R_Y|Z).$

To see this write

$$P(R_Y|X,Z) = E_{Y|X,Z}P(R_Y|X,Y,Z) = E_{Y|X,Z}P(R_Y|Z) = P(R_Y|Z),$$

because $P(R_Y|Z)$ is constant with respect to Y. Similarly,

$$P(R_Y|Y, Z) = E_{X|Y,Z} P(R_Y|X, Y, Z) = E_{X|Y,Z} P(R_Y|Z) = P(R_Y|Z),$$

because $P(R_Y|Z)$ is constant with respect to X. By Bayes' theorem,

$$P(Y|X, Z, R_Y) = P(R_Y|X, Y, Z)P(Y|X, Z)/P(R_Y|X, Z) = P(Y|X, Z).$$

Also note that

(B) $P(R_X|Y, Z, R_Y = 0) = P(R_X|X, Y, Z, R_Y = 0) = P(R_X|Z, R_Y = 0).$

To see this, write

$$P(R_X|Y, Z, R_Y = 0) = E_{X|Y,Z, R_Y=0} P(R_X|X, Y, Z, R_Y = 0)$$
$$= E_{X|Y,Z, R_Y=0} P(R_X|Z, R_Y = 0) = P(R_X|Z, R_Y = 0),$$

because $P(R_X|Z, R_Y = 0)$ is constant with respect to X. Then (16.48) is satisfied because

$$P(R_X|X, Y, Z) = P(R_X|X, Y, Z, R_Y = 1)P(R_Y = 1|X, Y, Z)$$
$$+ P(R_X|X, Y, Z, R_Y = 0)P(R_Y = 0|X, Y, Z)$$
$$= \underset{\text{[by (16.56)]}}{P(R_X|Y, Z, R_Y = 1)} \ \underset{\text{[by (A)]}}{P(R_Y = 1|Y, Z)}$$
$$+ \underset{\text{[by (B)]}}{P(R_X|Y, Z, R_Y = 0)} \ \underset{\text{[by (A)]}}{P(R_Y = 0|Y, Z)}$$
$$= P(R_X|Y, Z).$$

Problem 16.11. Given:
(a) $P(R_X|X, Y, Z) = P(R_X|Z),$
(b) $P(R_Y|X, Y, Z, R_X = 1) = P(R_Y|X, Z, R_X = 1)$, and
(c) $P(R_Y|X, Y, Z, R_X = 0) = P(R_Y|X, Z, R_X = 0).$
First note that

(A) $P(R_X|X, Z) = P(R_X|Y, Z) = P(R_X|X, Y, Z) = P(R_X|Z).$

Assumptions (a), (b), and (c) simply interchange the role of X and Y in (16.56). Use the same proof as in Problem 16.10, interchanging X and Y. This gives (16.48).

Also note that, again by interchange of the role of X and Y and the proof of Problem 16.10,

(B) $\quad P(R_Y|X, Z, R_X = 0) = P(R_Y|X, Y, Z, R_X = 0) = P(R_Y|Z, R_X = 0).$

Then by Bayes' theorem,

$$P(Y|X, Z, R_Y) = P(R_Y|X, Y, Z)P(Y|X, Z)/P(R_Y|X, Z) = P(Y|X, Z),$$

so it suffices to show $P(R_Y|X, Y, Z) = P(R_Y|X, Z)$. Again, this follows by interchange of X and Y in Problem 16.10. For a direct proof, write

$$
\begin{aligned}
P(R_Y|X, Y, Z) &= P(R_Y|X, Y, Z, R_X = 1)P(R_X = 1|X, Y, Z) \\
&\quad + P(R_Y|X, Y, Z, R_X = 0)P(R_X = 0|X, Y, Z) \\
&= \underset{\text{[by } (b)\text{]}}{P(R_Y|X, Z, R_X = 1)}\ \underset{\text{[by (A)]}}{P(R_X = 1|X, Z)} \\
&\quad + \underset{\text{[by (B)]}}{P(R_Y|X, Z, R_X = 0)}\ \underset{\text{[by (A)]}}{P(R_Y = 0|X, Z)} \\
&= P(R_Y|X, Z).
\end{aligned}
$$

Problem 17.1.

(a)

Hospital	n	Proportion Catatonic
1	112	0.286
2	154	0.506
3	31	0.419
4	151	0.364
5	124	0.298
Overall	$\overline{572}$	$\overline{0.376}$

(b) The value of chi squared for comparing these five proportions is 18.51.

(c) The critical value of chi squared with 4 df for the 0.001 significance level is 18.47. The standards for the differential diagnosis of catatonic and paranoid schizophrenia are significantly different ($p < 0.001$) across the five hospitals.

Problem 17.2.

(a) The value of P_L is 0.50, but that of p_L is $(0.75)(0.50) + (0.05)(0.50) = 0.40.$

(b) The value of P_B is 0.40, but that of p_B is $(0.9)(0.40) + (0.1)(0.60) = 0.42.$

(c) The value of $D = P_L - P_B$ is 0.10, but that of $d = p_L - p_B = -0.02.$ They are of opposite sign.

(d) The value of the odds ratio as a function of P_L and P_B is $(0.50)(0.60)/(0.40)(0.50) = 1.50$, but the value of the odds ratio as a function of p_L and p_B is $(0.40)(0.58)/(0.42)(0.60) = 0.92$. They are on opposite sides of unity.

Problem 17.3.

(a) $p_B = 60/200 = 0.30$, and the value of the odds ratio is $(0.44)(0.70)/(0.30)(0.56) = 1.83$.

(b) The value of n_{00}/n_0 is $18/18 = 1$, and that of n_{10}/n_1 is $2/32 = 0.06$. The resulting value of P_B is $(1)(0.30) + (0.06)(0.70) = 0.34$. The value of the odds ratio for the adjusted rates of smoking is $(0.51)(0.66)/(0.34)(0.49) = 2.02$. The association seems to be stronger than in (a).

(c) The values of n_{00}/n_0 is $16/18 = 0.89$ and that of n_{10}/n_1 is $7/32 = 0.22$. The resulting value of P_B is $(0.89)(0.30) + (0.22)(0.70) = 0.42$. The resulting value of the odds ratio is $(0.51)(0.58)/(0.42)(0.49) = 1.44$. The association seems to be weaker than in (a).

Problem 18.3.

(a)

Study	n	p_e	$\hat{\kappa}$	A	B	C	$\widehat{se}(\hat{\kappa})$
1	20	0.59	0.39	0.0742	0.0784	0.0009	0.21
2	20	0.71	0.48	0.0820	0.0393	0.0123	0.25
3	30	0.54	0.35	0.0714	0.1196	0.0000	0.17

The value of the numerator of (18.21) is $0.39/0.21^2 + 0.48/0.25^2 + 0.35/0.17^2 = 28.63$, and the value of the denominator is $1/0.21^2 + 1/0.25^2 + 1/0.17^2 = 73.28$. The overall value of kappa is $28.63/73.28 = 0.39$.

(b) The value of the chi squared statistic in (18.22) is $(0.39 - 0.39)^2/0.21^2 + (0.48 - 0.39)^2/0.25^2 + (0.35 - 0.39)^2/0.17^2 = 0.18$ with 2 df. The three estimates of kappa do not differ significantly.

(c) An approximate 95% confidence interval for the common value of kappa is $0.39 \pm 1.96 \times \sqrt{1/73.28}$, or the interval from 0.16 to 0.62. The overall value of kappa is significantly different from zero (the confidence interval does not contain the value 0), but the magnitude of kappa indicates little better than fair chance-corrected agreement (even the upper 95% confidence limit, 0.62, is low).

Problem 19.1.

(a) The rates of abnormal lung functioning in service industries are greater than or equal to those in manufacturing industries for employees aged 50 years, but are smaller for employees aged 50 or over.

(b) The only gain would be the simplicity of comparing just two adjusted rates. The major losses would be the failure to describe the crossover phenomenon and the strong dependence of the direction of the difference between the two adjusted rates on the age distribution of the standard.

(c)

	Adjusted Rates		
Standard	Manufac.	Service	Difference
1	3.98%	4.40%	Service > manufac.
2	8.37%	6.92%	Manufac. > service
3	3.87%	3.84%	Approximately equal

(d)

	Adjusted Rates		
Age Interval	Manufac.	Service	Difference
20–49	2.58%	3.37%	Service > manufac.
≥ 50	8.23%	7.14%	Manufac. > service

Author Index

Numbers in *italics* indicate pages where references appear.

Adelstein, S. J., 9, *16*

Advisory Committee to the Surgeon General of the Public Health Service, 123, 124, *143*

Afifi, A. A., 245, *282*

Agresti, A., 112, *140*, 245, *279*, 340, *371*, 619, 622, *623*

Ahlquist, D. A., *439*

Aickin, M., 619, 621, *623*

Albert, P. S., *439*, 476, *490*

Allison, T., 609, *623*

Altham, P. M. E., 95, *140*

Althouser, R. P., *403*

Altman, L. K., 179, *182*

Ament, R. P., 628, *647*

American Psychiatric Association, 565, *592*

Andersen, E. B., 408, *437*

Anderson, R. L., 58, *63*, 566, *595*

Anscombe, F. J., 102, *140*, 176, *182*

Anturane Reinfarction Trial Research Group, 160, *183*

Armitage, P., 160, *183*, *185*, 194, *230*, 602, 603, *623*

Armstrong, B., 589, *592*, 597, *623*

Arnold, J. C., 572, *593*

Arostegui, G. E., *158*

Ashford, J. R., 308, *338*

Assakul, K., 566, *592*

Azen, S. P., 621, *623*

Bagiella, E., *490*

Bahadur, R. R., 484, *488*

Bahn, A. K., 630, *647*

Bailey, K. R., 268, *279*, 535, *560*

Baker, S. G., 535, *558*

Bakwin, H., 565, *592*

Baldwin, I. T., *233*

Banerjee, M., 622, *623*

Banerjee, T., 216, *230*

Barlow, R. E., 198, *230*, 693, 694

Barlow, W., 619, 621, *623*

Barnard, G. A., *63*

Barnwell, G. M., *623*

Barron, B. A., 569, 570, 573, *592*

Bartholomew, D. J., 196, *230*, 694, 695, 696

Bartko, J. J., 604, 609, *623*

Bartlett, M. S., 106, *140*, 246, *279*

Statistical Methods for Rates and Proportions, Third Edition
By Joseph L. Fleiss, Bruce Levin, and Myunghee Cho Paik
ISBN 0-471-52629-0   Copyright © 2003 John Wiley & Sons, Inc.

Subject Index

WILEY SERIES IN PROBABILITY AND STATISTICS

ESTABLISHED BY WALTER A. SHEWHART AND SAMUEL S. WILKS

The **Wiley Series in Probability and Statistics** is well established and authoritative. It covers many topics of current research interest in both pure and applied statistics and probability theory. Written by leading statisticians and institutions, the titles span both state-of-the-art developments in the field and classical methods.

Reflecting the wide range of current research in statistics, the series encompasses applied, methodological and theoretical statistics, ranging from applications and new techniques made possible by advances in computerized practice to rigorous treatment of theoretical approaches.

This series provides essential and invaluable reading for all statisticians, whether in academia, industry, government, or research.

*Now available in a lower priced paperback edition in the Wiley Classics Library.

BENDAT and PIERSOL · Random Data: Analysis and Measurement Procedures, *Third Edition*

BERRY, CHALONER, and GEWEKE · Bayesian Analysis in Statistics and Econometrics: Essays in Honor of Arnold Zellner

BERNARDO and SMITH · Bayesian Theory

BHAT and MILLER · Elements of Applied Stochastic Processes, *Third Edition*

BHATTACHARYA and JOHNSON · Statistical Concepts and Methods

BHATTACHARYA and WAYMIRE · Stochastic Processes with Applications

BILLINGSLEY · Convergence of Probability Measures, *Second Edition*

BILLINGSLEY · Probability and Measure, *Third Edition*

BIRKES and DODGE · Alternative Methods of Regression

BLISCHKE AND MURTHY (editors) · Case Studies in Reliability and Maintenance

BLISCHKE AND MURTHY · Reliability: Modeling, Prediction, and Optimization

BLOOMFIELD · Fourier Analysis of Time Series: An Introduction, *Second Edition*

BOLLEN · Structural Equations with Latent Variables

BOROVKOV · Ergodicity and Stability of Stochastic Processes

BOULEAU · Numerical Methods for Stochastic Processes

BOX · Bayesian Inference in Statistical Analysis

BOX · R. A. Fisher, the Life of a Scientist

BOX and DRAPER · Empirical Model-Building and Response Surfaces

*BOX and DRAPER · Evolutionary Operation: A Statistical Method for Process Improvement

BOX, HUNTER, and HUNTER · Statistics for Experimenters: An Introduction to Design, Data Analysis, and Model Building

BOX and LUCEÑO · Statistical Control by Monitoring and Feedback Adjustment

BRANDIMARTE · Numerical Methods in Finance: A MATLAB-Based Introduction

BROWN and HOLLANDER · Statistics: A Biomedical Introduction

BRUNNER, DOMHOF, and LANGER · Nonparametric Analysis of Longitudinal Data in Factorial Experiments

BUCKLEW · Large Deviation Techniques in Decision, Simulation, and Estimation

CAIROLI and DALANG · Sequential Stochastic Optimization

CHAN · Time Series: Applications to Finance

CHATTERJEE and HADI · Sensitivity Analysis in Linear Regression

CHATTERJEE and PRICE · Regression Analysis by Example, *Third Edition*

CHERNICK · Bootstrap Methods: A Practitioner's Guide

CHERNICK and FRIIS · Introductory Biostatistics for the Health Sciences

CHILÈS and DELFINER · Geostatistics: Modeling Spatial Uncertainty

CHOW and LIU · Design and Analysis of Clinical Trials: Concepts and Methodologies, *Second Edition*

CLARKE and DISNEY · Probability and Random Processes: A First Course with Applications, *Second Edition*

*COCHRAN and COX · Experimental Designs, *Second Edition*

CONGDON · Bayesian Statistical Modelling

CONOVER · Practical Nonparametric Statistics, *Second Edition*

COOK · Regression Graphics

COOK and WEISBERG · Applied Regression Including Computing and Graphics

COOK and WEISBERG · An Introduction to Regression Graphics

CORNELL · Experiments with Mixtures, Designs, Models, and the Analysis of Mixture Data, *Third Edition*

COVER and THOMAS · Elements of Information Theory

COX · A Handbook of Introductory Statistical Methods

*COX · Planning of Experiments

CRESSIE · Statistics for Spatial Data, *Revised Edition*

*Now available in a lower priced paperback edition in the Wiley Classics Library.

*Now available in a lower priced paperback edition in the Wiley Classics Library.

*Now available in a lower priced paperback edition in the Wiley Classics Library.

*Now available in a lower priced paperback edition in the Wiley Classics Library.

MEERSCHAERT and SCHEFFLER · Limit Distributions for Sums of Independent Random Vectors: Heavy Tails in Theory and Practice

*MILLER · Survival Analysis, *Second Edition*

MONTGOMERY, PECK, and VINING · Introduction to Linear Regression Analysis, *Third Edition*

MORGENTHALER and TUKEY · Configural Polysampling: A Route to Practical Robustness

MUIRHEAD · Aspects of Multivariate Statistical Theory

MURRAY · X-STAT 2.0 Statistical Experimentation, Design Data Analysis, and Nonlinear Optimization

MURTHY, XIE, and JIANG · Weibull Models

MYERS and MONTGOMERY · Response Surface Methodology: Process and Product Optimization Using Designed Experiments, *Second Edition*

MYERS, MONTGOMERY, and VINING · Generalized Linear Models. With Applications in Engineering and the Sciences

NELSON · Accelerated Testing, Statistical Models, Test Plans, and Data Analyses

NELSON · Applied Life Data Analysis

NEWMAN · Biostatistical Methods in Epidemiology

OCHI · Applied Probability and Stochastic Processes in Engineering and Physical Sciences

OKABE, BOOTS, SUGIHARA, and CHIU · Spatial Tesselations: Concepts and Applications of Voronoi Diagrams, *Second Edition*

OLIVER and SMITH · Influence Diagrams, Belief Nets and Decision Analysis

PALTA · Quantitative Methods in Population Health: Extensions of Ordinary Regressions

PANKRATZ · Forecasting with Dynamic Regression Models

PANKRATZ · Forecasting with Univariate Box-Jenkins Models: Concepts and Cases

*PARZEN · Modern Probability Theory and Its Applications

PEÑA, TIAO, and TSAY · A Course in Time Series Analysis

PIANTADOSI · Clinical Trials: A Methodologic Perspective

PORT · Theoretical Probability for Applications

POURAHMADI · Foundations of Time Series Analysis and Prediction Theory

PRESS · Bayesian Statistics: Principles, Models, and Applications

PRESS · Subjective and Objective Bayesian Statistics, *Second Edition*

PRESS and TANUR · The Subjectivity of Scientists and the Bayesian Approach

PUKELSHEIM · Optimal Experimental Design

PURI, VILAPLANA, and WERTZ · New Perspectives in Theoretical and Applied Statistics

PUTERMAN · Markov Decision Processes: Discrete Stochastic Dynamic Programming

*RAO · Linear Statistical Inference and Its Applications, *Second Edition*

RENCHER · Linear Models in Statistics

RENCHER · Methods of Multivariate Analysis, *Second Edition*

RENCHER · Multivariate Statistical Inference with Applications

RIPLEY · Spatial Statistics

RIPLEY · Stochastic Simulation

ROBINSON · Practical Strategies for Experimenting

ROHATGI and SALEH · An Introduction to Probability and Statistics, *Second Edition*

ROLSKI, SCHMIDLI, SCHMIDT, and TEUGELS · Stochastic Processes for Insurance and Finance

ROSENBERGER and LACHIN · Randomization in Clinical Trials: Theory and Practice

ROSS · Introduction to Probability and Statistics for Engineers and Scientists

ROUSSEEUW and LEROY · Robust Regression and Outlier Detection

RUBIN · Multiple Imputation for Nonresponse in Surveys

RUBINSTEIN · Simulation and the Monte Carlo Method

RUBINSTEIN and MELAMED · Modern Simulation and Modeling

*Now available in a lower priced paperback edition in the Wiley Classics Library.

*Now available in a lower priced paperback edition in the Wiley Classics Library.

WOOLSON and CLARKE · Statistical Methods for the Analysis of Biomedical Data, *Second Edition*

WU and HAMADA · Experiments: Planning, Analysis, and Parameter Design Optimization

YANG · The Construction Theory of Denumerable Markov Processes

*ZELLNER · An Introduction to Bayesian Inference in Econometrics

ZHOU, OBUCHOWSKI, and McCLISH · Statistical Methods in Diagnostic Medicine